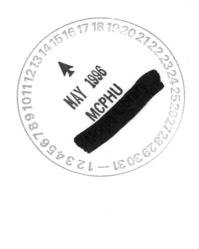

Advances in Pain Research and Therapy

Volume 22

Pain and the Brain
From Nociception to Cognition

Advances in Pain Research and Therapy
Series Editor: John J. Bonica, M.D., D.Sc., F.F.A.R.C.S. (Hon.)

Volumes not listed are out of print.

Advances in Pain Research and Therapy
Volume 22

Pain and the Brain
From Nociception to Cognition

Editors

Burkhart Bromm, M.D., Ph.D.
Institute of Physiology
University Hospital Eppendorf
Hamburg, Germany

John E. Desmedt, M.D., Ph.D.
Brain Research Unit
University of Brussels
Brussels, Belgium

RAVEN PRESS ◆ NEW YORK

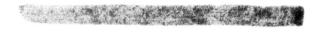

Raven Press, Ltd., 1185 Avenue of the Americas, New York, New York 10036

Made in the United States of America

Library of Congress Cataloging-in-Publication Data

Pain and the brain: from nociception to cognition / editors, Burkhart Bromm and John E. Desmedt.
    p.   cm. — (Advances in pain research and therapy ; vol. 22)
    Includes bibliographical references and index.
    ISBN 0-7817-0322-0
    1. Pain—Congresses. I. Bromm, Burkhart. II. Desmedt, John E. III. Series: Advances in pain research and therapy ; v. 22.
    [DNLM: 1. Pain—congresses. 2. Brain—physiology—congresses. 3. Cognition—congresses. 4. Nociceptors—physiology—congresses. W1 AD706 v.22 1995 / WL 704 P144366 1995]
    RB127.P332155   1995
    616.8'49—dc20
    DNLM/DLC
    for Library of Congress   95-3716

The material contained in this volume was submitted as previously unpublished material, except in the instances in which credit has been given to the source from which some of the illustrative material was derived.

Great care has been taken to maintain the accuracy of the information contained in the volume. However, neither Raven Press nor the editors can be held responsible for errors or for any consequences arising from the use of the information contained herein.

Materials appearing in this book prepared by individuals as part of their official duties as U.S. Government employees are not covered by the above-mentioned copyright.

9 8 7 6 5 4 3 2 1

Contents

III. Windows into Pain-Related Brain Activity

IV. Psychological Images of Pain

V. Abnormal Pain States

VI. Assessment of Drug-Induced Pain Relief

Contributing Authors

Ralph Adolfs
Department of Neurology
University of Iowa
Hospital and Clinics
200 Hawkins Drive
Iowa City, Iowa 52242-1053, USA

Allan L. Bernstein
Department of Neurology
Kaiser Permanente Medical Center
27400 Hesperian Boulevard
Hayward, California 94545-4297,
  USA

Jean-Marie Besson
INSERM -U 161
2, rue d' Alésia
F-75014 Paris, France

Peter Bieri
Institute of Philosophy
Free University of Berlin
Habelschwerdter Allee 30
D-14195 Berlin, Germany

Niels Birbaumer
Institute of Medical Psychology and
  Behavioral Neurobiology
University of Tübingen
Gartenstraβe 29
D-72074 Tübingen, Germany

Jörgen Boivie, M.D.
Department of Neurology
University Hospital
S-581 85 Linköping, Sweden

Didier Bouhassira
Department of Physiopharmacology
INSERM-U 161
2, rue d' Alésia
E-75014 Paris, France

Burkhart Bromm
Institute of Physiology
University Hospital Eppendorf
Martinistraβe 52
D-20246 Hamburg, Germany

Johannes Brüggemann
Neurosurgery Research Laboratory
Health Science Center
State University of New York
750 East Adams Street
Syracuse, New York 13210, USA

James N. Campbell
Department of Neurosurgery
Johns Hopkins University
600 North Wolfe Street
Baltimore, Maryland 21287, USA

J. Douglas Carroll
Department of Biopsychology
Rutgers University
Newark, New Jersey 07102, USA

Kenneth L. Casey
Neurology Services
Veteran's Affairs Medical Center
University of Michigan
2215 Fuller Road
Ann Arbor, Michigan 48104, USA

Fernando Cervero
Department of Physiology and
  Pharmacology
University Campus
University of Alcalá de Henares
E-28871, Madrid, Spain

C. Richard Chapman
Department of Anesthesiology
University of Washington
Seattle, Washington 98195, USA

Andrew C. N. Chen
Rheumatic Diseases Center
Clinical Sciences Building
Hope Hospital
University of Manchester
Eccles Old Road
Salford M6-8HD United Kingdom

W. Crawford Clark
Department of Psychiatry
College of Physicians and Surgeons
Columbia University
722 West 168th
New York, New York 10032, USA

Kenneth D. Craig
Department of Psychology
University of British Columbia
2136 West Mall
Vancouver, British Columbia V6T
  1Z4, Canada

Antonio R. Damasio
Department of Neurology
University of Iowa
Hospital and Clinics
200 Hawkins Drive
Iowa City, Iowa 52242-1053, USA

Stuart W. G. Derbyshire
Rheumatic Diseases Center
Clinical Sciences Building
Hope Hospital
University of Manchester
Eccles Old Road
Salford M6 8HD, United Kingdom

John E. Desmedt
Brain Research Unit
University of Brussels
20 rue Evers
B-1000 Brussels, Belgium

Hans Christoph Diener
Department of Neurology
University of Essen
Hufelandstraße 55
D-45122 Essen, Germany

Patrick M. Dougherty
Department of Neurosurgery
Johns Hopkins University
Meyer Building 7-113
600 North Wolfe Street
Baltimore, Maryland 21287-7713,
  USA

Diana K. Douglass
Neurobiology and Anesthesiology
  Branch
National Institute of Dental Research
Building 49
Bethesda, Maryland 21287-7713,
  USA

Thomas Elbert
Institute of Experimental Audiology
University of Münster
Kardinal-von-Galen-Ring 10
D-4819 Münster, Germany

J. David Fletcher
Department of Biopsychology
New York State Psychiatric Institute
New York, New York 10032, USA

Hertha Flor
Department of Psychology
Humboldt University, Berlin
D-10117 Berlin, Germany

Kirk A. Frey
Department of Internal Medicine
Division of Nuclear Medicine)
University of Michigan Medical
  Center
1103 East Huron Street
Ann Arbor, Michigan 48109, USA

Stephen J. Gibson
National Research Institute of
  Gerontology and Geriatric
  Medicine
North West Hospital
Poplar Road
Parkville, Victoria 3052, Australia

Peter J. Goadsby
Institute of Neurology
The National Hospital for Neurology
  and Neurosurgery
Queen Square
London WC 1N, United Kingdom

Gerald Granges
Department of Medicine
Monash Medical Center
246 Clayton Road
Clayton, Victoria 3168
Australia

Jan Gybels
Department of Neurosurgery
University of Leuven
UZ Gasthuisberg
Herestraat 49
B-3000 Leuven, Belgium

George Heidrich, III
Global Pharma Services, Inc.
2405 Oakridge Avenue
Madison, Wisconsin 53704, USA

Robert D. Helme
National Research Institute of
  Gerontology and Geriatric
  Medicine
North West Hospital
Poplar Road
Parkville, Victoria 3052, Australia

Werner M. Herrmann
Laboratory of Clinical
  Psychophysiology
Department of Psychiatry
Free University of Berlin
Spandauer Damn 130
D-10789 Berlin, Germany

Volker Höllt
Institute of Physiology
University of Munich
Pettenkoferstraße 12
D-808336 Munich, Germany

Raymond W. Houde
Memorial Sloan-Kettering Cancer
  Center
1275 York Avenue
New York, New York 10021, USA

Malvin N. Janal
Department of Biopsychology
New York State Psychiatric Institute
722 West 168th Street
New York, New York 10032, USA

Anthony K. P. Jones
Rheumatic Diseases Center
Clinical Sciences Building
Hope Hospital
University of Manchester
Eccles Old Road
Salford M6 8HD, United Kingdom

Robert F. Kaiko
The Purdue Frederick Company
100 Connecticut Avenue
Norwalk, Connecticut 06850-3590,
  USA

Oliver Kastrup
Department of Neurology
University of Essen
Hufelandstraβe 55
D-45122 Essen, Germany

Dan R. Kenshalo, Jr.
Neurobiology and Anesthesiology
  Branch
National Institute of Dental Research
Building 49
Besthesda, Maryland 20892

Klaus-D. Kniffki
Institute of Physiology
University of Würzburg
D-97070 Würzburg, Germany

Robert A. Koeppe
Department of Internal Medicine
Division of Nuclear Medicine
University of Michigan Medical
  Center
1103 East Huron Street
Ann Arbor, Michigan 48109, USA

Holger Kohlhoff
Institute of Physiology
University Hospital Eppendorf
Martinistraβe 52
D-20246 Hamburg, Germany

Klaus Kunze
Clinic of Neurology
University Hospital Eppendorf
Martinistraβe 52
D-20246 Hamburg, Germany

Ron Kupers
Department of Brain and Behaviour
  Research
UZ Gasthuisberg
University of Leuven
Herestraat 49
B-3000 Leuven, Belgium

Robert Laudahn
Institute of Physiology
University Hospital Eppendorf
Martinistraβe 52
D-20246 Hamburg, Germany

Daniel Le Bars
Department of Physiopharmacology
INSERM-U 161
2, rue d' Alésia
F-75014 Paris, France

Frederick A. Lenz
Department of Neurosurgery
Johns Hopkins University
Meyer Building 7-113
600 North Wolfe Street
Baltimore, Maryland 21287-7713,
  USA

Geoff O. Littlejohn
Department of Medicine
Monash Medical Center
246 Clayton Road
Clayton, Victoria 3168
Australia

Jürgen Lorenz
Institute of Physiology
University of Hospital Eppendorf
Martinistraβe 52
D-20246 Hamburg, Germany

Werner Lutzenberger
Institute of Medical Psychology and
*   Behavioral Neurobiology*
University of Tübingen
Gartenstraβe 29
D-72074 Tübingen, Germany

Mitchell B. Max
Clinical Trials Unit
Neurobiology and Anesthesiology
*   Branch*
National Institutes of Health
Building 10
Bethesda, Maryland 20892, USA

Ronald Melzack
Department of Psychology
McGill University
1205 Dr. Penfield Avenue
Montreal, Quebec H3A 1B1
Canada

Richard A. Meyer
Department of Neurosurgery
Johns Hopkins University
600 North Wolfe Street
Baltimore, Maryland 21287, USA

Satoshi Minoshima
Division of Nuclear Medicine
Department of Internal Medicine
University of Michigan Medical
*   Center*
1103 East Huron Street
Ann Arbor, Michigan 48109, USA

Panayiotis Mitsias
Department of Neurology
Ambulatory Headache Clinic
Henry Ford Hospital and Health
*   Sciences Center*
2799 West Grand Boulevard
Detroit, Michigan 48202-2689, USA

Thomas J. Morrow
Neurology Service
Veteran's Affairs Medical Center
University of Michigan
2215 Fuller Road
Ann Arbor, Michigan 48104, USA

Nabih M. Ramadan
Department of Neurology
Ambulatory Headache Clinic
Henry Food Hospital and Health
*   Sciences Center*
2799 West Grand Boulevard
Detroit, Michigan 48202-2689, USA

Eckehard Scharein
Institute of Physiology
University Hospital Eppendorf
Martinistraβe 52
D-20246 Hamburg, Germany

Rudolf van Schayck
Department of Neurology
University of Essen
Hufelandstraβe 55
D-45122 Essen, Germany

Barry J. Sessle
Faculty of Dentistry
University of Toronto
124 Edward Street
Toronto, Ontario M5G 1G6
Canada

Rainer Spanagel
Max-Planck-Institute of Psychiatry
Kraepelinstraβe 2
D-80804 München, Germany

Mircea Steriade
Laboratory of Neurophysiology
Department of Physiology
Laval University
Quebec G1K 7P4
Canada

Ronald R. Tasker
Division of Neurosurgery
The Toronto Hospital, Western
  Division
399 Bathurst Street
Toronto, Ontario M5T 2S8
Canada

Thomas R. Tölle
Max-Planck-Institute of Psychiatry
Kraepelinstraβe 2
D-80804 Munich, Germany

Claude Tomberg
Brain Research Unit
University of Brussels
20 rue Evers
B-1000 Brussels, Belgium

Rolf-Detlef Treede
Institute of Physiology and
  Pathophysiology
University of Mainz
Saarstraβe 21
D-55099 Mainz, Germany

Christiane Vahle-Hinz
Institute of Physiology
University Hospital Eppendorf
Martinistraβe 52
D-20246 Hamburg, Germany

Luis Villanueva
Department of Physiopharmacology
INSERM-U 161
2, rue d' Alésia
F-75014 Paris, France

Stanley L. Wallenstein
Memorial Sloan-Kettering Cancer
  Center
1275 York Avenue
New York, New York 10021, USA

Jean Claude Willer
Laboratory of Neurophysiology
Medical Faculty of Pitié-Salpêtrière
University Pierre et Marie Curie
91, Boulevard de l'Hôpital
F-75634 Paris, France

William D. Willis, Jr.
Department of Anatomy and
  Neurosciences
Marine Biomedical Institute
University of Texas Medical Branch
200 University Boulevard
Galveston, Texas 77555-0843

Walter Zieglgänsberger
Max-Planck-Institute of Psychiatry
Kraepelinstraβe 2
D-80804 Munich, Germany

Alexander Zimprich
Institute of Physiology
University of Munich
Pettenkoferstraβe 12
D-808336 Munich, Germany

Foreword

With 37 chapters written by well-known experts in their respective fields, this volume spans the wide arc of pain arising in specific sense organs distributed over the body and converging into the brain to make nociceptive activity conscious. While most books in the field of pain research so far refer to mechanisms of nervous transmission and neuronal processing at the peripheral level, the spinal cord or in lower brain structures, this volume describes the decisive role of consciousness, alertness, and integrative brain functions in the perception and experience of pain.

Some chapters discuss experimental data obtained in animals, but most of them are devoted to investigations in humans, in the healthy volunteer, as well as in the patient suffering from various pains. In fact, several non-invasive methods are available currently to measure higher brain functions; either classical methods, such as electroencephalography and evoked potential analyses, or more recently developed techniques such as positron emission tomography and magnetoencephalography, which appear very promising and certain to lead to the better understanding of complex pain problems.

A major and original feature of this volume is that it contains a considerable amount of information on the human brain at the thalamic, and more particularly, at the cortical level. Also, the psychological component of pain with its emotional, affective, and cognitive aspects is widely developed. As such, this book will stimulate further research in humans. This is crucial, since, despite the great progress in knowledge on basic mechanisms at the peripheral or spinal cord levels, only a few groups are involved in the study of pain processing in the brain. In fact, although there are already consistent data on the sensory discriminative component of pain in animals, it is obvious that most aspects of conscious pain experience remain to be considered. The difficulties of such approaches are reinforced by the multiplicity of ascending pain pathways, the multiplicity of cerebral structures involved in pain processing, and of course by ethical considerations.

Investigation of pain in humans has been in its infancy for a long time, as illustrated by numerous, often unsuccessful, attempts to lesion several nervous areas which are thought to be involved in pain circuitry. Even the reported effects of anterolateral cordotomy, a well-established surgical procedure which is performed less and less, are often contradictory.

The explosion of new exploratory methods will offer the clinicians the ability to make the diagnosis more precise and the therapeutics more appropriate. Moreover, these investigations, closely linked with basic research will be crucial for the understanding of the multiple complex pain syndromes. In fact, thanks to the late Professor J.J. Bonica, this has been the first goal of the International Association for the Study of Pain since it started in the early seventies.

It is certain that this volume, *Pain and the Brain*, will provide information of great interest to a variety of health professionals, students, neurologists, pharmacologists, neurosurgeons, clinical psychologists, pain clinicians and also basic researchers.

Jean-Marie Besson
President Elect of the
International Association
for the Study of Pain
Paris, France, March 1995

Preface

"To-day, then, since I have opportunely freed my mind from all cares, and since I am in the secure possession of leisure in a peaceable retirement, I will at length apply myself earnestly and freely to the general overthrow of all my former opinions. To this end, it will not be necessary for me to show that the whole of these are false—a point, perhaps, which I shall never reach; but, as even now my reason convinces me that I ought not the less carefully to withhold belief from what is not entirely certain and indubitable, than from what is manifestly false, it will be sufficient to justify the rejection of the whole if I shall find in each some ground for doubt.

Descartes[1]

Let us, then, make a fresh start and try to determine what the soul is and what will be its most comprehensive account

Aristotle[2]

Of course, refilling old wine into new pipes will not always improve its quality. But, there is no question that "Pain and the Brain—from Nociception to Cognition" will touch the mind–body problem—the greatest challenge in living memory of thinking. How can we explain conscious perception of certain neuronal impulse patterns elicited somewhere in the body? Do psychic states correspond to circumscript activity of the brain? Who is it who has knowledge about his own mental states and decides how to react and what to do next? At all times, these questions affected every thinking being in the attempt to qualify his private world as part of a whole; and at all times the answers described the contemporary background in science, belief, philosophy, and society.

For us who are involved in pain research and therapy, the mind-body problem has an immediate practical meaning, which has hitherto not been understood in all its consequences and extensions in the treatment of pain. Pain relief is generally based on effects upon both the body and the mind, upon nociception and consciousness. Under opiate, you may not drive a car because vigilance is reduced. Or during the operation, the surgeon elicits an enormous nociceptive impact into the brain; but the patient does not feel pain because his consciousness is suppressed by general anesthesia. Another example relevant to the often discussed problem of the

---

[1]R. Descartes, Meditation I, of the things of which we may doubt (Paris, 1641), in the translation by John Veitch, Renè Descartes, A Discourse on Method, published by J. M. Dent & Sons Ltd., London (1992).

[2]Aristotle (384–322 BC), De Anima, Book II, 412a 1, in the edition of M. Durrant, published by Routledge Inc., London 1993.

development of consciousness is the question at which state in ontogenesis does pain arise. The answer is of highest importance in infant surgery because neurons are destroyed by general anesthesia which has to be maximally avoided in the developing brain of newborns.

For these reasons, we brought together scientists, physiologists, clinicians and psychologists who are experts in their fields of research. We met in the most marvellous place in France, the middle-age city Beaune with the ancient Hospice de Dieu, most famous for medical care, as well as for the best wines—bearing in mind the Greek meaning of the word symposium, drinking and speaking together. Some contributions touched the borders of what can be described or known. But no work in science is more important for the human being than the investigation of the brain.

The book consists of 5 sections with different approaches of various disciplines, opening with an update of current concepts of nociception, pain, and consciousness, and proceeding to discuss practical clinical matters in the evaluation and management of pain states. It is the first volume to present an in-depth exploration of the mind-body problem in pain research and therapy and will, we hope, be of interest to a variety of health professionals, such as pharmacologists, physicians, nurses, neurobiological and biomedical scientists, and clinical psychologists. In spite of the multiple aspects of interdisciplinary roots, we tried to make the book valuable for the well-versed expert, as well as for the groping trainee. Each contribution starts with the fundaments of the respective fields, growing up to the clouds of future hopes; a brief introductory summary informs the reader what to expect next and what may be new to him. Complete lists of references and a thorough subject index make this volume a convenient and valuable reference source for years to come.

The symposium "From Nociception to Pain" was the breeding ground for this volume. The invited speakers left much time for discussion to foster the exchange of opinions. Many participants added their own ideas in the chapters; other authors joined us in a later stage. It is not easy to describe what exactly we are going to work out. Some contributions may touch the borders of what can be described or known. But no work in science is more important for the human being than the investigation of the brain.

Burkhart Bromm, M.D., Ph.D.
John E. Desmedt, M.D., Ph.D.

Acknowledgments

The symposium *From Nociception to Pain* (August 27–29, 1993, Beaune, France) was an official satellite symposium of the 7th World Congress on Pain in Paris, France 1993. We gratefully acknowledge that the symposium and this book were sponsored by the companies: Bayer, Boehringer Ingelheim, Byk Gulden, Cascan, Glaxo, Gödecke, Hoechst, Knoll, AG, Krewel, Lichtwer, Merck Darmstadt, Merck Sharp & Dohme, Mundipharma, Nordmark, Philips, Sandoz, and Schwarz Pharma.

We are especially grateful to Peter Bieri, Herbert Christoph Diener, Peter J. Goadsby, Anthony K. P. Jones, Dan R. Kenshalo, Jr., Frederick A. Lenz, Ronald Melzack, Barry J. Sessle, Walter Zieglgänsberger, for their contributions to this developing field, displaying their philosophical, neurological, pharmacological, and methodological aspects of cognitive brain functions in pain processing.

This book would not have been written without the help of many coworkers, especially of Eckehard Scharein, Rolf-Detlef Treede, Christiane Vahle-Hinz, Andrew C. N. Chen, Holger Kohlhoff, Robert Laudahn, and Jürgen Lorenz. They carefully read the manuscripts, discussed many questions with the authors, and gave valuable constructive arguments. This is the way research should be. We also thank Ute Phillipp for writing all the corresponding letters and many of the manuscripts, Krimhild Saha and Helga Geisser for doing the drawings, and last but not least and in particular, Craig Percy from Raven Press, for his great support, especially in forcing us to finish this book on time.

The Editors

Advances in Pain Research and Therapy
Volume 22

Pain and the Brain
From Nociception to Cognition

Pain and the Brain: From Nociception to Cognition, edited by Burkhart Bromm and John E. Desmedt, Advances in Pain Research and Therapy Vol. 22. Raven Press, Ltd., New York © 1995.

1

From Nociceptor to Cortical Activity

William D. Willis, Jr.

Department of Anatomy and Neurosciences, and Marine Biomedical Institute, University of Texas Medical Branch, Galveston, Texas 77555-1069, USA

SUMMARY

The pain system involves a set of ascending pathways that convey nociceptive information from peripheral nociceptors to higher levels of the central nervous system, as well as descending pathways that modulate that information. A variety of nociceptors has been found to innervate the skin, joints, muscles, and viscera. Activation of different types of nociceptors results in particular qualities of pain. Although the level of activity in nociceptors may not always be tightly coupled with pain, there is a clear causal relationship between the two. Some nociceptors are difficult to activate unless sensitized by inflammation. Nociceptive neurons in the dorsal horn include excitatory and inhibitory interneurons and cells of the ascending tracts. The interneurons may contribute to nociceptive reflexes or control the discharges of ascending-tract cells. Some of the latter, such as neurons of the spinothalamic tract, help to signal the sensation of pain, whereas others are more likely to activate descending control systems or to engage motivational–affective mechanisms. Nociceptive neurons in the ventrobasal thalamus and in the somatosensory areas of the cerebral cortex are likely to be involved in the perception of pain. Other diencephalic and telencephalic structures, including the medial thalamus, hypothalamus, amygdala, and limbic cortex, presumably play a role in a variety of motivational and affective pain reactions. Descending modulatory effects can be elicited by the activation of neurons in a number of brain-stem nuclei, including the anterior pretectal nucleus, periaqueductal gray, nucleus raphe magnus, medullary reticular formation, and parabrachial region.

INTRODUCTION

The sensation of pain usually depends on the activation of a set of neurons that includes primary afferent nociceptors, interneurons in the spinal cord (or brain stem, in the case of the trigeminal system), cells of the ascending tracts, thalamic neurons, and neurons of the cerebral cortex (Fig. 1; Willis 1985; Willis 1988). Together, these cells comprise a "pain system" that is analogous to other sensory systems, such as the visual and auditory systems (Perl 1971). A more comprehensive view of the pain system would include pathways descending from the brain that may reduce or even prevent nociceptive signals from reaching higher levels of the central nervous system (Fig. 1). All sensory systems are under the control of centrifugal pathways, but in the case of the pain system, the centrifugal control or "endogenous analgesia" system is of particular interest because of its clinical value in pain

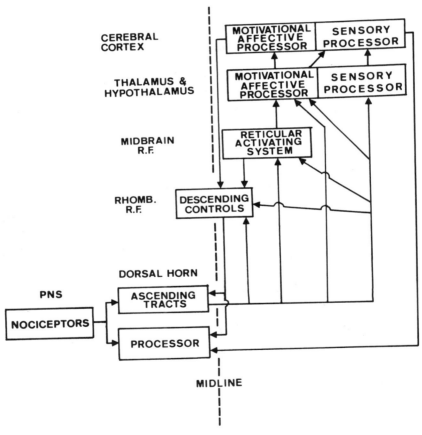

FIG. 1. Pathways of the pain system. The primary afferent nociceptors in the peripheral nervous system (PNS) convey nociceptive information to the dorsal horn, where the information is processed by interneurons and ascending-tract cells. Nociceptive information is then signaled to the reticular activating system and parts of the brain, including the thalamus and cerebral cortex, responsible for sensory and for motivational–affective processing. Descending controls originate at all levels and influence the processing of nociceptive information in the dorsal horn. (From Willis 1988, with permission.)

suppression (Willis 1982; Fields and Besson 1988). In addition to its sensory–discriminative component, pain has a motivational–affective component that is in part mediated by the same pathways, but is in part also mediated by additional pathways that access other brain structures, including the limbic system (Melzack and Casey 1968; Price and Dubner 1977).

The objective of this chapter is to review briefly the components of the pain system responsible for transmitting nociceptive signals from damaged tissue to higher levels of the central nervous system (CNS), and some of the descending systems that control such nociceptive transmission. Several issues that deserve more experimental attention will be emphasized.

NOCICEPTORS

Primary afferent fibers selectively responsive to stimuli that threaten or cause damage are classified as *nociceptors* (Sherrington 1906). Nociceptors have been described in the skin, joints, muscle, and some viscera (reviewed in Willis 1985; Willis and Coggeshall 1991). Experiments using microneurography have demonstrated that cutaneous Aδ- and C-nociceptors with characteristics similar to those observed in animals can be identified in human volunteers, and that activation of the Aδ-nociceptors by intraneural microstimulation causes pricking pain, while activation of the C-nociceptors causes burning or dull pain (Konietzny et al. 1981; Ochoa and Torebjörk 1989).

It is important to note that the threshold for activation of nociceptors is often well below the threshold for pain (Handwerker et al. 1984). Therefore, nociceptors can have a moderate level of activity before the perception of pain becomes conscious. This is consistent with Sherrington's definition of nociceptors, in that activity is initiated at stimulus intensities that only threaten damage rather than actually causing it. However, an increase in the discharge rate of nociceptors as the result of an increase in stimulus strength or sensitization of these cells may well produce pain. Furthermore, continued but decreasing rates of discharge of nociceptors may produce pain because of the central summation of nociceptor input (Adriaensen et al. 1984). Although nociceptor activity is not necessarily tightly coupled with pain, nociceptor discharge is still causally related to pain in the vast majority of episodes of the latter.

During the past decade, a special variety of nociceptor has been described in joints, skin, and viscera (Schaible and Schmidt 1988; Häbler et al. 1990; Handwerker et al. 1991; Davis et al. 1993). This type of nociceptor is very difficult to activate under normal circumstances, but when sensitized, such as by inflammation, it becomes very easy to activate. Nociceptors of this variety, often referred to by Schmidt and colleagues as "sleeping nociceptors" that are "awakened" by inflammation (Hanesch et al. 1992), may be a type of chemoreceptor that develops mechanical sensitivity as a result of the activation of second messenger systems by chemical agents, such as bradykinin, prostaglandins, serotonin, histamine, and

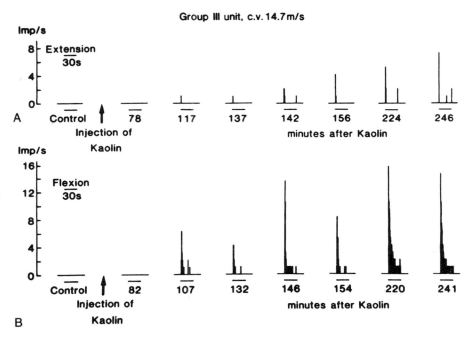

FIG. 2. Awakening of a sleeping nociceptor. The nociceptor was a Group III fiber that supplied the knee joint of a cat. Initially, the afferent failed to respond to either extension **(A)** or flexion **(B)** of the knee. Following the injection of kaolin and carrageenan (KAOLIN) into the joint capsule, the unit began to respond to joint movements in parallel with the development of acute arthritis. (From Schaible and Schmidt 1988, with permission.)

other substances released in damaged tissue (Dray et al. 1988; Birrell et al. 1993; Davis et al. 1993; Schepelmann et al. 1993). Fig. 2 shows the responses of such a receptor innervating the knee joint of a cat. The afferent fiber belonged to Group III, and failed to respond to innocuous extension of flexion of the knee during the control period. After the injection of kaolin and carrageenan into the joint capsule, however, the unit developed increasing responses to movements of the knee, especially flexion.

Another set of primary afferent fibers that belongs to the class of "sleeping" or "silent" nociceptor are tooth-pulp afferents, which presumably do not have a sensory function until dental pathology occurs (Silverman and Kruger 1987), after which they become a major source of pain. It has been proposed that the normally silent nociceptors may have an efferent function in the tissue they supply (Silverman and Kruger 1987; 1989; Kruger et al. 1989). This idea deserves further attention. It is, for example, possible that the release of peptides by these cells, such as calcitonin gene-related peptide (CGRP), could have some role in calcium metabolism in teeth or bone.

DORSAL-HORN NEURONS

Nociceptive information is transmitted synaptically to interneurons of the spinal cord and medullary dorsal horn (Willis 1985; Willis and Coggeshall 1991). The nociceptive input particularly evokes responses in neurons in laminae I, II, IV–VI, and X (plus flexor motor neurons). Neurons with nociceptive responses have been classified into several groups, including "wide-dynamic-range" (WDR) and "nociceptive-specific" (NS) neurons (Price and Dubner 1977). WDR neurons are defined as those that respond to innocuous stimuli but respond maximally to noxious stimuli, whereas NS neurons respond only to noxious stimuli. However, the exact criteria for this classification tend to vary between laboratories and with the kind of neuron under study; quantitative criteria are generally not specified. Furthermore, most investigators have no information about the functional effects of activation of the neurons being studied. Thus, for example, recordings from neurons in the superficial dorsal horn could come either from excitatory (e.g., glutamatergic) or inhibitory (e.g., GABAergic, enkephalinergic) interneurons (9). An increased discharge of inhibitory nociceptive interneurons might tend to produce analgesia rather than pain.

In our view, the discharges of ascending-tract cells are more likely to correlate well with pain sensation than are the discharges of local-circuit interneurons in the dorsal horn. However, particular types of ascending-tract cells may serve primarily to activate descending control systems rather than to signal pain sensation. Thus, in our laboratory, we prefer to record from neurons identified as spinothalamic-tract (STT) cells than from ascending-tract cells that project to areas known to be sources of analgesia pathways, on the assumption that STT cells are likely to signal the sensation of pain.

By recording the discharges evoked by graded mechanical stimulation of the skin from a large sample of STT cells that project to the ventral posterior lateral (VPL) nucleus of the thalamus, we were able to use a multivariate statistical analysis (cluster analysis) for the classification of STT cells. The cells could be divided into three groups, based on the selectivity of their responses to different intensities of mechanical stimuli applied to the skin (Owens et al. 1992). Fig. 3A is a three-dimensional plot showing the percentage of the summed total responses to brush, pressure, pinch, and squeeze stimuli that was produced by brush (x-axis), pinch (z-axis), and squeeze (y-axis) stimuli. The club symbols represent 14.3% of the neurons in our sample that were activated best by innocuous mechanical stimuli (see Fig. 3B, cluster 1); we suggest that such neurons contribute to touch, one of the sensory functions mediated by axons of the anterolateral quadrant of the spinal cord in humans (Noordenbos and Wall 1976). The remaining STT cells belonged to groups that were either best activated by a noxious mechanical stimulus of intermediate intensity (cylinders; 59.1%) or severe intensity (spades; 26.7%). Both of these groups of cells were excited slightly by innocuous mechanical stimuli (see Fig. 3B, clusters 2 and 3). Some STT cells that initially could not be activated by weak mechanical stimuli became very responsive to such stimuli following damage to the

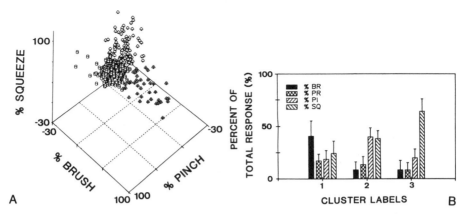

FIG. 3. Classification of primate spinothalamic-tract (STT) cells. The three-dimensional plot in **A** shows the proportions of the total responses of each of a population of STT cells to a series of four mechanical stimuli that were produced by brush, pinch, and squeeze stimuli. The clubs represent cluster 1 cells, the open cylinders cluster 2 cells, and the spades cluster 3 cells. The bar graph in **B** shows the mean (and SD) of the proportions of the total responses of the STT cells of clusters 1 through 3 that were evoked by brush (BR), pressure (PR), pinch (PI), and squeeze (SQ) stimuli. (From Owens et al. 1992, with permission.)

skin, indicating that these cells had subthreshold inputs from mechanoreceptors under normal conditions. Thus, on statistical grounds, the vast majority of the nociceptive STT cells in our sample would be classified as WDR neurons if such cells are defined as having any input at all from mechanoreceptors. We therefore suggest that most of the STT cells projecting to the VPL nucleus are nociceptive, and that their activity results in pain, provided that the discharge rate of these cells exceeds some threshold at higher levels of the CNS. We further suggest that the weak activity of these STT cells evoked by innocuous mechanical stimuli is normally insufficient to exceed the threshold of pain in the central pain system. When the STT cells (or excitatory interneuronal circuits affecting STT cells) are sensitized by peripheral or central damage, innocuous mechanical stimuli can evoke much larger responses in these cells, in which case tactile stimuli could provoke pain. This would be one mechanism underlying mechanical allodynia (Willis 1993).

Nociceptors also activate a number of other ascending pathways. These include at least some neurons belonging to the spinoreticular and spinomesencephalic tracts (SMT), that have axons in the anterolateral quadrant of the spinal cord; neurons of the spinocervical tract and postsynaptic dorsal-column pathway; and perhaps some STT and SMT neurons with axons in the dorsal part of the white matter of the spinal cord (Willis and Coggeshall 1991). We believe that the nociceptive pathways in the anterolateral quadrant other than the STT are likely to contribute to pain either by activating attentional mechanisms and arousal or by producing emotional and autonomic reactions through input to limbic structures by way of the medial thalamus, amygdala, and hypothalamus. The component of pain that involves responses in neurons of these structures would not be the sensory–discriminative but rather the motivational–affective component (Melzack and Casey 1968; Price and Dubner 1977). Clinically, this may well be the most relevant component of human pain, and so deserves more experimental attention than it has received. However, the neural basis of this aspect of pain is difficult to examine in experiméntal animals because of ethical constraints. It seems likely that the best chance for rapid progress in this area will come from studies of human subjects using imaging techniques (cf. Talbot et al. 1991).

Nociceptive pathways in the dorsal part of the spinal cord are not essential for human pain (Willis and Coggeshall 1991), although they may contribute to nociception in animals such as cats (Kennard 1954). Nociceptive neurons have been found in the dorsal-column nuclei in both monkeys and cats, and many of these neurons project to the VPL nucleus of the contralateral thalamus (Cliffer et al. 1992; Ferrington et al. 1988). For example, the receptive field (RF) and responses to mechanical stimuli of graded intensity of a neuron in the nucleus gracilis of a monkey are shown in Fig. 4. The best responses were to pinch and squeeze stimuli. This neuron could be activated antidromically from the contralateral VPL nucleus, and so was a gracilothalamic-projection neuron. The nociceptive responses of such neurons may depend on input to the dorsal-column nuclei from neurons of the postsynaptic dorsal-column pathway (Brown et al. 1983; Angaut-Petit 1975) or from fine primary afferent fibers that have recently been found to project directly to the dorsal-column nuclei (Conti et al. 1990; Patterson et al. 1990; 1992).

Nociceptive neurons are also present in the spinocervical tract (Cervero et al. 1977; Downie et al. 1988) and lateral cervical nucleus (Downie et al. 1988), and the latter in turn project to the contralateral VPL nucleus (see Willis and Coggeshall 1991). In animals other than cats, the sensory role of these nociceptive-tract neurons that project through the dorsal part of the spinal cord is unclear. One of their functions might be to activate descending control systems. For example, the dorsal-column nuclei and axons ascending in the dorsal lateral funiculus project to the anterior pretectal nucleus, which when stimulated produces analgesia without aversive side effects (Rees and Roberts 1993).

THALAMUS

In primates, including humans, the STT projects to a number of thalamic nuclei, including the VPL nucleus, the posterior complex, the centrolateral (CL) nucleus, and several other medial nuclei, including the nucleus submedius (see Willis 1985; Willis and Coggeshall 1991; see also chapter 11). In cats, the STT largely avoids the VPL nucleus itself, instead ending in a shell region dorsal and ventral to the VPL nucleus.

Recordings from neurons in the VPL nucleus of monkeys reveal that it contains WDR and NS neurons (Kenshalo et al. 1980; Casey and Morrow 1983; Chung et al. 1986). The neurons have restricted contralateral RFs, and their responses are robust;

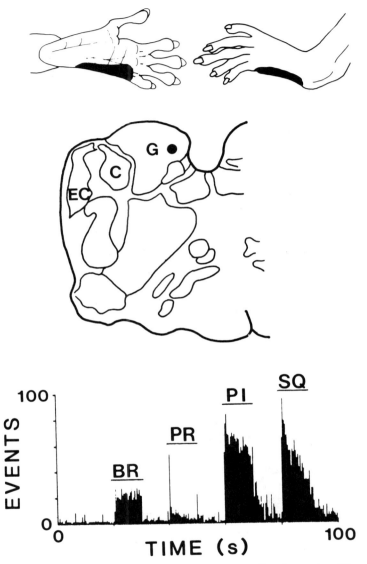

FIG. 4. Nociceptive responses of a neuron in the nucleus gracilis of a monkey. The receptive field is shown at the top and the location of the cell in the drawing at the center. The peristimulus-time histogram at the bottom shows that the cell responded better to pinch and squeeze than to brush or pressure stimuli. The neuron was antidromically activated from the contralateral ventral posterior lateral nucleus. (From Ferrington et al. 1988, with permission.)

they are somatotopically organized and project to the primary somatosensory cortex (SI) (Kenshalo et al. 1980). Some respond to both Aδ- and C-fiber volleys in peripheral nerves (Chung et al. 1986). The nociceptive input of these neurons generally ascends from the spinal cord in the lateral funiculus ipsilateral to the thalamic neuron (contralateral to the RF), although in some cases the input is transmitted in the dorsal quadrant ipsilateral to the thalamic neuron (Chung et al. 1986). However, nociceptive responses in monkeys depend on signals ascending in the anterolateral quadrant of the spinal cord, contralateral to the RF (ipsilateral to the thalamic target of the ascending projection), as shown by the reduction in nociceptive responses following cordotomy (Yoss 1953; Greenspan et al. 1986). For instance, the VPL neuron illustrated in Fig. 5A discharged strongly when the skin in the RF was stimulated with noxious heat. This response was unaffected when the dorsal quadrant of the spinal cord ipsilateral to the RF (contralateral to the thalamic neuron) was interrupted at a thoracic level (Fig. 5B). However, when a two-stage lesion of the contralateral lateral funiculus was made (Fig. 5C, D), the heat response was eliminated.

Similarly, nociceptive neurons are found in the VPL nucleus in rats (Guilbaud et al. 1980), and ventrolateral cordotomy eliminates nociceptive behavioral and electrophysiologic responses in these animals (Peschanski et al. 1985; 1986). Nociceptive neurons have also been described in the ventral posterior medial (VPM) nucleus of the thalamus in awake, behaving monkeys (Bushnell et al. 1993).

Recently, Lenz and colleagues (Lenz et al. 1993; see also chapter 11, this book) have reported that some neurons in the human nucleus ventralis caudalis (equivalent to the VPL nucleus in animals) respond to noxious heat stimuli. These nociceptive thalamic neurons were concentrated in regions that when stimulated electrically produced a painful sensation. Fig. 6A shows the responses of a neuron located in the cutaneous core of the nucleus ventralis caudalis to a noxious heat and to an innocuous mechanical stimulus. Fig. 6B shows in histogram and raster form the responses of the same neuron to noxious heat as well as to innocuous heat, mechanical, and cold stimuli. The greatest responses were to noxious heat (the application of a brass probe heated to 53°C to the skin) and the initial part of the cold stimulus. The locations of neurons responding to noxious heat stimuli in several subjects are shown in Fig. 6C in relation to the line connecting the anterior commissure (AC) to the posterior commissure (PC). Six of the nociceptive cells recorded were in the cutaneous core region and four were in the posteroinferior region.

CEREBRAL CORTEX

A longstanding debate centers on the involvement of the cerebral cortex in pain (see Kenshalo and Willis 1991). Several groups of investigators have proposed that pain is sensed at the thalamic rather than at the cortical level (Head and Holmes 1991; Holmes 1927; Penfield and Boldrey 1937). However, others have provided evidence for a cortical involvement in pain sensation (see Kenshalo and Willis 1991).

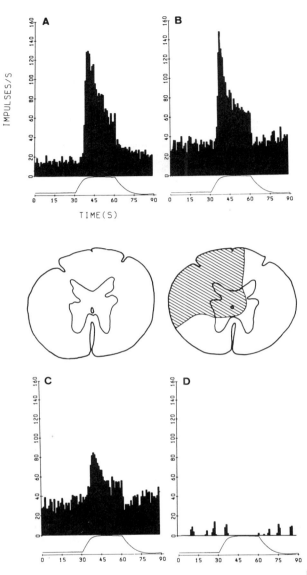

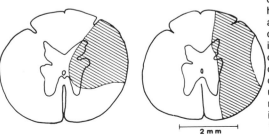

FIG. 5. Responses of a nociceptive neuron in the ventral posterior lateral nucleus of the thalamus of a monkey to noxious heat pulses. **A–D:** Responses before and after the lesions of the spinal cord indicated by the hatched areas on the drawing of a spinal-cord section. Interruption of the anterolateral quadrant of the spinal cord on the side contralateral to the receptive field (ipsilateral to the thalamic unit) eliminated the response and also markedly reduced the background activity of the cell **(D)**. (From Kenshalo et al., 1980, with permission.)

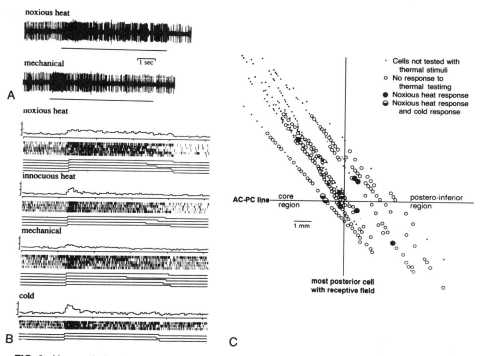

FIG. 6. Human thalamic neuron responding to noxious heat and innocuous mechanical stimulation. **A:** Recordings of the response of a neuron in the cutaneous core of the human thalamic nucleus ventralis caudalis to noxious heat and to innocuous mechanical stimulation in its receptive field. The horizontal lines below the records indicate the duration of the stimuli. **B:** Histograms and raster displays of the spikes evoked by several stimulation trials. The best responses were to noxious heat and, at least initially, to cold. The deflections of the lower traces show when stimuli were applied. **C:** The response properties of units recorded along tracks through the thalamus in several different subjects. The tracks are viewed as if in a parasagittal plane; the anterior commissure–posterior commissure (AC–PC) line is indicated, and the zones occupied by the cutaneous core and the posteroinferior regions are indicated. The key shows the symbols used to represent neurons having different response properties. (From Lenz et al. 1993, with permission.)

For example, recordings from single neurons in the SI cortex of monkeys, particularly in area 1, have revealed the presence of both WDR and high-threshold (HT) neurons in the middle layers of the cortex (Kenshalo and Isensee 1983). The RFs of these nociceptive cortical neurons were often small and located in a somatotopically appropriate region on a contralateral extremity. In some cases, however, the neurons' receptive fields were large and bilateral. The neurons often responded to both strong mechanical and thermal stimuli, and repeated strong heat stimuli caused their responses to increase, presumably because of sensitization of cutaneous thermal nociceptors.

Similarly, nociceptive neurons of both the WDR and (HT) type have been found in the somatosensory cortex of the rat (Lamour et al. 1983a,b). The RFs of these neurons often covered the entire surface of the body. As in monkeys, the neurons responded to both noxious mechanical and thermal stimuli. In contrast to monkeys, the nociceptive cortical neurons in rats were concentrated in the deep layers of the cortex. Nociceptive responses have also been recorded from neurons in the second-ary somatosensory cortex (SII) and area 7b (Robinson and Burton 1980; Dong et al. 1989), as well as in the cingulate gyrus (Sikes and Vogt 1992).

The stimulus–response functions of nociceptive neurons in the SI cortex in awake monkeys have been compared with the speed of detection of small increments in noxious heat stimuli applied to the animals' faces (Kenshalo et al. 1988). A signifi-cant correlation was found between the peak firing rates of WDR neurons and the speed of detection of increments in the heat stimulus. Furthermore, the peak firing rate for a given neuron was greater when near-threshold noxious heat stimuli were detected than when they were not.

Functional inactivation of area 2 in the primary sensory cortex (S1) by cooling has been reported to result in deficits in the ability of monkeys to respond to pin-prick stimuli applied to the hand (Brinkman et al. 1985). Furthermore, bilateral lesions of the S1 cortex reduced the ability of monkeys to detect noxious heat stim-uli applied to the face, as well as to discriminate between two heat stimuli differing by less than 1°C (Kenshalo et al. 1989).

Late and ultra-late evoked brain potentials have been recorded from the vertex of the skull in humans following laser stimulation of the skin (Bromm et al. 1983; Bromm and Treede 1987; 1991). Examples of these potentials are shown in Fig. 7. The ultra-late evoked potential was not clearly seen in records of the late evoked potential, but appeared when the late evoked potential was blocked by pressure applied to the appropriate peripheral nerve. The late evoked responses reflect the activity in Aδ- heat nociceptors, while the ultra-late responses reflect the activity in C-nociceptors. This is shown by the disappearance of the late evoked potential following application of the pressure block (Fig. 7, A-fiber block) and the disap-pearance of the ultra-late evoked potential when C-fibers were blocked by injection of a local anesthetic (Fig. 7, lidoc.). The evoked potentials correlated with first and second pain reports in the subjects. These electroencephalographically (EEG) re-corded potentials originated from the vertex of the skull, exending parietally; they presumably arose from the vicinity of the S1 cortex (Treede and Bromm 1988; Bromm and Treede 1991).

Recently, imaging studies using positron-emission tomography (PET) have re-vealed that painful heat stimuli applied to one arm in human subjects activate the S1 and secondary (S2) somatosensory cortices and anterior cingulate gyrus on the side contralateral to the stimulus (Talbot et al. 1991). Presumably, more regions of the cerebral cortex, particular those with limbic function, would have been involved if the stimulus had not been restricted to a minimally painful level.

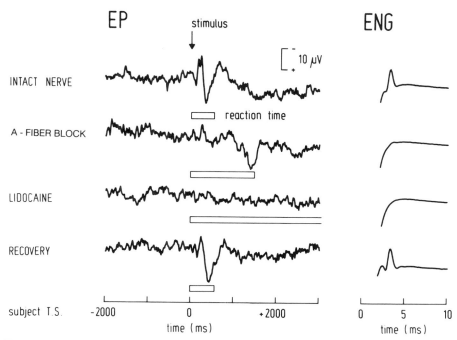

FIG. 7. Ultra-late laser-evoked brain potentials in response to C-fiber activation. Brief radiant heat pulses (20 msec, 8 W, 10.8 μm wavelength) were applied to the hairy skin of the left hand. Evoked brain potentials (EP, vertex, negativity upward) were built by averaging over 40 stimulus repetitions with painful intensities; in addition, motor reaction times and the usual peripheral electroneurogram (ENG) were measured. With intact A-fibers ENG was normal, reaction times were approximately 500 msec, and late EPs appeared (N260 = negativity at 260 msec, and P400 = positivity at 400 msec). After mechanical A-fiber block, C-fibers mediated the information toward the brain: the ENG disappeared, the reaction times were prolonged to 1,400 msec, and ultra-late EPs emerged with N1,250 and P1,400 msec. Injection of lidocaine (1%) wiped out all EPs. After release of the pressure block, the changes were rapidly reversible. (From Bromm and Treede 1991, with permission.)

DESCENDING CONTROL SYSTEMS

When stimulated, many areas of the brain stem produce analgesia or antinociception (Willis 1982). Some of these areas are the periaqueductal gray (PAG), the nucleus raphe magnus, and the medullary reticular formation; others will be mentioned below. However, most of these areas also produce aversive responses. An exception to this is the anterior pretectal nucleus of rats, which when stimulated produces a purely antinociceptive effect (Rees and Roberts 1993). The descending pathways responsible for this effect appear to relay in the ventrolateral medulla and parabrachial area of the pons (Terenzi et al. 1991; 1992).

The descending pathways from such regions as the PAG have proven to be very complex. There are nociceptive projections ascending directly to the PAG from the spinal cord through the spinomesencephalic tract (Yezierski et al. 1987; Yezierski and Broton 1991), as well as collateral projections to the PAG from the STT (Yezierski et al. 1987; Harmann et al. 1988; Zhang et al. 1990). However, the consequences of nociceptive input to the PAG are likely to be mediated by projections descending both to the pons and to the medulla, as well as by projections ascending to the thalamus and hypothalamus (Cameron et al. 1993a,b). Furthermore, neurons of the PAG seem to be organized in longitudinal columns having different functions (Bandler and Depaulis 1991; Lovick 1991). For example, stimulation of a dorsolateral column in the PAG not only causes antinociception but also an increase in blood pressure and heart rate, whereas stimulation of a ventrolateral column causes antinociception accompanied by a decrease in blood pressure and heart rate. These different functions are likely to be mediated by connections with different sets of brain-stem nuclei.

Another important concentration of neurons that is undoubtedly involved in pain-related activity is nuclei in the parabrachial region of the rostral pons. There is a direct spinal projection to this area (Bernard et al. 1989; Kitamura et al. 1993), and neurons of the parabrachial region receiving spinal input project to both the amygdaloid nucleus (Bernard and Besson 1990) and to the intralaminar nuclei of the thalamus (Fulwiler and Saper 1984). It has been proposed that the parabrachial region is involved in relaying nociceptive information that contributes to the emotional and autonomic responses to painful events (Bernard and Besson 1990). Stimulation of the dorsolateral pons, including the parabrachial region, results in antinociception. However, at least part of this effect probably depends on the activation of catecholaminergic projections to the spinal cord from the locus coeruleus and subcoeruleus (Jones and Gebhart 1986).

Recently, Le Bars and colleagues have examined the possible antinociceptive role of neurons in the dorsal reticular nucleus of the medulla (Bouhassira et al. 1992; Roy et al. 1992; see also chapter 34, this book). These cells receive a largely crossed spinal projection through the ventral lateral quadrant (Bing et al. 1990), and in turn project to the dorsal horn of the spinal cord through the dorsal lateral funiculus (Bernard et al. 1990). This nucleus appears to play a major role in the "diffuse noxious inhibitory controls" described by Le Bars and this group. Evidently, the rostral ventromedial medulla, including the nucleus raphe magnus, does not play such a role (Bouhassira et al. 1993).

CONCLUSIONS

It can be concluded from the findings discussed in this chapter that:

1. The system that mediates the sensation of pain includes primary afferent nociceptors, interneurons of processing circuits of the dorsal horn, cells of ascending tracts, thalamic neurons, and neurons of the cerebral cortex. In addition, the pain system can be considered to include the endogenous analgesia system, as well as neurons involved in the motivational–affective component of pain.

2. Nociceptors are sensory receptors that signal damage or the threat of damage to the body. A recently discovered type of nociceptor is normally difficult to activate unless sensitized by inflammation. Such receptors may have efferent as well as chemoreceptive functions.

3. Nociceptive neurons in the dorsal horn may have sensory, motor, or inhibitory actions. Nociceptive tract cells, such as those belonging to the STT, typically respond to both innocuous and noxious stimuli. When these neurons are sensitized, their enhanced responses to innocuous stimuli may cause allodynia.

4. A number of ascending pathways, including the dorsal column–medial lemniscus system contain nociceptive neurons. The sensory role of nociceptive neurons whose axons ascend in the dorsal part of the spinal cord is unclear. These neurons may serve to activate descending inhibitory systems.

5. The ventrobasal (VB) complex of the thalamus contains nociceptive neurons that project to the S1 cortex. These include WDR and high-threshold neurons. They are somatotopically organized and respond to volleys in both Aδ- and C-fibers.

6. Noxious heat stimuli activating Aδ- and C-fibers evoke late and ultra-late potentials that can be recorded from the vertex region of the skull in human subjects. Both the S1 and S2 areas of the somatosensory cortex and the anterior cingulate gyrus are activated by noxious stimuli in human subjects, as determined by PET. Nociceptive neurons have been identified in the S1 and S2 cortices and anterior cingulate gyrus of animals. These observations suggest that the sensory–discriminative processing of nociceptive information, and presumably of pain, involves the somatosensory thalamus and cortex. Many other structures, including the medial thalamus, hypothalamus, amygdala, and limbic cortex are likely to be involved in the motivational–affective component of pain.

7. The endogenous analgesia system involves a number of brain-stem structures. When stimulated, several of these structures also cause aversive reactions and are likely to convey nociceptive information to higher centers concerned with emotion and autonomic adjustments. The anterior pretectal nucleus seems to be exceptional in that its action seems to be limited to analgesia.

ACKNOWLEDGMENTS

The experiments done in the author's laboratory were supported by Grants NS 09743 and NS 11255 from the NIH and by an unrestricted grant from the Bristol-Myers Squibb Co.

REFERENCES

Adriaensen H, Gybels J, Handwerker HO, Van Hees J. Nociceptor discharges and sensations due to prolonged noxious mechanical stimulation—a paradox. *Hum Neurobiol* 1984;3:53–58.

Angaut-Petit D. The dorsal column system: II. Functional properties and bulbar relay of the postsynaptic fibres of the cat's fasciculus gracilis. *Exp Brain Res* 1975;22:471–493.

Bandler R, Depaulis A. Midbrain periaqueductal gray control of defensive behavior in the cat and rat. In:

Depaulis A, Bandler R, eds. *The midbrain periaqueductal gray matter.* New York: Plenum Press, 1991;175–198.

Bernard JF, Besson, JM. The spino(trigemino)pontoamygdaloid pathway: electrophysiological evidence for an involvement in pain processes. *J Neurophysiol* 1990;63:473–488.

Bernard JF, Peschanski M, Besson JM. A possible spino(trigemino)-ponto-amygdaloid pathway for pain. *Neurosci Lett* 1989;100:83–88.

Bernard JF, Villanueva L, Carroué J, Le Bars D. Efferent projections from the subnucleus reticularis dorsalis (SRD): A *Phaseolus vulgaris* leucoagglutinin study in the rat. *Neurosci Lett* 1990;116:257–262.

Bing Z, Villanueva L, Le Bars D. Ascending pathways in the spinal cord involved in the activation of subnucleus reticularis dorsalis neurons in the medulla of the rat. *J Neurophysiol* 1990;63: 424–438.

Birrell GJ, McQueen DS, Iggo A, Grubb BD. Prostanoid-induced potentiation of the excitatory and sensitizing effects of bradykinin on articular mechanonociceptors in the rat ankle joint. *Neuroscience* 1993;54:537–544.

Bouhassira D, Bing Z, Le Bars D. Studies of brain structures involved in diffuse noxious inhibitory controls in the rat: the rostral ventromedial medulla. *J Physiol* 1993;463:667–687.

Bouhassira D, Villanueva L, Bing Z, Le Bars D. Involvement of the subnucleus reticularis dorsalis in diffuse noxious inhibitory controls in the rat. *Brain Res* 1992;595:353–357.

Brinkman J, Colebatch JG, Porter R, York DH. Responses of precentral cells during cooling of post-central cortex in conscious monkeys. *J Physiol* 1985;368:611–625.

Bromm B, Treede RD. Human cerebral potentials evoked by CO_2 laser stimuli causing pain. *Exp Brain Res* 1987;67:153–162.

Bromm B, Treede RD. Laser-evoked cerebral potentials in the assessment of cutaneous pain sensitivity in normal subjects and in patients. *Rev Neurol* 1991;146:625–644.

Bromm B, Neitzel H, Tecklenburg A, Treede RD. Evoked cerebral potential correlates of C-fiber activity in man. *Neurosci Lett* 1983;43:109–114.

Brown AG, Brown PB, Fyffe REW, Pubols LM. Receptive field organization and response properties of spinal neurons with axons ascending the dorsal columns in the cat. *J Physiol* 1983;337:575–588.

Bushnell MC, Duncan GH, Tremblay N. Thalamic VPM nucleus in the behaving monkey. I. Multimodal and discriminative properties of thermosensitive neurons. *J Neurophysiol* 1993;69:739–752.

Cameron AA, Khan IA, Westlund KN, Cliffer KD, Willis WD. The efferent projections of the periaqueductal gray in the rat: a *Phaseolus vulgaris* leucoagglutinin (PHA-L) study. 1. Ascending projections. *J Comp Neurol* 1995a;351:568–584.

Cameron AA, Khan IA, Westlund KN, Willis WD. The efferent projections of the periaqueductal gray in the rat: a *Phaseolus vulgaris*-leucoagglutinin (PHA-L) study. II. Descending projections. *J Comp Neurol* 1995b;351:585–601.

Casey KL, Morrow TJ. Ventral posterior thalamic neurons differentially responsive to noxious stimulation of the awake monkey. *Science* 1983;221:675–677.

Cervero F, Iggo A, Molony V. Responses of spinocervical tract neurones to noxious stimulation of the skin. *J Physiol* 1977;267:537–558.

Chung JM, Lee KH, Surmeier DJ, Sorkin LS, Kim J, Willis WD. Response characteristics of neurons in the ventral posterior lateral nucleus of the monkey thalamus. *J Neurophysiol* 1986;56:370–390.

Cliffer KD, Hasegawa T, Willis WD. Responses of neurons in the gracile nucleus of cats to innocuous and noxious stimuli: basic characterization and antidromic activation from the thalamus. *J Neurophysiol* 1992;68:818–832.

Conti F, De Biasi S, Giuffrida R, Rustioni A. Substance P-containing projections in the dorsal columns of rats and cats. *Neuroscience* 1990;34:607–621.

Davis, KD, Meyer, RA, Campbell JN. Chemosensitivity and sensitization of nociceptive afferents that innervate the hairy skin of monkey. *J Neurophysiol* 1993;69:1071–1081.

Dong WK, Salonen LD, Kawakami Y, Shiwaku T, Kaukoranta EM, Martin RF. Nociceptive responses of trigeminal neurons in SII-7b cortex of awake monkeys. *Brain Res* 1989;484:314–324.

Downie JW, Ferrington DG, Sorkin LS, Willis WD. The primate spinocervicothalamic pathway: responses of cells of the lateral cervical nucleus and spinocervical tract to innocuous and noxious stimuli. *J Neurophysiol* 1988;59:861–885.

Dray A, Bettaney J, Forster P, Perkins MN. Bradykinin-induced stimulation of afferent fibres is mediated through protein kinase C. *Neurosci Lett* 1988;91:301–307.

Ferrington DG, Downie JW, Willis WD. Primate nucleus gracilis neurons: responses to innocuous and noxious stimuli. *J Neurophysiol* 1988;59:886–907.

Fields HL, Besson JM, eds. Pain modulation. *Progress in brain research*, vol. 77. Amsterdam: Elsevier, 1988;

Fulwiler CE, Saper CB. Subnuclear organization of the efferent connections of the parabrachial nucleus in the rat. *Brain Res Rev* 1984;7:229–259.

Greenspan JD, Vierck CJ, Ritz LA. Sensitivity to painful and nonpainful electrocutaneous stimuli in monkeys: effects of anterolateral chordotomy. *J Neurosci* 1986;6:380–390.

Guilbaud G, Peschanski M, Gautron M, Binder D. Neurones responding to noxious stimulation in VB complex and caudal adjacent regions in the thalamus of the rat. *Pain* 1980;8:303–318.

Häbler HJ, Jänig W, Koltzenburg M. Activation of unmyelinated afferent fibres by mechanical stimuli and inflammation of the urinary bladder in the cat. *J Physiol* 1990;425:545–562.

Handwerker HO, Adriaensen H, Gybels JM, Van Hees J. Nociceptor discharges and pain sensations: results and open questions. In: Bromm B, ed. *Pain measurement in man. Neurophysiological correlates of pain.* Amsterdam: Elsevier, 1984;55–64.

Handwerker HO, Kilo S, Reeh PW. Unresponsive afferent nerve fibres in the sural nerve of the rat. *J Physiol* 1991;435:229–242.

Hanesch U, Heppelmann B, Messlinger K, Schmidt RF. Nociception in normal and arthritic joints. In: Willis WD, ed. *Hyperalgesia and allodynia.* New York: Raven Press, 1992;81–106.

Harmann PA, Carlton SM, Willis WD. Collaterals of spinothalamic tract cells to the periaqueductal gray: a fluorescent double-labeling study in the rat. *Brain Res* 1988;441:87–97.

Head H, Holmes G. Sensory disturbances from cerebral lesions. *Brain* 1911;34:102–254.

Holmes G. Disorders of sensation produced by cortical lesions. *Brain* 1927;50:413–427.

Jones SL, Gebhart GF. Characterization of coeruleospinal inhibition of the nociceptive tail-flick reflex in the rat: Mediation by spinal α_2-adrenoreceptors. *Brain Res* 1986;364:315–330.

Kennard MA. The course of ascending fibers in the spinal cord of the cat essential to the recognition of painful stimuli. *J Comp Neurol* 1954;100:511–524.

Kenshalo DR Jr, Anton F, Dubner R. The detection and perceived intensity of noxious thermal stimuli in monkey and man. *J Neurophysiol* 1989;62:429–436.

Kenshalo DR Jr, Chudler EH, Anton F, Dubner R. SI nociceptive neurons participate in the encoding process by which monkeys perceive the intensity of noxious thermal stimulation. *Brain Res* 1988;454: 378–382.

Kenshalo DR Jr, Giesler GJ, Leonard RB, Willis WD. Responses of neurons in primate ventral posterior lateral nucleus to noxious stimuli. *J Neurophysiol* 1980;43:1594–1614.

Kenshalo DR Jr, Isensee O. Responses of primate SI cortical neurons to noxious stimuli. *J Neurophysiol* 1983;50:1479–1496.

Kenshalo DR, Willis WD. The role of the cerebral cortex in pain sensation. In: Peters A, Jones EG, eds. *Cerebral cortex. Normal and altered states of function*, vol. 9. New York: Plenum Press, 1991;153–212.

Kitamura T, Yamada J, Sato H, Yamashita K. Cells of origin of the spinoparabrachial fibers in the rat: a study with fast blue and WGA-HRP. *J Comp Neurol* 1993;328:449–461.

Konietzny F, Perl ER, Trevino D, Light A, Hensel H. Sensory experiences in man evoked by intraneural electrical stimulation of intact cutaneous afferent fibers. *Exp Brain Res* 1981;42:219–222.

Kruger L, Silverman JD, Mantyh PW, Sternini C, Brecha NC. Peripheral patterns of calcitonin-gene-related peptide general somatic sensory innervation: cutaneous and deep terminations. *J Comp Neurol* 1989;280:291–302.

Lamour Y, Guilbaud G, Willer JC. Rat somatosensory (SmI) cortex: II. Laminar and columnar organization of noxious and non-noxious inputs. *Exp Brain Res* 1983a;49:46–54.

Lamour Y, Willer JC, Guilbaud G. Rat somatosensory (SmI) cortex: I. Characteristics of neuronal responses to noxious stimulation and comparison with responses to non-noxious stimulation. *Exp Brain Res* 1983b;49:35–45.

Lenz FA, Seike M, Lin YC, Baker FH, Rowland LH, Gracely RH, Richardson RT. Neurons in the area of the human thalamic nucleus ventralis caudalis respond to painful heat stimuli. *Brain Res* 1993;623: 235–240.

Lovick TA. Interactions between descending pathways from the dorsal and ventrolateral periaqueductal gray matter in the rat. In: Bandler R, Carrive P, eds. *The midbrain periaqueductal gray matter.* New York: Plenum Press, 1991;101–120.

Melzack R, Casey KL. Sensory, motivational and central control determinants of pain. In: Kenshalo DR Jr, ed. *The skin senses.* Springfield, IL: Charles C. Thomas, 1968;423–439.

Noordenbos W, Wall PD. Diverse sensory functions with an almost totally divided spinal cord. A case of spinal cord transection with preservation of part of one anterolateral quadrant. *Pain* 1976;2:185–195.

Ochoa J, Torebjörk E. Sensations evoked by intraneural microstimulation of C nociceptor fibres in human skin nerves. *J Physiol* 1989;415:583–599.

Owens CM, Zhang D, Willis WD. Changes in the response states of primate spinothalamic tract cells caused by mechanical damage of the skin or activation of descending controls. *J Neurophysiol* 1992; 67:1509–1527.

Patterson JT, Chung K, Coggeshall RE. Further evidence for the existence of long ascending unmyelinated primary afferent fibers within the dorsal funiculus: effects of capsaicin. *Pain* 1992;49:117–120.

Patterson JT, Coggeshall RE, Lee WT, Chung K. Long ascending unmyelinated primary afferent axons in the rat dorsal column: immunohistochemical localizations. *Neurosci Lett* 1990;108:6–10.

Penfield W, Boldrey E. Somatic motor and sensory representation in the cerebral cortex of man as studied by electrical stimulation. *Brain* 1937;60:389–443.

Perl ER. Is pain a specific sensation? *J Psychiatr Res* 1971;8:273–287.

Peschanski M, Briand A, Gautron M, Guilbaud G. Electrophysiological evidence for a role of the anterolateral quadrant of the spinal cord in the transmission of noxious messages to the thalamic ventrobasal complex in the rat. *Brain Res* 1985;342:77–84.

Peschanski M, Kayser V, Besson JM. Behavioral evidence for a crossed ascending pathway for pain transmission in the anterolateral quadrant of the rat spinal cord. *Brain Res* 1986;376:164–168.

Price DD, Dubner R. Neurons that subserve the sensory-discriminative aspects of pain. *Pain* 1977;3: 307–338.

Rees H, Roberts MHT. The anterior pretectal nucleus: a proposed role in sensory processing. *Pain* 1993; 53:121–135.

Robinson CJ, Burton H. Somatic submodality distribution within the second somatosensory (SII), 7b, retroinsular, postauditory, and granular insular cortical areas of M. fascicularis. *J Comp Neurol* 1980; 192:93–108.

Roy JC, Bing Z, Villanueva L, Le Bars D. Convergence of visceral and somatic inputs onto subnucleus reticularis dorsalis neurones in the rat medulla. *J Physiol* 1992;458:235–246.

Schaible HG, Schmidt RF. Time course of mechanosensitivity changes in articular afferents during a developing experimental arthritis. *J Neurophysiol* 1988;60:2180–2195.

Schepelmann K, Messlinger K, Schmidt RF. The effects of phorbol ester on slowly conducting afferents of the cat's knee joint. *Exp Brain Res* 1993;92:391–398.

Sherrington CS. *The integrative action of the nervous system*, 2nd ed. New Haven, CT: Yale University Press, 1947;1–147.

Sikes RW, Vogt BA. Nociceptive neurons in area 24 of rabbit cingulate cortex. *J Neurophysiol* 1992;68: 1720–1732.

Silverman JD, Kruger L. An interpretation of dental innervation based upon the pattern of calcitonin gene-related peptide (CGRP)-immunoreactive thin sensory axons. *Somatosens Res* 1987;5:157–175.

Silverman JD, Kruger L. Calcitonin gene-related peptide-immunoreactive innervation of the rat head with emphasis on specialized sensory structures. *J Comp Neurol* 1989;280:303–330.

Talbot JD, Marrett S, Evans AC, Meyer E, Bushnell MC, Duncan GH. Multiple representations of pain in human cerebral cortex. *Science* 1991;251:1355–1358.

Terenzi MG, Rees H, Morgan SJS, Foster GA, Roberts MHT. The antinociception evoked by anterior pretectal nucleus stimulation is partially dependent upon ventrolateral medullary neurones. *Pain* 1991; 47:231–239.

Terenzi MG, Rees H, Roberts MHT. The pontine parabrachial region mediates some of the descending inhibitory effects of stimulating the anterior pretectal nucleus. *Brain Res* 1992;594:205–214.

Treede RD, Bromm B. Reliability and validity of ultra-late cerebral potentials in response to C-fibre activation in man. In: Dubner R, Gebhart GF, Bond MR, eds. *Proceedings of the Vth World Congress on Pain*. Amsterdam: Elsevier, 1988;567–573.

Willis WD. Control of nociceptive transmission in the spinal cord. In: Ottoson D, ed. *Progress in sensory physiology*, vol. 3. Berlin: Springer-Verlag, 1982;1–159.

Willis WD. *The pain system*. Basel: Karger, 1985;1–346.

Willis WD. Physiology of pain perception. In: Takagi H, Oomura Y, Ito M, Otsuka M, eds. *Biowarning system in the brain*. Tokyo: University of Tokyo Press, 1988.

Willis WD. Mechanical allodynia. A role for sensitized nociceptive tract cells with convergent input from mechanoreceptors and nociceptors? *Amer Pain Soc Journal* 1993;2:23–33.

Willis WD, Coggeshall RE. *Sensory mechanisms of the spinal cord*, 2nd ed. New York: Plenum Press, 1991;1–575.

Yezierski RP, Broton JG. Functional properties of spinomesencephalic tract (SMT) cells in the upper cervical spinal cord of the cat. *Pain* 1991;45:187–196.

Yezierski RP, Sorkin LS, Willis WD. Response properties of spinal neurons projecting to midbrain or midbrain-thalamus in the monkey. *Brain Res* 1987;437:165–170.

Yoss RE. Studies of the spinal cord. 3. Pathways for deep pain within the spinal cord and brain. *Neurology* 1953;3:163–175.

Zhang D, Carlton SM, Sorkin LS, Willis WD. Collaterals of primate spinothalamic tract neurons to the periaqueductal gray. *J Comp Neurol* 1990;296:277–290.

Pain and the Brain: From Nociception to Cognition, edited by Burkhart Bromm and John E. Desmedt, Advances in Pain Research and Therapy Vol. 22. Raven Press, Ltd., New York 1995.

2

The Role of the Cerebral Cortex in the Experience of Pain

Dan R. Kenshalo, Jr. and Diana K. Douglass

Neurobiology and Anesthesiology Branch, National Institute of Dental Research, National Institutes of Health, Bethesda, Maryland 20892

SUMMARY

In the early 1900s, Head and Holmes observed that damage to the parietal lobes produced at most a temporary loss in pain sensation. On this basis they suggested that the cerebral cortex plays little role in the experience of pain. Evidence from more recent studies has reversed this belief. The technique of positron-emission tomography (PET) has been used in humans to show that several cortical areas exhibit a response to acute painful stimuli that is not seen with neutral, warm, or vibrotactile stimuli, suggesting that these areas are indeed involved in the perception of pain. These cortical areas include the primary somatosensory cortex (SI), secondary somatosensory cortex (SII), insula, and cingulate cortex. The primary somatosensory cortex appears to be involved in the sensory–discriminative aspect of pain. Clinical lesions in humans and experimental lesion studies in primates have shown that SI is involved in the ability to detect and discriminate changes in the intensity of painful stimuli. Electrophysiological studies in monkeys and rats have demonstrated neurons in SI that respond to and can encode the intensity of noxious stimuli. Other cortical areas that have been implicated in pain perception appear to be involved in aspects of pain other than the sensory–discriminative component. Nociceptive neurons in SII and Area 7b tend to have large, sometimes bilateral receptive fields (RFs) and often respond to auditory and visual stimuli. These data suggest that these areas may be important in spatially directed attention to noxious stimuli. The anterior cingulate cortex is considered part of the medial pain system, and there is evidence from both clinical observations and animal studies that it may be concerned with the affective–motivational aspect of pain perception, though this has yet to be directly tested. Nociceptive neurons in the ventrolateral orbital cortex have been shown to respond to noxious stimulation of skin, viscera, and joints; to have large, often bilateral RFs and to lack somatotopic organization. It is suggested that this area may also play a role in the affective–motivational component of pain perception.

INTRODUCTION

The notion that the cerebral cortex does not play a role in pain sensation can be traced to the observations of Head and Holmes (1911; Head 1920; Holmes 1927). They observed that damage to the parietal lobes sometimes produced a loss of pain sensation, but that the deficits were almost always temporary. Head and Holmes thought that pain reached conscious levels of sensation in the "essential organ" of the thalamus, and believed that SI participated only in the localization of a painful stimulus. Later observations by Penfield and Boldrey (1937) supported these beliefs, in that electrical stimulation of SI rarely evoked pain sensations in conscious patients.

Noxious stimuli applied to the body elicit a complex sequence of sensations and physiologic events. The characteristics of painful stimulation are divided into sensory–discriminative and motivational–affective components. The sensory–discriminative components are closely linked to the sensory aspects of the stimulus and make the "pain-sensing system" comparable to other sensory systems (Melzack and Casey 1968; Price and Dubner 1977). The sensory–discriminative components include the ability to judge the quality of the stimulus and location, intensity, and duration. The motivational–affective components of painful stimulation include the somatic and autonomic reflexes, endocrine changes, arousal, discomfort, and unpleasantness that accompany it.

The purpose of this chapter is to examine the role of the cerebral cortex in the experience of pain. The data available from neurophysiological studies employing microelectrode techniques and analyses of electroencephalographic (EEG) data; from functional morphologic studies such as positron-emission tomography (PET) and functional magnetic resonance imaging (fMRI); and from regional cerebral blood flow (rCBF) measurements (see Part IV of this book) suggest that multiple areas of the cerebral cortex are involved in the experience of pain. It seems likely that these areas are SI, SII, area 7b, the anterior cingulate cortex, and the orbital frontal cortex.

PRIMARY SOMATOSENSORY CORTEX

Despite the observations of Head and Holmes, many other clinical investigators found that lesions of the parietal cortex produce hypalgesia, and in some patients a discrete lesion in the postcentral gyrus has been associated with a highly localized area of contralateral analgesia (Davison and Shick 1935; Dejerine and Mouzon 1915; Foerster 1927; Marshall 1951; Russell 1945; Stone 1950; Talairach et al. 1960; White and Sweet 1969; for reviews see Kenshalo and Willis 1991; Sweet 1982). These observations led Russell to suggest that small excisions of the postcentral gyrus often produce a permanent loss of all forms of sensation in a contralateral limb, and that large incisions in the same area permanently destroy discriminative functions. By contrast, other investigators have found that cortical lesions may also produce hyperalgesia (Sweet 1982). These findings suggest that either analgesia or hyperalgesia may result from a lesion of the primary somatosensory cortex. They further suggest that the region near the central sulcus may contain an area that is important for pain sensation, whereas more caudal portions of the primary somatosensory cortex contain a region that exerts inhibitory control over pain sensation (Kenshalo and Willis 1991). Marshall (1951) documented that small lesions that destroy the area around the postcentral gyrus produce analgesia. Conversely, damage to more caudal portions of the somatosensory cortex, in areas known to inhibit the discharge of spinothalamic tract (STT) neurons in response to innocuous and noxious stimuli (Coulter et al. 1974; Yezierski et al. 1983), produce hyperalgesia.

Few studies have examined the influence of excision of the somatosensory cortex on pain sensation in primates. Peele (1944) found that lesions of areas 2, 5, and 7 of the parietal cortex of monkeys resulted in increased thresholds and delayed responses to pinprick stimuli. Furthermore, the monkeys were unable to localize either pinprick or tactile stimuli applied to the contralateral side of the body. A year after the lesion, the responses to pinprick appeared to be exaggerated. More restricted lesions of SI produced an initial insensitivity to both tactile and pinprick stimuli. After 3 weeks, the monkeys responded to pinprick stimuli, but the responses were much slower than normal and the monkeys could not localize the stimuli. The ability to localize pinprick had not returned to normal after a year of testing (Peele 1944).

Porter (1987) examined the ability of monkeys to make temperature discriminations after lesions in the parietal cortex. The monkeys were taught to discriminate between 24°C and a comparison temperature of 58°C, or a variable temperature between 25° and 58°C. Following various cortical lesions, including bilateral and unilateral excisions of SI and SII, all of the lesioned animals relearned the discrimination, although more trials were required to learn the discrimination postoperatively. Cortical lesions did not affect the monkeys' accuracy in making the 24°C versus 50°C or 24°C versus 58°C temperature discrimination. For comparisons involving a smaller difference in temperature not within the noxious temperature range, an impairment was found in the monkeys' discrimination ability. These experiments led Porter to conclude that the parietal cortex plays little role in the perception of noxious thermal stimulation of the hand. In contrast, Brinkman et al. (1985) found that transient cooling of area 2 in awake monkeys eliminated the animals' orienting responses to pinprick stimuli applied to the hand.

We recently examined the effects of SI ablation on the reactions of monkeys to noxious thermal stimuli (Kenshalo et al. 1991). The monkeys were trained either to detect small increases in temperature superimposed on noxious levels of thermal stimulation, or to discriminate the intensity of noxious thermal stimulation. In the detection task the monkeys detected increases of 0.2°, 0.4°, 0.6°, or 1.0°C (T2) superimposed upon temperatures of 45°, 46°, or 47°C (T1). In the discrimination task the skin temperatures were increased to between 48° and 49°C in 20% of the trials. The monkeys were required to recognize that the stimulus intensity was higher than the normal range of T1 stimuli and to escape the stimulus by releasing a key. During sets when T1 was 45° and 46°, the discrimination temperatures were 47° (difficult), 48° (moderate), and 49°C (easy). The speed of key release was used as a measure of the monkeys' perceived intensity of sensation (Kenshalo et al. 1988).

After bilateral ablation of areas 3a, 3b, and 1, the monkeys exhibited deficits in both the detection and the discrimination tasks. In the detection task, the decreases in detection speed for one monkey were statistically significant for all T2 intensities for 3 weeks following the lesion. The same general trends were found for the other monkey, but the decrease in detection speed reached statistical significance only for a T2 of 0.4°. For both animals the deficits in detection speed returned to near-preoperative levels by the end of 24 weeks. In the discrimination task both monkeys exhibited statistically significant decreases in discrimination speed for the difficult, moderate, and easy discrimination temperatures. Both monkeys' discrimination speeds exhibited a tendency to return to near-preoperative levels at 24 weeks. The deficits produced by the SI lesion could not be ascribed to changes in the motor, attentional, or motivational component of the monkeys' behavior, since their ability to detect cold stimuli or visual stimuli did not change. These data suggest that SI is involved in the detection of noxious thermal stimulation. In the monkeys in our study, this area appeared to be more concerned with the ability to extract particular features of either an innocuous or noxious stimulus.

Electrophysiological studies of neuronal activity in the somatomotor cortex of anesthetized rats (Lamour et al. 1983a,b) and the primary somatosensory cortex of monkeys (Chudler et al. 1989; Kenshalo et al. 1988; Kenshalo et al. 1992) revealed the existence of neurons that encode the intensity of noxious thermal stimulation applied to the skin. Stimulation of the tooth pulp at intensities sufficient to produce pain in humans has also been shown to activate SI neurons (Anderson et al. 1977; Biedenbach et al. 1979; Iwata et al. 1987; Iwata et al. 1988; Matsumoto et al. 1987; Roos et al. 1983a,b). Manipulations that alter the intensity of pain sensation in humans, such as varying the interstimulus interval, produce concomitant changes in the discharge frequency of nociceptive SI neurons in monkeys (Chudler et al. 1989). Moreover, the discharge rate of wide-dynamic-range (WDR) neurons in the SI of monkeys is correlated with their ability to detect changes in noxious thermal stimuli (Kenshalo et al. 1988).

The RFs of nociceptive neurons in the primate SI are somatotopically organized, similar to low-threshold mechanoreceptive neurons in the same region of the cortex (Kenshalo et al. 1992). The locations of nociceptive neurons with receptive fields on the foot are located more medially than are those with receptive fields on the hand. In the foot representation, the recording sites were near the boundary between areas 3b and SI, whereas the neurons with RFs in the hand showed a tendency to be located more caudally, in area 1. Nociceptive-specific neurons (NS) responsive only to noxious stimulation tended to be located in the rostral portion of the distribution of WDR neurons. Both classes of neurons are distributed in layers II through V. Nociceptive neurons were not encountered in layer VI of SI.

Nociceptive neurons tended to be organized in aggregations within the SI. However, low-threshold neurons were found intermingled with nociceptive neurons. The organization of nociceptive neurons in area 1 may be analogous to the segregation of rapidly and slowly adapting neurons in area 3b (Sur et al. 1984). Rapidly adapting neurons are found in all cortical layers, whereas cells with slowly adapting responses are found only in the middle layers. The pattern of distribution of slowly adapting mechanoreceptive neurons suggested that there were bands or clusters of such neurons oriented in a rostrocaudal direction within the middle cortical layers. Columns of nociceptive neurons of a single, pure modality probably do not exist, since: (a) such neurons were not found in layer VI; and (b) nociceptive neurons are intermingled with low-threshold cells having RFs in matching locations. This conclusion does not agree with the findings of Matsumoto et al. (1987). They concluded, based on peripheral and pulpal RFs, and response latencies to electrical stimulation, that tooth-pulp-driven neurons were arranged in vertical columns in the cat SI cortex.

A number of differences are evident between the response characteristics of nociceptive neurons found in the monkey and those found in the rat. Lamour et al. (1983b) observed that neurons responsive to noxious stimuli in the rat somatosensory cortex were intermingled with neurons responsive to innocuous stimuli. However, in their study the nociceptive neurons were primarily located in layers V and VI. NS neurons were found almost exclusively in layers Vb. and VI, whereas the majority of WDR neurons were found in layer V, with only a few located in layer VI. By contrast, the majority (80%) of nociceptive neurons in macaque monkeys are located in the middle layers (III and IV) of SI (Kenshalo et al. 1992). Differences also exist in the RFs of nociceptive neurons in macaques and in the rat. For instance, the RFs of NS neurons in the rat often cover large areas of the body surface (Lamour et al. 1983a), whereas in the monkey the RFs of NS neurons are limited to one digit or a part thereof. In the primate, the RFs of WDR neurons are considerably larger than those of NS neurons. These observations suggest considerable species differences in the organization of nociceptive neurons in the rat and primate SI.

Much information has accumulated about the responses and organization of nociceptive neurons in SI in the anesthetized animal, but the studies yielding this information did not address the participation of these neurons in pain sensation. Furthermore, the use of anesthetics limits any conclusion about the participation of SI neurons in the perceived intensity of noxious thermal stimulation. Kenshalo et al. (1988) recorded the activity of nociceptive, primary somatosensory neurons while monkeys detected small increases in skin temperature superimposed on noxious levels of thermal stimulation. Two-thirds of the neurons that responded to noxious thermal stimulation increased their discharge frequency with increases in the intensity of the thermal stimulation. The remaining neurons responded to noxious thermal stimulation but did not exhibit graded responses that varied with the intensity of the stimulus. The responses of nociceptive SI neurons that encoded the intensity of noxious thermal stimulation were significantly correlated with the monkeys' detection speed. These data suggest that the discharges of nociceptive SI neurons are involved in the encoding process by which monkeys perceive the intensity of noxious thermal stimulation.

In summary, the primary somatosensory cortex appears to play a role in the sensory–discriminative characteristics of pain. Neurons in SI are capable of encoding the location and intensity of noxious thermal stimulation. Furthermore, lesions of SI produce deficits in the ability of humans and nonhuman primates to detect and discriminate noxious thermal stimulation. The most pronounced deficits are found when primates are required to extract specific features of noxious thermal stimulation. We conclude that for pain sensation, as in the case of touch, SI is more concerned with specific features of stimulation than with the noxious nature of the stimulation.

SECONDARY SOMATOSENSORY CORTEX

The SII cortex has been divided into a rostral and a caudal zone (Whitsel et al. 1969). Neurons in the rostral region of SII of awake, paralyzed monkeys were characterized by their responses to light tactile stimuli rather than noxious mechanical stimuli. A large percentage (90%) of the neurons in the rostral zone had bilateral RFs that crossed the midline, and another group had smaller RFs that were often discontinuous. Neurons in the caudal region responded to cutaneous, auditory, and visual stimuli. The cutaneous RFs were often large, bilateral areas, and the responding cells required noxious intensities of stimulation for activation. Whitsel et al. (1969) noted that the response properties of neurons in the caudal region of SII resembled those of the neurons in the posterior thalamic nuclei described by Poggio and Mountcastle (1960). It seems unlikely that neurons with polysensory input and large RFs are involved in the sensory–discriminative aspects of pain sensation.

More recent data suggest that SII, as defined by Whitsel et al. (1969), probably includes neurons located in SII, area 7b, and the retroinsular cortex. Whereas Whitsel et al. (1969) defined SII according to the responses of cells to low-intensity tactile stimulations, Friedman et al. (1980) and Robinson and Burton (1980a,b,c) used thalamic connectivity to define the extent of SII. However, it now appears that the major pathway for nociceptive information via the spinothalamic tract is through ventroposterior lateral (VPL) nucleus to SI. A smaller nociceptive pathway to SI is provided by the spinothalamic tract through the ventroposterior inferior nucleus and centrolateral nucleus. (Gingold et al. 1991). The major pathway for SII to receive nociceptive information from the spinothalamic tract is through the ventroposterior inferior, ventroposterior lateral and posterior nucleus (Stevens et al. 1993). These data further suggest that SI and SII may receive and process nociceptive information in a parallel fashion.

Using a more restrictive definition of SII, Robinson and Burton (1980c) found that most of the neurons in this area responded to innocuous mechanical stimuli and had restricted contralateral RFs. However, some had large, bilateral RFs. Only a few neurons (less than 3%) in SII cortex responded to noxious stimulation. The response properties of the nociceptive neurons were not characterized. Given that nociceptive neurons appear to be clustered in restricted areas in SI, the low percentage of nociceptive neurons found in SII is probably of little significance.

In the primate, WDR and NS neurons were reported in area 7b by Robinson and Burton (1980c). Noxious stimulation activated these neurons from a wider area than did innocuous stimuli. These neurons appeared to be clustered in localized regions, particularly in the whole-body representation of area 7b. The neurons were subdivided into two groups. One group had large RFs and a slowly-adapting discharge that was graded with the intensity of the noxious stimulus. The other group of neurons had large RFs and did not encode the intensity of noxious thermal stimuli. Dong et al. (1989) reported a cluster of NS neurons with small trigeminal RFs located on the border between SII and area 7b. These high-threshold neurons did not encode the intensity of noxious thermal stimuli, but did provide information about the duration of the stimulus. More recently, Dong et al. (1994) expanded their population of nociceptive neurons in area 7b of awake, trained primates. Approximately 9% of the neurons with trigeminal receptive fields were responsive to noxious thermal stimulation. This percentage agrees with that found by Robinson and Burton (1980c). Nociceptive neurons were divided into subpopulations of neurons that either encoded or did not encode the intensity of noxious thermal stimulation. The discharge of nociceptive neurons that encoded the intensity of noxious thermal stimulation was found to be significantly correlated with the escape frequency of the monkey in response to thermal stimulation. Many of the neurons responsive to noxious thermal stimulation also responded to threatening visual stimuli, such as a syringe approaching the monkey. These data suggest that area 7b of the monkey cortex is an important area for integration of visual and somatosensory information, particularly nociceptive information, that is necessary for spatially directed attention.

Clinical evidence suggests that SII and area 7b participate in pain sensation. Greenspan and Winfield (1992) examined a patient with a cerebral tumor compressing the posterior insula and parietal operculum. On the side contralateral to the tumor, the patient exhibited higher mechanical and heat-pain thresholds, increased cold-pain tolerance, and a decreased ability to discriminate roughness. After removal of the tumor the patient regained normal sensitivity in the affected hand. Other deficits have been reported in patients with lesions located in the posterior insula and the parietal operculum (Berthier et al. 1988); a large percentage of these patients exhibited a higher level of tolerance to pain stimuli presented on either side of the body. In addition, many of the patients exhibited deficits in the motivational–affective component of pain. Dong et al. (1994) suggested that these pain-related deficits may be a sign of unilateral neglect that develops after lesions of the posterior parietal cortex.

Neither the clinical literature nor the response characteristics and RFs sizes of the nociceptive neurons that have been found in SII and area 7b suggests an involvement of these neurons in the sensory–discriminative aspects of pain. The posterior parietal cortex may play an important role in spatially directed attention to noxious thermal stimuli.

ANTERIOR CINGULATE CORTEX

The anterior cingulate cortex is thought to be part of the medial pain system, and appears to be involved in the affective aspect of pain sensation (Vogt 1985). Anatomically, the medial and the lateral pain systems divide at the level of the thalamus, where nociceptive neurons in the lateral nuclei project to the primary and secondary somatosensory cortices, while nociceptive neurons from the medial and intralaminar thalamic nuclei project to limbic cortices, including the anterior cingulate cortex (Vogt et al. 1992). The medial pain system also involves connections to the midbrain periaqueductal gray, orbitofrontal and precentral agranular cortices, and the amygdala (Vogt et al. 1992).

Much evidence for the involvement of the anterior cingulate cortex in chronic pain comes from neurosurgical observations. Surgical lesions of the cingulate cortex and/or the cingulum bundle have been reported to alleviate chronic pain (Foltz and White 1962; 1968; Ballantine et al. 1967; Faillace et al. 1971; Sharma 1973; Hurt and Ballantine 1974; Corkin 1980; Pillay and Hassenbusch 1992). In psychiatric surgeries, patients with varying emotional disturbances reported fair to excellent relief of pain following cingulotomy (Foltz and White 1962, 1968). While cingulotomy has been reported to be more effective in patients who have additional symptoms of anxiety and depression (Foltz and White 1962), other studies report relief of pain in a significant percentage of nonpsychiatric patients as well (Ballantine et al. 1967; Hurt and Ballantine 1974; Corkin 1980). Corkin and Hebben (1981) using results from the McGill Pain Questionnaire, reported that bilateral cingulotomy reduced the emotional but not the sensory component of chronic pain for at least a short period after surgery.

More direct information for understanding the role of the cerebral cortex in human pain has come through the use of positron-emission tomography (PET). This technique offers the opportunity to study changes in regional cerebral blood flow (rCBF) produced by painful cutaneous stimulation in human subjects. PET studies consistently reveal increases in rCBF during noxious thermal stimulation in SI, SII, the insula, and the cingulate cortex (Talbot et al. 1991; Casey et al. 1994; Coghill et al. 1994). While clinical PET studies have found no evidence of changes in local cerebral blood flow in the cingulate cortex in patients with chronic pain (Di Piero et al. 1991; Katayama et al. 1986), all recent studies involving acute painful heat stimuli have shown some level of activation in the anterior cingulate cortex (Jones et al. 1991; Talbot et al. 1991; Coghill et al. 1994; Casey et al. 1994; see also Chapters 13 and 14).

Jones et al. (1991; see also Chapter 14) measured rCBF in response to thermal stimuli. When painful heat was compared with nonpainful heat, activity was seen in the contralateral anterior cingulate cortex but not in the primary somatosensory cortex. They interpreted their results as being consistent with the concept of pain as a predominantly emotional experience that might be expected to cause greater activity in the medial system. Talbot et al. (1991) used subtractive PET to measure rCBF in response to painfully hot versus warm stimuli. They found that painful stimuli caused significant increases in contralateral activity in the anterior cingulate and somatosensory cortices. Using a similar technique, Coghill et al. (1994) assessed potential differences in activity with painful heat versus robust vibrotactile stimulation. They found that painful as compared to neutral stimuli produced significant contralateral activation in the anterior cingulate cortex as well as the somatosensory and other cortices. The cortical areas activated by pain overlapped extensively with those activated by vibration, but the vibrotactile stimulus did not cause any significant activation in the anterior cingulate cortex, suggesting that the activation observed in this region with heat was not due to mechanical stimulation but was specific to the painful stimulus.

Although PET studies offer the unique opportunity to study the metabolic changes that occur in the human brain during painful stimulation, these studies also have limitations. First, it has yet to be shown that the changes it reveals in blood flow, which presumably reflect changes in synaptic activity, depend on the intensity of painful stimulation. It is therefore difficult to determine whether the changes in blood flow seen during noxious stimulation are related to the sensory components or motivational-affective components of stimulation, or to both. A second major problem with PET has recently been pointed out by Sergent (1994). Changes in blood flow in the cingulate cortex may be the result of the subject's inability to withdraw his hand during painful stimulation. Therefore, activation of the cingulate cortex might be the result of the suppression of an automatic motor reaction, with the changes in blood flow being only indirectly related to the painful stimulus.

In addition to PET, electrical and magnetic brain signals elicited by various noxious stimuli have been used to study cortical activity during acute pain in humans. With both approaches, localization of the sources of multiple spatial-temporal dipoles involved in pain processing is currently under investigation. Activity has been found in primary and secondary somatosensory cortices, the frontal lobe, and deep brain structures, presumably at the location of the anterior cingulate gyrus in response to painful heat pulses delivered by infrared laser (Bromm et al. 1995). The following chapters, especially in Part V of this book, summarize the findings of these noninvasive techniques as new windows into the brain.

Few animal studies have directly examined the involvement of the cingulate cortex in nociception and pain. Vaccarino and Melzack (1989) studied the effect of lidocaine injected into the bundle of the anterior cingulum on the formalin test in rats. The cingulum contains projection fibers that run from thalamic nuclei to the anterior cingulate cortex, temporal cortex, and hippocampus, and fibers from the frontal cortex to the cingulate cortex and hippocampus. They found that injection of lidocaine into the cingulum bundle attenuated responses to tonic (formalin injection) but not phasic (hot water foot-flick test) pain. Vaccarino and Melzack argue that because formalin pain has a significantly longer duration than brief phasic pain, it may have a greater affective component, and that the observed effect of lidocaine on formalin pain therefore reflects a role of the anterior cingulum bundle in the affective–motivational component of pain perception.

In a rat model of peripheral neuropathy, Mao et al. (1993) used the ^{14}C-2-deoxyglucose (2-DG) autoradiographic technique to measure the local glucose utilization rate. In animals exhibiting thermal hyperalgesia and spontaneous pain behavior, increases in the metabolism of 2-DG were seen in the cingulate and somatosensory cortices, as well as in noncortical brain structures known to be involved in pain processing.

Sikes and Vogt (1992) have recorded directly from units in area 24 of the anterior cingulate cortex in rabbits. They found neurons that responded to noxious mechanical and thermal stimuli; and which had response properties similar to those of neurons in the parafascicular, centrolateral, and submedial nuclei of the thalamus. These neurons responded primarily to noxious stimuli, had little or no somatotopic organization, and had broad receptive fields, although some had a significant lateral preference. Sikes and Vogt gave further evidence that the nociceptive responses seen in the anterior cingulate cortex are transmitted through the medial and intralaminar thalamic nuclei by showing that lidocaine injections into the medial thalamus virtually abolished the responses seen in the cingulate. They also made surgical lesions to remove input from other cortical regions, including the somatosensory, insula, parietal, and posterior cingulate cortices, with no effect on nociceptive responses in the anterior cingulate cortex. They concluded that in light of the connections and the response properties of anterior cingulate neurons, the anterior cingulate cortex may be directly involved in affective and/or autonomic responses to noxious stimuli.

VENTROLATERAL ORBITAL CORTEX

Interest in the role of the ventrolateral orbital cortex (VLO) in the processing of nociceptive information has increased in the past few years. The increased interest is based on the observation that this cortex receives major afferent input from the nucleus submedius (Craig and Burton 1981; Yoshida et al. 1992), which is known to have a large population of neurons responsive to noxious stimulation. The principal termination of thalamocortical afferents from the nucleus submedius is in layer III, but terminals of these afferents are also located in layers I, V, and VI (Craig et al. 1982).

The majority of neurons in VLO respond to noxious stimulation of skin, viscera, and joints (Snow et al. 1992). These neurons are characterized by large receptive fields that may cover the entire body. There is no evidence for a somatotopic organization of the nociceptive neurons in VLO, given the large degree of spatial convergence. In the cat, nociceptive neurons in VLO are relatively unresponsive to low-threshold tactile stimulation (Snow et al. 1992), whereas in the rat, many neurons in VLO appear to grade their response with the intensity of the stimulus (Bakonja and Miletic 1991). The greatest excitation of nociceptive neurons was produced by intense, prolonged noxious visceral or cutaneous stimulation applied for up to 30 sec (Snow et al. 1992; Bakonja and Miletic 1991).

Other evidence also suggests that VLO participates in the processing of nociceptive information. Electrical stimulation of the sciatic nerve at sufficient strengths to activate C-fibers increased local blood flow in VLO (Tsubokawa et al. 1981). Conversely, the application of procaine, a local anesthetic, to VLO appeared to reduce aversive reactions of rats to electrical stimulation. In humans, lesioning of the inferomedial orbital cortex, thought to be homologous to VLO, is known to provide pain relief to patients with chronic pain (Grantham 1951).

In summary, the lack of somatotopic organization and the convergence of cutaneous, visceral, and joint-related information on nociceptive neurons suggests that VLO neurons are more likely to play a role in the motivational-affective component of pain. Activation of VLO may be responsible for the unpleasant experience that causes the organism to attempt escape from prolonged painful stimulation.

REFERENCES

Anderson SA, Keller O, Roos A, Rydenhag B. Cortical projection of tooth pulp afferents in the cat. In: Anderson DJ, Mathews B, eds. *Pain in the trigeminal region*. Amsterdam: Elsevier, 1977;355–364.

Bakonja M, Miletic V. Responses of neurons in the rat ventrolateral orbital cortex to phasic and tonic nociceptive stimulation. *Brain Res* 1991;557:353–355.

Ballantine HT Jr, Cassidy WL, Flanagan NB, Marino R Jr. Stereotaxic anterior cingulotomy for neuropsychiatric illness and intractable pain. *J Neurosurg* 1967;26:488–495.

Berthier M, Starkstein S, Leiguarda R. Asymolia for pain: a sensory limbic disconnection syndrome. *Ann Neurol* 1988;24:41–49.

Biedenbach MA, van Hassel HJ, Brown AC. Tooth pulp-driven neurons in somatosensory cortex of primates: role in pain mechanisms including a review of the literature. *Pain* 1979;7:31–50.

Brinkman J, Colebatch JG, Porter R, York DH. Responses of precentral cells during cooling of the postcentral cortex in conscious monkeys. *J Physiol* 1985;368:611–625.

Bromm B, Chen ACN, Treede RD. Brain electrical source analysis of laser evoked potentials in response to painful trigeminal nerve stimulation in man. *Electroencephalogr Clin Neurophysiol*. (*in press*).

Casey KL, Minoshima S, Berger KL, Koeppe RA, Morrow TJ, Frey KA. Positron emission tomographic analysis of cerebral structures activated specifically by repetitive noxious heat stimuli. *J Neurophysiol* 1994;71:802–807.

Chudler EH, Anton F, Dubner R, Kenshalo DR Jr. Responses of nociceptive SI neurons in monkeys and pain sensation in humans elicited by noxious thermal stimulation: Effects of interstimulus interval. *J Neurophysiol* 1989;63:559–569.

Coghill RC, Talbot JD, Evans AC, Meyer E, Gjedde A, Bushnell MC, Duncan GH. Distributed processing of pain and vibration by the human brain. *J Neurosci* 1994;14:4095–4108.

Corkin S. A prospective study of cingulotomy. In: Valenstein ES, ed. *The psychosurgery debate*. San Francisco: W. H. Freeman, 1980.

Corkin S, Hebben N. Subjective estimates of chronic pain before and after psychosurgery or treatment in a pain unit. *Pain* 1981;(Suppl 1):S150.

Coulter JD, Maunz RA, Willis WD. Effects of stimulation of sensorimotor cortex on primate spinothalamic neurons. *Brain Res* 1974;65:351–356.

Craig AD, Burton H. Spinal and medullary lamina I projection to nucleus submedius in medial thalamus: a possible pain center. *J Neurophysiol* 1981;45:443–466.

Craig AD, Wiegand SJ, Price JL. The thalamo-cortical projection of the nucleus submedius in the cat. *J Comp Neurol* 1982;206:28–48.

Davison C, Schick W. Spontaneous pain and other subjective sensory disturbances. *Arch Neurol Psychiatr* 1935;34:1204–1237.

Dejerine J, Mouzon J. Un nouveau type de syndrome sensitif cortical observe dans un cas de monoplegie corticale dissociée. *Rev Neurol* 1915;14:521–532.

Di Piero V, Jones AKP, Iannotti F, Powell M, Perani D, Lenzi GL, Frackowiak RSJ. Chronic pain: a PET study of the central effects of percutaneous high cervical cordotomy. *Pain* 1991;46:9–12.

Dong WK, Salonen LD, Kawakami Y, Shiwaku T, Kaukoranta EM, Martin RF. Nociceptive responses of trigeminal neurons in SII-7b cortex of awake monkeys. *Brain Res* 1989;484:314–324.

Dong WK, Chudler EH, Sugiyama K, Roberts V, Hayashi T. Somatosensory, multisensory and task-related neurons in cortical area 7b (PF) of unanesthetized monkeys. *J Neurophysiol* 1994;72:542–564.

Faillace LA, Allen RP, McQueen JD, Northrup B. Cognitive deficits from bilateral cingulotomy for intractable pain in man. *Dis Nerv Syst* 1971;32:171–175.

Foerster O. Die Leitungsbahnen des Schmerzgefuchls und dischirurgische Behandlung der Schmerzzustaende. Berlin: Urban & Schwarzenberg, 1927;360.

Foltz EL, White EL. Pain "relief" by frontal cingulotomy. *J Neurosurg* 1962;19:98–100.

Foltz EL, White EL. The role of rostral cingulumotomy in "pain" relief. *Int J Neurol* 1968;6:353–373.

Friedman DP, Jones EG, Burton H. Representation pattern in the second somatic sensory area of the monkey cerebral cortex. *J Comp Neurol* 1980;192:21–41.

Gingold SI, Greenspan JD, Apkarian AV. Anatomic evidence of nociceptive inputs to primary somatosensory cortex: relationships between spinothalamic terminals and thalamocortical cells in squirrel monkeys. *J Comp Neurol* 1991;308:467–490.

Grantham EG. Prefontal lobotomy for relief of pain with a report of a new operative technique. *J Neurosurg* 1951;8:405–410.

Greenspan JD, Winfield JA. Reversible pain and tactile deficits associated with a cerebral tumor compressing the posterior insula and parietal operculum. *Pain* 1992;58:29–39.

Head H. *Studies in neurology*, vol. 2. London: Oxford University Press, 1920.

Head H, Holmes G. Sensory disturbances from cerebral lesions. *Brain* 1911;34:102–254.

Holmes G. Disorders of sensation produced by cortical lesions. *Brain* 1927;50:413–427.

Hurt RW, Ballantine HT Jr. Stereotactic anterior cingulate lesions for persistent pain: a report on 68 cases. *Clin Neurosurg* 1974;21:334–351.

Iwata K, Itoga H, Muramatsu H, Toda K, Sumino R. Responses of bradykinin sensitive tooth-pulp-driven neurons in the cat cerebral cortex. *Exp Brain Res* 1987;66:435–439.

Iwata K, Muramatsu H, Tsuboi Y, Sumino R. Responses of thermoreceptive tooth-pulp-driven neurons in the cat cerebral cortex. In: Dubner R, Gebhart G, Bond MR, eds. *Proceedings of the Vth World Congress on Pain*. Amsterdam: Elsevier, 1988;560–566.

Jones AKP, Brown WD, Friston KJ, Qi LY, Frackowiak RSJ. Cortical and subcortical localization of response to pain in man using positron emission tomography. *Proc R Soc Lond* [B] 1991;244:39–44.

Katayama Y, Tsubokawa T, Hirayama T, Kido G, Tsukiyama T, Iio M. Response of regional cerebral blood flow and oxygen metabolism to thalamic stimulation in humans as revealed by positron emission tomography. *J Cereb Blood Flow Metab* 1986;16:637–641.

Kenshalo DR Jr, Chudler EH, Anton F, Dubner R. SI cortical nociceptive neurons participate in the encoding process by which monkeys perceive the intensity of noxious stimulation. *Brain Res* 1988;454:378–382.

Kenshalo DR Jr, Isensee O. Responses of primate SI cortical neurons to noxious stimuli. *J Neurophysiol* 1983;50:1496–1497.

Kenshalo DR Jr, Thomas DA, Dubner R. Primary somatosensory cortical lesions reduce the monkeys' ability to discriminate and detect noxious thermal stimulation. *Soc Neurosci Abstr* 1991;17:206.

Kenshalo DR Jr, Iwata K, Thomas DA. Differences in the distribution of nociceptive neurons in SI cortex of the monkey. In: Inoki R, Shigenaga Y, Tohyama T, eds. *Processing and inhibition of nociceptive information*. Amsterdam: Excerpta Medica, 1992;141–146.

Kenshalo DR Jr, Willis WD Jr. The role of the cerebral cortex in pain sensation. In: Jones EG, Peters A, eds. *Cerebral cortex*. New York: Plenum Press, 1991;153–212.

Lamour Y, Guilbaud G, Willer JC. Rat somatosensory (SmI): II. Laminar and columnar organization of noxious and non-noxious inputs. *Exp Brain Res* 1983a;49:35–45.

Lamour Y, Willer JC, Guilbaud G. Rat somatosensory (SmI): I. Characteristics of neuronal responses to noxious stimulation and comparison with responses to non-noxious stimulation. *Exp Brain Res* 1983b;49:35–45.

Marshall J. Sensory disturbances in cortical wounds with special reference to pain. *J Neurol Neurosurg Psychiatry* 1951;14:187–204.

Mao J, Mayer DJ, Price DD. Patterns of increased brain activity indicative of pain in a rat model of peripheral mononeuropathy. *J Neurosci* 1993;13:2689–2702.

Matsumoto N, Sato T, Yahata F, Suzuki T. Physiological properties of tooth pulp-driven neurons in the first somatosensory cortex (SI) of the cat. *Pain* 1987;31:249–362.

Melzack R, Casey KL. Sensory, motivational, and central control determinants of pain: a new conceptual model in pain. In: Kenshalo DR Jr, ed. *The skin senses*. Springfield, IL: Charles C. Thomas, 1968;423–439.

Peele TL. Acute and chronic parietal lobe ablations in monkeys. *J Neurophysiol* 1944;7:269–286.

Penfield W, Boldrey E. Somatic motor and sensory representation in the cerebral cortex of man as studied by electrical stimulation. *Brain* 1937;60:389–443.

Pillay PK, Hassenbusch SJ. Bilateral MRI-guided stereotactic cingulotomy for intractable pain. *Stereotact Funct Neurosurg* 1992;59:33–38.

Poggio GF, Mountcastle VB. A study of the functional contribution of the lemniscal and spinothalamic systems to somatic sensibility. *Bull Johns Hopkins Hosp* 1960;106:266–316.

Porter L. Experimental investigation of the parietal lobes and temperature discrimination in monkeys. *Brain Res* 1987;412:54–67.

Price DD, Dubner R. Neurons that subserve the sensory–discriminative aspects of pain. *Pain* 1977; 3:307–338.

Robinson CJ, Burton H. Somatotopic organization in the second somatosensory cortex of M. fascicularis. *J Comp Neurol* 1980a;192:43–67.

Robinson CJ, Burton H. Organization of somatosensory receptive fields in cortical areas 7b, retroinsular, postauditory, and granular insula of M. fascicularis. *J Comp Neurol* 1980b;192:69–92.

Robinson CJ, Burton H. Somatic submodality distribution within the second somatosensory (SII) 7b, retroinsular, postauditory, and granular insular cortical areas of M. fascicularis. *J Comp Neurol* 1980c;192:93–108.

Roos A, Rydenhag B, Anderson SA. Activity in cortical cells after stimulation of tooth-pulp afferents in the cat: Intracellular analysis. *Pain* 1983a;16:49–60.

Roos A, Rydenhag B, Anderson SA. Activity in cortical cells after stimulation of tooth-pulp afferents in the cat: extracellular analysis. *Pain* 1983b;16:61–72.

Russell WR. Transient disturbances following gunshot wounds of the head. *Brain* 1945;68:79–97.

Sergent J. Brain-imaging studies of cognitive functions. *Trends Neurosci* 1994;17:221–227.

Sharma T. Absence of cognitive deficits from bilateral cingulotomy for intractable pain in humans. *Texas Med* 1973;69:79–82.

Sikes RW, Vogt BA. Nociceptive neurons in area 24 of rabbit cingulate cortex. *J Neurophysiol* 1992;68:1720–1732.

Snow PJ, Lumb BM, Cervero F. The representation of prolonged and intense, noxious somatic and visceral stimuli in the ventrolateral orbital cortex of the cat. *Pain* 1992;48:89–99.

Stevens RT, London SM, Apkarian AV. Spinothalamocortical projections to the secondary somatosensory cortex (SII) in squirrel monkey. *Brain Res* 1993;631:241–246.

Stone TT. Phantom limb pain and central pain. *Arch Neurol Psychiatry* 1950;63:739–748.

Sur M, Wall JT, Kaas JH. Modular distributions of neurons with slowly adapting and rapidly adapting responses in area 3b of somatosensory cortex in monkeys. *J Neurophysiol* 1984;51:724–744.

Sweet WH. Cerebral localization of pain. In: Thompson RA, Green JR, eds. *New perspectives in cerebral localization*. New York: Raven Press, 1982;205–242.

Talairach J, Tournoux P, Bancaud J. Chirugie parietale de la douleur. *Acta Neurochir* 1960;8:153–250.

Talbot JD, Marrett S, Evans AC, Meyer E, Bushnell MC, Duncan GH. Multiple representations of pain in human cerebral cortex. *Science* 1991;251:1355–1358.

Tsubokawa T, Katayama Y, Ueno Y, Moriyasu N. Evidence for involvement of the frontal cortex in pain-related cerebral events in cats: increase in local cerebral blood flow by noxious stimulation. *Brain Res* 1981;217:179–185.

Vaccarino AL, Melzack R. Analgesia produced by injection of lidocaine into the anterior cingulum bundle of the rat. *Pain* 1989;39:213–219.

Vogt BA. Cingulate cortex. In: Peters A, Jones EG, eds. *Cerebral cortex*, vol. 4. New York: Plenum Press, 1985;89–149.

Vogt BA, Sikes RW, Vogt LJ. Anterior cingulate cortex and the medial pain system. In: Vogt BA, Gabriel M, eds. *The neurobiology of cingulate cortex and limbic thalamus*. Boston: Birkhauser, 1993.

White JC, Sweet WH. *Pain and the neurosurgeon. A forty-year experience*. Springfield, IL: Charles C. Thomas, 1969.

Whitsel BL, Perucelli LM, Werner G. Symmetry and connectivity in the map of the body surface in somatosensory area II of primates. *J neurophysiol* 1969;32:170–183.

Yezierski RP, Gerhart KD, Schrock BJ, Willis WD. A further examination of effects of cortical stimulation on primate spinothalamic tract cells. *J Neurophysiol* 1983;49:424–441.

Yoshida A, Dostrovsky JO, Chiang CY. The afferent and efferent connections of the nucleus submedius in the rat. *J Comp Neurol* 1992;324:115–133.

Pain and the Brain: From Nociception to Cognition, edited by Burkhart Bromm and John E. Desmedt, Advances in Pain Research and Therapy Vol. 22. Raven Press, Ltd., New York © 1995.

3

Consciousness, Pain, and Cortical Activity

Burkhart Bromm

Institute of Physiology, University Hospital Eppendorf, University of Hamburg, D-20246 Hamburg, Germany

SUMMARY

A discussion of consciousness, subjectivity, and self-cognition inherent in the experience of pain encounters methodologic limitations arising from reasoning at different levels. These limitations can be treated by following the thinking of Descartes, who divided the world into objective and subjective components with borders that cannot be transcended even with Feigl's imagined method of "autocerebroscopy." In accord with this concept, pain is contrasted with nociception. Nociception is neuronal activity in the pain-mediating nervous system, whereas pain is a subjective experience based on cognitive mechanisms that depend on its level of arousal. This differentiation has particular meaning in the discussion of antinociceptive or sedative modes of analgesic drug action. A number of examples of long-latency brain potentials in response to noxious stimuli reflect the subjective experience of pain and pain-related cognitive processes. The relevant brain generators of these components are triggered and modified by both nociceptive and nonspecific inputs, the latter arising from brain-stem structures involved in mechanisms of attention, cognition, and arousal. In a first example of long-latency brain potentials, the influence of attention on brain-potential amplitudes is shown from experiments using laser stimuli that activate both Aδ- and C-fibers. Because of the very different conduction velocities of these fibers (14 msec vs. 1 msec), a single laser pulse evokes two pain sensations and two, late and ultra-late brain potentials which depend on whether the subject concentrates on the first or the second pain. In another example, principal components of spontaneous and evoked electroencephalographic (EEG) potentials are shown to differentiate between sedative and analgesic effects of centrally acting drugs. Brain potentials can be used in assessing analgesic states in unconscious patients, particularly during light anesthesia with low-dose ketamine.

DESCARTES AND THE LIMITS OF SCIENCE

The Preface to this book cites a statement by Descartes (1641) about his "secure possession of leisure in a peaceable retirement" as a prerequisite for reconsidering the fundamental aspects of contemporary philosophy and science. We are tempted to ask for the results of his meditations. Philosophers respect Descartes for his excellent line of argumentation leading to the dualism in which the world is split into an external *res extensa* and internal *res intensa*. Scientists appreciate his deductive construction of physics and mathematics, resulting in fundamental laws of mechanics, optics, and geometry. Pain researchers like to quote Descartes' physical analysis of perception, in particular his ideas about man functioning as a "machine." The logo of the International Association for the Study of Pain (IASP) is a figure by Descartes of a child with a foot near a fire and nerves shown projecting this information toward the brain.

In order to generalize his experiences, beliefs, and insights into his internal world ("sum res cogitans," *Meditation* IV), Descartes began with a proof for the existence of a "good" god who will not "cause me to err, in particular in matters where I think I possess the highest evidence" (*Meditation* III). For example, if we accept mathematical statements like "a = a," or "a = b and b = c means a = c," then it appear to be evidently correct "prima luce," or in an elementary light[1]. At the end of his meditations, Descartes accepts the existence of *a priori* truths. These truths are eternal and innate in human thinking, and provide logically independent axioms. All scientific explanation of the world means a logical deduction down to these basic truths, which are experienced "clearly and distinctly" in each individual.

Clearly, this is not the place to argue the pro and con of Descartes' ideas; thousands of philosophers and neurobiologists have written treatises on these ideas over the course of centuries (e.g., Damasio 1994; see also Chapter xx, Adolph's and Damasio). But in my opinion, the most essential outcome of Descartes' work, at least for our topic, is seldom discussed. It is his deduction of the basic impossibility, as a matter of principle, to solve the mind-body problem with methods of science. Descartes is widely accepted as the founder of modern science, since he elaborated the importance of a strict differentiation between object (which is contemplated) and subject (which contemplates) in order to explain the world on the basis of general mechanisms acceptable for each human principle—a scientific basis. It became a law in science, not to mix observer and object or thoughts and facts. It was exactly this careful separation between the "thinking self" and the "surrounding world" to be inspected that delivered the essential methodologic prerequisite for the elaboration of valid and universal insight and knowledge of the world, common for all, over centuries. Thinking is the method the self uses to explore its surroundings. Applying this method to the mind–body problem therefore means nothing other than that we try to think about thinking. Is this possible, and may we expect universally valid results from it? I think not.

A method cannot be applied to study itself. One of the oldest examples of this occurs in the Greek story of the man from Crete who says that all Cretans are liars.

---

[1]Descartes' proof of the existence of God or "some being, by whatever name I may designate him," who causes thoughts that are true, is excellent for his time and meaningful for the issue of this book. In brief, he argues that our reasoning may be "correct" or "wrong," but that in any case we can ourselves conceive an idea of completeness, and that absolute completeness will not deceive. However, the only imagined completeness is less complete than the truly existent completeness; in other words, completeness must exist and may be called God; God will not deceive us in our experiences of logical evidences "prima luce."

The literature of operant logistics is full of such examples, which sound correct but are absolutely meaningless. Following the thinking of Descartes: *res cogitans* cannot be *res extensa*. It is true that modern physics broke down the borders between object and subject: the result of an experiment depends on the question the experimenter asks (light turns out to be particle or wave according to the respective method applied to studying it); given Heisenberg's principle, the behavior of elementary quantum particles is undetermined. But these findings, derived with Descartes' method of strict separation between object and subject, demonstrate the divergence between the complexity of the real world and the simplified use of logical reasoning, rather than constituting a criticism of methodologic lines of argumentation from elementary evidence.

A modern holder of the dualistic view is Eccles (e.g., 1986) who separates conscious experience into morphologic cerebral substrates denoted "dendrons," consisting of aggregates of spinal synapses of dendrites (world I), and elementary units of mental processes denoted "psychons" (world II). The two structures are assumed to have a dualistic interaction (Popper and Eccles 1977). Eccles (1986) further suggests that mental events interact with neural events analogous to the probability fields of quantum statistics. Most of us surely agree that activity in certain brain areas is related to consciousness. Consciousness, however, means knowledge about one's own mental states (mental representation) and the ability to decide how to react to a situation and what to do next (intentionality). But who is it that experiences and decides? It is precisely with this question that we leave Descartes' dualistic postulation to distinguish strictly between object and subject in scientific research, and I fear that monistic approaches that assume mental states to be epiphenomena of or even identical with cerebral states run into logically incoherent conclusions; they leave argumentation at the level of chains of objective statements accepted consensually "in an elementary light."

Perhaps the most distinct hypothetical experiment in this context is "autocerebroscopy," as conceived by Feigl (1958). In this, the subject, while introspectively attending to his feelings (of anger, love, or intention) simultaneously observes a vastly magnified computer display of his own cerebral neurologic activities, obtained by perfect neurophysiologic and morphologic measurements. But does this approach solve the mind–body problem? Observing the picture will change neuronal activity, which in turn will change the picture—altogether providing an impressive example of the difficulties arising if Descartes' rule is violated, and subject and object are mixed.

In my opinion, brain science should continue to isolate basic neuronal mechanisms that can be generalized from what is called self-consciousness, thus enlarging *res extensa* into the central nervous system and into the brain. These experiments should continue until new questions require new kinds of thinking (Crick and Koch 1990). The chapters of this book follow this line of experimental research and reasoning with regard to pain. We will leave Descartes with a comment made in a letter to Elisabeth of Böhmen from May 21, 1643: "Our senses let us feel that there is an interaction between mind and body, but our intellect is unable to understand how this interaction can happen."

NOCICEPTION AND PAIN

Pain is widely agreed to result from an altered neuronal activity somewhere within the nociceptive nervous system. Enhanced nociceptive activity causes pain, pain-relevant behavior, and nocifensive reactions. The nociceptive system has so far been as well investigated as other afferent sensory channels. Our knowledge of this system is reviewed by Willis (see Chapter 1), in the chapter pursuing the neuronal impulse pattern elicited by noxious stimuli through the peripheral Aδ- and C-afferents into the spinal cord, and ascending into the thalamus and cortex. Most information about this system has been gathered from animal experiments, but no major differences in basic mechanisms of nociceptors, nociceptive afferents, or spinal-cord transmission and projection tracts to the thalamus and cortex have been found between humans and the animals most often investigated in pain research, such as mice, rats, cats, and monkeys. The same is true, starting at upper levels of the central nervous system (CNS) including the brain, for efferent mechanisms in pain processing, such as descending noxious inhibitory control (DNIC, see in particular Chapters 34 and 35) or the action of opioids at different levels of the nociceptive system (see Chapter 35).

Similarly, pain-relieving treatments, such as the application of pharmacologic substances, physical procedures, and surgery, are mainly evaluated in animal experiments. This is particularly true for the development of novel drugs. By law, the analgesic efficacy of such drugs has to be demonstrated in the laboratory animal, using motor or vegetative reactions to pain-inducing stimuli, the hot-plate test, withdrawal reflexes, skin-twitch reactions (for a review, see e.g., Hammond 1989), or, at a higher CNS level, by evaluating complex animal behaviors that allow the differentiation between sensory, motor, and attentional aspects in processing noxious stimulation (e.g., Vierck et al. 1989).

Nociception, however, is neither a necessary nor a sufficient condition for pain. Even if we knew all about nociception and the pain-processing nervous system up to the cerebral cortex, we wouldn't be able to explain pain in a general way. The intense nociceptive impulse pattern elicited, for example, by an injury during a sporting competition, will not necessarily induce pain, at least not at the time of the accident. Many examples are known of wounds that do not hurt during battle; even severe damage to the body is not always accompanied by pain. And vice versa, an imagined wound can lead to excruciating pain. Taken together, pain is seen to be a "complex experience that involves emotions, previous experiences with pain, and what the pain means to us at any time." The borderline between the physiology and psychology of pain is confused. But on the other hand, the differentiation between nociception and pain has particular meaning for the development and evaluation of treatments for relieving pain. Relief from pain means only that brain activity has changed in those structures that are involved in its conscious experience, not that changes have necessarily occurred in the nociceptive system summarized by Willis (see Chapter 1).

The experience of pain is essentially coupled with consciousness and with all the characteristics of mind, including mental representation as characterized by immediate knowledge of one's own mental states, with self-relation and time integration as well as intentionality (the decision to act or to react by free will; see, e.g., Searle 1993). Without consciousness there is no pain. The anatomic substrate of the experience of pain is the brain, even though pain is usually felt at the site of injury in the body. The decapitated animal, such as the spinal frog in laboratory experiments, or the beheaded cock, exhibits all of the nociceptive behavioral reactions used in the laboratory animal to indicate effects of pain-relieving drugs, particularly motor responses to noxious stimuli. Yet there is no question among physicians that these animals do not feel any pain at all.

These examples insistently demonstrate that nociceptive reactions as measured in the laboratory animal do not necessarily indicate pain. Noxious stimuli, such as injury, tissue damage, or alterations in tissue metabolism clearly induce nociceptive activity, but this neuronal activity is only the initiator for the pain felt by the subject. In other words, the nociceptive impulse pattern only opens the door to the conscious experience of pain; whether the subject really feels pain is a different matter. Several contributions to this volume show that nociceptive projection must occur with a sufficiently high state of arousal to produce the sensation of pain. Conversely, both the attenuation of nociceptive activity and the manipulation of arousal can relieve pain.

Since the beginning of this century, states of consciousness have been attributed to functions of the brain stem, thalamus, and cerebral cortex. There is no controversy about the existence of an activating system in the brain stem and midbrain. Electrical stimulation in the medial bulbar reticular formation, in the pontile and midbrain tegmentum, and in the locus coeruleus leads to an arousal reaction with desynchronization of EEG activity (for a review see Kandel et al. 1992). In other words, the brain stem contains areas of neurons that modulate the momentary arousal level, the state of consciousness, the rhythm of wakefulness and sleep, and other circadian rhythms, as well as autonomic functions governing cardiovascular and respiratory function (e.g., Peschanski et al. 1983; Redfern et al. 1985). Stimulation of the brain-stem reticular formation affects both arousal and sleep, depending on the specific neuronal populations (rostral or caudal) activated. Clinically, lesions in these areas usually result in permanent sleep and coma (e.g., Cairns 1952; Buser and Rougeul-Buser 1978).

Since these changes occur diffusely over the entire cortex, they are thought to be mediated by an "unspecific" ascending system, in contrast to the "specific" projection tracts of sensory channels into primary sensory cortical areas. However, the concepts relating to a coherent and unique ascending reticular activating system (ARAS) discussed in the important and now classical paper by Moruzzi and Magoun (1949), although still in use, especially in the anesthesiologic and forensic literature (e.g., McQuillen 1991), have to be modified, especially with regard to the authors' assumption about the anatomic substrate of the system (see, e.g., Brodal 1981). The reticular formation is a network of neurons of all sizes, extending from the medulla through the pons to the midbrain and tegmentum, and it is a physiologically and anatomically inhomogeneous structure. It surely has centers that lead to a desynchronization of EEG activity in the sense of increased attention. But other centers attenuate the state of alertness. Moreover, the projections of these neuronal areas do not accord with the anatomically defined reticular formation. Last but not least, the same structures that activate the cortex in an ascending manner may also activate the spinal cord, such as through descending noxious inhibitory control (for details see Chapter 34). For these reasons the term "ascending reticular activating system" is misleading, and modern brain research argues against the ARAS as a unique and coherent system. We still do not know much about these mechanisms, which can hardly be investigated in the anesthetized laboratory animal.

Essential neurotransmitters discussed in the control of arousal are serotonin and noradrenalin (norepinephrine). Serotonin is found in the raphe nucleus and noradrenalin in the locus coeruleus; both nuclei belong to the rostral brain stem. Release of serotonin decreases the state of arousal and induces sleep, presumably controlling specific "sleep substances." Contrastingly, the release of noradrenalin is associated with an alert, attentive state, probably due to modulation of the threshold of activation centers in the brain stem and midbrain (for details see, e.g., Ganten and Pfaff 1982). When under stress we surely are not drowsy. In any case, serotonin and noradrenalin release in the brain stem are the most often mentioned mechanisms in modern discussions of the mode of anesthetic action.

Still the question remains as to how nociceptive activity becomes conscious and induces feelings of pain. This is the mind–body problem. As already argued using Descartes' line of reasoning, this problem cannot in my opinion be answered in any general way with the usual methods of science. But this negative attitude does not mean that the question of conscious experience is in fundamental contrast to physical or physiologic processes, as if these two levels of discussion were principally independent. As shown in several chapters of this book, careful inspection and examination of patients with circumscriptive deficits in the pain system, especially those resulting from well-defined neurosurgical operations, provides some evidence for a close relationship between localizable cerebral activity and mental processes.

Evidence for the congruence between mental and cerebral states can also be obtained noninvasively by evaluating spontaneous and evoked EEGs. Power-spectrum analysis of the spontaneous EEG is often used for estimating arousal states. As already formulated in the classical paper of Moruzzi and Magoun (1949), transitions from drowsiness to alertness are characterized by a "breaking up of the synchronization of discharges of elements of the cerebral cortex," marked in the EEG by the "replacement of high-voltage slow waves with low-voltage fast activity." Conversely, a decrease in the arousal level of the brain is typically reflected by a shift in EEG activity toward lower frequencies (cf. Matejcek 1982; Gray et al. 1989; Steriade 1991; see also Chapter 8). The changes in EEG activity accompanying different sleep states are well known (e.g., Ganten and Pfaff 1982). Meanwhile, the spontaneous EEG is also widely used to monitor psychotropic effects of drugs (pharmaco-EEG; see, e.g., Herrmann Irrgang 1984, and Chapter 31).

With respect to pain, no systematic investigations have so far been reported about alterations of spontaneous EEG activity concomitant with different pain states. In fact, pain itself is an arousal stimulus that can, for example, break through the sedative effects of analgesics, and this is an important fact in the discussion of how to use opioids in patients with pain (see Chapters 30 and 32). In contrast, many investigations have been published on stimulus-induced changes in the spontaneous EEG evoked by appropriate noxious stimulation. Our experiments have led us to infer that it is the late brain potential in particular that can be used as an electrophysiologic correlate of conscious pain experience, as will be shown in the following sections.

PAIN-RELEVANT BRAIN POTENTIALS

Evoked brain potentials are stimulus-induced changes in the EEG, and as such are the most central signs of sensory perception measurable by noninvasive electrophysiologic methods (Fig. 1). The stimulus-evoked changes are small and hardly observable in the spontaneous EEG; therefore, repeated stimulation and averaging techniques are required to increase the signal-to-noise ratio. However, the spontaneous EEG is by no means noise. It reflects states of attention, arousal, sleep, narcosis, and mental processes (see below). In the past decade especially the 40-Hz rhythm has been discussed as a possible correlate of states of consciousness (Gray et al. 1989, see also Chapter 8). In any case, continuous prestimulus EEG activity should be included in the analysis of evoked brain potentials as stimulus-induced changes.

The earliest components recorded over the cortex are far-field potentials with noncortical sources, arising, for example, from stimulus-induced activity in the primary afferents or in the brain stem. They are followed by the early cortical (near-field) potentials, which are interpreted as summated electrical fields of postsynaptic potentials occurring synchronously with the earliest arrival of the nervous impulse pattern activated by the stimulus (for a review see, e.g., Picton 1988). Their latencies depend on the fiber-spectrum that is activated and on the neuronal distance to be conducted. In the case of median nerve stimulation the far-field potentials do not appear before about 20 msec (for review see Desmedt 1988). The earliest cortical potentials in response to selective activation of nociceptive Aδ afferents in the back of the hand are expected at 80 msec (with a mean conduction velocity in humans of 14 msec), while the earliest cortical potentials in response to pure C-fiber activation (0.86 msec) do not occur before 1,000 msec, as will be discussed in more detail below (for conduction velocities in humans see Vallbo et al. 1979; Bromm et al. 1994; Treede et al. 1988a). However, none of these "early" brain potentials in response to noxious stimuli has so far been observed. Because of the low signal-to-noise ratio, up to 1,000 stimulus repetitions are necessary to extract early potentials from the spontaneous EEG, a requirement that seems impossible in the case of pain-inducing stimuli. In addition, repeated stimuli normally activate different fibers with slightly different conduction velocities. In the case of the slowly conducting nociceptive afferents, this means that the latencies of single-trial brain responses are too large to allow conventional averaging.

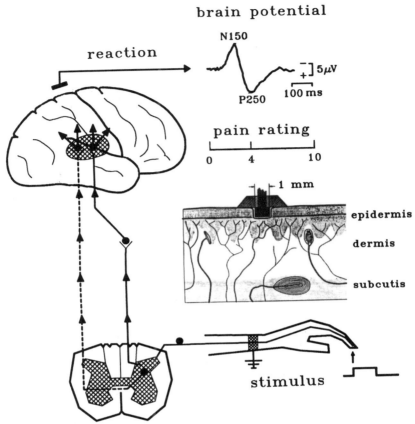

FIG. 1. The measurement of pain-related cerebral potentials. Pain-inducing stimuli, such as the intracutaneous shock (lower right) or the laser heat pulse, specifically activate nociceptive afferents, which conduct information in anterolateral and dorsal tracts to the thalamus, and from there to the cortex. Sensation is estimated on an analogue scale with values of 4 and more denoting increasing pain. In the surface EEG, stimulus-induced brain potentials appear, which are visible after averaging more than 40 stimulus repetitions. The negativity (*upward deflection*) at 150 msec (N150) after stimulus onset, and the positivity at 250 msec (P250) are late components of the evoked potential that reflect, among other essentials, the painfulness of the stimulus applied.

Whereas the early cortical potentials can best be recorded with scalp electrodes over the corresponding primary sensory cortical areas, later brain potentials are maximal at the vertex. Since their amplitudes are much larger, only about 40 stimulus repetitions may be sufficient for signal averaging. It is widely accepted that the long-latency brain potentials coincide with cognitive-processing mechanisms of arriving information induced by the stimulus, such as stimulus recognition, magnitude estimation, quality of sensation (e.g., painfulness), and the cortical initiation of a movement in reaction to the event (for a review see Vaughan and Arezzo 1988;

McCallum 1988; for the differentiation between sensory and motor potentials in response to noxious stimuli see Tarkka et al. 1992). Consequently, the late brain potentials depend on the experimental surroundings, background noise, stress situation, the subject's attention to the stimulus, distraction, stimulus expectance, vigilance level, and many other factors (e.g., Hillyard 1978; Picton 1988).

Because of their nonspecificity, it is difficult to extract pain-relevant components from the late brain potentials. Nevertheless, many papers have reported a good correlation between late-potential amplitudes and the painfulness of the applied stimulus (for a review see Chudler and Dong 1983; Bromm 1989; Handwerker and Kobal 1993). This is expected, since there is an inherent correlation between stimulus intensity and pain, and it is well known that brain-potential amplitudes increase with increasing stimulus intensities. For these reasons we performed a study with stimuli of different qualities and intensities (electrical and mechanical skin stimuli below and above the individual threshold of pain) applied to the hand of a particular subject, and evaluated the resulting data by multivariate factor analysis, separating the effects of stimulus intensity from those of painfulness (Bromm and Scharein 1982a; see also Becker et al. 1993). The main result was that two principal components could be identified, each of which varied in a highly significant manner with the painfulness of the applied stimuli, and with maxima arising at 150 and 250 msec (Fig. 1). These components provide a sensitive measure of pain states in normal subjects and in patients with altered pain sensibility (for a review see Bromm and Treede 1991, and Chapters 25 and 27), and reflect the relief of pain from efficient analgesic drugs (Bromm 1989; Chapter 32).

Essentially important for the investigation of pain-relevant brain potentials is the choice of the most appropriate stimulus. This stimulus should clearly induce pain with a minimum of other sensations, be suitable for repeated application with minimal adaptation or habituation, and not cause tissue damage. To apply averaging techniques, a well-defined trigger time for nociceptor activation is also required. There are no specific pain stimuli that activate only nociceptors, and low-threshold mechanoreceptors are always coactivated with them (for a detailed discussion see Bromm 1985; 1989). After many years of experimenting with various kinds of stimuli, we now use two types of pain-inducing stimuli in our laboratory. One type is the short radiant-heat pulse emitted by an infrared laser, which is invisible, inaudible, and does not contact the skin. Because of the long wavelength of the radiation (CO_2 laser: 10.6 μm; Carmon et al. 1976; thulium YAG laser: 1.8 μm; Kazarians et al. 1995), the heat pulse is absorbed by the very superficial skin layers within less than 100 μm, thus predominantly reaching the thinnest nerve terminals of the nociceptive Aδ- and C-afferents (see below). The second type of stimulus we use is intracutaneous electrical shock. This involves perforating the most superficial skin and delivering brief electrical pulses. With this procedure the stimulus again reaches the thinnest nerve terminals directly, and causes a stabbing, hot, sharp sensation of pain very similar to tooth-pulp stimuli (see Chapter 25).

Further experimental conditions must be fulfilled if late brain potentials are used to quantify pain, as has been discussed in detail elsewhere (e.g., Bromm 1989). In any case, the stimuli used to evoke these potentials must be randomized with respect to both stimulus interval and intensity, inducing unpredictably painful and nonpainful sensations. In this manner the subject is kept at a high and constant state of arousal even in long-lasting experimental sessions (Bromm and Scharein 1982b). Under highly constant experimental conditions, late brain potentials can in fact become powerful tools for quantifying experimentally induced pain (Chapter 32).

The following three examples are given to prove the usefulness of evoked brain potentials in the assessment of pain, and to illuminate the milieu of conscious experience from different points. The first example refers to the evoked brain potential as an objective measure of attentional states of pain. The second describes the combined analysis of spontaneous and evoked EEGs to differentiate between analgesic and sedative components of pain-relieving drugs. The third example provides results in patients and volunteers under general anesthesia that allow the assessment of analgesia in varying states of unconsciousness. Other chapters in this book summarize results of the application of brain potentials in identifying cerebral centers involved in pain processing through the use of multi-channel EEG (see Chapter 16) or magnetoencephalography (Chapter 17), the analysis of deficits in patients with pain (Chapters 25 and 27), and the quantitative evaluation of analgesic efficacy (Chapters 31 and 32).

ATTENTION, PAIN, AND BRAIN POTENTIALS

The brief radiant heat pulses emitted by the infrared laser induce reliable pain sensations. According to the fiber spectrum activated, a single laser stimulus applied to the back of the hand, for example, elicits a double pain sensation. The first pain to appear has a mean latency of 240 msec and is described as a sharp and stinging, well localizable pinprick pain, as induced by Aδ-fiber activity (mean velocity: 14 msec). This is followed by a second, more diffuse, burning component with a mean latency of 1,200 msec, which can be ascribed to C-fiber conduction (with a velocity of approximately 1 msec). Similarly, late and ultra-late brain potentials have been found with comparable waveforms and scalp distributions, with the former consisting of a negativity at 240 msec (N240) and a positivity at 370 msec (P370), and the latter consisting of a negativity at 1,180 msec (N1180) and a positivity at 1,300 msec (P1300), as described by Bromm et al. 1983 and Treede and Bromm 1988.

Fig. 2 illustrates the influence of attention on the amplitudes of late and ultra-late brain potentials. An inexperienced subject directs his attention only to the first painful sensation, thus missing the second, but with increasing experience the subject is able to differentiate between both kinds of pain: he then distinctly feels the different pain components and the time delay between them. As shown in Fig. 2, if the skilled subject focuses his attention on the second painful sensation, he exhibits ultra-late cerebral potentials as well. The more the subject concentrates on the appearance of the second pain, the more distinct are the ultra-late cerebral potentials.

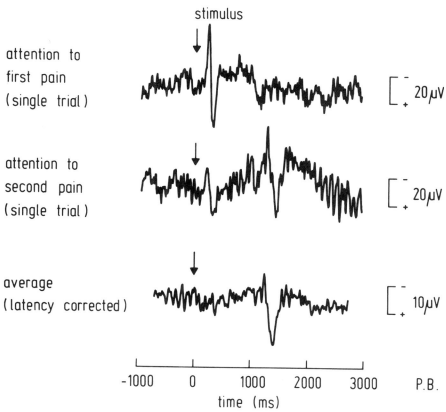

FIG. 2. First and second pain and their electrical brain correlates modulated by shift in attention. Late and ultra-late cerebral potentials are given in response to CO_2 laser stimuli of 20 msec duration and 18 W/20 mm², applied to the upper surface of the left foot. The stimulus activates both myelinated Aδ- and unmyelinated C-fiber nociceptors, and accordingly induces two pain sensations with a delay of approximately 1,000 msec. If the experienced subject shifts attention from the first to the second pain sensation, the ultra-late potential as a correlate of the C-fiber-mediated second pain is increased. (From Bromm 1989, with permission.)

The two pain sensations elicited by a single stimulus, as well as their neurophysiologic correlates, depend on many factors, and can emerge to a very different degree in patients with a special loss in nerve conduction, such as that due to syphilis (Treede et al. 1988b) or neuropathy (Lankers et al. 1991; see also Chapter 25). Moreover, the ultra-late potentials seem to be differentially sensitive to analgesic drugs. In preliminary experiments we found a considerably greater responsiveness of ultra-late potentials to opiates. In a recent investigation with multilead EEG, it has been shown that the late brain potentials described here can clearly be separated from the well-known P300 and later cognitive brain potentials (Becker et al.

1993). In fact, the design of experiments with repetitive pain-inducing stimuli differs from the "odd-ball" design used to elicit the P300 potential. Considered together, experiments like these give some evidence that the late (or ultra-late) cerebral potentials depend on attention and cognition, and reflect conscious pain experience.

The latencies of the first and second pain sensations were estimated by measurements of the reaction time to laser stimuli in intact nerves and nerves with their A-fibers mechanically blocked. Mean reaction times were found at 480 msec and 1,430 msec, respectively (Bromm et al. 1983). In a study with healthy volunteers, we compared the late brain potentials in response to noxious and auditory stimuli with movement-related cortical potentials, including the "Bereitschafts-potentials" in self-paced voluntary movements (Tarkka et al. 1992). In this way we estimated the conduction latencies for the different loops involved in performing a motor reaction. The main result was that the long-latency vertex negativity coincides with the beginning of a cortical reaction in response to the stimulus. With auditory stimuli the latency of this negativity is 105 msec (see also Starr and Don 1988), while with median nerve stimuli it is 150 msec (see also Treede et al. 1988a), and with laser heat stimuli 240 msec, or even 1,180 msec if the A-fibers are blocked (see also Bromm and Treede 1991).

The coincidence of the vertex negativity with the beginning of a cortical reaction to a stimulus does not necessarily mean that this negativity is a correlate of conscious experience of the sensory input. It can instead be a signal of subconscious processing of the received stimulus; the conscious evaluation of the event may follow. This concept is particularly supported by the finding that the subsequent positivity correlates most strongly with the subject's estimation of stimulus intensity and painfulness (Carmon et al. 1976; Miltner et al. 1989). In patients with a lack of cutaneous sensitivity to pain, the P240 potential was especially found to be abnormal (Bromm and Treede 1991). In other words, the discrimination between nonpainful and painful stimuli may be attributed to brain processes that are reflected in the late vertex positivity at 370 msec, or at 1,300 msec if the A-fibers are blocked or disturbed.

The latencies in the afferent loop consist of the nociceptor activation time (approximately 50 msec); conduction from the dorsal surface of the hand to the cervical spinal cord, which is probably at least 60 msec, using 14 msec as an estimate of Aδ-fiber conduction velocity and 85 cm as an estimate of the distance traveled by the impulse; and another 10 msec, which may be added for conduction from the cervical spinal cord to the cortex (for references regarding these estimates, see Tarkka et al. 1992). Earliest cortical potentials in response to Aδ-fiber stimulation with radiant heat pulses are therefore not expected before 120 msec. In the case of selective C-fiber activation, we found a conduction velocity of 0.86 ± 0.28 msec (Bromm et al. 1983), resulting in a conduction time of 990 msec for the 85 cm distance of impulse travel and a peak latency of 1,050 msec for the earliest cortical potentials in response to laser-emitted heat pulses applied to the back of the hand, if the other parameters were the same as given above.

Estimations like these are of course unsatisfactory, but suggest that: (a) the further cortical processing of Aδ- and C-fiber inputs seems to be similar; and (b) at least 100 msec seem to be needed by the brain to make information conscious after its arrival. The first statement is confirmed by multilead recordings of scalp topography of the negativity of the potentials evoked by painful stimuli, which show a bilateral symmetrical distribution with a maximum at the vertex for both the late and ultra-late brain potentials (Treede and Bromm 1988). To a first approximation, this is true for all sensory modalities, including auditory, visual, and somatosensory evoked potentials (for a review see Picton 1988). But closer inspection reveals considerable differences in the late-potential distributions for different sensory modalities. The negativity of the late auditory potential N105 has a more frontal accentuation (for a review see Starr and Don 1988), the negativity of the visual evoked potential N100 is maximal in the parietocentral region (Pz), arising from neuronal activity in areas 18 and 19 (Jeffreys 1977), and negativity of the N240 potential in response to laser stimuli exhibits its maximum between the cortical (Cz) and Pz regions (Treede et al. 1988a).

Many studies about the time interval necessary for cognitive processing mechanisms, especially in the literature of experimental psychology have been reported. The reader is referred to the excellent review by Fraisse (1963). The 100 msec estimated above agrees well with the mean range reported, which depends strongly, however, on the sensory modality activated. Stimuli applied successively to neighboring receptive fields (RFs) can elicit a phantom movement if, in case of the tactile system, the time interval between the stimuli is below 100 msec, or, in case of the retina, below 60 msec. Longer interstimulus intervals create an impression of separate stimuli. In patients with cortical injuries these intervals are considerably prolonged (e.g., Brenner 1956). Furthermore, the estimated 100 msec needed for rendering impulse information conscious depends on attention to the specific stimulus and on practice. If the same mechanical stimulus is applied simultaneously to the knee and the temple, the neuronal impulse patterns arrive at the cortex with a delay of 20 to 35 msec; with sufficient training this delay can be perceived consciously (Klemm 1925). The effect of optimal practice was estimated to shorten the brain processing time by 50 msec (Frankenhaeuser 1959; Fraisse 1963). Generally, humans perceive information through several sensory channels: we both see and hear a person coming, or we are both hit and injured by a flying stone (with tactile, nociceptive, and visual information). Within 100 to 200 msec the brain blends all of this different information together into one conscious experience. However, the more we concentrate upon single sensory channels, the more we are able to experience the time delays between different information sources.

In the case of pain, the spectrum of fibers that are activated is largely inhomogeneous: Aβ-fibers transmit tactile information, Aδ- and C-fibers inform about different components of pain. However, we perceive all of this differently conducted information as being simultaneous, or as an integrated entity. The example given above with the laser stimulus activating both Aδ- and C-fibers indicates that incoming information sources with a time interval of 1 sec between them can still be interpreted as being simultaneous. Comparable experiments have been performed with repeated pain stimuli. If the interstimulus intervals are below 1 sec, a sustained persistent pain is felt, and as a consequence, the late brain potentials relevant for phasic pain decrease (Chapman et al. 1981). Yet as shown in Fig. 2, with some practice the brain separates the different times of impulse arrival, as can be clearly documented by measurements of evoked brain potentials. In other words, cognitive brain potentials in response to pain-inducing stimuli are an efficient tool for the investigation of conscious pain experience, including questions relating to time integration and spatial resolution.

ANALGESIA: ANTINOCICEPTION OR SEDATION?

The second example concerns the evaluation of the pharmacological treatment of pain using evoked brain potentials. As extensively discussed by Beecher (1957), pharmacologically induced pain relief should be documented by showing a reduction of experimentally increased nociceptive activity toward normality. Similarly, Bonica (1979) defined analgesia as "the absence of experimentally induced pain." If the reduction in neuronal activity can be specified selectively within the nociceptive system, we would like to call this effect "antinociceptive." Lidocaine acts by reversibly blocking nerve conduction, but it does not exclusively inhibit nociceptive afferents. Aspirin is usually called an antinociceptive drug, but it does not act on the nociceptive nervous system. The analgesic effect of aspirin is based on its antiinflammatory action through its inhibition of prostaglandin biosynthesis, thus treating prostaglandin-enhanced nociceptive activity causally. Most animal experiments in algesimetry are designed to prove the antinociceptive effects of drugs, such as by stimulating nociceptive afferents and measuring nocifensive reactions. However, it is not easy to interpret the results obtained from such studies as documenting specific antinociceptive efficacy (for a detailed discussion see Chapman and Loeser 1989).

On the other hand, analgesic states can also be achieved by drugs that nonspecifically decrease the state of arousal. A typical example of this is the pain relief that occurs under general anesthesia (see below). Other examples are the analgesic states that occur with sedatives, hypnotics, tranquilizers, or alcohol, all of which can attenuate pain to some degree. These drugs do not exert specific effects on the nociceptive system; they are instead assumed to act on the ascending reticular afferent system (see p. 39), making the patient sleepy and drowsy. Consequently, we do not call these substances analgesics (for details of this see Chapter 33). However, most efficient analgesics, and not only the narcotic analgesics, exhibit at least some sedative properties by decreasing the state of arousal and as a consequence the conscious experience of pain. Under the influence of strong analgesics one should not drive a car. There is no question that the antinociceptive action of opiates results from specific receptors in the pain system (Chapters 30 and 34); the question is whether the hypnotic and euphoric components of opiates are only "side effects" of their analgesic action.

As already mentioned, the spontaneous EEG activity occurring immediately before a stimulus must be evaluated in the analysis of evoked brain potentials. One approach to this is the single-trial analysis of peristimulus EEG epochs, including both the spontaneous and the evoked EEG, immediately before and after stimulation. The activity in the spontaneous EEG is commonly described by spectral-power analysis in discrete frequency bands. Because evoked-potential measurements are usually analyzed for periods of only 500 msec, parametric spectral estimators have to be used, since the Fourier transformation provides an insufficient resolution of frequency that is inversely related to the length of the EEG periods used (2 Hz for segments of 1/2 sec). The greatest success has been achieved by adopting the autoregressive moving average filter or the maximum entropy method (for details see, e.g., Scharein et al. 1984). These techniques yield power-density functions by modelling the process that generated the data.

An essential observation about stimulus-induced EEG alterations in the frequency domain is given in Fig. 3. For simplification, a single trial EEG of 500 msec before stimulation (spontaneous EEG) and 500 msec after stimulation (stimulus-induced brain potential) in response to a brief laser stimulus is shown at the top of the figure. Each of these single-trial segments was subjected to spectral analysis by the maximum entropy method, after which averages over blocks of 80 stimuli (random intensities of two- and threefold greater than the individual pain threshold) were generated (middle line). To the left, the power spectra of the spontaneous EEG before stimulation can be seen with a clear alpha-peak and some power accumulated in the delta frequency range. To the right, the effects of the painful stimulus are seen in an enormous increase of power in the delta band. This low-frequency activity might be deduced from the late-potential waveforms. Interestingly, however, the same frequency bands originally derived from the spontaneous EEG (Berger 1938) also proved valid for the description of stimulus-evoked responses, with distinct borders between the known frequency bands. Moreover, we have deduced from single-trial analyses of peristimulus EEG segments (Bromm and Scharein, unpublished results) that precisely those generators that define the momentary delta frequency immediately before a stimulus is applied are triggered by the stimulus. In other words, the single-trial waveforms of the late brain potentials can be defined by the generators of the spontaneous EEG immediately before stimulus onset. In any case, the stimulus enhances low-frequency activity, whereas it exerts little influence on alpha and beta activity. This is demonstrated again in the lower graph of Fig. 3, which shows the grand-mean power-density functions before and after stimulation for all subjects participating in this study. To the right are shown the factors by which the powers of the different frequency bands were enhanced by the pain-inducing stimulus.

In order to specify, through EEG measures, the degree of sedation produced by opioid analgesia, the strong narcotic-analgesic meperidine (100 mg, p.o.) was tested against the tranquilizer diazepam (50 mg, p.o.) in a placebo-controlled, repeated-measures design (Bromm et al. 1989). Decreases in pain and brain potentials were measured to document analgesic effects, whereas reaction times, mood scales, and changes in EEG activity were recorded to estimate changes in alertness. Princi-

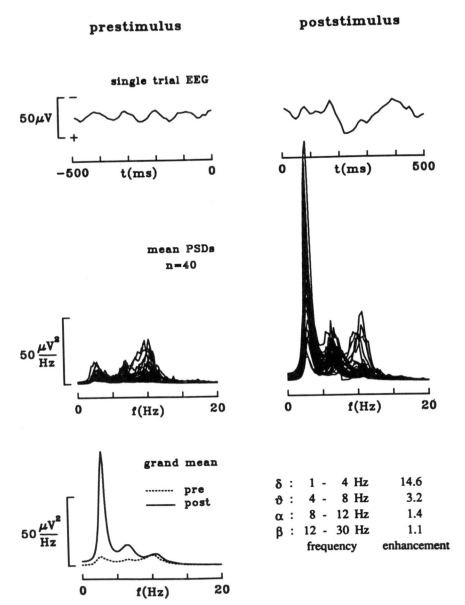

FIG. 3. The effect of the pain-inducing stimulus on EEG activity. Top row: Single-trial peristimulus EEG segment of 500 msec before (spontaneous EEG) and 500 msec after stimulation (stimulus-induced change). Middle row: Mean power spectra density functions over 80 segments for 21 subjects. Left: spontaneous EEG. Right: stimulus-induced EEG alterations; the stimulus increases low-frequency activity. The same frequency bands, which were originally derived from the spontaneous EEG, also proved valid for the description of stimulus-evoked responses. Bottom row: Grand-mean averages over the 21 subjects (*left*), and frequency bands with stimulus-induced amplification factors (*right*). (Modified from Bromm et al. 1989.)

pal-component analysis revealed four major components that accounted for 92% of total variance. The principal component PC1 described low-frequency activity in the prestimulus EEG, while the PC2 component described that of the poststimulus EEG. The components PC3 and PC4 referred to alpha and beta activity of the entire peristimulus EEG segment, before and after stimulation, in accord with the finding that higher EEG frequencies were little affected by the stimulus.

Obviously the scores of these four PCs were able to differentiate between the sedative and analgesic effects of the two drugs tested. Fig. 4 summarizes the correlation of the scores of these four PCs with subjective pain relief (left) and with sedation (right). PC2, comprising the poststimulus delta and theta power, correlated particularly strongly with the subjectively reported decrease in pain ratings, whereas PC3, the alpha activity of both the spontaneous and evoked EEGs, correlated best with sedation as measured by an increase in reaction times. The correlation between PC2 and pain relief was significantly ($r = 0.82$) greater than that between PC3 and sedation ($r = 0.57$). In summary, spectral analysis of the peristimulus EEG, in both the spontaneous and evoked situation, is a tool for the quantitative differentiation between drug-induced analgesia and drug-induced sedation.

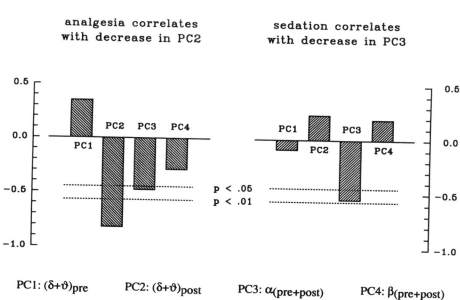

PC1: $(\delta + \vartheta)_{pre}$ PC2: $(\delta + \vartheta)_{post}$ PC3: $\alpha_{(pre+post)}$ PC4: $\beta_{(pre+post)}$

FIG. 4. Factors in brain potentials differentiating between analgesia and sedation. Principal-component analysis of spontaneous and evoked EEG activity in 24 subjects under an opioid (meperidine) and a tranquilizer (diazepam) yielded factors that distinguish between specific analgesic and nonspecific sedative components. Analgesia was measured by pain ratings and delta activity in brain potentials; sedation was measured by reaction times and mood scales. (From Scharein and Bromm 1991, with permission.)

PAIN RELIEF UNDER GENERAL ANESTHESIA

The goal of general anesthesia is loss of consciousness (White 1987), but how can we be sure that nociceptive acitivity elicited under surgery is not felt by the patient? This question is of special interest because we know that most anesthetics do not inhibit nociceptive activity (i.e., they do not have antinociceptive properties). With most anesthetics, the nociceptive input elicited by surgery continues to occur and reaches central structures in the midbrain, thalamus, and cortex, as has been shown in many animal experiments (see, e.g., Willis 1985, and Chapter 1). Many experiments, mainly in laboratory animals, have meanwhile demonstrated that it is the ascending reticular afferent system (see pp. 39 and 40) in particular that is modulated by anesthetics, causing a decrease in alertness and inducing unconsciousness (for a review see Angel 1991).

The action of anesthetics is therefore nonspecific. Anesthesia causes loss of sensory experience, particularly experience of pain, as well as loss of memory and loss of consciousness. In addition, anesthetic agents influence motor control and autonomic nervous mechanisms, and modulate cardiac and respiratory functions, blood pressure, and blood circulation in the brain and body. Although these effects on vegetative parameters are "side effects" that accompany the main effect of an anesthetic, they are used clinically to monitor the depth of anesthesia. Yet the question of which of these parameters, if any, reflect the degree of pain relief remains unanswered.

In the past decade, spectral analysis of the spontaneous EEG has been proposed for monitoring the depth of narcosis. It is well known that the EEG is characteristically modified in deep sleep (see Chapter 31) and gives some evidence about the state of arousal or alertness and about the vigilance level of the subject under medication. In fact, EEG changes are directly related to changes in electrical activity of the cortex. However, the rhythmic potential fluctuations in cortical cells are driven by excitatory input from specific thalamic nuclei, and these thalamic generators are in turn influenced by the midbrain and brain-stem reticular formation. The main site of action of anesthetics in these regions is currently being discussed (for a detailed review see Rubin et al. 1991). Many anesthetics presumably act by modulating the serotonine and noradrenaline release control mechanism in the nuclei Raphé and ceruleus (see pp. 40). For these reasons it is likely that the power-spectral density of the continuously recorded EEG gives information about the actual functional state of the brain under general anesthesia (Prior 1979). Although different anesthetic agents produce different EEG patterns, the power in the spontaneous EEG is usually shifted toward lower frequencies (e.g., Schulte am Esch and Kochs 1994; see also Fig. 6). On-line EEG analysis in the operating room may therefore facilitate the individual tailoring of anesthetics to specific surgical and patient needs (e.g., Schwilden and Stoeckel 1993).

On the basis of the observation that factors in the spontaneous and evoked EEGs differentiate between specific pain-reducing and nonspecific sedative modes of analgesic action, we investigated peristimulus EEG segments with intracutaneous stimuli in patients (Kochs et al. 1991) and healthy volunteers under general anesthesia (Bromm et al. 1994). The main result was again that long-latency brain potentials evoked by pain-inducing stimuli can clearly document the degree of analgesia under general anesthesia. These potentials were completely eliminated under deep narcosis (e.g., induced by halothane and nitrous oxide), reappeared to some degree if general anesthesia was flattened (e.g., by omitting N_2O), and varied in a highly sensitive manner with the narcotic-analgesic fentanyl (for a detailed discussion see Kochs and Bischoff 1994).

The results of a placebo-controlled study of 20 healthy volunteers under ketamine are given in Fig. 5 (single case) and Fig. 6 (grand means). Ketamine, a phencyclidine derivative, is a so-called dissociative anesthetic that induces a state of sedation, immobility, and amnesia as well as a marked analgesia, and a brief state of unconsciousness (for a review see Marshall and Wollman 1985). Subjects given the drug often complain of unpleasant hallucinations and disagreeable dreams (e.g., White et al. 1982). Because it does not induce respiratory depression, low-dose

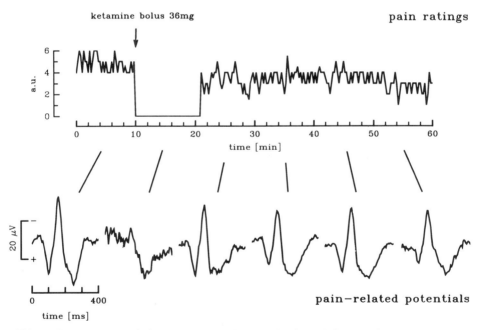

FIG. 5. Pain ratings and pain-related cerebral potentials after a bolus injection of 36 mg ketamine (single case). Top row: Pain ratings in response to intracutaneous stimuli of two- and threefold greater than the pain threshold strength (randomly applied). Immediately after ketamine injection (0.5 mg/kg), a brief state (11 min) of unconsciousness occurs. Later the pain ratings reappeared but remained decreased by approximately 25%. Bottom row: Brain potentials in response to the painful stimuli averaged over time periods of 10 min. They were reduced but present during the state of unconsciousness; in the steady state they were also reduced by approximately 25% at the end of the period of measurement. (From Bromm et al. 1994, with permission.)

KETANEST: mean single trial spectra of spontaneous EEG activity (N=10)

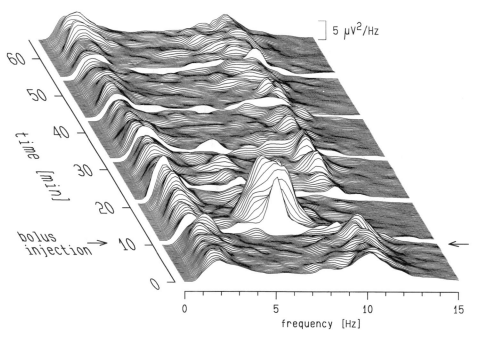

FIG. 6. Power spectra of spontaneous EEG activity after a bolus injection of 0.5 mg/kg ketamine (grand means over 10 subjects). Each peristimulus EEG segment of 5-sec duration was subjected to Fourier transformation. The single-trial power spectra were then smoothed and averaged over all 10 subjects. Immediately after bolus injection the alpha rhythm (8–12 Hz) is eliminated and a large increase in theta power (4–7 Hz) appears. The duration of these effects differed between individuals. The duration of the period of increased theta power correlates highly ($p<0.001$) with the duration of unconsciousness. (From Bromm et al. 1994, with permission.)

ketamine (0.25 to 0.50 mg/kg) is often used clinically to provide adequate postoperative analgesia without inducing major anesthetic effects.

The upper line in Fig. 5 illustrates the effects of ketamine on pain ratings in response to randomly applied intracutaneous stimuli of intensities two- and threefold greater than the individual pain threshold. Before medication, the stimuli were clearly within the pain range (ratings between 4 and 6). Injection of 0.5 mg/kg ketamine hydrochloride immediately induced a state of unconsciousness during which pain ratings were not to be made. Eleven minutes later, the subject came out of anesthesia and was again able to rate the intensity of the induced pain. However, the ratings in the latter case were reduced by at least 25% from their premedication levels. A comparable attenuation was found in the pain-relevant brain potentials (lower traces). Immediately after ketamine injection, the mean peak-to-peak amplitude difference, an estimate of analgesic efficacy, was reduced until the end of the period of measurement, again by approximately 25%. The analgesic component of 36 mg of ketamine as described in both variables corresponds to that of 100 mg of tramadol, a weak opioid (for the comparative evaluation of analgesics, see Chapter 32).

Interestingly, the pain-relevant brain potentials did not completely disappear during the ketamine-induced state of unconsciousness. During this period without verbal reports of pain, the brain potentials indicated an incomplete analgesic state under low-dose ketamine, comparable to that under 1% halothane alone, if the usual N_2O admixture was omitted (Kochs et al. 1991). In other words, the subjects might have perceived nociceptive activity but could not report it, and in all cases could not remember it. This is an example of the use of evoked brain potentials to assess pain states in cases in which verbal reports of pain are unavailable, such as in coma patients. Whether these methods can also be used to explore pain experience in newborns needs further research, since cerebral pain-processing mechanisms in this population are expected to be different from those of adults because of the incomplete myelinization of nociceptive afferents and projection tracts.

The brain potential in the unconscious state shown in Fig. 5 is superimposed on slow waves. The reason for this is that ketamine produces distinct effects in the spontaneous EEG (for a review see Tatsuno et al. 1990), described by an immediate destruction of the alpha rhythm and an increase in theta-frequency power (Fig. 6). In our study the effect on theta activity vanished within about 10 minutes, whereas the recovery of alpha activity required a longer period (50 min on the average). No ketamine effect was observed on delta and beta activity. With these findings we were able to compare the ketamine-induced periods of unconsciousness with periods of altered neurophysiologic and cardiovascular parameters. The results indicate that the duration of unconsciousness in each individual corresponds to the period of increased theta activity in the spontaneous EEG. Clearly, the ketamine-induced enhancement of theta power can be used to predict the duration of unconsciousness ($r = 0.96$) with great accuracy. In contrast, the changes over time in the cardiovascular variables, such as blood pressure, heart rate, and cerebral blood flow, occurred in parallel with changes in alpha activity of the spontaneous EEG.

In summary, the amplitudes of the brain potentials evoked by pain-inducing stimuli varied with the state of analgesia. Under flat narcosis with incomplete analgesia these potentials are attenuated but not completely eliminated, whereas pain ratings cannot be obtained if unconsciousness is induced. These findings again underline the relevance of the components of the late brain potential discussed in this chapter to the assessment of pain. In particular, combined analysis of the spontaneous and evoked EEGs is recommended in the assessment of both the analgesic and anesthetic components of anesthesia.

CONCLUSIONS

Pain cannot be defined in a general way. This fact may be illustrated by an analogy with vision: The usual scientific approach to investigating the visual system is to present a brief monochromatic flash and to measure the neuronal responses at different levels of the CNS, including cortical areas. This approach is analogous to the assessment of nociception by neurophysiologic methods. However, completely different brain-processing mechanisms occur during the contemplation of a famous painting. With the description of these brain mechanisms we enter a very subjective area. Judgement of the visual input is based on the individual's education in arts, intelligence, age, sex, race, social and cultural background, and immediate mood. To experience a visual impression we do not even necessarily need our eyes; we could, for example, merely dream of it. Comparable brain processes are assumed to be involved in pain experience.

In this chapter I have attempted to demonstrate that late brain potentials in response to pain-inducing stimuli may be particularly appropriate for investigating conscious pain perception. They reflect the subject's pain ratings and vary sensitively with many manipulations that alter pain experience. Pain-relevant brain potentials also respond, as does pain, to placebo. They are sensitive to the momentary arousal of the subject. In a drowsy subject, brain potentials evoked by similar stimulus intensities are less pronounced, and the same is true for the corresponding pain ratings. As a consequence, late brain potentials are increasingly used to document the analgesic potency of drugs, and to monitor the depth of analgesia in unconscious subjects under anesthesia.

REFERENCES

Angel A. Adventures in anaesthesia. *Exp Physiol* 1991;76:1–38.

Becker, DE, Yingling CD, Fein G. Identification of pain, intensity, and P300 components in the pain evoked potential. *Electroencephalogr Clin Neurophysiol* 1993;88:290–301.

Beecher HK. The measurement of pain. Prototype of the quantitative study of subjective responses. *Pharmacol Rev* 1957;9:59–209.

Berger H. Über das Elektroenkephalogramm des Menschen. *Nova Acta Leopoldina* 1938;6 6–173.

Bonica JJ. The need of a taxonomy. *Pain* 1979;6:247–252.

Brenner WM. The effect of brain damage on the perception of apparent movement. *J Pers* 1956;25:202–212.

Brodal A. *Neurological anatomy in relation to clinical medicine.* New York: Oxford University Press, 1981;427–459.

Bromm B, ed. *Pain measurement in man: neurophysiological correlates of pain.* Amsterdam: Elsevier, 1984;291–300.

Bromm B. Evoked cerebral potentials and pain. In: Fields HL, Dubner R, Cervero F, eds. *Proceedings of the IVth World Congress on Pain. Advances in pain research and therapy*, vol. 9. New York: Raven Press, 1985;305–330.

Bromm B. Laboratory animals and human volunteers in the assessment of analgesic efficacy. In: Chapman CR, Loeser JD, eds. *Issues in pain measurement. Advances in pain research and therapy*, vol. 12. New York: Raven Press, 1989;117–143.

Bromm B. The evoked brain potential as over-all control of sensory channels. In: Schulte Am, Esch J, Kochs E, eds. *Central nervous system monitoring in anesthesia and intensive care.* New Delhi: Macmillan, 1994;115–126.

Bromm B, Scharein E. Principal component analysis of pain related cerebral potentials to mechanical and electrical stimulation in man. *Electroencephalogr Clin Neurophysiol* 1982a;53:94–103.

Bromm B, Scharein E. Response plasticity of pain-evoked reactions in man. *Physiol Behav* 1982b;28:109–116.

Bromm B, Treede RD. Laser evoked cerebral potentials in the diagnosis of cutaneous pain sensitivity. *Rev Neurol* (Paris) 1991;147:625–643.

Bromm B, Meier W, Scharein E. Pre-stimulus/post-stimulus relations in EEG spectra and their modulation by an opioid and an antidepressant. *Electroencephalogr Clin Neurophysiol* 1989;73:188–197.

Bromm B, Neitzel H, Tecklenburg A, Treede RD. Evoked cerebral potential correlates of C-fibre activity in man. *Neurosci Lett* 1983;43:109–114.

Bromm B, Scharein E, Kochs E, Schulte am Esch J. Dissociation between analgesia and anaesthesia under ketamine. In: Gebhart GF, et al. eds. *Proceedings of the VIIth World Congress on Pain*, Paris. Seattle: IASP Publications, 1994;657–668.

Buchsbaum MF. Quantification of analgesic effects by evoked potentials. In: Bromm B, ed., *Pain measurement in man: Neurophysiological correlates of pain*. Amsterdam: Elsevier, 1984;291–300.

Buser PA, Rougeul-Buser A, eds. *Cerebral correlates of conscious experience*. Amsterdam: Elsevier, 1978.

Cairns W. Disturbances of consciousness with lesions of the brainstem and diencephalon. *Brain* 1952;8:75–92.

Carmon A, Mor J, Goldberg J. Evoked responses to noxious thermal stimulations. *Exp Brain Res* 1976;25:103–107.

Chapman CR, Loeser JD, eds. *Issues in pain measurement. Advances in pain research and therapy*, vol. 12. New York: Raven Press, 1989.

Chapman CR, Colpitts YH, Mayeno JK, Gagliardi GJ. Rate of stimulus repetition changes evoked potential amplitude: dental and auditory modalities compared. *Exp Brain Res* 1981;43:246–252.

Chudler EH, Dong WK. The assessment of pain by cerebral evoked potentials. *Pain* 1983;16:221–244.

Crick F, Koch C. Towards a neurobiological theory of consciousness. In: *Seminars in the neurosciences*, vol. 2. Cambridge, MA: Cold Spring Harbor Laboratory Press, 1990;263–275.

Damasio AR. *Descartes' error*. New York: Putnam (*in press*).

Descartes R. Meditations. In: Veitch J, Transl. *Renè Descartes: A discourse on method*. (1641). London: J. M. Dent & Sons Ltd, 1992.

Desmedt JE. Somatosensory evoked potentials. In: Picton TW, ed. *Human event-related potentials. Handbook of electroencephalography and clinical neurophysiology*, vol. 3. Amsterdam: Elsevier, 1988; 245–360.

Eccles JC. Do mental events cause neural events analogously to the probability fields of quantum mechanics? *Proc R Soc (Lond* [B]) 1986;227:411–428.

Feigl H. The mental and the physical. In: Feigl H, Screven M, Maxwell G, eds. *Minnesota studies in the philosophy of science*, vol. 2. Minneapolis, MN: University of Minnesota Press, 1958;370–497.

Fraisse P. Perception et estimation du temps. In: Fraisse P, Piaget J, eds. *Traité de psychologie experimentale*, vol. 6. Paris: Presses Universitaires, 1963;60–95.

Frankenhaeuser M. *Estimation of time*. Stockholm: University Press, 1959.

Ganten D, Pfaff D, eds. *Sleep. Clinical and experimental aspects*. Berlin: Springer, 1982.

Gray CM, König P, Engel AK, Singer W. Oscillatory responses in cat visual cortex inhibit intercolumnar synchronization which reflects global stimulus properties. *Nature* 1989;33:334–337.

Hammond DL. Inference of pain and its modulation from simple animal behaviors. In: Chapman CR, Loeser JD, eds. *Issues in pain measurement. Advances in pain research and therapy*, vol. 12. New York: Raven Press, 1989;69–92.

Handwerker HO, Kobal G. Psychophysiology of experimentally induced pain. *Physiol Rev* 1993;73:639–671.

Herrmann, WM, Irrgang, U. Characterization and classification of psychoactive drugs on a functional electrophysiological level. In: Bromm B, ed. *Pain measurement in man. Neurophysiological correlates of pain*. Amsterdam: Elsevier, 1984;167–188.

Hillyard SA. Sensation, perception and attention: analysis using ERPs. In: Callaway E, Tueting P, Koslow SH, eds. *Event-related brain potentials in man*. New York: Academic Press, 1978;223–321.

Jeffreys DA. The physiological significance of pattern visual evoked potentials. In: Desmedt J, ed. *Visual evoked potentials in man*. Oxford: Clarendon Press, 1977;134–167.

Kandel ER, Schwartz JH, Jessel TM, eds. *Principles of neural science*, 3rd ed. Amsterdam: Elsevier, 1991.

Kazarians H, Scharein E, Bromm B. Laser-evoked brain potentials in response to painful trigeminal nerve activation. *Intern J Neurosci* 1995;81:111–122.

Klemm O. Über die Wirksamkeit kleinster Zeitunterschiede. *Arch Ges Psychol* 1925;50:204–220.

Kochs E, Schulte am Esch J, Treede RD, Bromm B. Modulation of pain-related somatosensory evoked potentials by general anesthesia. *Anesth Analg* 1991;71:225–230.

Kochs E, Bischoff P. Anesthesia and somatosensory evoked potentials. In: Schulte am Esch J, Kochs E, eds. *Central nervous system monitoring in anesthesia and intensive care.* New Delhi: Macmillan, 1994;146–175.

Landers J, Frieling A, Kunze K, Bromm B. Ultralate cerebral potentials in a patient with hereditary motor and sensory neuropathy type I indicate preserved C-fibre function. *J Neurol Neurosurg Psychiat* 1991;54:650–652.

Marshall BE, Wollman H. General anesthetics. In: Goodman LS, Gilman A, Rall TW, Murad F, eds. *The pharmacological basis of therapeutics.* New York: MacMillan, 1985;276–301.

Matejcek M. Vigilance and the EEG: psychological, physiological and pharmacological aspects. In: Herrmann WM, ed. *Electroencephalography in drug research.* Stuttgart: Fischer, 1982;405–508.

McCallum WC. Potentials related to expectancy, preparation and motor activity. In: Picton TW, ed. *Human event-related potentials. Handbook of electroencephalography and clinical neurophysiology,* vol 3. Amsterdam: Elsevier, 1988;427–534.

McQuillen MP. Can people who are unconscious or in the "vegetative state" perceive pain? *Iss Law Med* 1991;6:373–383.

Melzack R. Measurement of the dimension of pain experience. In: Bromm B, ed. *Pain measurement in man: Neurophysiological correlates of pain.* Amsterdam: Elsevier, 1984;327–348.

Miltner W, Johnson R, Braun C, Larbig W. Somatosensory event-related potentials to painful and non-painful stimuli: effects of habituation. *Pain* 1989;38:303–312.

Moruzzi G, Magoun HW. Brainstem reticular formation and activation of the EEG. *Electroencephalogr Clin Neurophysiol* 1949;1:455–473.

Peschanski M, Ralston HJ, Roudier F. Reticularis thalami afferents to the ventrobasal complex of the rat thalamus. *Brain Res* 1983;270:325–339.

Picton TW, ed. *Human event-related potentials. Handbook of electroencephalography and clinical neurophysiology,* vol. 3. Amsterdam: Elsevier, 1988.

Popper KR, Eccles JC. *The self and its brain.* Berlin, Heidelberg, London, New York: Springer, 1977.

Prior PF. *Monitoring cerebral function.* Amsterdam: Elsevier, 1979.

Redfern PH, Campbell IC, Davies JA, Martin KF, eds. *Circadian rhythms in the central nervous system.* Weinheim: VCH, 1985.

Regan D. Human visual evoked potentials. In: Picton TW, ed. *Human event-related potentials. Handbook of electroencephalography and clinical neurophysiology,* vol. 3. Amsterdam: Elsevier, 1988; 159–244.

Rubin E, Miller KW, Roth SH, eds. Molecular and cellular mechanisms of alcohol and anesthetics. *Ann NY Acad Sci* 1991;625:1–848.

Scharein E, Bromm B. Spectral principal components of spontaneous and pain-related EEG activity. *Eur J Neurosci* 1991;(Suppl 4):38.

Scharein E, Häger F, Bromm B. Spectral estimators for short EEG segments. In: Bromm B, ed. *Pain measurement in man: Neurophysiological correlates of pain.* Amsterdam: Elsevier, 1984;189–202.

Schulte am Esch J, Kochs E, eds. *Central nervous system monitoring in anesthesia and intensive care.* New Delhi: Macmillan, 1994.

Schwilden H, Stoeckel H. Closed-loop feedback controlled administration of alfentanil during alfentanil-nitrous oxide anaesthesia. *Br J Anaesth* 1993;70:389–393.

Searle J. The problem of consciousness. *Consc Cogn* 1993;2:310–319.

Starr A, Don M. Brain potentials evoked by acoustic stimuli. In: Picton TW, ed. *Human event-related potentials. Handbook of electroencephalography and clinical neurophysiology,* vol. 3. Amsterdam: Elsevier, 1988;97–157.

Steriade M. Alertness, quiet sleep, dreaming. *Cereb Cortex* 1991;9:279–357.

Tarkka IM, Treede RD, Bromm B. Sensory and movement-related cortical potentials in nociceptive and auditory reaction time tasks. *Acta Neurol Scand* 1992;86:359–364.

Tatsuno J, Kawakami Y, Suzuki H, Fujita M. Ketamine induced changes in the electroencephalogram (EEG). Investigated by two-dimensional maps. In: Domino EF, ed. *Status of ketamine in anesthesiology.* Ann Arbor, MI: NPP Books 11. 1990;167–180.

Treede RD, Bromm B. Reliability and validity of ultra-late cerebral potentials in response to C-fibre activation in man. In: Dubner R, Gebhart GF, Bond MR, eds. *Proceedings of the VIth World Congress on Pain.* Amsterdam: Elsevier, 1988;567–573.

Treede RD, Kief S, Hölzer T, Bromm B. Late somatosensory evoked cerebral potentials in response to cutaneous heat stimuli. *Electroencephalogr Clin Neurophysiol* 1988a;70:429–441.

Treede RD, Meier W, Kunze K, Bromm B. Ultralate cerebral potentials as correlates of delayed pain perception. A clinical observation in a case of neurosyphilis. *J Neurol Neurosurg Psychiatry* 1988b; 51:1330–1333.

Vallbo AB, Hagbarth KE, Torebjörk HE, Wallin BG. Somatosensory, proprioceptive, and sympathetic activity in human peripheral nerves. *Physiol Rev* 1979;59:919–957.

Vaughan HG, Arezzo JC. The neural basis of event-related potentials. In: Picton TW, ed. *Human event-related potentials. Handbook of electroencephalography and clinical neurophysiology, vol. 3.* Amsterdam: Elsevier, 1988;45–96.

Vierck CJ, Cooper BY, Ritz LA, Greenspan JD. Inference of pain sensitivity from complex behaviors of laboratory animals. In: Chapman CR, Loeser JD, eds. *Issues in pain measurement. Advances in pain research and therapy*, vol. 12. New York: Raven Press, 1989;93–115.

White DC. Anesthesia: a privation of the senses. A historical introduction and some definitions. In: Rosen M, Lunn JN, eds. *Consciousness, awareness and pain in general anesthesia.* London: Butterworths, 1987;1–9.

White PF, Way WL, Trevor AJ. Ketamine—its pharmacology and therapeutic uses. *Anesthesiology* 1982;56:119–136.

Willis WD. The pain system; the neural basis of nociceptive transmission in the mammalian nervous system. *Pain Headache* 1985;8:341–346.

Pain and the Brain: From
Nociception to Cognition,
edited by Burkhart Bromm and
John E. Desmedt, Advances in Pain
Research and Therapy Vol. 22.
Raven Press, Ltd., New York © 1995.

4

Consciousness and Cognitive Brain Potentials

John E. Desmedt and Claude Tomberg

Brain Research Unit, University of Brussels, B-1000 Brussels, Belgium

The study of the distribution of consciousness shows it to be exactly as we might expect in an organ added for the sake of steering a nervous system grown too complex to regulate itself.

William James, *The Principles of Psychology*, p. 141

SUMMARY

Consciousness offers a major challenge to the neurosciences. Even though consciousness is by definition subjective, we consider it to be an intrinsic feature of biologic processes in the brain. It should be viewed in the Darwinian perspective of natural selection, which implies that conscious brain functions have survival value and cannot be mere epiphenomena. In a neurophysiologic approach in humans, we show that the P300 potential manifests nonspecific inhibitory deactivation after perceptual decision making, and has limited use for analyzing the brain processing of somatic or pain signals. We found that short-latency cortical potentials preceding P300 were strongly enhanced for finger stimuli that were given the subject's attention, thus manifesting a remarkable cognitive potentiation of specific representations in the receptive regions of the parietal cortex. Subsequently, the dorsolateral prefrontal cortex showed enhanced electrical activity reflecting an activation of somatic representations in the working memory. A functional linkage between these critical areas was revealed by the transient selective phase locking of 40-Hz oscillations recorded in the parietal and prefrontal cortices contralateral to the stimulated finger. We consider such reentrant interactions at 40 Hz to be an essential part of the conscious somatic brain mechanisms that achieve object identification (in this example, a finger) and the decision to generate a motor-behavioral response.

CONSCIOUSNESS

Although a meaningful philosophical stance is important with respect to the problem of consciousness, it is not sufficient for significant progress in understanding the neurophysiology of consciousness. One must approach this formidable challenge from a realistic vantage point so as to enhance the feasibility of the necessary studies. Philosophers, even when citing findings in the neurosciences, are generally not primarily concerned with experimental designs that might help resolve any particular item in their lists of problems. Some even appear somewhat suspicious of experimentation in the neurosciences, and may in fact deny any operational function to consciousness even when using its name to provide a catchy title for a book (Dennett 1991).

Consciousness is by definition subjective and private to the organism concerned; it cannot be dealt with as a third-person objective phenomenon; it is fairly continuous during the waking state, and includes, at any time in a unified conscious experience, various items that can either be within the focus or at the periphery of attention, such as nondescript emotional tones (Searle 1993). Along with Searle, we consider consciousness to be an intrinsic feature of biologic processes in the brain. This view is at variance both with Descartes' dualism and with modern black-box functionalism, with its claim that computer programs running on nonbiologic hardware could emulate brain operations (Johnson-Laird 1988).

EVOLUTION OF CONSCIOUSNESS

The relevance of an evolutionary approach to the problem of consciousness is clear. Every burst of evolution in which phenotypes underwent change was followed by a flurry of extinctions, raising the major question of why certain organisms survived while others disappeared. Obviously any change in molecular features at the gene level (microevolution) makes sense only in the context of higher-order systems, such as organisms living in their environments (macroevolution). In fact, highly developed organisms impose severe restrictions in terms of those genetic variations that might actually be helpful (Diamond 1993; Noble and Boyd 1993).

Essential in biologic design are the bodily functions responsible for the constancy and adaptive regulation of the "milieu intérieur," as documented by Claude Bernard (1865). Moreover, the continued adequate functioning of an organism's physiological machinery depends crucially on adaptive control of the organism's behavior through appropriate central nervous system operations.

While inherited patterns of responses (such as instincts) lacking any foresight of consequences can meet certain stereotyped environmental challenges (Tinbergen 1952), a hard-wired nervous system makes no sense when organisms have to adapt to various or changing living conditions.

In the context of the Darwinian process of natural selection, one can envision in the brain the emergence and development of conscious mechanisms allowing meaningful flexibilities in behavior, whereby organisms such as early mammals were endowed with a decisive advantage for survival in a hostile environment.

We know that consciousness is a manifest feature of higher organisms and the human species. Like any trait, it must have evolved through natural selection. If it has indeed been so selected, it is because it served a useful function, such as to upgrade perceptual decisions and behavioral choices. If the conscious functions of the brain had lacked any survival value, they would have failed to develop through Darwinian evolution and would not now exist (Darwin 1871; James 1890).

This evolutionary approach is totally incompatible with the view of consciousness as a mere epiphenomenon (Huxley 1874). It also implies that the full-blown consciousness generally discussed in the current literature (Baars 1988; Marcel and Bisiach 1988; Donald 1991) did not suddenly appear by any magic stroke, either in humans or at a particular stage in evolution. A conscious function of the brain should rather be viewed as developing over many millennia, like other brain mechanisms, from elementary levels to increasingly sophisticated levels of efficiency.

Nor should the notion of consciousness adding critically assistive components to behavior control be taken as compatible with any suggestion that the mind would be able to escape from the deterministic neurophysiology of the brain, as James (1890) and Popper (1978) seem to have considered and even apparently hoped. The added utility of conscious brain mechanisms rests only in biologic processes that add flexibility and sophistication to behavior (and survival at initial stages), thereby enabling upgraded features of behavior to meet environmental challenges.

RATIONALE

We believe that an efficient experimental approach to the conscious function of the brain requires refraining at this stage from considering the actual neurophysiology of the most sophisticated features of consciousness, such as language and self-consciousness. Nevertheless, we believe that humans are preferable to other animals as subjects for such (noninvasive) experiments because they can speak to the experimenter and describe their conscious experience in elaborate detail during the course of the experimentation.

The pain inputs to the brain do not yet appear to readily lend themselves to the precise correlations that we are now seeking, if only because of the rather blurred onset/offset timing of most pain perceptions and the complex organization of their central projections (see chapters by Bromm; Willis; Chen et al.).

A further consideration is that experimental designs be precisely definable so as to help assess specific interventions of a conscious mechanism during the fraction of a second in which the brain is processing a simple sensory input and a behavioral decision is elaborated and executed.

EVENT-RELATED POTENTIALS OF THE BRAIN

The noninvasive recording of brain potentials through a set of electrodes applied to the skin of the head (scalp mapping) has established itself as a major methodology for analyzing cognitive and perceptual functions in humans. One class of studies with this technique has concentrated on event-related potentials (ERP) elicited by a well-defined event, such as a sensory stimulus with controlled features that are separated by sufficient intervals to allow completion of their perceptual elaboration.

One can identify several main points of entry in the design of ERP studies. One of these has to do with the analysis of cortical potentials elicited by a sensory event in the so-called primary receiving cortical areas. This was done in the classical work on primates of Marshall et al. (1941), Arezzo et al. (1981), and Kaas et al. (1983), and has now been considerably elaborated in humans for the visual (Heinze et al. 1990; Zeki 1993) and somatosensory (Desmedt 1988; Desmedt and Tomberg 1989) modalities, among others.

Another major breakthrough has been the demonstration that in addition to generating potentials reflecting the detailed hard-wired sensory projections in receiving cortical areas, the brain generates potentials related to cognitive operations, the best known examples of which are the surface-positive P300 potential (with a peak latency between 300 and about 800 msec, depending on the duration of perceptual evaluation) (Sutton et al. 1965; Desmedt et al. 1965), and the surface-negative contingent negative variation (CNV) (Walter et al. 1964) (see Hillyard and Picton 1987; Luck and Hillyard 1990).

The controversy about whether P300 and CNV were distinct has now been resolved by several experimental designs showing that one of these components could be elicited in the absence of the other (Donchin et al. 1975; Desmedt and Debecker 1979a). However, questions remain about the true significance of these relatively slow components, which have become important to the neurosciences and neuropsychiatry (Timsit-Berthier et al. 1973; Pritchard 1981; Knight et al. 1881; Hillyard and Picton 1987; Smith et al. 1990; Goodin 1990; Polich 1991). Both CNV and P300 are sizeable electrical events in their duration, voltage (a few hundredths of one volt), and extensive brain topography. They are influenced to only a relatively small extent by the sensory modality of the event being processed, which is one argument for considering them to be in some way "invoked" in the course of brain processing, rather than being "evoked" by the sensory event itself.

All of these features favor the view that the widespread CNV and P300 do not directly reflect any of the specific cognitive brain operations that ceaselessly analyze the environment in order to make sense of a myriad of sensory events and attempt to control behavior appropriately.

We proposed that in contrast to then prevalent interpretations, P300 was not related to any specific cognitive operation for the actual identification of a sensory event, but rather that P300 reflected an extensive inhibitory brain deactivation that followed perceptual identification of the event. Consequently, we designated P300 by coining the term *post-decision closure* and suggested that it performed an essential "brain housekeeping function" by deactivating the sets of brain circuits that had been active in processing the event, and which were to be cleared before upcoming events could make use of appropriate brain resources for their own perceptual processing (Desmedt and Debecker 1979a,b; Desmedt 1980).

It is now agreed that most brain potentials recorded from the scalp reflect extracellular fields generated by coherent shifts of membrane potential in the apical dendrites of the large pyramidal neurons making up the cortical columns (Mountcastle 1979). More succinctly, neuromodulatory mechanisms regulating excitability and synaptic transactions in cortical neuron assemblies tend to depolarize superficial parts of the pyramidal dendrites (see Skinner and Yingling 1977; Steriade 1981; Colonnier 1981; Bloom 1981; Desmedt 1981), resulting in surface-negative scalp potentials such as the CNV. By contrast, P300 manifests a transient reduction in that depolarizing pressure and it is seen as widespread surface-positive potentials on the scalp (see discussion in Desmedt and Debecker 1979a). The dynamics of slow potential shifts (SPS) have been analyzed in mammals (Caspers 1963; Wurtz 1966; Rowland 1968). In this physiologic perspective, essential features of P300 are the widespread (cortical and subcortical) inhibitory shifts that can phase out and interrupt ongoing specific cognitive activities in order to achieve a more consistent use, with time, of the (limited) brain resources available for perceptual processing (Desmedt 1980).

Fig. 1 provides an example of scalp potentials recorded in a young normal human from the right parietal cortex. The sensory stimulus was a brief, near-threshold (about 90% detection by the subject) electrical pulse delivered to the left index finger. The finger stimuli were randomly intermixed with acoustic clicks. Because the interval between each stimulus was fixed at 2.5 sec, the subject rapidly became able to predict the time at which the next stimulus would appear. In the experimental runs in which the finger stimulus was designated to be mentally counted by the

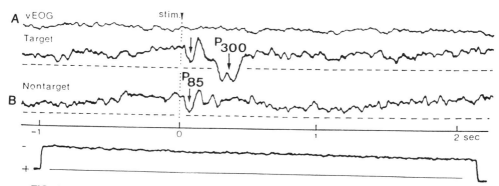

FIG. 1. Averaged event-related potentials (ERP) evoked by a brief near-threshold electrical pulse delivered to the left index finger (*arrow and vertical dots*). The finger stimuli are randomly intermixed with near-threshold acoustic clicks of equal probability. The interstimulus intervals are fixed at 2.5 sec. The active electrode was on the right (contralateral) parietal scalp at 7 cm from the midline and 3 cm behind the vertex (Cz). The linked mastoids were used as a reference. The system bandpass was 0.02 to 2,000 Hz (3 dB down) and the bin width 3.2 msec. A square calibration pulse of 3 μV and about 3-sec duration shows the low-frequency fidelity of the recording system (*bottom*). **A:** Vertical electro-oculogram (*upper trace*) and ERP to target finger stimuli counted mentally by the subject. The large P300 is preceded by positive (P85) and negative phasic components. **B:** ERPs to identical index-finger stimuli that were designated as nontargets to the subject, who was mentally counting the acoustic clicks (other runs of the same experiment). Notice the slow negative shift of both ERP traces before the time of delivery of the stimuli. (From Desmedt and Debecker 1979b, with permission.)

subject, a clear positive P300 was recorded (Fig. 1A), whereas P300 failed to occur when identical finger stimuli were designated in other runs as nontargets that the subject was to ignore (Fig. 1B). It was remarkable that in both cases the stimulus was preceded by a progressive surface-negative shift of about 2 μV, which reflected a neuromodulatory cortical preparation in this situation in which the subject could anticipate the sensory events. Furthermore, the target and nontarget finger stimuli were followed by transient surface-positive (we now call them P85) and -negative potentials that manifested cognitive-processing operations before the occurrence of P300 (Fig. 1).

In other words, an inhibitory P300 was recorded in the experimental trials in which the attended signal had been identified by the subject and the selective attention task had thus actually been fulfilled (Desmedt and Debecker 1979b). However, a surface-negative neuromodulatory shift appeared in both situations in conjunction with the ability of the subject to predict (in this paradigm with fixed interstimulus intervals) the approximate time of the next event, even though the subject could not know whether the event would be task-relevant (a target finger signal) or not task-relevant (a nontarget acoustic signal).

This example of selective attention between two distinct sensory modalities has been elaborated for selective attention within a single modality. When brief electrical stimuli of similarly low intensity were delivered in randomly intermixed sequences to two adjacent fingers of both the left and the right hands, the subject had a very difficult selective attention task in identifying the single target finger designated in a particular experimental run. For the response to the finger designated as the target (shown in black in the figurine in Fig. 2), there was a large P300 preceded by positive (P40 and P85) and negative (N140) cognitive potentials (Fig. 2B) (Desmedt and Robertson 1977). These enhanced responses were estimated by comparison with the response to an identical stimulation of the same finger when that finger had been designated as nontarget in another experimental run, in which the target finger was on the opposite hand (thin superimposed trace in Fig. 2).

The remarkable finding was that the brain response to the finger adjacent to the target finger did not disclose any P300, even though it presented sizeable P40 and N140 potentials (Fig. 2E). These latter short-latency components manifested the cortical processing that had obviously been necessary for the subject to distinguish the nontarget finger from the adjacent target finger stimulated at other times in the same experiment (Desmedt and Robertson 1977).

Recently, experimental analyses of ERPs have increasingly shown that the cognitive brain potentials preceding P300 closure are highly significant and manifest achievement of the processing tasks essential for perceptual identification and environmental monitoring (Desmedt and Tomberg 1989; Tomberg et al. 1989.

This is an important consideration for the future development of pain-perception research, in which the analysis of early cortical events has so far proved more difficult than for skin somatic tactile sensations. We consider it an important matter to clearly distinguish P300-like responses from those brain potentials that could more

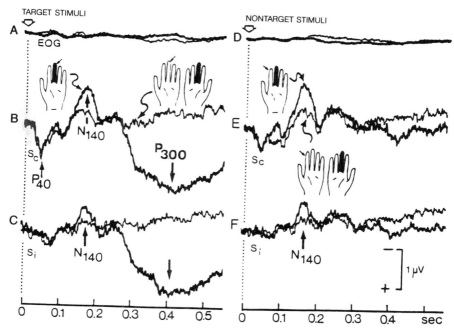

FIG. 2. Averaged ERPs during somatosensory selective attention to randomly intermixed sequences of near-threshold electrical stimuli delivered to four fingers (fingers II and III of the left and right hands). One of the fingers was designated as a target in which the stimuli were to be mentally counted in any given experimental run. Subjects counted target stimuli to the third finger of either the left hand (*thicker traces*) or the right hand (*thinner traces superimposed*). The attended finger is represented in black in the figurines. The *small arrows* point to the stimulated finger that evokes the ERP in question. **A** and **D**: Vertical electrooculogram controls showing absence of eye-movement artifact. **B** and **E**: Somatosensory ERPs recorded from contralateral scalp (Sc) and elicited by stimuli applied either to the third **(B)** or second **(E)** finger of the left hand. **C** and **F**: ERPs recorded simultaneously from ipsilateral (Si) parietal scalp electrode. The negative (upward) N140 is larger contralaterally for both target and nontarget stimuli to the left hand. The P300 is symmetrical but occurs only for target stimuli **(B–C)**. The shorter-latency P40 appears only contralaterally in **B** and **E**. (From Desmedt and Robertson 1977, with permission.)

genuinely reflect pain perception. It appears useful at this stage to elaborate on the experimental results in this area and to distinguish, in experimental designs, P300 itself, which we do not believe reflects any specific step in sensory processing.

Nevertheless, research on P300 remains valuable because P300 is obviously under the control of the cognitive prefrontal systems involved in organizing goal-directed behavior (Milner 1964; Luria 1973). We certainly agree that the timing of negative shifts and of positive P300s during sequential behavior can provide important clues about the dynamics of cognitive brain operations.

NEUROPHYSIOLOGY OF CONSCIOUSNESS

The results and concepts summarized above suggest that the critical brain activities involved in conscious perception should become manifest within the interval between the arrival of the relevant sensory input to the cortex and the onset of a P300.

With regard to this, we have studied somatic sensations, and particularly the tactile and joint inputs from fingers. These appeared rather manageable because they involve brief volleys of impulses traveling rapidly in the dorsal column and lemniscal pathways to a set of well-defined cortical areas that have been charted in detail by scalp mapping over the brain convexity (Desmedt 1988). We used an oddball type of experimental paradigm in which fingers were stimulated in random sequences with a brief, near-threshold electrical pulse. During the test, the subject had to identify the sensory input from one designated finger (the target) and respond by a key press (with the right big toe), neglecting the sensory inputs from other finger(s). Details of the methods used are available elsewhere (Desmedt and Tomberg 1989; Tomberg et al. 1989).

With this technique, a target-finger stimulus activates the primary receiving somatic cortex in the contralateral parietal areas 3b, 1, and 2 of Brodmann, where the features of the sensory input are analyzed and represented in detail (Kaas et al. 1983; Desmedt 1988). We found that in conjunction with target perceptual processing, these somatic representations were strongly enhanced, as manifested by remarkable cognitive P30–P40 potentials in areas 1 and 2 (Desmedt and Tomberg 1989; Tomberg et al. 1989, 1990). From about 120 msec after the finger stimulus, the activities of the parietal areas (including posterior areas 5 and 7b) were joined by potentials evoked in the dorsolateral prefrontal cortex (N140), which are believed to reflect the activation of somatic representations in the working memory (Goldman-Rakic 1990), consisting of contextual information and stored experiences including, in this example, "body-image" items. These prefrontal areas have reciprocal cortico-cortical connections with the posterior parietal areas (Petrides and Pandya 1984; Selemon and Goldman-Rakic 1988) whereby the activities in the parietal cortex are projected to the prefrontal areas, from which they can in turn be "re-entrantly" (Edelman 1989) fed back to the parietal neuronal assemblies involved in processing the immediately incoming information.

We recently provided direct evidence for a functional linkage between these critical areas by showing a transient and selective phase locking of 40-Hz oscillations recorded in the cortical areas of the parietal and prefrontal cortices (Fig. 3A) (Desmedt and Tomberg 1994). Remarkable features of this transient 40-Hz phase locking were: (a) its selectivity for these areas on the side contralateral to the target finger, (b) its characteristic frequency (there was no concomitant synchrony at other frequencies), (c) the large distance (about 90 mm) over which the synchrony was recorded, and (d) the critical timing of the synchrony, which occurred 100 to 200 msec after the finger stimulus, at about the time when perceptual processing directed at object identification must have been in progress.

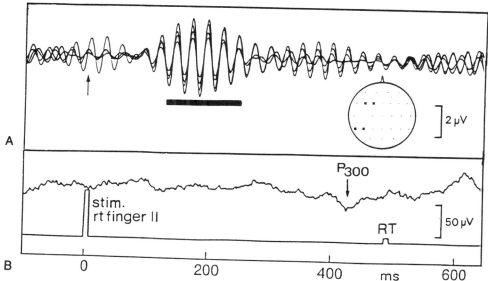

FIG. 3. A: Transient phase locking of 40-Hz oscillations in the left parietal and prefrontal cortex (see scalp figurine with the 32 electrode positions and larger dots for the traces shown). Superimposed traces filtered at 35 to 45 Hz with non-recursive finite-impulse-response digital filter. The transient phase locking is indicated by a solid horizontal bar. **B:** Non-averaged, unfiltered left parietal recording showing P300 (*upper trace*) and technical channel showing time of delivery of a target near-threshold electric stimulus to the right index finger and the subject's reaction time (RT). (From Desmedt and Tomberg 1994, with permission.)

Microphysiologic studies in cats and monkeys have documented transient synchronies of 30- to 50-Hz action potentials discharged by neurons of the visual cortex when these cells were analyzing distinct features of a given visual object (Gray et al. 1989).

Our finding of transient 40-Hz phase locking that can achieve a functional linkage of parietal and prefrontal areas offered direct evidence for reciprocal and reentrant interactions between live detailed representations in the primary projection cortex and the stored representations called upon by the working-memory mechanism in the prefrontal cortex. We consider these interactions to be an essential part of the conscious brain mechanisms achieving identification of an object or event (in this example, a finger) that can lead to the decision to express an appropriate motor behavioral response (in this example, the reaction time response) (Fig. 3).

Interestingly, the 40-Hz phase locking clearly preceded the simultaneously recorded P300 component (Fig. 3B) that we had interpreted as an inhibitory postdecision closure (Desmedt and Debecker 1979a,b). Such critical timing therefore documented a conscious brain process that was not epiphenomenal (it occurred before the perceptual decision) and which was not delayed with respect to the behavioral response of the subject.

We conclude that the transient and selective 40-Hz binding thus disclosed in humans subserves a conscious brain mechanism that is directly involved in the perceptual and behavioral decisions relating to a sensory object or event (Desmedt and Tomberg 1994).

REFERENCES

Arezzo JC, Vaughan HG, Legatt AD. Topography and intracranial sources of somatosensory evoked potentials in the monkey. *Electroencephalogr Clin Neurophysiol* 1981;51:1–18.

Baars BJ. A cognitive theory of consciousness. Cambridge, MA: Cambridge University Press, 1988.

Bernard C. *Introduction à l'étude de la médecine expérimentale*. Paris: Baillière, 1865.

Bloom FE. Chemical signaling and cortical circuitry: integrative aspects. In: Schmitt FO, Worden FG, Adelman G, Dennis SG, eds. *The organization of the cerebral cortex*. Cambridge, MA: MIT Press, 1981;359–372.

Caspers H. Relations of steady potentials shifts in the cortex to the wakefulness-sleep spectrum. In: Brazier M, ed. *Brain function*, vol. 1. Los Angeles: University of California Press, 1963;177–214.

Colonnier M. The electron-microscopic analysis of neuronal organization of the cerebral cortex. In: Schmitt FO, Worden FG, Adelman G, Dennis SG, eds. *The organization of the cerebral cortex*. Cambridge, MA: MIT Press, 1981;125–152.

Darwin C. *The descent of man and selection in relation to sex*. London: Murray, 1871.

Dennett DC. *Consciousness explained*. Boston: Little, Brown, 1991.

Desmedt JE. P300 in serial tasks: an essential post-decision closure mechanism. *Progr Brain Res* 1980; 54:682–686.

Desmedt JE. Scalp recorded cerebral event-related potentials in man as points of entry into the analysis of cognitive processing. In: Schmitt FO, Worden FG, Adelman G, Dennis SG, eds. *The organization of the cerebral cortex*. Cambridge, MA: MIT Press, 1981;441–476.

Desmedt JE. Somatosensory evoked potentials. In: Picton T, ed. *Human event-related potentials. Handbook of EEG and clinical neurophysiology*, vol. 3 (Revised Series). Amsterdam: Elsevier, 1988;245–360.

Desmedt JE, Debecker J. Waveform and neural mechanism of the decision P300 elicited without prestimulus CNV or readiness potential. *Electroencephalogr Clin Neurophysiol* 1979a;47:648–670.

Desmedt JE, Debecker J. Slow potential shifts and decision P300 interactions with random sequences of near-threshold clicks and finger stimuli delivered at regular intervals. *Electroencephalogr Clin Neurophysiol* 1979b;47:671–679.

Desmedt JE, Debecker J, Manil J. Mise en évidence d'un signe électrique cérébral associé à la détection par le sujet d'un stimulus sensoriel tactile. *Bull Acad Roy Médicine Belg* 1965;5:887–936.

Desmedt JE, Robertson D. Differential enhancement of early and late components of the cerebral somatosensory evoked potentials during forced-paced cognitive tasks in man. *J Physiol* (Lond) 1977; 271:761–782.

Desmedt JE, Tomberg C. Mapping early somatosensory evoked potentials in selective attention: critical evaluation of control conditions used for titrating by difference the cognitive P30, P40, P100 and N140. *Electroencephalogr Clin Neurophysiol* 1989;74:321–346.

Desmedt JE, Tomberg C. Transient phase-locking of 40-Hz electrical oscillations in prefrontal and parietal human cortex reflects a conscious somatic perception process. *Neurosci Lett* 1994;168:126–129.

Diamond JM. Evolutionary physiology. In: Boyd CAR, Noble D, eds. *The logic of life*. Oxford: Oxford University Press, 1993;89–112.

Donald M. *Origins of the modern mind*. Cambridge, MA: Harvard University Press, 1991.

Donchin E, Tueting P, Ritter W, Kutas M, Heffley E. On the independence of the CNV and P300 components of the human averaged evoked potentials. *Electroencephalogr Clin Neurophysiol* 1975; 38:449–461.

Edelman GM. *The remembered present*. New York: Basic Books, 1989.

Goldman-Rakic PS. Cellular and circuit basis of working memory in prefrontal cortex of non-human primates. *Progr Brain Res* 1990;85:325–335.

Goodin DS. Clinical utility of long latency ERPs (P3). *Electroencephalogr Clin Neurophysiol* 1990; 76:2–5.

Gray CM, König P, Engel AK, Singer W. Oscillatory responses in cat visual cortex exhibit intercolumnar synchronization which reflects global stimulus properties. *Nature* 1989;338:334–337.

Heinze HJ, Luck SJ, Mangun GR, Hillyard SA. Visual event-related potentials index focused attention within bilateral stimulus arrays: evidence for early selection. *Electroencephalogr Clin Neurophysiol* 1990;75:511–527.

Hillyard SA, Picton TW. Electrophysiology of cognition. In: Plum F, ed. *Handbook of physiology*, vol. 5. Bethesda, MD: American Physiological Society, 1987;519–584.

Huxley TH. On the hypothesis that animals are automata and its history. *Fortnightly Rev* 1874;22:555–589.

James W. *The principles of psychology*, New York: Holt, 1890.

Johnson-Laird PN. *The computer and the mind*. Cambridge, MA: Harvard University Press, 1988.

Kaas JH, Merzenich MM, Killackey HP. Changes in the organization of somatosensory cortex following peripheral nerve damage in adult and developing mammals. *Annu Rev Neurosci* 1983;6:325–356.

Knight J, Hillyard SA, Woods DL, Neville HJ. The effects of frontal cortex lesions on event-related potentials during auditory selective attention. *Electroencephalogr Clin Neurophysiol* 1981;52:571–582.

Luck SJ, Hillyard SA. Electrophysiological evidence for parallel and serial processing during visual search. *Percept Psychophys* 1990;48:603–617.

Luria AR. *The working brain*. New York: Penguin Books, 1973.

Marcel AJ, Bisiach E, eds. *Consciousness in contemporary science*. Oxford: Clarendon Press, 1988.

Marshall WH, Woolsey CN, Bard P. Observations on cortical somatic sensory mechanisms in cat and monkey. *J Neurophysiol* 1941;4:1–24.

Milner B. Some effects of frontal lobectomy in man. In: Warren JM, Akert K. eds. *The frontal granular cortex and behavior*. New York: McGraw Hill, 1964;313–334.

Mountcastle VB. An organizing principle for cerebral function: the unit module and the distributed system. In: Edelman GM, Mountcastle VB, eds. *The mindful brain*. Cambridge, MA: MIT Press, 1979;7–50.

Noble D, Boyd CAR. The challenge of integrative physiology. In: Boyd CAR, Noble D, eds. *The logic of life*. Oxford: Oxford University Press, 1993;1–14.

Petrides M, Pandya DN. Projections to frontal cortex from posterior parietal region in rhesus monkey, *J Comp Neurol* 1984;228:105–116.

Polich J. P300 in clinical applications. *Am J EEG Technol* 1991;31:201–231.

Popper K. Natural selection and the emergence of mind. *Dialectica* 1978;32:339–355.

Pritchard WS. Psychophysiology of P300. *Psychol Bull* 1981;89:506–540.

Renault B, Ragot R, Lesèvre N, Rémond A. Onset and offset of brain events as indices of mental chronometry. *Science* 1982;215:1413–1415.

Rowland V. Cortical steady potential in reinforcement and learning. *Progr Physiol Psychol* 1968;2:1–77.

Searle J. The problem of consciousness. *Consc Cognit* 1993;2:310–319.

Selemon LD, Goldman-Rakic PS. Common cortical and subcortical targets of the dorsolateral prefrontal and posterior parietal cortex in rhesus monkey. *J Neurosci* 1988;8:4049–4068.

Skinner JE, Yingling CD. Central gating mechanisms that regulate event-related potentials and behavior: a neural model for attention. In: Desmedt JE, ed. *Progress in clinical neurophysiology*, vol. 1. Basel: Karger, 1977;28–68.

Smith ME, Halgren E, Sokolik M, Baudena P, Musolino A, Liégeois-Chauvel C, Chauvel P. The intracranial topography of P3 event-related potential elicited during auditory oddball. *Electroencephalogr Clin Neurophysiol* 1990;76:235–248.

Steriade M. Mechanisms underlying cortical activation. In: Pompeiano O, Ajmone-Marsan C, eds. *Brain mechanisms and perceptual awareness*. New York: Raven Press, 1981;327–377.

Sutton S, Braren M, Zubin J, John ER. Evoked potentials correlates of stimulus uncertainty. *Science* 1965;150:1187–1188.

Timsit-Berthier M, Delaunay J, Konincks N, Rousseau JC. Slow potential changes in psychiatry: CNV. *Electroencephalogr Clin Neurophysiol* 1973;35:355–361.

Tinbergen N. *The study of instinct*. Oxford: Oxford University Press, 1952.

Tomberg C, Desmedt JE. A method for identifying short-latency cognitive potentials in single trials by scalp mapping. *Neurosci Lett* 1994;168:123–125.

Tomberg C, Desmedt JE, Ozaki I, Nguyen TH, Chalklin V. Mapping somatosensory evoked potentials to finger stimulation at intervals of 450 to 4000 msec and the issue of habituation when assessing early cognitive components. *Electroencephalogr Clin Neurophysiol* 1989;74:347–358.

Tomberg C, Noel P, Ozaki I, Desmedt JE. Inadequacy of the average reference for the topographic mapping of focal enhancements of brain potentials. *Electroencephalogr Clin Neurophysiol* 1990;77: 259–265.

Walter WG, Cooper R, Aldridge VJ, McCallum WC, Winter AL. Contingent negative variation: an electric sign of sensory-motor association and expectancy in the human brain. *Nature London* 1964;203:380–384.

Wurtz RH. Steady potential correlates of intracranial reinforcement. *Electroencephalogr Clin Neurophysiol* 1966;20:59–67.

Zeki S. *A vision of the brain*. London: Blackwell, 1993.

*Pain and the Brain: From
Nociception to Cognition,*
edited by Burkhart Bromm and
John E. Desmedt, Advances in Pain
Research and Therapy Vol. 22.
Raven Press, Ltd., New York 1995.

5

Phantom-Limb Pain and the Brain

Ronald Melzack

Department of Psychology, McGill University, Montreal, Quebec, H3A 1B1 Canada

SUMMARY

A phantom limb is universally experienced after a limb has been amputated or its sensory roots have been destroyed. A complete break of the spinal cord also often leads to a phantom body below the level of the break. Severe pain is frequently experienced in the phantoms of amputees and paraplegics, and is usually attributed to peripheral factors such as neuromas or to long-lasting spinal processes. Clinical evidence, however, points to the important role of the brain in phantom-limb pain. It suggests that neural networks in the brain generate all the qualities of experience —including pain—that are felt to originate in the body, so that inputs from the body may trigger or modulate the output of the networks, but are not essential for any of the qualities of experience. A new theory has been developed to explain this conclusion. It is proposed that humans are born with a widespread neural network, known as the *neuromatrix*, for the body-self, and that this is subsequently modified by experience. The neuromatrix imparts a pattern, called the *neurosignature*, on all inputs from the body, so that experiences of one's own body have a quality of self and are imbued with affective tone and cognitive meaning. The following discussion describes recent research on pain mechanisms that derives from the theory and supports it.

INTRODUCTION

Three kinds of phantom-limb phenomena have been reported: the experience of a limb (or other body part) after it has been amputated, the experience of an arm after its sensory roots to the spinal cord have been destroyed, and the experience of the legs and body below the level of a complete break of the spinal cord (examples are given in Fig. 1). Melzack and Loeser (1978) described severe pains in the phantom bodies of paraplegics with verified total sections of the spinal cord, and proposed a central "pattern-generating mechanism" above the level of the section. Recently, I have explored new theoretical concepts to explain phantom-body experiences, from

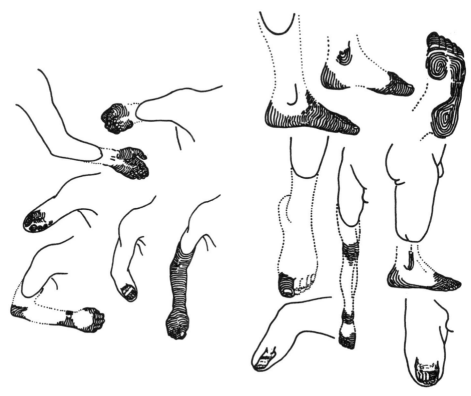

FIG. 1. Drawings of phantom arms and legs based on patient reports. Phantom sensation is indicated by a dotted line, with solid lines to show the most vividly experienced parts. Note that some of the phantoms are telescoped into the stump. (From Solonen 1962, with permission.)

pain to orgasm, in people with total spinal sections (Melzack 1989, 1990). Because the brain in these individuals is completely disconnected from the spinal cord, these experiences reveal important features of brain function.

Brain activity related to pain involves more than just the spinal projection systems to the thalamus and cortex. These are important, of course, but they mark only the beginning of the psychological processes that underlie perception. The cortex, as White and Sweet (1969) have made amply clear, is not the pain center, and neither is the thalamus (Spiegel and Wycis 1966). The areas of the brain involved in pain experience and behavior are very extensive. They must include somatosensory projections as well as the limbic system. Furthermore, because body perceptions include vestibular mechanisms as well as cognitive processes, widespread areas of the brain must be involved in pain. However, we do not know how the neural activity in these widespread areas is integrated to produce coherent perceptual experience with inherent affect and meaning.

PHANTOM LIMBS AND THE CONCEPT OF A NEUROMATRIX

My analysis of phantom-limb phenomena (Melzack 1989, 1990), particularly in paraplegics with a complete spinal cord section at high thoracic levels, has led to four conclusions that point to a new concept of the nervous system. First, because the phantom limb (or other body part) feels as real as the physical limb, it is reasonable to conclude that the body as normally felt is subserved by the same neural processes in the brain; these brain processes are usually activated and modulated by inputs from the body, but can also act in the absence of any inputs. Second, all of the qualities normally experienced from the body, including pain, are also felt in the absence of inputs from the body. From this we may conclude that the patterns that underlie the qualities of experience originate in neural networks in the brain; stimuli may trigger the patterns but do not produce them. Third, the body is perceived as a unity and is identified as the "self," distinct from other people and the surrounding world. The experience of a unity of such diverse feelings, including the self as the point of orientation in the surrounding environment, is produced by central neural processes and cannot derive from the peripheral nervous system or spinal cord. Fourth, the brain processes that underlie the body-self are, to an important extent that can no longer be ignored, "built-in" by genetic specification, although this built-in substrate must clearly be modified by experience. These conclusions provide the basis of the new conceptual model of the nervous system.

OUTLINE OF THE THEORY

I will first present an outline of the theory and then deal with each of its components.

I propose that the anatomic substrate of the body-self is a large, widespread network of neurons that consists of loops between the thalamus and the cortex as well as between the cortex and limbic system. I have labeled the entire network, whose spatial distribution and synaptic links are initially determined genetically and are later sculpted by sensory inputs, as a *neuromatrix*. The loops diverge to permit parallel processing in different components of the neuromatrix, and converge repeatedly to permit interactions between the output products of processing. The repeated cyclical processing and synthesis of nerve impulses through the neuromatrix imparts a characteristic pattern, the *neurosignature*, on all nerve-impulse patterns that flow through the neuromatrix. The neurosignature is produced by the patterns of synaptic connections in the entire neuromatrix. All inputs from the body undergo cyclical processing and synthesis, so that characteristic patterns are impressed on them in the neuromatrix. Portions of the neuromatrix are specialized to process information related to major sensory events (such as injury, temperature change, and stimulation of erogenous tissue), and may be designated as *neuromodules* that impress subsignatures on the larger neurosignature.

The neurosignature, which is a continuous outflow from the body-self neuromatrix, is projected to areas in the brain, known as the *sentient neural hub* (SNH), in which the stream of nerve impulses (the neurosignature modulated by ongoing inputs) is converted into a continually changing stream of awareness. Furthermore, the patterns of the neurosignature may also activate a neuromatrix to produce movement. This occurs through a bifurcation of the signature patterns so that a particular pattern proceeds to the sentient neural hub (where the pattern is converted into the experience of movement) while a similar pattern proceeds through a neuromatrix that eventually activates neurons in the spinal cord to produce patterns of muscle activity for complex actions.

Thus, the four components of the new concept of the nervous system are: (a) the body-self neuromatrix; (b) cyclical processing and synthesis in which the neurosignature is produced; (c) the sentient neural hub, which converts (transduces) the flow of neurosignatures into the flow of awareness; and (d) activation of an action neuromatrix to provide the pattern of movements that will bring about the desired goal.

THE BODY-SELF NEUROMATRIX

The body is experienced as a unity, with different qualities at different times. I believe that the brain mechanism underlying this experience also comprises a unified system that acts as a whole and produces the neurosignature pattern of a whole body. The conceptualization of this unified brain mechanism lies at the heart of the new theory, and I believe that the term "neuromatrix" best characterizes it. "Matrix" has several definitions in Webster's dictionary, and some of them imply precisely the properties of the neuromatrix as I conceive of it. First, a matrix is defined as "something within which something else originates, takes form or develops." This is exactly what I wish to imply: that the neuromatrix (not the stimulus, peripheral nerves, or "brain center") is the origin of the neurosignature; the neurosignature originates and takes form in the neuromatrix. Although the neurosignature may be triggered or modulated by input, the input is only a "trigger," and does not produce the neurosignature itself. A matrix is also defined as a "mold" or "die" that leaves an imprint on something else. In this sense, the neuromatrix "casts" its distinctive signature on all inputs (nerve-impulse patterns) that flow through it. Finally, matrix is defined as "an array of circuit elements . . . for performing a specific function as interconnected." I propose that the array of neurons in the neuromatrix is genetically programmed to perform the specific function of producing the signature pattern. The final, integrated neurosignature pattern for the body-self ultimately produces awareness and action.

For these reasons, the term neuromatrix seems appropriate for the brain mechanism by which the body is experienced as a unity. The neuromatrix, distributed throughout many areas of the brain, comprises a widespread network of neurons that generates patterns, processes information that flows through it, and ultimately produces the pattern that is felt as a whole body. The stream of neurosignature output, with constantly varying patterns riding on the main signature pattern, produces the sensations of the whole body with their constantly changing qualities.

PSYCHOLOGICAL REASONS FOR A NEUROMATRIX

The way in which individual bits of information from skin, joints, and muscles can all come together to produce the experience of a coherent, articulated body seems incomprehensible. At any instant, millions of nerve impulses are arriving at the brain from all of the body's sensory systems, including the proprioceptive and vestibular systems. How can all of this information be integrated to create a constantly changing unity of experience? Where does it all come together?

Although I cannot imagine how all these bits of data are added to produce a whole, I can conceive that the genetically built-in neuromatrix for the whole body generates a characteristic neurosignature of the body that carries with it patterns for the myriad qualities we experience. In my concept, the neuromatrix produces a continuous message that represents the whole body and which differentiates details within the whole as inputs come into it. According to this concept the neuromatrix is a template of the whole that provides the characteristic neural pattern for the whole body (the body's neurosignature) as well as subsets of signature patterns (from neuromodules) that relate to events at (or in) different parts of the body.

These views are in sharp contrast to the classical specificity theory, in which the qualities of experience are presumed to be inherent in peripheral nerve fibers. Pain is not injury; the quality of pain experiences must not be confused with the physical event of breaking skin or bone. Warmth and cold are not "out there"; temperature changes occur "out there," but the qualities of experience of warmth or cold must be generated by structures in the brain. There are no external equivalents to stinging, smarting, tickling, or itching; the qualities of these sensations are produced by built-in neuromodules whose neurosignatures innately produce the qualities.

We do not learn to feel qualities of experience: our brains are built to produce them. The inadequacy of the traditional peripheralist view becomes especially evident when we consider paraplegics with high-level complete spinal breaks. Despite the absence of inputs from the body, these individuals experience virtually every quality of sensation and affect. It is known that the absence of input produces hyperactivity and abnormal firing patterns in spinal cells above the level of the break (Melzack and Loeser 1978). But how, from this jumble of activity, do we get the meaningful experience of movement, the coordination of limbs with other limbs, cramping pain in specific (nonexistent) muscle groups, and so on? This must occur in the brain, in which neurosignatures are produced by neuromatrixes that are triggered by the output of hyperactive cells.

When all sensory systems are intact, inputs modulate the continuous output of the neuromatrix to produce the wide variety of our experiences. We may experience position, warmth, and several kinds of pain and pressure all at once. The feeling accompanying this is a single unitary feeling, just as an orchestra produces a single unitary sound at any moment, even though the sound comprises violins, cellos, horns, and so forth. Similarly, at a particular moment in time we experience complex qualities in all parts of the body. In addition, our experience of the body includes visual images, affect, "knowledge" of the self (versus not-self), and the meaning of body parts in terms of social norms and values. I cannot comprehend how all these bits and pieces come together to produce a unitary body-self, but I can visualize a neuromatrix that impresses a characteristic signature on all the inputs that converge on it, and thereby produces the never-ending stream of feeling from the body.

The experience of the body-self involves sensory, affective, evaluative, postural, and many other dimensions. The sensory dimensions are subserved, at least in part, by portions of the neuromatrix that lie in the sensory projection areas of the brain; presumably, the affective dimensions are subserved by areas in the brain stem and limbic system. The particular portion of the neuromatrix designated as a neuro-module subserves each major psychological dimension (or quality) of experience, contributing a distinct portion of the total neurosignature. To again use the analogy of a symphony orchestra, each neuromodule is like the string section, tympani, woodwinds, or brasses, each of which comprises a "module" of the whole orchestra, making its unique contribution yet constituting an integral part of the orchestra, capable of immense and continuous variation in the music it makes.

The neuromatrix resembles Hebb's "cell assembly" in being a widespread network of cells that subserves a particular psychological function. However, Hebb (1949) conceived of the cell assembly as a network developed by gradual sensory learning, while I propose that the structure of the neuromatrix is predominantly determined by genetic factors, although its eventual synaptic architecture is influenced by sensory inputs. This emphasis on the genetic contribution to the brain does not diminish the importance of sensory inputs. The neuromatrix is a psychologically meaningful unit, developed by both heredity and learning, that represents an entire unified entity.

ACTION PATTERNS: THE ACTION-NEUROMATRIX

The output of the body neuromatrix is directed at two systems: (a) the neuromatrix that produces awareness of the output, and (b) a neuromatrix involved in overt action patterns. In this discussion, it is important to keep in mind that just as there is a steady stream of awareness (even during the dream episodes of sleep), there is also a steady output of behavior (including movements during sleep).

It is important to recognize that behavior occurs only after the input has been at least partially synthesized and recognized. For example, when we respond to the experience of pain or itch, it is evident that the body-self neuromatrix (or relevant neuromodules) has sufficiently synthesized the experience to have imparted the neurosignature patterns that underlie the quality of experience, affect, and meaning. Apart from a few reflexes (such as withdrawal of a limb, eye-blink, and so on), behavior occurs only after inputs have been sufficiently analyzed and synthesized to produce meaningful experience. When we reach for an apple, a neuromatrix has clearly synthesized the visual input from the apple, so that it has three-dimensional shape, color, and meaning as an edible, desirable object. All of these effects are produced by the brain and are not in the object itself. When we respond to pain (by withdrawal or even by telephoning for an ambulance), we respond to an experience that has sensory qualities, affect, and meaning as a dangerous (or potentially dangerous) event to the body.

I propose that after inputs from the body undergo transformation in the body neuromatrix, the appropriate action patterns are activated concurrently (or nearly so) with the neuromatrix for experience. Thus, in the action-neuromatrix, cyclical processing and synthesis (CPS) produces activation of several possible patterns and their successive elimination until one particular pattern emerges as the most appropriate for the existing circumstances. In this way, input and output are synthesized simultaneously and in parallel, rather than in series. This permits a smooth, continuous stream of action patterns.

The command that originates in the brain to execute a pattern such as running activates the neuromodule, which then produces firing in sequences of neurons that send precise messages through ventral horn neuron pools to appropriate sets of muscles. At the same time, the output patterns from the body neuromatrix that engage the neuromodules for particular actions are also projected to the sentient neural hub and produce experience. In this way the commands from the brain may produce the experience of movement of phantom limbs even though there are no limbs to move and no proprioceptive feedback. Indeed, reports by paraplegics of terrible fatigue caused by persistent bicycling movements (like the painful fatigue in a tightly clenched phantom fist reported by arm-amputees) indicate that feelings of effort and fatigue are produced by the signature of a neuromodule rather than by particular input patterns from muscles and joints.

IMPLICATIONS OF THE NEW CONCEPT

Phantom-Limb Pain

The new theory of brain function proposed on the basis of phantom-limb phenomena provides an explanation for phantom-limb pain. Amputees suffer burning, cramping, and other qualities of pain in their phantom limbs. An excellent series of studies (Krebs et al. 1984; Jensen et al. 1985) found that 72% of amputees had phantom-limb pain a week after amputation, and that 60% had pain 6 months later. Even 7 years after amputation, 60% continued to suffer phantom-limb pain, which means that only about 10 to 12% of amputees obtain pain relief. The pain is remarkably intractable; although more than 40 forms of treatment for it have been tried, none has proved particularly efficacious (Sherman et al. 1980).

Why is there so much pain in phantom limbs? I believe that the active body neuromatrix, in the absence of modulating inputs from the limbs or body, produces a signature pattern that is transduced in the sentient neural hub into a hot or burning quality. The cramping pain experienced in phantom limbs may be due to messages from the action-neuromatrix to move muscles in order to produce movement. In the absence of the limbs, the messages to move the muscles become more frequent and stronger in the attempt to move the limb. The end result of the output message may be felt as cramping muscle pain. Shooting pains may have a similar origin, in which the action-neuromatrix attempts to move the body and send out abnormal patterns that are felt as shooting pain. The origins of these pains, then, lie in the brain.

Recent Research

Surgical removal of the somatosensory areas of the cortex or thalamus fails to relieve phantom-limb pain (White and Sweet 1969). However, the new theory conceives of a neuromatrix for the body-self that extends throughout selective areas of the whole brain, and to destroy this neuromatrix, which generates the neurosignature pattern for pain, is impossible. Nevertheless, if the neurosignature for pain is generated by cyclical processing and synthesis, it may be possible to block it by injecting a local anesthetic into a discrete area. Such an injection would be relatively easy to accomplish and harmless and could bring relief that extends beyond the duration of action of the anesthetic.

In our first study of this problem, my students and I (Tasker et al. 1987) injected the local anesthetic lidocaine into the lateral hypothalamus, an area we considered strategic for a neuromatrix for the body-self and pain. We found that freely moving rats given the injection showed a significant reduction of pain in the formalin test, which produces moderately intense pain for 1 to 2 hours and has many of the characteristics of the pain produced by injury in humans. However, the injection had no effect on tail-flick pain, which is primarily a spinally mediated reflex. Moreover, lidocaine injected into adjacent hypothalamic structures (including the medial hypothalamus) had no effect on the pain caused by the formalin test, indicating that the analgesia achieved in this case was produced by local anesthesia in a specific group of neurons. Since the analgesia was bilateral, it is reasonable to assume that the lateral hypothalamus contains neurons that are important for producing the neurosignature for pain in both sides of the body.

Recently, Vaccarino and I (Vaccarino and Melzack 1992) injected lidocaine into the cingulum bundle and other limbic and reticular areas that seem to be strategically located in the neuromatrix for synthesis of the neurosignature for pain. The results showed that the lidocaine produces striking decreases in pain in the formalin test as well as in self-mutilation produced by pain or dysesthesia after peripheral nerve lesions. McKenna and I (1992) obtained similar results after injecting lidocaine into the dentate nucleus, which has major connections with the hippocampus. We (McKenna and Melzack 1994) have also shown that lidocaine injected into the medial and intralaminar thalamus significantly reduced pain-related behaviors in the formalin test, while a similar injection of lidocaine into the ventrobasal thalamus had no effect in the formalin test but produced enhanced sensitivity in the tail-flick test, which measures brief, threshold-level pain.

My students and I have also gathered some direct evidence for the suggestion that the brain—and by implication, the neuromatrix—can by itself generate sensation.

The formalin test produces an "early" pain that rapidly rises and falls in intensity during the first 5 min after the formalin injection, followed by a "late" pain that begins about 15 min after the injection and persists for about an hour. By means of this test, Coderre, Vaccarino, and I (1990) found that an anesthetic block of the paw completely obliterates the late pain, but only if the anesthetic is delivered in time to prevent the early response. Once the early pain occurs, the drug only partly reduces the later response. This observation of pain continuing even after the nerves carrying pain signals are blocked implies that long-lasting pain (such as that in phantom limbs) is determined not only by sensory stimulation during the discomfort, but also by brain processes that persist without continual priming.

In a related study, Katz et al. (1991) showed that injury to a rat's paw before it is totally denervated leaves a lasting memory that influences the rat's later perception of pain in the "phantom" of the denervated paw. These "pain memories" are consistent with earlier observations that the pain felt in phantom limbs in humans often resembles the pain of injuries to these limbs prior to their amputation (Katz and Melzack 1990).

Because my model of brain function posits that the neuromatrix as a whole may contribute to pain, the model also suggests that altering the activity of pathways outside the somatosensory system may be important, either alone or in combination with other treatments, in relieving pain. One place in which to begin work on this is the limbic system. Until now, limbic structures have been relegated to a secondary role in efforts to treat pain, because injurious stimuli do not directly active them. Yet, if the limbic system contributes to output by the neuromatrix, as I have proposed, it may well contribute to the pain felt in phantom limbs. The results of the studies cited above of the effects of lidocaine injection into the cingulum, dentate nucleus, and other limbic areas support this proposal.

The phenomenon of phantom limbs has allowed me to attack some fundamental assumptions in psychology. One of these is that sensations are produced only by stimuli, and that perceptions in the absence of stimuli are psychologically abnormal. The experience of phantom limbs, as well as phantom sight (Schultz and Melzack 1991), indicate that this assumption is wrong. The brain does more than detect and analyze inputs: it generates perceptual experience even when no external inputs occur.

Another entrenched assumption is that perception of one's body results from sensory inputs that leave a memory in the brain, and that the sum of these signals becomes the body image. However, the occurrence of phantom-limb phenomena in people born without a limb or who have lost a limb at an early age suggests that the neural networks for perceiving the body and its parts are built into the brain. The absence of inputs does not stop these networks from generating messages about missing body parts; they continue to produce such messages throughout life. In short, phantom limbs are a mystery only if we assume that the body sends sensory messages to a passively receiving brain. Phantoms become comprehensible when we recognize that the brain generates the experience of the body. Sensory inputs merely modulate that experience; they do not cause it.

REFERENCES

Coderre TJ, Vaccarino AL, Melzack R. Central nervous system plasticity in the tonic pain response to subcutaneous formalin injection. *Brain Res* 1990;535:155–158.

Hebb DO. *The organization of behavior*. New York: Wiley, 1949.

Jensen TS, Krebs B, Nielsen J, Rasmussen P. Immediate and long-term phantom limb pain in amputees: incidence, clinical characteristics and relationship to preamputation limb pain. *Pain* 1985;21:267–278.

Katz J, Melzack R. Pain "memories" in phantom limbs: review and clinical observations. *Pain* 1990;43: 319–336.

Katz J, Vaccarino AL, Coderre TJ, Melzack R. Injury prior to neurectomy alters the pattern of autotomy in rats. *Anesthesiology* 1991;75:876–883.

Krebs B, Jensen TS, Kroner K, Nielsen J, Jorgenssen HS. Phantom limb phenomena in amputees 7 years after limb amputation. *Pain* 1984;(Suppl. 2):S85.

McKenna JE, Melzack R. Analgesia produced by lidocaine microinjection into the dentate gyrus. *Pain* 1992;49:105–112.

McKenna JE, Melzack R. Dissociable effects of lidocaine injection into medial versus lateral thalamus in formalin and tail-flick pain tests. *Pathophysiology* 1994;1:205–214.

Melzack R. Phantom limbs and the concept of a neuromatrix. *Trends Neurosci* 1990;13:88–92.

Melzack R. Phantom limbs, the self and the brain (The D. O. Hebb Memorial Lecture). *Can Psychol* 1989;30:1–14.

Melzack R, Loeser JD. Phantom body pain in paraplegics: evidence for a central "pattern generating mechanism" for pain. *Pain* 1978;4:195–210.

Schultz G, Melzack R. The Charles Bonnet syndrome: "phantom visual images." *Perception* 1991;20: 809–825.

Sherman RA, Sherman CJ, Gall NG. A survey of current phantom limb pain treatment in the United States. *Pain* 1980;8:85–90.

Solonen KA. Phantom limbs. *Acta Orthop Scand* 1962;(Suppl. 54):6–37.

Speigel EA, Wycis HT. Present status of stereoencephalotomies for pain relief. *Conf Neurol* 1966;27: 7–17.

Tasker RAR, Choinière M, Libman SM, Melzack R. Analgesia produced by injection of lidocaine into the lateral hypothalamus. *Pain* 1987;31:237–248.

Vaccarino AL, Melzack R. Temporal processes of formalin pain: differential role of the cingulum bundle, fornix pathway and medial bulboreticular formation. *Pain* 1992;49:257–271.

White JC, Sweet WH. *Pain and the neurosurgeon*. Springfield, IL: Charles C. Thomas, 1969.

*Pain and the Brain: From
Nociception to Cognition,*
edited by Burkhart Bromm and
John E. Desmedt, Advances in Pain
Research and Therapy Vol. 22.
Raven Press, Ltd., New York © 1995.

6

Consciousness and Neuroscience

Ralph Adolphs and Antonio R. Damasio

Department of Neurology, University of Iowa College of Medicine, Iowa City, Iowa 52242

SUMMARY

On the one hand we know that we have experiences about entities, and that we think about states of affairs of the world external to us. On the other hand, we are made of matter and appear to obey the laws of physics and biochemistry. How can these two sets of facts be reconciled? Our text singles out two specific properties of conscious mental events: intentionality and subjectivity. Conscious phenomena relate to objects or events in the world, and are thus *intentional*, while the experience of conscious events is *subjective*. We propose that intentionality can be understood by two properties of perception: a topographic neural representation on which mental images are based, and memory. The claim for these two properties suggests that the neural events that constitute our perception of objects in the world can represent those objects in a sufficiently strong sense to be called "intentional." Mental subjectivity may be a more difficult problem. Part of the difficulty resides in our current formulation; we suggest the need for an analysis that takes account of the relations between neural representations and representations of the organism ("self-representations"). In our view, mental phenomena are subjective by virtue of involving relations to the self: when we see something, we feel that it is ourselves that is doing the seeing. This view is not homuncular, because we do not envisage that object representations are *presented* to organism representations, but rather that these two kinds of representations are linked in a neural network whose collective activity generates subjective experience. Although these are only rough sketches of neurobiologic ideas about consciousness, we believe that it is from a neuroscientific perspective that a real understanding of these processes is likely to come.

INTRODUCTION

The terms "mind" and "consciousness," as currently discussed in the literature of the fields that comprise the cognitive sciences, are used to describe an extremely heterogeneous set of objects and events. We intend here to restrict our focus to a subset of mental events that exhibit two special features: they are representational and they are subjective. The understanding of either feature poses a serious hurdle to any theory of consciousness. First, we will outline our analytical approach and frame the problems that we wish to discuss. After a brief introduction to the philosophers' view of mental representation and subjectivity, we will indicate how theories from systems neuroscience might inform these issues.

There is disagreement about whether consciousness is an intrinsic or a relational property of certain brain states. For example, could the isolated visual neocortices, if they were to exhibit the right kind of neural activity patterns, be said to be conscious? Or would their activity have to be presented to other neural systems in order for conscious visual experience to occur? The answers to these questions depend in part on a theory of personhood and in part on a framework of what constitutes the subject of the visual experience, among other foundations. We take the view that the predicate "is conscious of" can usefully be said to hold true only for a complete and embodied nervous system. Nonetheless, it may well be that a restricted set of parts of the neuraxis is sufficient to support mental events; the problem is that we have no idea what to say about either the subjective qualities or the references of such mental events, since they are not properties of the whole person. Our commonsensical concepts and vocabulary apply, and presumably evolved to apply, to intact persons. Thus, when we speak of the mental properties of parts of the brain, it should be understood that we view these parts of the brain functioning *in situ*, as components of a conscious person. We can certainly analyze the functions of such components in generating the mind, without thereby being committed to cutting into pieces the mental events in which they participate.

By way of introduction, consider the philosophers' favorite example: You have hit your thumb with a hammer and are suddenly in pain. We can agree that you are in a conscious state of experiencing pain in your thumb, at least under ordinary circumstances. Is this the same as saying that a certain neural event occurred in your brain a few milliseconds after the hammer struck your thumb?

We shall begin with the mental description of the event. At a certain point in time, and for some time thereafter, you had pain in your thumb. Under a mental description, the causal dependencies for your pain run roughly as follows. Sensory input eventually causes sensations or perceptions, which are neural processes that can be described as mental. Sensation (or perception) is in turn inferential and determines the content of propositional attitudes, such as beliefs. Thus, for example, a sensory input of sudden pain leads to a sensation/perception of pain, which leads you to believe that your thumb has been hit with a hammer. Finally, intentional states such as beliefs lead to action. Notice that, as would be the case in this example, there are sensory-motor loops of varying complexity; accordingly, there would no doubt also be a reflex of pain input leading to rapid withdrawal of the arm. However, this does not involve anything mental; it is not perceptual and it involves neither belief nor conscious agency.

In the mental description, the pain is a property of you, as a person, and is located in your thumb, not in your brain. Now you might describe this very same event with the vocabulary of physics, chemistry, and neurobiology by saying that some very complex pattern of changes in biochemical and biophysical state has occurred over a large number of neurons in your brain. What, one might ask, happened to the reference to person and thumb in the physical description? And what happened to the particular quality of the experience of pain that you had? These puzzles constitute two of the main issues in the philosophy of mind: the intentionality of the mental and the subjectivity of the mental. With respect to our example, how is it that your pain is *about* something? It is about your thumb, and about an injury that occurred at that location. And how is it that you do not only know that you are in pain (as if someone had informed you of a fact), but that you actually *feel* pain? We address these two issues in turn.

MENTAL AND NEURAL REPRESENTATION

The question of how your pain can be *about* something has been picked up with fervor by the cognitive-science community under the rubric of "representation." Even on the topic of representation, the literature presents a motley batch of arguments that do not obviously all refer to the same thing. Hard-core philosophers typically take the problem to be rather deeper and less tractable than do cognitive scientists and those working in the neurosciences. Philosophers talk of intentionality, the property of mental events that relates them to states of affairs in the world. Traditionally, intentionality has been viewed as a specific intrinsic property that can belong only to mental events; an often quoted slogan is, "intentionality is the mark of the mental" (Brentano 1874; for a review see Putnam 1981, 1988; Searle 1983). However, modern usage in both philosophy and cognitive science often treats mental representation as simply a special case of representation in general. Our concern will be with the way in which neural events can represent objects, events, and their conjunctions that have been experienced, and with the special properties those neural events must exhibit in order to account for the features of mental representation.

One modern philosopher who has forcefully argued for a mechanism of representation that relates certain states of the brain to certain events in the world is Fodor. His argument runs as follows (Fodor 1992): Suppose that you see a cow in broad daylight. After the information on your retina has become available to many cortical regions, and after much processing of this information, you will recognize the animal as a cow. The reason that you recognize the animal is that you have a history of seeing instances of it before. As a consequence of having seen cows before, you can categorize what you see as a cow; you will remember that this is what cows look like. Now suppose that you are confronted on a dark night with a horse, and that you mistake it for a cow. Do the neural events occurring in your brain at that moment correctly represent a horse, or do they incorrectly represent a cow? We would want to say that they represent a cow, since this is what you take the animal to be. But how could your brain represent a cow if the neural events in it are actually caused by a horse? Shouldn't the neural events represent whatever actually caused them? After all, if you take a photograph with a camera, it will necessarily represent whatever you took a picture of, or whatever caused the photo. How could it possibly represent anything else? But the brain is not a camera.

Fodor's solution, in rough and abbreviated form,[1] is that the only reason you mistook the horse for a cow was that you had previously (correctly) seen cows as cows on some occasions. You knew what a cow looked like, and thought the horse looked like one of those. Were you not able to recognize cows, you would not have thought that the horse was a cow. Fodor insists that on the dark night you are really —although incorrectly—representing a cow, and that you can do so because you have previously and correctly seen cows as cows on several occasions. Moreover, this situation is asymmetrical: If you couldn't recognize a cow, you couldn't mistake a horse for one; on the other hand, if you can't mistake horses for cows, your ability to represent cows is unaffected, all else being equal.

We agree with the general scope of this argument. Events in the brain can stand only for events in the world, provided that: (a) our representations depend on what it is that they represent in the correct way (they are asymmetrically and causally dependent on these objects), and (b) we have the appropriate experience with the world. A perspective from systems neuroscience can shed some light on this discussion by suggesting that perception and memory are closely linked. In our view, point (b) above, together with causal dependence, strongly suggests asymmetry. Our mistaken representation of a cow is in fact not caused solely by visual input from the horse; rather, the neural events that stand for the cow in our brain are also a result of activity evoked from memory. We have stored information about the features of cows, and this stored information represents cows dispositionally. Such a memory of cows is dispositional in that it is not itself a currently active representation, but is capable of bringing about the latter. Seeing the horse causally influences these dispositional representations; they in turn lead to an active representation of a cow, which is not, however, solely a causal consequence of seeing the horse. The brain can mistake horses for cows only because of such "top-down" causal effects. At the level of Fodor's description, these effects translate into asymmetric causal dependence of the representation on the stimulus. Although the history of Fodor's discussion focuses mainly on so-called propositional attitudes (e.g., believing, hoping, desiring that something is the case), it is really a species of the more general "symbol-grounding problem" (Harnad 1990; see also Searle 1980; Dennett 1987).

For any thought (any mental event) to be about anything in the world, it must ultimately be composed of primitives that intrinsically refer to objects or events in the outside world. The property by virtue of which these primitives achieve such reference has been hard to identify; Fodor's asymmetrical causal dependence is one recent candidate. This solution aside, the physical properties that might create a pattern of neural activity with the ability to represent an object in the world remain a question. Our hunch is that images provide one possible answer: Images represent by

---

[1] Our gloss on Fodor does not accurately state his position, which is too technical for present purposes. Fodor's argument is specifically a solution to the disjunction problem of informational semantics. There is disagreement over Fodor's theory; the interested reader is referred to Loewer and Rey (1991).

resembling, which is to say that there are isomorphisms between (mental or neural) transformations of images and the physical transformations of the objects they represent. This suggestion is made more general by the finding, all over the brain, of neural representations that map dimensions of what it is that they represent. Early sensory cortices (which include primary sensory cortices and "low-order" sensory cortices), all motor cortices, and many of their thalamic-projection nuclei display neuronal activity in a topographically organized fashion that is consistent with the shape of entities as we experience them in the world. The neural organization of these cortical regions mirrors the way in which what they represent appears to us.[2]

There is similarity of structure at three separate levels: The neural maps exhibit a topographic structure similar to the structure of the mental sensations of an object in perceptual space; and both in turn are similar to some aspects of the actual structure of the distal-stimulus properties of the object being represented. We believe that isomorphism between the properties of neural, mental, and external events is a very general finding: There may be similarities in the structure of time (e.g., discharges in auditory neural tissue may correlate temporally with amplitude changes at the ear), function (verbs are represented in sectors of the brain more closely tied to motor actions; nouns are represented in separate regions), or space (topography). Topographic similarities are most easily conceptualized; spatial vision is a clear example. Visual cortices contain topographic maps of the location of a stimulus in extrapersonal space: Adjacent stimuli are represented in adjacent neural tissue and other, distinct stimuli are represented in separated regions in the brain. As a consequence, the spatial relations of proximity, contiguity, and separation that hold between objects also hold between the neural representations of those objects. Consequently, our mental visual images exhibit similar relationships among one another: An object in a particular external position is represented at a corresponding neural locus, and gives rise to a visual sensation that is invariant with respect to spatial location.

Compelling examples also come from the very well understood sensory maps of other animals. The barn owl computes a neural map of auditory space in its midbrain (cf. Konishi et al. 1988). Similarly, bats synthesize maps of the distance to and relative velocity of targets in their auditory cortex (Nachtigall and Moore 1988; Dear et al. 1993). In both cases, the cues available to owls or bats at the periphery (binaural time and intensity disparities for the former; echo delays and Doppler shifts for the latter) are not spatially topographic. In order to generate neural maps that literally "re-present" the spatial relationships of auditory objects, owls and bats need to translate temporal and amplitude information contained in a stimulus into topographic activity patterns in neural tissue. It is also important to note that maps

[2] As far as we are aware, the first person to point this out explicitly was Roger Shepard, whose experiments on rotational transformations of visual mental images well illustrate the point (Shepard 1989; see also Merzenich et al. 1988; Georgopoulos et al. 1989, 1993; Kosslyn et al. 1993). These ideas, and a more explicit discussion of the distinction between mapped representations that constitute conscious experience and other representations that do not, are given by Damasio (1994). In general, the number of dimensions of the parameter spaces that are mapped are much greater than the dimensionality of cortex (two-dimensional), leading to discontinuous mappings (cf. Durbin and Mitchison 1990).

are a property of neural tissue on a relatively macroscopic scale. In many cases, microscopic examination reveals a breakdown of strict topography (see, e.g., Schieber and Hibbard 1993).

Although neural, mental, and external structures covary in this way, only neural and mental events are coextensive. External reality both contains events that we cannot represent (ultraviolet light reflectance that bees can see but that is invisible to us, sounds that only bats can hear, electrical fields that electroreceptive fish can detect, etc.) and consists of structures to which our representations are only approximations (the spatial location and translation of macroscopic objects as we experience them are Newtonian approximations that are not reflected in the microscopic quantum-mechanical descriptions of these objects). From an evolutionary perspective, it appears that neural and mental representations construct a model of precisely those aspects of objective reality about which the organism needs to know. Consequently, the objective properties that our nervous system assigns to objects in the world must be veridical descriptions of those objects (or else we could not have evolved), but they need not be complete descriptions.

The richness and versatility of our experience of the world require more than only a topographic representation of distal-stimulus properties. They also require that this representation be linked to other neural processes to yield an integrated experience of a scene. One of us has previously (Damasio 1989a, b) given a systems-level account of such multilevel neural processing. This account provides a picture in which topographic representation in sensory and motor cortices participates in a neural ensemble that includes many high-order neural regions. Not only does the hierarchy of feed-forward information processing have such a very distributed nature (see, e.g., Felleman and van Essen 1991), but higher regions provide extensive feedback that yields a tightly coupled, dynamic system with detailed temporal structure. The function of higher regions, such as temporal and frontal association cortices, is to link neural activity in many different places, enabling the resulting composite brain activity to encompass an experience that involves many objects and events, each with multiple features, values, and associations to memory. Pain is a particularly good example of a mental event that requires the activation of multiple neural representations, as will be discussed elsewhere in this volume.

HOW CAN THE STRUCTURE OF NEURAL EVENTS EXPLAIN SENSORY EXPERIENCE?

So much for representation. While many conscious events are also representational events, not all representations are necessarily conscious, although we agree with Searle (e.g., 1990) that any representation that is mental must be at least in principle accessible to consciousness. Some philosophers have supposed that one of the factors responsible for this difference is that conscious events essentially involve *subjectivity*. It is somewhat unclear what they mean by this word, but Nagel has tried to articulate the idea with the phrase, "what it is like to be someone" (Nagel

1974; the clearest formulation of the problem of subjectivity can be found in Nagel 1986). There seems to be a difference between objective information about a system and the subjective states of the system. The knowledge that we have is always obtained from a particular point of view, and in the case of conscious systems, our point of view as observers apparently does not allow us to know what it is like to be the system being observed.

The issue is clarified by examples, with one of the best known from philosophy coming from Jackson (1982). Jackson has us imagine that we know all that there is to know about the brain. He gives us the example of a brilliant neuroscientist named Mary, who can thus tell us exactly what happens in the brains of people when they see a red sunset, smell a rose, hear one of Bach's Brandenburg concertos, or feel pain. She can tell us all of this in neural terms even though, according to Jackson's story, she has actually been born and raised in a room that presents only black and white. She can talk to the outside world, and she watches TV and works on her computer terminal, but her screens show pictures only in black and white. Jackson's thought experiment now asks us to imagine what would happen if Mary were to step out of her black-and-white room and see a red sunset for the first time in her life. Would she have learned anything new? She already knew what seeing a red sunset was: She knew what happened in the brains of people when they saw red sunsets. But it seems that she would now know something that she did not know before: having had the experience of the sunset, she knows what it is like to see the color red. The example would therefore seem to suggest that the mental experience of seeing the color red cannot be the same as a neural event in the brain.

We do not need Jackson's thought experiment to realize this. Suppose that there is a taste or a smell that we have never experienced before. Will any amount of knowledge about the gustatory or olfactory system allow us to know what it is like to actually taste or smell the novel item? It surely will not. According to this, one would be forced to conclude that whatever happens in the brain cannot in fact tell us everything there is to know about the mind, not even in principle.

However, there are problems with this conclusion. The philosopher Dennett has argued that the premises are misleading because they suppose that one knows "everything" there is to know about the brain (see, e.g., Dennett 1991, p. 398). What could this possibly mean? If it is supposed to mean that we know what it is like to have a certain conscious neural event (e.g., to see red or smell a rose), there is no problem. It only seems counterintuitive that any amount of knowledge coming from neuroscience could include that sort of information. Nonetheless, Dennett warns us that intuitions are not sound foundations for thought experiments of this sort.

There is another answer, and one that we favor. There is indeed a difference between knowing what it is like to see in color and merely having a neuroscientific description of what happens in the brain when we see color. But the difference is not as mysterious as it at first seems. It amounts to the difference between an event and its description. What happens in Mary's brain, in Jackson's thought experiment, is quite different in the two cases of the sunset. In the first case she has a description of what happens in the brain when we see red; in the second case her visual cortex and associated neural structures are properly engaged so that she actually sees red. In the first case, the only way in which she could actually see red would be by causing herself to hallucinate. The conclusion is simply that the knowledge of conscious neural events is not analogous to the knowledge of any nonconscious event. If we have all of the physical information about a rock, or about a spinal reflex, that is all that can be said about it. But having all of the objective (external) information about someone's seeing a red sunset is not the same as having the experience. It is not that the amount of information differs; the difference is in how the information is known and in how it can be used. These considerations suggest that consciousness is a particular way of handling information, one that allows us (inter alia) to examine relationships between many things at the same time (cf. Baars 1988). It seems probable that the evolutionary advantages of consciousness pertain to its processing capabilities.

What exactly is it about some neural events that makes them conscious events? Numerous neural events take place in the spinal cord, or, for that matter, in the neural plexus of the gut. But they are not conscious. Although we do not yet know enough about the brain to have a full theory of the neural basis of consciousness, we have some leads. First, conscious events must contain information in a way that makes them subjective: The organism must know immediately that it is experiencing a sensation. Second, the brain must coordinate activity in many disparate regions. Third, each of these regions must represent and process information in a particular way. With regard to the last two points, we have suggested that the following features are necessary to support a conscious event (Damasio 1989a, b):

1. A large number of neurons must be involved.
2. Neocortical structures must be engaged.
3. There must be an integrative causal structure supported by loops of feed-forward and feedback.
4. The activity in all structures causing a conscious event must be temporally coherent (correlated in time).

These views are consistent with what we know from neuroscience: that the brain uses distributed representations based on cell assemblies, rather than local representations based on "grandmother" neurons; that those organisms to which we are most inclined to attribute consciousness have neocortices; and that the brain is a dynamic system with a very large number of feedback loops, so that the flow of information is not one-way but recursive. The picture that emerges is of a very highly interconnected system. It contains many multidirectional links, and its input and output pathways are small by comparison to its internal connectivity. As a result, the dynamics of the system are essentially "creative" rather than "reactive": The brain is always "on," and input serves to alter its activity patterns rather than to initiate them. As the reader may already have guessed, these facts about the brain make us doubt that conventional computer systems provide an appropriate analogy to the brain.

A brief examination of the brain system about which we know most—the visual system—will serve to illustrate the picture we have in mind. The retina gives rise to many central projections, of which the major component goes to the thalamus, and thence to V1, the primary visual cortex. A common account of information processing explains that from the primary cortex, information is shipped to higher-order cortical areas in a parallel and hierarchical fashion across approximately six levels (Felleman and van Essen 1991). Ultimately, information ends up in such structures as the hippocampus, amygdala, or frontal cortex. These structures thus sit at an apex of hierarchical processing, yet lesions in them do not abolish perception, sensation, or consciousness. This is because the flow of information is much more multidirectional and distributed than simple hierarchical processing schemes would suggest. The picture of information flowing from station to station in a hierarchical scheme does not do justice to the complex way in which the brain handles information. At the highest levels, hierarchy breaks down altogether. For example, the cingulate, frontal, and parietal cortices are connected in a network of interdigitating columns or alternate layers that defies any feed-forward or feedback architecture (Selemon and Goldman-Rakic 1988); and much of the connectivity of the limbic system also defies any easy categorization.

The importance of feedback is illustrated by the finding of neurons with complex response properties even at low levels: V4 and the inferotemporal visual cortex contain neurons whose responses are modulated by attention (Moran and Desimone 1985); the end-stopping of some cells in V1 is abolished by lesioning a high structure, the claustrum. Feedback comes from many places: almost all connections between visual areas are reciprocal (although different layers are involved in feed-forward or feedback), and there are indirect routes for feedback via thalamic relays (e.g., reticular nuclei) or via the amygdala (which projects back to all visual areas, including V1). Another example of activation by feedback is the activation of V1 during visual imagery (Damasio et al. 1993; Kosslyn et al. 1993). Mignard and Malpeli (1991) clearly illustrate that lower neural regions can be driven directly by higher regions. This architecture makes any attempt to trace the flow of information in the brain difficult, and it leads to a very rich temporal structure of the neural events that result from sensory input.

The second important feature of neural connectivity manifests itself at the level of the single neuron: Connectivity is sparse and distributed. Again taking a neuron in the primary visual cortex as our example, the thalamic input to the neuron constitutes only about 20% of the total excitatory input; most of the excitatory inputs are cortico-cortical (e.g., Douglas and Martin 1991). Connections between single neurons are very weak: A cortical pyramidal cell receives tens of thousands of inputs, but the input from any particular thalamic or cortical neuron constitutes perhaps as few as only one or two connections. Thus, not only is the activity in a single (or even a few hundred) neurons generally insufficient for consciousness, it is also insufficient to cause any other neuron in the brain to fire (although there may be exceptions to this in some regions, such as the area of the brain concerned with processing visual motion).

These examples suggest the necessary features for consciousness that were enumerated earlier: that many neocortical neurons must be active in a large-scale, multidirectionally interconnected network. Also of great importance is temporal coherence in the activity of such a network. Support for this phenomenon comes from studies of the so-called binding problem. It has turned out that one way of solving this problem is to have synchronous firing in neurons that are processing information about different features of the same object or event (von der Mailsburg and Schneider 1986; Eckhorn et al. 1988; Singer et al. 1990; Engel et al. 1991; Bressler et al. 1993; for a review, see Stryker 1991). In this way, high-order brain regions could unambiguously bind together all of the different features of an object; otherwise, in a complex scene composed of multiple objects, we would not know which features (colors, shapes, etc.) would go with which objects (an apple, a banana, an orange, etc.). The same solution has been proposed for the recall of events (Damasio 1989a,b).

While there is now good evidence that synchrony in the firing of spatially distant neurons contributes to the binding together of features of various objects within the visual system, it is less clear how this relates to consciousness. Koch and Crick (1991) have argued that synchronous oscillations are in fact the basis of consciousness. In their view, an event is conscious if it consists of a very large number of the right neurons firing in synchrony and in the right structures. What the right neurons and right structures are is an unanswered empirical question. Consequently, this hypothesis somewhat begs the question; it also fails to explain why synchrony should be essential to consciousness. In all theories of consciousness we must always ask ourselves: What are the necessary and sufficient conditions? If neural synchrony is merely the way in which the brain happens to solve the binding problem, saying that synchrony can lead to consciousness may be no more profound than saying that having a brain can lead to consciousness. Is synchrony sufficient for consciousness? Presumably not: When we hear a tone, very many axons in the eighth nerve fire in synchrony; similarly, the thalamus and hippocampus show synchronous oscillations, as does the whole brain during epilepsy. Are synchronous oscillations necessary for consciousness? Saying that they are will render nonconscious all states in which attention is low, perhaps including dreaming; it will also rule out all forms of consciousness that happen to solve the binding problem in ways other than by a synchrony of processing elements.

We have discussed some of the dynamic and architectural features that brains and their component systems ought to exhibit to generate conscious events. Yet while these features may describe the neural mechanics of consciousness, they leave open some puzzling questions. We began this section with the problem of subjectivity. How can the neural account that we have sketched explain the subjective nature of conscious events?

One component of subjectivity appears to be a referral of the mental content of an event to its owner, the person experiencing that event. When you hit your thumb with a hammer, the pain is your pain and the thumb hit is your thumb. This reference to self is an important feature of what it is like to experience pain or to see a red sunset. In our view, a neural implementation of the concept of "self" is required for such experience.

We propose that an active representation produces a subjective mental event when it participates in a distributed neural event with the following features:

1. The active sensory representation indicates that something has happened to the organism or that something has changed in its surroundings (its thumb was hit; the rays of a sunset struck its eye).
2. There is a representation of the organism itself. This representation is distributed across brain sectors that process somatosensory information (e.g., parietal and insular cortex). A representation of the organism's body is constructed in the brain.
3. There is a highly distributed representation of the organism's history, future plans, and relations to its social and physical environment. Components of such a self-representation include autobiographical memory, memory of intentions and plans, current information about the organism's interactions with the environment, and representations of past body states and interactions. In humans, such a representation amounts to a model of how we view ourselves. Moreover, this model is continuously updated. The neural sectors involved in it will include those in section 2 of this list as core components, along with virtually the entire set of tissues required for memory.
4. Crucial for subjectivity are relations between the events given in section 1 of this list and the factors that represent the organism (sections 2 and 3). Linking a sensory representation that might involve visual cortical regions to the bodily representations in sections 2 and 3 makes it possible to construct a meta-representation (involving sections 1, 2, and 3) that not only represents objects and events in the external environment, but that also represents how these objects and.events relate to the organism. Such a comprehensive network activity could potentially generate the reference to self that subjective mental events possess.

THE FEATURES OF CONSCIOUSNESS

We have identified two topics, mental representation and subjectivity, that a theory of consciousness would seemingly have to address. The fundamental belief of neuroscience, which we have assumed but for which we have not argued, is that all conscious events are in fact neural events, although not all neural events are conscious. Those neural events that are conscious, directly give rise to consciousness, or cause consciousness, should be capable of supporting either representation and/or subjectivity. Finally, conscious neural events must bear causal relationships one to another, such that an individual ends up thinking a train of thoughts or having a succession of images or an association of memories.

Although the associationists of the early 20th century conceived of conscious progressions in the neural state as largely "flowing" from one association to another, more recent proposals include the concept of a "language of thought" (a summary is provided by Fodor 1987) that mirrors the structure of logical argumentation. We believe that both accounts are plausible, and that the progression of thoughts can be explained by appeals to a variety of paradigms.

In summary, then, consciousness is a property of neural events:

(a) that can represent objects/events in the world;
(b) there is something it is like to have such a neural event, and
(c) neural events are causally interconnected so as to yield adaptive thought and behavior.

We have focused our discussion on condition (a), the mental representation, and (b), the sensory experience and subjectivity. Condition (a) may have at its rock bottom a physical property of neural events, perhaps something like structural/functional isomorphism with denotata (i.e., mapped representation). At a mechanistic level of this explanation, representation may be the result of asymmetrical causal dependence of neural representations on the object or event that they represent. The causal dependence of consciousness could be provided by the upward flow of information in perception, while the asymmetry may result from the involvement of memory as a top-down effect. These primitive properties are necessary only if one is a realist about intentionality. However, regardless of one's views on this issue, primitive neural symbols must engage a composition that involves large-scale neural ensembles linked by both feed-forward and feedback causal architectures. Such a composition can explain the productivity and flexibility of the mind; it is also supported by neuroscience (cf. Damasio 1989a, b). Simple reflex arcs lack this feature (they are rigid) and are not intentional (they do not really know anything about the world, they merely react). Thus, a crucial component of perception is memory: mental representation is possible only because it engages the vast knowledge accumulated in the distributed neural networks that subserve it.

Condition (b) is arguably the most mysterious feature of consciousness, as has been stressed by Nagel (e.g., 1974). We believe that subjectivity is a real issue, and that somehow the experience of certain types of neural events demonstrates that such events have specific qualities. Our hunch is that the explanation for this will require a neurobiologic account in which many representations are simultaneously active across large regions of the brain (Adolphs and Damasio 1994). It seems that many structures, provided they are sufficiently centrally located, participates in sensations. It does not seem likely that the retina or the spinal cord participate in sensations, since sensations can be produced in the absence of activity in these tissues. More centrally, stimulation of the visual cortex certainly can generate visual sensations (independent of activity on the retina), and the phenomenon of blind sight may indicate that early visual cortices are necessary (though perhaps not sufficient) for visual sensations (Brindley and Lewin 1968; Halgren 1978; Richer et al. 1991). Although interpretations of the abilities of blind-sighted patients are controversial, it seems clear that their deficits (lack of visual sensation) result from the absence of visual cortical tissue. A similar argument holds, for example, for patients with damage to the cortical area responsible for processing color vision; these patients do not have sensations of color, nor can they imagine color (or dream in color). These tissues are therefore necessary, but perhaps not sufficient, for sensation. These cases further suggest that sensation may be distinct from perception in some (perhaps only pathologic) cases. Blind-sighted patients may discriminate among visual stimuli without seeing that they are there; and some achromatopsic patients may discriminate hues without seeing color. At the motor end, stimulation of the motor cortex, while leading to movement, does not necessarily lead to sensation, although stimulation of the more central premotor cortex does appear to give rise to sensations and urges to move (Fried et al. 1991).

Lastly, a theory of consciousness would need to account for the dynamics of human mental life (condition [c]), and particularly for the twists and turns of thoughts that occur during thinking. Physically, the causal relations revealed through anatomic and electrophysiologic studies of the brain will explain its dynamics. Reasoning, planning, and decision-making are the paradigmatic mental phenomena that supervene on the brain's causal architecture.[3] However, we do not believe that all reasoning proceeds by a rational "language of thought," but that dynamics of a more analogous and less language-like nature, such as gut feelings, intuitions, and hunches, play a crucial role in reasoning in complex domains. The arguments and detailed neuropsychological evidence for our position can be found in Damasio et al. (1991), with a later complete discussion (Damasio 1994). Of particular relevance is reasoning in the social domain, the subvenient mechanisms of which are likely to involve extracerebral tissues.

Evidence from neuropsychology suggests that systems of the body (musculoskeletal, visceral, and endocrine) participate importantly in reasoning under the guise of what we commonly refer to as emotion and feeling. Consequently, it may be possible to usefully investigate representation by restricting one's scope to the sensory neocortex; however, the transformations of such representations in reasoning and thinking also require an account of their value: One must go outside the neocortex to include other neural structures and, perhaps, structures that are not neural at all. In our view, only a restricted set of neural tissues (e.g., neocortex) may suffice to support representations and subjectivity. But this is a static picture. What we do with those subjective representations, and how they change, will depend on relations to structures outside the cortex, relations to body states, and, no doubt, relations to culture.

ACKNOWLEDGMENT

We wish to thank Jamie Mazer, Dan Tranel, and Dave Hilbert for helpful comments on the manuscript. Some of the ideas in this chapter arose from work sup-

---

[3] The problem of free will is close at hand here. Although we don't propose to have a full solution for it, our view is that agency depends on one's point of view. Described as mental, our thoughts and actions must be free; described as physical, they must be deterministic. The difference may lie in the fact that psychological laws are not strict, and do not allow for unequivocal prediction, whereas physical laws are strict. The real problem is, however, still deeper, and amounts to worrying whether or not mental events are causally efficacious. The interested reader is referred to Heil and Mele (1993).

ported by NINDS Program Project Grant NS 19632, to A.R.D. Dr. Adolphs is a Burroughs-Wellcome Fund Fellow of the Life Sciences Research Foundation.

REFERENCES

Adolphs R, Damasio AR. Real Qualia (in prep.).

Baars BJ. *A cognitive theory of consciousness.* Cambridge: Cambridge University Press, 1988.

Brentano F. The distinction between mental and physical phenomena. In: Brentano F, ed. *Psychology from an empirical standpoint.* (English translation edited by Kraus O, McAllister L) London: Routledge and Kegan Paul, 1874/1973.

Bressler SL, Coppola R, Nakamura R. Episodic multiregional cortical coherence at multiple frequencies during visual task performance. *Nature* 1993;366,153–156.

Brindley GS, Lewin WS. The senations produced by electrical stimulation of the visual cortex. *J Physiol* 1968;196,479–493.

Crick F, Koch C. Towards a neurobiological theory of consciousness. *Semin Neurosci* 1990;2:263–277.

Damasio AR. *Descartes' error: reason, emotion, and the human brain.* New York: Putnam's, 1994.

Damasio AR. The brain binds entities and events by multiregional activation from convergence zones. *Neur Comput* 1989a;1:123–132.

Damasio AR. Time-locked multiregional retroactivation: A systems-level proposal for the neural substrates of recall and recognition. *Cognition* 1989b;33:25–62.

Damasio AR, Tranel D, Damasio H. Somatic markers and the guidance of behavior: Theory and preliminary testing. In: Levin HS, Eisenberg HM, Benton AL, eds. *Frontal lobe function and dysfunction.* New York: Oxford University Press, 1991.

Damasio H, Grabowski TJ, Damasio A, Tranel D, Boles-Ponto L, Watkins GL, Hichwa RD. Visual recall with eyes closed and covered activated early visual cortices. *Soc Neurosci* 1993;19:1603.

Dear SP, Simmons JA, Fritz J. A possible neuronal basis for representation of acoustic scenes in auditory cortex of the big brown bat. *Nature* 1993;364:620–623.

Dennett DC. *Consciousness explained.* New York: Little and Brown, 1991.

Dennett DC. Evolution, error, and intentionality. In: Dennett DC, ed. *The intentional stance.* Cambridge, MA: MIT Press, 1987;287–323.

Douglas RJ, Martin KAC. A functional microcircuit for cat visual cortex. *J Physiol* 1991;440:735–769.

Durbin R, Mitchison G. A dimension reduction framework for understanding cortical maps. *Nature* 1990;343:644–647.

Eckhorn R, Bauer R, Jordan W, Brosche M, Kruse W, Munk M, Reitboek HJ. Coherent oscillations: A mechanism of feature linking in the visual cortex? *Biol Cybernetics* 1988;60:121–130.

Engel, AK, Kreiter, AK, Koenig P. Synchronization of oscillatory neuronal responses between striate and extrastriate visual cortical areas of the cat. *Proc Nat Acad Sci USA* 1991;88: 6048–6052.

Felleman D, Van Essen DC. Distributed hierarchical processing in the primate cerebral cortex. *Cereb Cortex* 1991;1:1–48.

Fodor JA. Psychosemantics. Cambridge, MA: MIT Press, 1987.

Fodor, JA. *A theory of content.* Cambridge, MA: MIT Press, 1992.

Fried I, Katz A, McCarthy G, Sass KJ, Williamson P, Spencer SS, Spencer DD. Functional organization of human supplementary motor cortex studied by electrical stimulation. *J Neurosci* 1991;11:3656–3666.

Georgopoulos AP, Lurito JT, Petrides M, Schwartz AB, Massey JT. Mental rotation of the neuronal population vector. *Science* 1989;243:234–236.

Georgopoulos AP, Taira M, Lukashin A. Cognitive neurophysiology of the motor cortex. *Science* 1993; 260:47–52.

Halgren E. Mental phenomeny evoked by electrical stimulation of the human hippocampal formation and amygdala. *Brain* 1978;101:83–117.

Harnad S. The symbol-grounding problem. *Physica D.* 1990;42,335–346.

Heil J. and Mele A. *Mental causation.* Oxford: Oxford University Press, 1993.

Jackson F. Epiphenomenal qualia. *Philos Q* 1982;32:127–136.

Konishi M, Takahashi T, Wagner H, Sullivan WE, Carr CE. Neurophysiological and anatomical substrates of sound localization in the owl. In: Edelman G, Gall W, Cowan W, eds. *Auditory function.* New York: John Wiley, 1988.

Kosslyn SM, Alpert NM, Thompson WL. Visual mental imagery activated topographically organized visual cortex: PET investigations. *J Cogn Neurosci* 1993;5:263–287.

Loewer B, Rey G. *Meaning in mind: Fodor and his critics*. Oxford: Basil Blackwell, 1991.

Merzenich MM, Recanzone G, Jenkins WM, Allard TT, Nudo RJ. Cortical representational plasticity. In: Racik P, Singer W, eds. *Neurobiology of neocortex*. New York: Wiley, 1988.

Mignard M, Malpeli JG. Paths of information flow through visual cortex. *Science* 1991;251:1249–1251.

Moran J, Desimone R. Selective attention gates visual processing in the extrastriate cortex. *Science* 1985;229:782–811.

Nachtigall PE, Moore PB. *Animal biosonar: Processes and performance*. New York: Plenum Press, 1988.

Nagel T. What is it like to be a bat? *Phil Rev* 1974;83:435–450.

Nagel T. *The view from nowhere*. Oxford: Oxford University Press, 1986.

Putnam H. *Reason, truth and history*. Cambridge: Cambridge University Press, 1981.

Putnam H. *Representation and reality*. Cambridge: Cambridge University Press, 1988.

Richer F, Martinez M, Cohen H, Saint-Hilaire J-M. Visual motion perception from stimulation of the human medial parieto-occipital cortex. *Exp Brain Res* 1991;87:649–652.

Roland P. Cortical representation of pain. *Trends Neurosci* 1992;15:3–5.

Schieber MH, Hibbard LS. How somatotopic is the motor cortex hand area? *Science* 1993;261:489–491.

Searle JR. Consciousness, explanatory inversion, and cognitive science. *Behav. Brain Sci* 1990;13:585–642.

Searle J. *Intentionality*. Cambridge, MA: MIT Press, 1983.

Searle J. Minds, brains, and programs. *Behav. Brain Sci* 1980;3:417–457.

Selemon LD, Goldman-Rakic PC. Common cortical and subcortical targets of the dorsolateral prefrontal and posterior parietal cortices in the rhesus monkey: Evidence for a distributed neural network subserving spatially guided behavior. *J Neurosci* 1988;8:4049–4068.

Shepard R. Neural connections and mental computation. Cambridge, MA: MIT Press, 1989;104–135.

Singer W, Gray C, Engel A, Koenig P, Artola A, Broecher S. Formation of cortical cell assemblies. *Cold Spring Harbor Symp Quant Biol* 1990;55:939–953.

Stryker MP. Seeing the whole picture. *Curr Biol* 1991;1:252–253.

Von der Malsburg C, Schneider W. A neural cocktail-party processor. *Biol Cybernet* 1986;54:29–40.

*Pain and the Brain: From
Nociception to Cognition,*
edited by Burkhart Bromm and
John E. Desmedt, Advances in Pain
Research and Therapy Vol. 22.
Raven Press, Ltd., New York © 1995.

7

Pain: A Case Study for the Mind-Body Problem

Peter Bieri

Department of Philosophy, Free University Berlin, D-1495 Berlin, Germany

SUMMARY

A personal and a subpersonal level are distinguished for the description and explanation of pain. Three explanatory projects are sketched, two of them within a single level of conception and the third across two levels. It is shown that even after the satisfactory completion of these projects there would remain a fundamental puzzle about the experience of pain. From a specific viewpoint of consciousness, the relation between conscious pain at the personal level and the corresponding neural processes at the subpersonal level remains conceptually hard to grasp. Considered in terms of causation, the relation creates the danger of an inacceptable epiphenomenalism. Conceived of as identity, the relation becomes unintelligible. When discussed in terms of supervenience or emergence, the relation in effect remains unexplained, and the danger of epiphenomenalism tends to recur. The discussion ends with warnings of false conclusions.

PERSONAL AND SUBPERSONAL LEVELS IN THE DESCRIPTION OF HUMAN BEINGS

I want to discuss a puzzle about pain which may be called a *philosophical* puzzle because it is very general and probably cannot be solved by empirical means, at least not by experiments as they are performed in empirical research on pain.[1] The puzzle is an aspect or facet of the larger mind-body problem, and has to do with the role and nature of consciousness.

---

[1] The qualification is necessary for general epistemologic reasons: Once we stop drawing a fixed and rigid line between "empirical" and "nonempirical" or "synthetic" and "analytic" discoveries or truths, there remains no firm and absolute distinction between "empirical" and "philosophical" ("conceptual") puzzles, either. What remains is merely the distinction between more or less general puzzles, and between questions that can be addressed by experiments and those which must be answered on overall theoretical grounds. I have in mind here the epistemologic discussion initiated by W.V. Quine (1953).

My point of departure, following Dennett (1969, 1978, 1987, 1991), is the distinction between two fundamentally different levels on which we can, and do, give descriptions, analyses, and explanations of human beings. The first of these levels may be called the *personal level*. Here we are talking about an organic system as a whole. We represent and treat this system as a person in the sense that we attribute to it not only bodily properties and capacities but also mental or psychological capacities, features, and states. Thus, a person is a system that has beliefs and thoughts, desires, emotions, and bodily sensations such as pain. The logical subject of such psychological ascriptions is always the whole system: It is you and me (i.e., whole persons) who believe and think, perceive and dream, have emotions and pain. The ascriptions of common sense or folk psychology essentially belong to the personal level of description, analysis, and explanation.

There is a second, lower[2] level on which to approach human beings, which may be called the *subpersonal level*. On this level we focus on the various subsystems that together make up the whole system. Here we are talking, for example, about the nervous system, the brain, neuronal assemblies, single neurons and their parts, and electrochemical processes and their constituents, down to the molecular, atomic, or even subatomic level. If we want, we may say that this subpersonal level is in itself a hierarchy of levels, depending on what we choose as our unit or logical subject of study, whether the whole brain, single neurons, or biologic molecules, for example. The essential conceptual point about this entire subpersonal level is that the mental concepts of common sense or personal psychology are out of place in it. These concepts may not, strictly speaking, be applied to subsystems of the human being. It is, for example, not our nervous system, our brain, or our neurons that think, have beliefs and emotions, and feel pain. It is, rather, ourselves as whole persons who do and suffer all these things. Concepts such as "thought," "emotion," or "pain" are not "made" for the subpersonal level. To transport them from the personal level down to the subpersonal one inevitably leads to categorical mistakes.

EXPLANATORY PROJECTS WITHIN AND BETWEEN THE LEVELS

Given this observation, we can now, very roughly, distinguish three explanatory projects:

1. To know how the features and states we ascribe to the personal level are causally or in some other way[3] relevant to a person's behavior. When this is applied to pain, we get the project of finding out how the experience of pain in its various

---

[2]The spatial suggestion embodied in talk about "higher" and "lower" levels is, of course, purely metaphorical and must not be taken literally. Talking about "levels" of description and explanation is merely a use of different vocabularies, descriptive systems, and explanatory strategies. The spatial connotation is entirely gratuitous (for a discussion, see Goodman 1978).

[3]I have in mind a very important class of personal states, namely *intentional* states, that are so related to a person's behavior as to rationalize it. Viewed in this perspective, the intentional states are the *reasons* a person has for his or her behavior, although the same states may, from a different perspective, be described as *causes* of behavior. I do not believe that pain is an intentional state and I therefore confine myself here to the causal perspective.

modes and degrees leads to various patterns of pain-related behavior. It is also part of this project to establish how the various psychological states of a person interact, or, in other words, how the personal level is structured in itself. In the case of pain we are examining how various psychological variables influence the experience of pain: how, for example, motivational, cognitive, and emotional factors determine whether we feel any pain at all, or to what degree, or the extent of our tolerance of pain.

2. To understand how the subpersonal level of a human being is organized. Here we are looking for the detailed neurobiologic picture of certain organisms. We can, again very roughly, distinguish two forms of this picture: (a) it may be a neurobiologic picture in the strict sense of charting "hardware" structures on various macro- and microscopic levels; or it may be (b) a more abstract picture in terms of the purely functional structure of the subpersonal level, specifying the pathways of subpersonal information processing.

Each of these first two projects is confined to a single level of description, analysis, and explanation: the personal or the subpersonal level. A third project cuts across these two levels:

3. To know how elements and structures specified on the personal level are related to elements and structures specified on the subpersonal level. We may call the explanations we are seeking *instantiation explanations* (for detailed comments of the entire cross-level project see Cummins 1983). An instantiation explanation is, quite formally, an answer to the question: "What is it for a system to instantiate (carry, have) property P?", or "How is it possible for a system to instantiate P?" To answer a question like this is, again quite formally, to explain a system's having property P by accounting for it in terms of the system's elements (subsystem) and their topologic and functional organization. A relatively simple example of an instantiation explanation is the kinetic theory of gases, which explains the phenomenologic temperature of a gas by reference to its molecules and their mean kinetic energy. If we look for instantiation explanations of psychological properties by moving from the personal level down to a subpersonal level, things become immensely more complicated; but the explanatory structure is, I suggest, the same. Take the case of pain: We want, within this project, to make the fact that a person can feel pain intelligible in terms of what we know about the physical and functional composition of the human system. We are telling a complicated subpersonal story, like that of the gate-control theory (see in particular Chapter 5), in order to answer the question: "How is it possible to feel pain?"

Instantiation explanations are what join the first and the second explanatory projects. Looking for instantiation explanations is a top-down strategy: One begins with phenomena on the personal level and moves on to subpersonal structures that will, hopefully, explain their instantiation within the whole system of the person. In that sense the personal level of description has methodologic priority: One would not know what to seek on the subpersonal, neurobiologic level without an explanandum on the personal, psychological level. The items on the personal level are what fixes our point of reference. But, as we have learned in many cases, this top-down strategy will not lead to satisfactory results if the items on the personal level are treated in isolation.

PAIN AT THE INTERSECTION OF THE PERSONAL AND SUBPERSONAL LEVELS

If I have correctly understood the empirical literature I had time to scan, pain is an excellent case for studying the intersection of the personal and subpersonal levels of human experience. The old specificity theory of pain, for example, held that specific pain receptors in body tissue project via pain fibers and pain pathways to a pain center in the brain, and assumed that the activation of specialized neurons is both a necessary and sufficient condition for the experience of pain. Most workers in the field seem to agree that this theory is largely false because it can neither explain the occurrence of chronic pain (phantom-limb pain, causalgia, and the neuralgias) nor the influence of motivational, cognitive, and emotional variables on both chronic and acute pain. Where, then, did this unsatisfactory or downright false instantiation explanation of pain go wrong? One reason may be that it erred from a myopic concentration on obvious but isolated cases of acute pain caused by injury. Had the authors of the theory more closely examined the way in which pain is, on the personal level, interwoven with many other phenomena on that level, the specificity theory would have looked unpromising from the start.

The moral of this is that instantiation explanations of our conscious life ought to do justice to the holistic nature of that life. If we want to make the conscious life of an organism intelligible in terms of subpersonal science, we need a neurobiologic account that preserves the inherent complexities of the personal level.

Suppose now, counterfactually, that we had such an account, which could identify in every detail the subpersonal counterparts of whatever capacities, features, and states we experience on the personal level. Suppose, in other words, that the project of giving top-down instantiation explanations for our personal psychology could be considered closed. What would that mean? Would the mind-body problem be solved?

In one sense it would be, in that there would be no *empirical* problem left. There would be no questions left that could or would have to be answered by experiments. Knowing everything that is going on at the subpersonal level, and knowing exactly how it relates to the features of our conscious, personal life, we could close our laboratories. But would the situation be clear in every other respect, too? Above all, would it provide a conceptually clear (for the distinction between "empirical" and "conceptual" see footnote 1) explanation of the relationship between items on the personal and items on the subpersonal level?

No, it would not, and in the remainder of this discussion I shall focus on one important respect in which there would still remain a puzzle. Consider pain. What we have in our hypothetical, ideal state of science are various truths couched in the vocabulary of subpersonal science (i.e., neurobiology). The point of an instantiation explanation of pain is that the psychological truths about it are determined by the neurobiologic truths. It is true that we feel pain of a certain sort, in a certain place, and of a certain intensity *because* certain subpersonal processes and not others are taking place in certain of our subsystems. This dependence of personal facts on subpersonal facts may be rephrased to say that there could, by necessity, be no difference on the personal level between two systems without there also being some difference between these systems on the subpersonal level. In other words, the perfect subpersonal duplicate of a system would necessarily also be a personal duplicate; hence, no psychological difference without a neurobiologic difference.

That much seems clear. But what does it mean? How is this relationship between the personal and subpersonal level of pain to be interpreted? I will discuss three options that have been taken in doing this.

1. We say that there is a systematic variation between events on the personal level and events on the subpersonal level because the latter events *cause* the former events. Thus, certain patterns of neural processes cause a person to feel a specific pain.
2. We say that psychological truths about a system vary systematically with variations in its neurobiologic truths because the phenomena on the personal and the subpersonal levels are *identical*, being one and the same phenomenon. A certain specified pain, for example, **is** simply a certain pattern of neural processes described on the subpersonal level.
3. We invoke a third notion in addition to identity and causation, and claim that phenomena on the personal level *emerge from* or *supervene* phenomena on the subpersonal level. Thus, pain as a property of a whole system supervenes or emerges from a certain pattern of processes in the subsystems that subserve the experience of pain.

PAIN AS A "CONSCIOUS" PHENOMENON

I shall now show how all of these proposals lead to puzzles. In order to do this I shall point out next a feature of pain (and of some other psychological states, such as emotions) that philosophers have come to call its *phenomenal nature*. This can be set out by three closely connected observations:

1. To be in a phenomenal state such as pain is to be in a state with respect to which we may ask the questions: *"How is it* to be in pain?", or: *"What is it like* to be in pain?"[4] Thus, a man may ask a woman: "What is it like to have labor pain?" It is, therefore, to be in a specific state called pain that differs, for example, from the

---

[4] This way of characterizing phenomenal states was introduced by Farrell (1950), and was made famous by Nagel's (1979) question: "What is it like to be a bat?" Cf. Bieri (1982).

state of having green eyes or blood type AB. Furthermore, it is specific for the person who is in pain. This phenomenal aspect of pain is what workers in pain research sometimes call the "subjective" aspect of pain.

2. It is a conceptual truth that pain, considered on the personal level, exists only as long as it is felt. The notion of an unfelt pain is, as far as the personal level of description is concerned, an incoherent notion. Once a sensation of pain falls below the pain threshold, it ceases to exist as pain (i.e., as the phenomenal state it essentially is). Thus, unlike most other entities in the world, the *esse* of pain (and of other phenomenal states) is *percipi* or, rather, *sentiri*. This is not an assumption about data. Rather, it spells out the very point of the concept of pain.[5]

3. Regarding phenomenal states like pain, there is no room for distinguishing between appearance and reality. Although this distinction applies to the counterpart of pain on the subpersonal level, it does not apply to pain itself. A pain is as it appears (i.e., in how it feels). For this reason the notion of a "pain hallucination" would be an incoherent notion. To hallucinate is to imagine, by means of a phenomenal state (e.g., a pattern of visual sense impressions), something as real that is not real. But just as the visual phenomenal state exists in a case of hallucination, so would the imagination of pain by means of the phenomenal state mean to actually be in pain.

The phenomenal character of pain that I have been triangulating by these observations is sometimes epitomized by saying that pain is essentially a *conscious* phenomenon, or a phenomenon of which we are consciously aware. Now the concept of consciousness is an intricate concept, and the main thing to remember about it is that it involves many different concepts rather than a single, uniform concept. I do not have the time to discuss all of the conceptual phenomenology necessary to disentangle this cluster of concepts. It must suffice here to distinguish two importantly different senses in which a state such as pain can be conscious. In the first sense, to say that pain is conscious is simply to say that it is a phenomenal state as characterized earlier—a state that when present is essentially felt to be present. In this sense pain is, as we have seen, necessarily conscious. Let me term this *phenomenal consciousness*. In a second sense of consciousness, to be conscious of sensation or object "X" is to be aware that there is an "X," which in turn means to have the belief that there is an "X." This form of consciousness or awareness involves concepts that entail propositions. It is what philosophers call a "propositional attitude," and it may therefore be termed *propositional consciousness*. Obviously, only beings capable of dealing with concepts are capable of this form of consciousness. Only if I possess the concept "pain" can I be aware that I am in "pain," even though I can feel pain without the concept of "pain."

How are these two forms of consciousness or awareness of pain factually related

---

[5]This claim is not uncontested among philosophers; the reader may refer, for example, to the influential paper by Pitcher (1970). But even if my claim about the way our notion of pain works were false, so that it would make sense to talk about unfelt pain, that would still leave us to explain by way of an instantiation explanation the phenomenal feature that pain has when it is felt. Usually this is granted (see, however, Dennett 1978, 1991).

in human beings? Both the empirical literature and the philosophical literature have a tendency to claim that there is a necessary covariation between phenomenal and propositional awareness—that if and only if a person *feels* pain is he or she also aware of *being* in pain (i.e., in the state called "pain"). I think this is a mistake, for I see no reason to postulate a logical connection between my being in pain (and feeling it) and my believing that I am in pain. True, we are as a matter of empirical fact relatively reliable in generating beliefs about our phenomenal states, once we have been trained to have such beliefs at all. But I see no reason why some of these beliefs could not be plainly false. If I understand the empirical data correctly, pain patients' cognitive self-management often involves systematic self-deception both in the sense of believing themselves to be in pain when they are not and refusing to believe that they are in pain when they feel it. It is admittedly tricky to conclude any of this from behavioral evidence (i.e., from outside observation), but even if none of this evidence were conclusive, another, more general consideration shows that there may be a gap between phenomenal and propositional awareness. This consideration is that the subpersonal mechanisms subserving the two forms of consciousness are presumably different, and it may therefore simply be that the empirical tie between them is occasionally or even frequently broken. There can, after all, be false belief about one's own pain, so why should there not also be total lack of belief? Although pain cannot be phenomenally unconscious, it can be propositionally unconscious. Pain is necessarily the object of phenomenal consciousness but not necessarily the object of propositional consciousness.

CAUSATION: THE PUZZLE

Despite their apparent logic, all three models of the relationship between the personal level and the subpersonal level lead to puzzles.[6]

Let us first look more closely at the idea that the phenomenal states of a person, like pain, are *caused* by a complicated pattern of neurobiologic states described at the subpersonal level. What makes this idea puzzling is that once we enter the subpersonal level by looking for neurobiologic mechanisms, we take this level to be causally closed. What this means is that the causal properties we ascribe to an item at the subpersonal level hold with respect to other items that are also specified at this level. Take, for example, an electrochemical process at a synapse. Both its causal antecedents and its causal consequences are neuronal processes, such as the production and absorption of neurotransmitters, the buildup or discharge of action potentials, the transmission of impulses, and so forth. Once we start moving on the subpersonal level, the only causal analyses that matter or are recognized as valid are those described in terms of subpersonal entities. We try to knit as dense and tight a causal net as possible, but none of its knots will involve any entities mentioned at the personal level. Even if we knew all of the causal chains existing at the subper-

---

[6] I have further developed these puzzles in Bieri (1992a,b).

sonal level, and knew them fully, there would, within that realm of subpersonal causal explanations, be no mention of the entities ascribed at the personal level. All of the links of all of the chains would be neurobiologic. How, then, could it be that the *phenomenal* state of pain is caused by subpersonal processes?

The same point may be put in a slightly different way: Explaining an event B as the causal effect of another event A means specifying a causal chain between A and B. Specifying such a chain means describing the *modus operandi* of the cause vis-à-vis the effects. It means answering the question: "How does A work to bring about B?" Now suppose we claim that certain neurobiologic events cause the phenomenal experience of pain. How can we answer the *modus operandi* question? We cannot, since all of the links of the causal chain that we can mention will be subpersonal links, whereas we want to know how such links produce phenomenal pain; thus, for fundamental reasons, it seems that no progress can be made in this area.

The reason for this apparent disjuncture is that the notion of causation or causality is implicitly bound or restricted to levels of description and explanation. It works properly only within levels and not across them. We tend to forget this because, when beginning a project of causal explanations, we have usually already committed ourselves to a certain level and, as a rule, we stick to it. We don't notice the level-dependence of the notion of causation until we try to cross levels and run into puzzles of the sort discussed above.[7]

Consequently, there does not appear to be any upward causation between subpersonal and personal states such as phenomenal pain, and there also and for the same reason appears to be no downward causation either. Just as a neurobiologic process subserving pain does not cause the pain but causes other subpersonal processes, so are the neurobiologic processes subserving pain not caused by the experience of pain but by other subpersonal processes. This conclusion, incidentally, could not be avoided by saying that subpersonal processes both cause and are caused by other subpersonal processes and phenomenal states like pain, since doing so would mean that the branch of the causal tree involving phenomenal pain would pose the same problem all over again.

Suppose that the foregoing suggestion is true. Where does that leave us? At first, it would seem to leave us with the puzzle of epiphenomenalism. Let us suppose once again that we already had the complete subpersonal account of what happens to human beings who are in pain, both in terms of what they do and what they suffer; that we knew, in other words, the complete causal, explanatory story for their pain in terms of subpersonal science. Given what I have so far said, it would

---

[7] The observation in this paragraph is a consequence of the fact that the context "A explains B causally" is intentional (i.e., it holds for A and B not under *any* true description of these events, but only under those descriptions that succeed in specifying their causally relevant features). Working causal explanations, in other words, presuppose the choice of an appropriate descriptive system or vocabulary which, by the very fact of its explanatory success, counts as a single level of description. It comes as no surprise, then, that cross-level causal explanations do not seem to get off the ground. We owe most of the insights in this area to Donald Davidson's work (Davidson 1980). A head-on attack against this doctrine was launched by Searle (1983), who sees no problems with cross-level causation. I think Searle confuses the claim that (a) "Knowledge of causation does not presuppose knowledge of laws" with the claim that (b) "Knowledge of causation is neutral as to the level of description of the events involved." Point (a) does not entail point (b); point (a) is, I believe, true, whereas (b) is false.

then seem that the entire domain of phenomena described at the personal level is causally completely irrelevant. The picture we get is that of an immensely complicated subpersonal machinery doing all of the causal work without being seen. What happens at the personal level and the level of awareness is, as far as the causal structure of the world is concerned, completely gratuitous, negligible, and irrelevant. Phenomenal pain, for example, would be no more than a causally free-floating state, having no causal impact whatsoever. It would, in a sense, be completely *unnecessary*. And so would be all phenomenal and, for that matter, all propositional consciousness.

Most people find this hard to believe, and I am no exception. Yet I cannot resist raising a question that is in the line of epiphenomenalism and which I find very difficult to answer. Pain, it is said in the empirical literature, has the function of making people learn to avoid harm and to behave so as to support the healing of injuries. I am aware that a functional account such as this does not cover all kinds of pain, and particularly not chronic pain, which is puzzling precisely because chronic pain *is* dysfunctional. Still, phenomenal pain is said to be functionally necessary for survival, and accounts of pain often amount to evolutionary explanations of it. My question is: Why do an organism's states, which serve this function, have to be *phenomenal* states which are *experiences* in the sense that an organism can be in these states? Suppose there were such people as "biologic engineers" who built biologic organisms from scratch, and suppose you were one of them. Your task would be to build a biologic system flexible enough to get along in the world by adapting to a certain environment. Is there any reason why you would want to endow such a system with phenomenal, subjective states like pain? Why would such states require phenomenal consciousness?

You might want to say that the organism needs phenomenal pain because it must be able to register certain stimuli, namely injuries. The system, you may say, must be kept informed about what is happening to it. All that is, of course, true. You could not solve your task unless you built into the organism an information-processing system with lots of control and feedback mechanisms. But again, why would that system have to operate on a phenomenal, conscious level? After all, there are countless ways in which we adapt to the world every second of our lives without noticing it. We each register a huge amount of information that has no phenomenal quality whatsoever and of which we are completely unaware. Why could a biologic system—including the guiding function that phenomenal pain has for our behavior—not then be run on the basis of unconscious, subpersonal information processing alone, with as many feedback loops as you like? Indeed, is it not actually the case that the subpersonal counterparts of felt pain are playing this role?

IDENTITY: THE PUZZLE

It seems that we can free ourselves from this cluster of puzzles at one stroke if we opt for our second model and say that phenomena at the personal level are to be *identified* with processes at the subpersonal level. Feeling pain or being conscious of pain is just being in a certain complicated state of one's nervous system. We do not have two states, the neural and the phenomenal, as in the first model; we have only one state. This proposal amounts to saying that instantiation explanations are straightforward identity statements. It is an attractive proposal because, first, it explains why truths on the personal level vary systematically with subpersonal truths. Second, it does not run into the puzzle of cross-level causation, and third, it avoids in an obvious way the puzzle of epiphenomenalism.

But the proposal carries its own puzzles. To put these briefly, we do not understand how a phenomenal, conscious state like pain can be identical to a neural state of a system that is not a phenomenal, conscious state. If there is this crucial difference between the two states, how could the first state possibly *be* the second? A subpersonal account of a human being is an objective account in the sense in which all science strives for objectivity: a representation of the facts that is as free as possible of subjectivity. Phenomenal consciousness, on the other hand, is, as we saw, essentially linked to a subjective perspective: the move away from appearance to reality is a move that doesn't seem to make sense in the case of phenomenal states like pain. Rather than bringing us closer to the real nature, the essence of felt pain, moving away from subjectivity is likely to lose the phenomenon altogether. For what would pain be without the subjective viewpoint that defines its phenomenal nature?[8]

If the identity theory were true, it would solve many intricate problems. And it is deceptively easy to *say*: "Pain is simply a complicated neural state," or "Phenomenal consciousness is just a complicated feedback mechanism in the brain." It is much less easy to find such a proposition truly intelligible. The progress made in the measurement of pain does not help us with this problem. Measuring pain is an objectivizing step in the sense that it provides more precise information about the quality and intensity of pain (see Chapters 3, 25, 32), and may therefore make it appear that we had begun to understand phenomenal pain in objective terms. But this would seem not to be the case because we still do not understand how a complicated neural mechanism can be identical to phenomenal consciousness, which is by its very nature an irreducibly subjective phenomenon. Being able to measure the nature and intensity of pain still leaves the crucial question of how pain can have an objective nature at all.

Notice, furthermore, that it is of no help to say that pain has "two aspects," one neurobiologic and the other phenomenal, and that "they are aspects of one and the same phenomenon." To say this is not to solve our problem but merely to restate it, since what we are trying to understand is precisely how something can at the same time have both of these aspects. We are still left with the question: "How is phenomenal consciousness possible in a biologic organism?" To answer this question it is not enough to know how the subpersonal machinery works in detail. For even if we knew that whole story we would still not understand how perfectly objective, neurobiologic facts can be reflected as phenomenal consciousness.

---

[8] Nagel (e.g. 1979 and 1986) has long pressed such questions.

SUPERVENIENCE: THE PUZZLE

Finally, let us turn to the third and last model, based on the concept of the emergence or supervenience of phenomena on the personal level from phenomena on the subpersonal level. Roughly speaking, we get this notion when we want neither identity or reduction nor cross-level causation. Basically, it involves referring back to what is generally granted: that the subpersonal level determines the personal level in the sense that there could be no change at the second level without a change at the first. This determination is what constitutes emergence or supervenience.[9] But whereas the model of cross-level causation and the identity theory can be seen as an explanation for why this relationship holds, the model of emergence or supervenience is in a sense a refusal to explain its existence any further. Proponents of this position are likely to simply maintain that once you have said that whole systems have properties determined by subsystems that do not themselves have these properties, you have said all that can intelligibly be said.

Perhaps this is true. But I want to point out briefly why I think the proposal leads back to the puzzles so far outlined. First, it brings us back to the observation leading to epiphenomenalism: If the subpersonal level is causally closed, does it not follow that the domain of emergent or supervenient states, such as pain, is causally irrelevant, floating freely without being captured in a causal net? The model of emergence may be defended against this argument by claiming that although phenomenal pain is not causally relevant on the subpersonal level, it is causally relevant on the personal level.[10] This reply fits my earlier claim that the notion of causation is level-bound. But the epiphenomenalist has another move left: He will point out that on the personal level we do not get any specification of causal chains leading from pain behavior. What, for example, is the *modus operandi* of phenomenal pain that causes us to move in response to it? To get a detailed causal chain, we must, it seems, descend to the subpersonal level. And doesn't this mean that the causal role ascribed to phenomenal pain on the personal level is merely spurious? How do we meet that challenge?

A second problem is that the question I raised about the identity theory also tends to recur, although in a slightly modified form. For although the third proposal does not pose the problem of understanding how a phenomenal state could be a neural state, it still leaves the question of how a system consisting of perfectly objective, biologic elements can, once it has reached a certain complexity, produce states that are essentially subjective. This case is different from an object's displaying macroproperties by virtue of certain microcomponents being organized in a certain way. The emergence of consciousness is much harder to understand because its phenomenal aspect is so completely unlike anything we find on the subpersonal level.

---

[9] The canonical papers on the notion of supervenience can be found in Kim (1993).
[10] A position like this is defended by Kim (1993).

NO FALSE CONCLUSIONS

I want to conclude these inconclusive remarks by warding off a possible misunderstanding. I have not been trying to establish some sort of metaphysical gulf between neurobiology and phenomenologic psychology, or between the personal and the subpersonal level in the experience of pain. In particular, I do not think that a distinction between the "physical" and the "nonphysical" aspects of a human being would be necessary, helpful, or even intelligible for this purpose. Traditional ontologic dualism turned out long ago to be a blind alley. On the contrary, I think we need both empirical, naturalistic instantiation explanations of phenomenal consciousness and a conceptually coherent and convincing commentary on such explanations. Progress in the first task does not automatically mean progress in the second one. But only when both tasks have been mastered will we have understood how we can, at the same time, be biologic organisms and conscious persons.

ACKNOWLEDGMENT

Major aspects of this contribution have been published in *Acta Neurochirurgica* 1987; Suppl. 38: 157–164. The author thanks the Springer Publishing Company, Heidelberg, Germany, for granting permission to include them in this discussion.

REFERENCES

Bieri P. Nominalism and inner experience. *Monist* 1982;65:68–87.
Bieri P. Was macht Bewußtsein zu einem Rätsel? *Spekt Wissensch* 1992b;Oktober,48–56.
Bieri P. Trying out epiphenomenalism. *Erkenntnis* 1992a;36:283–309.
Cummins R. *The nature of psychological explanation.* Cambridge, MA: MIT Press, 1983.
Davidson D. *Essays on actions and events.* Oxford: Clarendon Press, 1980.
Dennett DC. *Content and consciousness.* London: Routledge and Kegan Paul, 1969.
Dennett DC. *Brainstorms.* Hassocks, UK: Harvester Press, 1978.
Dennett DC. *The intentional stance.* Cambridge, MA: MIT Press, 1987.
Dennett DC. *Consciousness explained.* Boston: Little, Brown & Company, 1991.
Farrell BA. Experience. *Mind* 1950;59:170–198.
Goodman N. *Ways of worldmaking.* Hassocks, UK: Harvester Press, 1978.
Kim J. *Essays on mind and supervenience.* Cambridge: Cambridge University Press, 1993.
Nagel T. What is it like to be a bat? In: Nagel T, ed. *Mortal questions,* Cambridge: Cambridge University Press, 1979;165–180.
Nagel T. *The view from nowhere.* Oxford: Oxford University Press, 1986.
Pitcher G. Pain perception. *Philos Rev* 1970;79:368–393.
Quine WV. Two dogmas of empiricism. In: Quine WV, ed. *From a logical point of view.* Cambridge, MA: Harvard University Press, 1953;20–46.
Searle J. *Intentionality.* Cambridge: Cambridge University Press, 1983.

*Pain and the Brain: From
Nociception to Cognition,*
edited by Burkhart Bromm and
John E. Desmedt, Advances in Pain
Research and Therapy Vol. 22.
Raven Press, Ltd., New York © 1995.

8

Slow (<14 Hz) and Fast (20–40 Hz) Oscillations of Intralaminar Thalamic Neurons in the Sleeping and Aroused Brain

Mircea Steriade

*Laboratoire de Neurophysiologie, Faculté de Médecine, Université Laval,
Quebec, Canada G1K 7P4*

SUMMARY

The intrinsic cellular properties and synaptic networks underlying the three major sleep oscillations (spindles, the delta rhythm, and slow rhythms), and the modulation of these sleep rhythms by arousing systems with generalized actions, are described by means of intracellular recordings *in vivo*. The slow oscillation (<1 Hz) arises in cortical networks and has the virtue of grouping thalamically generated spindle (7–14 Hz) and delta (1–4 Hz) oscillations. All these sleep rhythms are blocked by ascending activating cholinergic systems which: (a) decouple the neurons of the reticular thalamic nucleus, the spindle pacemaker; (b) depolarize thalamocortical cells and shift them out of the voltage-range at which intrinsic delta potentials are generated; and (c) disrupt the long-lasting hyperpolarizations in neocortical cells, a major substrate of the slow oscillation. In addition to blocking sleep rhythms, arousing cholinergic systems in the mesopontine region and basal forebrain elicit fast rhythms of around 40 Hz in thalamocortical systems. A subgroup of intralaminar thalamocortical neurons discharge fast (20–40 Hz) spike-bursts at unusually high frequencies (900–1,000 Hz) during both brain-active states of wakefulness and rapid-eye-movement (REM; dreaming) sleep. This activity pattern is regarded as playing a role in the generalized 40-Hz activity described during the dreaming state of humans. I speculate that these high-frequency spike-bursts of centrolateral intralaminar thalamic neurons with cortical projections are sources for the transformation, during dreaming, of non-noxious somatosensory signals into pain or for the transfer to the neocortex of long-stored memory of pain.

INTRALAMINAR THALAMIC NEURONS,
PAIN SIGNALS, AND BRAIN AROUSAL

Accumulating evidence indicates that the rostral intralaminar centrolateral-para-central (CL-PC) nuclei relay afferents of pain pathways in their route to the cerebral cortex. Spinothalamic axons arise from high-threshold or wide-dynamic-range (WDR) neurons and, in addition to terminating in the ventroposterior (VP) complex, distribute within the large-celled part of the CL nucleus (Giesler et al. 1981; Kenshalo and Willis 1991). It is thought that the discriminative system of pain passes through VP cells, while CL neurons are mainly concerned with the affective state generated by a noxious stimulus. This assumption seems to be supported by a high concentration of opiate receptors in the intralaminar region of termination of spinothalamic fibers (Pert et al. 1976). The role played by CL-PC neurons in the sensation of pain is corroborated by reports of diffuse aching pain after stimulation of the intralaminar region adjacent to the nucleus limitans (Hassler 1970) and relief of intractable pain by intralaminar thalamotomy (Sano 1977).

The involvement of CL-PC intralaminar nuclei in the sensation of pain is related to the crucial role of this thalamic territory in brain arousal. The identification beyond hypothesis of the final corticipetal link in the substratum of diffuse cortical arousal elicited by activation of the brain stem reticular core was made possible by demonstrating monosynaptic excitation of antidromically identified CL-PC thalamocortical neurons from the midbrain reticular formation in animals with chronic pontine lesions, to produce degeneration of passing fibers (Steriade and Glenn 1982). Subsequent studies, combining retrograde tracing and immunohistochemistry for choline acetyltransferase, have demonstrated projections of mesopontine cholinergic neurons as well as of more rostral, midbrain noncholinergic (presumably glutamatergic) cells to the CL-PC nuclei (Paré et al. 1988). The intralaminar nuclei are targets of converging inputs from spinothalamic fibers as well as from a series of brain-stem core structures ranging from the giganto- and magnocellular bulbar nuclei to the upper mesencephalic tegmentum, as indicated by morphologic and electrophysiologic studies (Bowsher et al. 1968; Steriade et al. 1984b; Paré et al. 1988). Investigation of state-dependent activities in medullary, mesopontine, and rostral midbrain reticular neurons having physiologically identified projections to the CL-PC thalamic nuclei have revealed that these brain-stem core elements increase their firing rates during brain-active states of wakefulness and rapid-eye-movement (REM) sleep, with signs of increased discharge frequencies reliably preceding the time 0 (EEG activation) of these behavioral states (Steriade et al. 1982, 1984b, 1990a). The CL-PC thalamocortical neurons that are the preferential targets of brain-stem-activating cells display tonic firing patterns associated with enhanced antidromic and orthodromic responsiveness during both brain-active states of waking and REM sleep, as opposed to their burst firing, which reflects membrane hyperpolarization during EEG-synchronized sleep (Glenn and Steriade 1982). This change in the functional mode of CL-PC thalamic cells accompanying a transition from quiescent sleep to either arousal or REM sleep is similar to that observed in most thalamocortical neurons recorded from other dorsal thalamic nuclei (Steriade et al. 1990b).

In this chapter I first discuss the main features of low-frequency (<14 Hz) oscillations occurring in thalamocortical neurons during the state of resting sleep. I then summarize the actions of neuromodulatory systems that block sleep oscillations, thus promoting neuronal activities characteristic of the aroused brain. Last, I present recent data on the electrophysiologic properties of a peculiar subpopulation of thalamocortical cells, recorded from the large-celled part of the CL nucleus in which spinothalamic axons distribute, that discharge rhythmic, fast (20–40 Hz) spike-bursts at unusually high frequencies (900–1,000 Hz) during both waking and REM sleep. This finding led me to speculate that these thalamocortical cells are implicated in the sensation of pain during waking as well as during the dreaming state.

SLEEP OSCILLATIONS IN THALAMOCORTICAL SYSTEMS

Three types of sleep oscillations occur in thalamic and cortical networks (Steriade 1993). Spindles (7–14 Hz) are the epitome of EEG synchronization at sleep onset. Their prevalence in the rostral intralaminar thalamic nuclei and the corresponding neocortical areas is attributable to the massive afferentation of CL-PC nuclei from the reticular thalamic (RE) nuclear complex (Steriade et al. 1984a). Indeed, the pacemaking role played by RE neurons in the genesis of spindles was demonstrated by the abolition of spindles in thalamocortical systems after lesions of the RE nuclear complex (Steriade et al. 1985) and by the preservation of spindles in RE neurons isolated from their cortical and thalamic inputs (Steriade et al. 1987). The fact that CL thalamocortical cells spend most of their spindling time in inhibitory postsynaptic potentials (IPSPs), generated by rhythmic spike-bursts of GABAergic RE cells, explains the greatly reduced synaptic transmission of afferent signals through the CL-PC nuclei during EEG-synchronized sleep (Glenn and Steriade 1982). This is the major factor behind forebrain deafferentation from the very onset of sleep.

The delta rhythm (1–4 Hz) appears during later stages of sleep. This oscillation is generated in thalamocortical cells by the interplay between two intrinsic currents: the hyperpolarization-activated cation current I_h and the low-thresold transient Ca^{2+} current I_t (McCormick and Pape 1990; Steriade et al. 1991a). However efficiently intrinsic currents may generate delta potentials in thalamocortical cells, this oscillation would not be expressed at the macroscopic EEG level without the synchronization of neuronal pools in dorsal thalamic nuclei. The most potent stimuli for the potentiation and synchronization of thalamocortical cells within this rhythm are corticothalamic volleys impinging on RE thalamic cells. By virtue of their GABAergic nature and widespread projections to the dorsal thalamus, RE neurons set the membrane potential (V_m) of thalamocortical cells at the required level for delta-rhythm generation and synchronize otherwise independent oscillators (Steri-

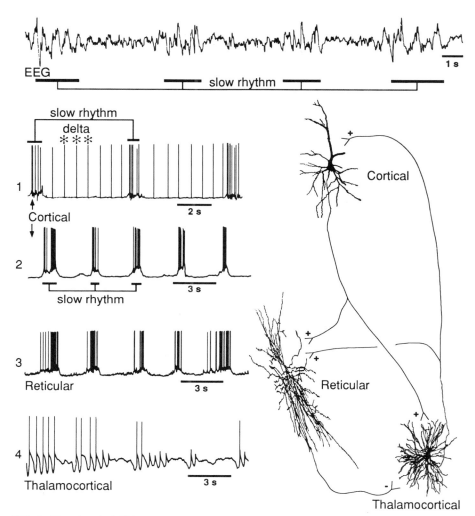

FIG. 1. The slow (<1 Hz) neocortical oscillation and its reflection in thalamic neurons. At top, surface EEG recording of the slow rhythm (≈0.2 Hz) of delta waves (1–1.5 Hz) in the naturally sleeping cat; periodic sequences of delta waves are marked by horizontal bars. Below, intracellular recordings of four neurons (two neocortical [1–2], reticular thalamic [3], and thalamocortical [4]) in anesthetized cats. Intracellularly stained cortical, reticular thalamic, and thalamocortical neurons (Modified from Steriade and Deschênes 1984, Steriade et al. 1993d). Cortical neuron 1 displays the slow rhythm (≈0.16 Hz) and, between the slow depolarizing events, clocklike action potentials (*asterisks*) recurring at the delta frequency (≈1.6 Hz), arising in thalamocortical cells. Cortical neuron 2 exhibits the slow rhythm at ≈0.3 Hz. Reticular thalamic neuron 3 oscillates at ≈0.3 Hz, a frequency similar to the slow cortical rhythm. Thalamocortical neuron 4 oscillates with the rhythm of delta potentials (≈2.5 Hz) that tend to dampen and are periodically revived, within the frequency range of the slow rhythm (≈0.2–0.3 Hz). (Modified from Steriade et al. 1993b, d, e.)

ade et al. 1991a). Since delta potentials occur at a V_m that is more negative than that for spindles (Steriade et al. 1991a), it was postulated that with the deepening of sleep, the V_m of thalamocortical cells undergoes a progressive hyperpolarization (Steriade et al. 1991a) due to the diminished firing rates in activating cholinergic and monoaminergic neurons (Steriade and McCarley 1990).

Recently, we discovered a slow rhythm (<1 Hz) of neocortical cells with anti-dromically identified thalamic and callosal projections (Fig. 1). The slow oscillation consists of prolonged depolarizations, on which trains of action potentials are super-imposed, separated by long-lasting hyperpolarizing components (Steriade et al. 1993d). This oscillation survives total lesions of thalamic nuclei projecting to the recorded cortical cells (Steriade et al. 1993e). However, the slow rhythm is re-flected in RE and thalamocortical neurons (Fig. 1), thus grouping the thalamically generated spindles and delta oscillations into wave sequences that recur periodically every 2 to 5 sec (Steriade et al. 1993b). Multi-site extra- and intracellular recordings revealed a dramatic synchronization of neocortical, RE, and thalamocortical neu-rons within the frequency range of slow and other sleep oscillations, with time lags ranging from 10 msec to more than 100 msec (Fig. 2). The coherence between cortical and thalamic cells varies in parallel with the synchronization state of the EEG (Steriade and Contreras 1993).

The foregoing variety of sleep rhythms is explained by different intrinsic and network properties of RE, thalamocortical, and neocortical neurons, resulting in different frequency ranges of oscillation. However, all of these oscillations have in common prolonged IPSPs (spindles) and Ca^{2+}-dependent K^+ conductances (corti-cal slow rhythm), or are generated at a hyperpolarized V_m (delta oscillation). Con-sequently, they all may lead to a convergent outcome consisting of the obliteration of messages from the outside world during a behavioral state in which the large-scale coherent thalamocortical activities associated with rhythmic spike-bursts may be used to reorganize networks and/or to systematically sift and consolidate infor-mation acquired during the waking state.

CONTROL OF SLEEP OSCILLATIONS BY NEUROMODULATORY SYSTEMS

The tonic discharge patterns of single spikes in thalamocortical and long-axoned neocortical cells during waking develop during EEG-synchronized sleep into spike-bursts interspersed with periods of silence, whereas during the subsequent stage of REM sleep the firing patterns are very similar to those during wakefulness (Steriade 1978; Glenn and Steriade 1982). The comparison of this picture, resulting from extracellular studies in animals with chronically implanted electrodes, with the in-tracellular data from *in vivo* and *in vitro* experiments (Llinás 1988; Steriade et al. 1990b; McCormick 1992a) allows us to consider waking and dreaming sleep as behavioral states associated with a relative depolarization of thalamic and cortical neurons, whereas the same cells become hyperpolarized and much less responsive during EEG-synchronized sleep.

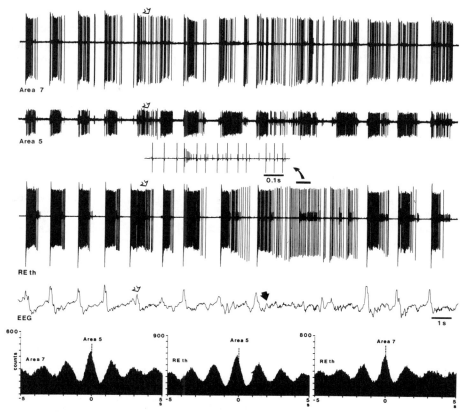

FIG. 2. Synchronization of slow rhythm (≈0.6 Hz) in cortical and thalamic cells and its disruption during short periods of EEG activation occurring spontaneously. Simultaneous extracellular recordings in cortical areas 5 and 7 and in the reticular thalamic (RE th) nucleus under ketamine and xylazine anesthesia. Note two synchronously oscillating cells, recorded by the same microelectrode, in both area 5 and RE th. EEG is depicted below. The synchronous spike barrages in three neurons (an area-7 cell and neurons with high-amplitude spikes in area 5 and RE th) are documented by cross-correlograms between cortical cells (area-5 neuron is the reference, time 0), as well as between RE th neuron and either area-5 or area-7 neurons. Slight change in the EEG synchrony (*empty arrow*) was associated with slight changes in unit firing (tendency to tonic discharges, indicated by *empty arrows* on all cellular traces). A period of more pronounced EEG activation (starting at *filled arrow*) was associated with more marked tonic firing disrupting the slow rhythm; however, the RE th cell discharging low-amplitude spikes remained in a burst-firing pattern and continued the slow rhythm (*oblique arrow* indicates the expanded inset; larger spikes were truncated). (From Steriade et al. 1993a, with permission.)

These changes from the sleeping to the aroused brain are due to the actions of brain-stem, posterior hypothalamic, and basal forebrain neuromodulatory systems releasing acetylcholine (ACh), serotonin, noradrenaline, histamine, and glutamate. Obviously the best candidates for subserving the modulation of thalamic and cortical neurons are those systems whose fluctuations in state-dependent activities parallel the similarly enhanced forebrain excitability during waking and dreaming sleep, consisting of cholinergic and glutamatergic brain-stem core neurons that increase their firing rates and excitability during both of these brain-active states (Steriade et al. 1982, 1990a). Stimulation of mesopontine cholinergic neurons induces a prolonged ($\approx$20 sec) depolarization with spike discharges in thalamocortical neurons, accompanied by an EEG-activated response having a similar time-course. (Curró Dossi et al. 1991). This effect is biphasic. It consists of an early, relatively short-lasting depolarizing component associated with an increase in membrane conductance and sensitive to nicotinic antagonists, followed by a secondary, long-lasting component associated with an increase in apparent input resistance and sensitive to blockers of muscarinic receptors. The cholinergic depolarization of thalamic relay cells results from the reduction of a specialized, K^+ leak conductance, I_{KL}, that is coupled through G-proteins to muscarinic (as well as α_1-adrenergic) receptors (McCormick 1992b). The association between a prolonged depolarization and an increase in input resistance provides the necessary mechanism for the passage from the oscillatory state of quiescent sleep to an activated brain state characterized by enhanced responsiveness to incoming volleys. This is indeed what is observed by testing CL-PC and other thalamocortical cells with ortho- and antidromic stimuli during natural states of vigilance (Glenn and Steriade 1982; Steriade et al. 1990b).

The cholinergic modulation of the thalamocortical oscillatory state is effective in blocking all sleep rhythms and therefore in promoting activity patterns such as those seen during waking and REM sleep. Spindles are blocked by cholinergic stimulation because this system, arising in mesopontine and basal forebrain neurons, hyperpolarizes RE thalamic cells by activating a K^+ conductance (McCormick and Prince 1986; Hu et al. 1989), and therefore decouples the spindle-pacemaking RE network. The intrinsic delta oscillation of thalamocortical cells is also blocked by brain-stem cholinergic stimulation that depolarizes these neurons and shifts them out of the voltage range at which delta potentials are generated (Steriade et al. 1991a). In addition to this, the cortical slow rhythm is blocked by cholinergic and noradrenergic stimulation, leading to tonic firing through a disruption of rhythmic, long-lasting hyperpolarizations (Steriade et al. 1993a). A similar disruption of the slow rhythm recorded from multiple thalamic and cortical sites is observed during spontaneous episodes of EEG activation (Fig. 2).

It should be emphasized that arousing stimulations do not activate brain electrical activity only by blocking low-frequency oscillations; such stimuli also elicit fast EEG waves at $\approx$40 Hz (Steriade et al. 1991a,b, 1993a), revealing coherent activities of neuronal groups in the thalamus and cerebral cortex. In the next section, I deal with fast (20–40 Hz) spike-bursts in CL thalamic neurons that may be relevant to the main topic of this symposium.

FAST SPIKE-BURSTS IN INTRALAMINAR THALAMIC NEURONS DURING WAKING AND REM SLEEP: POSSIBLE RELATIONS WITH PAIN IN DREAMS

A special cellular population recorded from the dorsolateral, large-celled part of the CL nucleus (Fig. 3A) displays unusually high-frequency spike-bursts ($\approx$1,000 Hz), not only during EEG-synchronized sleep but also during waking and REM sleep (Glenn and Steriade 1982; Steriade and Glenn 1982; Steriade et al. 1993c; Fig. 3C), two states in which other thalamocortical cells fire single spikes (Steriade et al. 1990b). The large-celled CL district receives spinothalamic axons (Jones 1985). The neurons recorded within this dorsolateral CL area can be antidromically activated from cortical association area 5 at latencies of 0.4 to 0.5 msec (Fig. 3B), indicating conduction velocities of 40 to 50 msec, which are much greater than those of any other class of thalamocortical cell. The antidromic response is followed by a burst of five to six spikes at 900 to 1,000 Hz. The synaptic responses of these CL cells to stimulation of the midbrain reticular formation also takes the form of a spike-burst at $\approx$1,000 Hz (Fig. 3B).

The exceedingly high-frequency bursts in these dorsolateral, large-size CL cells (Steriade et al. 1993c) is probably due to the absence of a K^+-mediated afterhyperpolarizing potential (AHP), higher absolute values and steeper slopes for the rate functions of Na^+ and K^+ conductances, and other kinetic parameters required to achieve such firing rates (Traub 1977).

Another remarkable characteristic of this group of CL neurons is their rhythmic burst firing at 20 to 40 Hz during natural behavioral states of waking and REM sleep. In these CL cells, depolarizing current pulses at the resting V_m (around -60 mV) elicit fast oscillations in intracellular recordings, consisting of spike doublets or triplets, with interspike intervals of 1.1 msec, corresponding to an intraburst frequency of $\approx$900 Hz (Fig. 4A). This pattern corroborates the data obtained in naturally behaving animals, showing that repetitive spike-bursts occur during waking and REM sleep (see Fig. 3C), two states in which thalamic cells are depolarized (Steriade et al. 1990b). Upon steady hyperpolarization, bringing the V_m to -68 mV, a low-threshold Ca^{2+} spike (LTS; see (Llinás 1988) is de-inactivated, and depolarizing current pulses trigger an oscillation at 40 to 60 Hz, with spike-bursts at 800 to 900 Hz that are sculptured by one or two hyperpolarizations. Eventually, at around -80 mV, the LTS dominates the cell behavior, and a single, fully developed spike-burst at 900 Hz is triggered (Fig. 4A). Similar patterns occur spontaneously at the same V_ms (Fig. 4B).

These data on voltage-dependent $\approx$40-Hz oscillations in CL thalamocortical neurons are of importance because the CL nucleus as a whole (but not single CL cells)

FIG. 3. REM; instead, during both of these EEG-desynchronized behavioral states, short (5 msec) bursts with an intraburst frequency of 800 to 1,000 Hz recurred at 20 Hz. (Modified from Steriade et al. 1993c.)

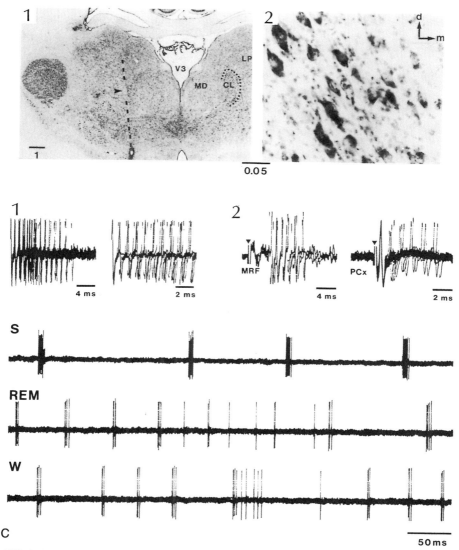

FIG. 3. Large-dorsolateral CL thalamocortical neurons of cats discharging rhythmic (20–40 Hz) spike-bursts with unusually high (≈1,000 Hz) frequencies during waking and REM sleep in chronic experiments. **A1:** Frontal section with microelectrode track (interrupted line) through the lateral part of the CL (*arrowhead*). A small electrolytic lesion was made ≈3 mm ventral to the CL nucleus to allow localization of recorded neurons. In the contralateral thalamus, some thalamic nuclei are indicated, and the dorsolateral part of the CL is marked by dots. Abbreviations: LP = lateroposterior nucleus; MD = mediodorsal nucleus; V3 = third ventricle. **A2:** Cell population in the large-celled CL area, with darkly stained neurons. *Arrows* indicate dorsal (d) and medial (m). *Horizontal line* indicates millimeters. **B1:** Expanded spike-bursts (intraburst frequency ≈1,000 Hz) fired by CL thalamocortical cells during EEG-synchronized sleep. **B2:** Synaptic burst (1,000 Hz) elicited by stimulating (*arrowhead*) the midbrain reticular formation (MRF), and antidromic spike (0.4 msec) followed by burst (1,000 Hz) in response to stimulation (*arrowhead*) of area 5 in the parietal association cortex (PCx). **C:** Discharge patterns during EEG-synchronized sleep (S), REM sleep, and waking (W). The patterns were recorded in this order. Note that high-frequency (900–1,000 Hz) spike-bursts during S did not change into tonic, single-spike firing during W and

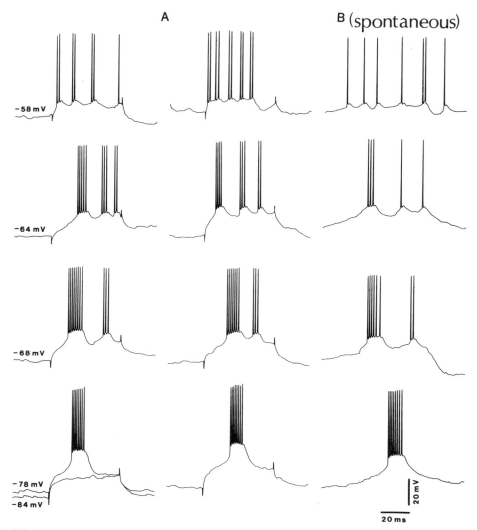

FIG. 4. Fast oscillatory patterns of dorsolateral CL cell induced by depolarizing current pulses and occurring spontaneously. **A:** Activities triggered by depolarizing current pulse (+ 1.2 nA, 50 msec) at different V_ms (indicated at left). Two examples are illustrated for each V_m level. At bottom, LTS leading to high-frequency (800 Hz) spike-burst at −78 mV, and its absence at −84 mV. **B:** Oscillatory patterns similar to those elicited by current injection occurred spontaneously at similar V_ms (from top to bottom: −58, −64, −68, and −78 mV). (From Steriade et al. 1993c, with permission.)

projects to widespread cortical territories, including limbic areas (Jones 1985). The unusually high-frequency spike-bursts exhibited by these cells may then exert powerful influences on cortical cells as compared to other thalamocortical cells, including the transfer of 40-Hz rhythms to broad cortical regions during both waking and REM sleep. Indeed, a coherent 40-Hz oscillation was found to characterize the magnetoencephalographic activity of humans during waking as well as in the dreaming state (Llinás and Ribary 1993). It was hypothesized that this generalized rhythm involves the participation of intralaminar thalamic nuclei in the resonant process.

Let me finally make a leap of faith and speculate that these high-frequency spike-bursts in CL cells with cortical projections may be a source of internally generated pain, and that pain sensations may also occur during the dreaming state. In the introductory section of this chapter I mentioned some data indicating that pain may be elicited by stimulation of the intralaminar region (Hassler 1970), and that intralaminar thalamotomy was found effective in alleviating intractable pain (Sano 1977). Although dreamed pain is usually not mentioned in reports of dream content (Snyder 1970; McCarley and Hobson 1979; Hobson 1988), other observations and more recent studies (Nielsen 1993; Nielsen et al. 1993) indicate that not only can pain sensations be integrated directly into the dream content of REM sleep, but that pain feeling may occur in the dreaming state without any corresponding external noxious stimuli. Indeed, non-noxious somatosensory stimuli can be amplified and elaborated within a pain dream, as suggested by one subject in Maury's study who reported a frightening dream in which a mask of pitch was pulled off of the face ripping off the skin; this dream occurred while the subject's lips and nose were being gently tickled with a feather (see Nielsen 1993). Other subjects report imaginary pain in dreams after long-past traumatic experiences (Nielsen et al. 1993) or even without any history of injury. Could the unusually high-frequency spike-bursts of CL thalamocortical cells, oscillating at fast rates, account for the transformation during dreaming of somatosensory signals into pain, or for the transfer to the cerebral cortex of long-stored memories of pain?

ACKNOWLEDGMENTS

My own experiments mentioned in this chapter were supported by the Medical Research Council of Canada.

REFERENCES

Bowsher D, Mallart A, Petit D, Albe-Fessard D. A bulbar relay to the centre médian. *J. Neurophysiol* 1968;31:288–300.

Curró Dossi R, Paré D, Steriade M. Short-lasting nicotinic and long-lasting muscarinic depolarizing responses of thalamocortical neurons to stimulation of mesopontine cholinergic nuclei. *J Neurophysiol* 1991;65:393–406.

Giesler GJ, Yezierski RP, Gerhart KD, Willis WD. Spinothalamic cells that project to medial and/or lateral thalamic nuclei: evidence for a physiologically novel population of spinal cord neurons. *J Neurophysiol* 1981;46:1285–1308.

Glenn LL, Steriade M. Discharge rate and excitability of cortically projecting intralaminar thalamic neurons during waking and sleep states. *J Neurosci* 1982;2:1387–1404.

Hassler R. Dichotomy of facial pain conduction. In: Hassler R, Walker AE, eds., *Trigeminal neuralgia*. Philadelphia: WB Saunders, 1970;123–138.

Hobson JA. *The dreaming brain*. New York: Basic Books, 1988, pp .

Hu B, Steriade M, Deschênes M. The effects of brainstem peribrachial stimulation on perigeniculate neurons: the blockage of spindle waves. *Neuroscience* 1989;31:1–12.

Jones EG. *The thalamus*. New York: Plenum Press, 1985; pp .

Kenshalo DR, Willis WD. The role of cerebral cortex in pain sensation. In: Peters A, Jones EG, eds. *Cerebral cortex*, vol 9. New York: Plenum Press, 1991;153–212.

Llinás RR. The intrinsic electrophysiological properties of mammalian neurons: a new insight into CNS function. *Science* 1988;242:1654–1664.

Llinás RR, Ribary U. Coherent 40-Hz oscillation characterizes dream state in humans. *Proc Natl Acad Sci USA* 1993;90:2078–2081.

McCarley RW, Hobson JA. The form of dreams and the biology of sleep. In: Wolman BB, ed. *Handbook of dreams. Research, theory and applications*. New York: Van Nostrand Reinhold, 1979;76–130.

McCormick DA. Neurotransmitter actions in the thalamus and cerebral cortex and their role in neuro-modulation of thalamocortical activity. *Progr Neurobiol* 1992a;39:337–388.

McCormick DA. Cellular mechanisms underlying cholinergic and noradrenergic modulation of neuronal firing mode in the cat and guinea pig lateral geniculate nucleus. *J Neurosci* 1992b;12:278–289.

McCormick DA, Pape HC. Properties of a hyperpolarization-activated cation current and its role in rhythmic oscillation in thalamic relay neurones. *J Physiol (Lond)* 1990;431:291–318.

McCormick DA, Prince DA. Acetylcholine induces burst firing in thalamic reticular neurones by activating a potassium conductance. *Nature* 1986;319:402–405.

Nielsen TA. Changes in the kinesthetic content of dreams following somatosensory stimulation of leg muscles during REM sleep. *Dreaming* 1993;3:99–113.

Nielsen TA, McGregor DL, Zadra A, Ilnicki D, Ouellet L. Pain in dreams. *Sleep* 1993;16:490–498.

Paré D, Smith Y, Parent A, Steriade M. Projections of upper brainstem cholinergic and non-cholinergic neurons of cat to intralaminar and reticular thalamic nuclei. *Neuroscience* 1988;25:69–88.

Pert CB, Kuhar MJ, Snyder SH. Autoradiographic localization of opiate receptors in rat brain. *Proc Natl Acad Sci USA* 1976;73:3729–3733.

Sano K. Intralaminar thalamotomy (thalamolaminotomy) and postero-medial hypothalamotomy in the treatment of intractable pain. *Progr Neurol Surg* 1977;8:50–103.

Snyder F. The phenomenology of dreaming. In: Madow H, Snow LH, eds. *The psychodynamic implication of the physiological studies of dreams*. Springfield, IL: Charles C Thomas, 1970;124–151.

Steriade M. Cortical long-axoned cells and putative interneurons during the sleep-waking cycle. *Behav Brain Sci* 1978;3:465–514.

Steriade M. Cellular substrates of brain rhythms. In: Niedermeyer E, Lopes da Silva F, eds., *Electroencephalography: basic principles, clinical applications, and related fields*. Baltimore: Williams & Wilkins, 1993;27–62.

Steriade M, Amzica F, Nuñez A. Cholinergic and noradrenergic modulation of the slow ($\approx$0.3 Hz) oscillation in neocortical cells. *J Neurophysiol* 1993a;70:1385–1400.

Steriade M, Contreras D. Synchronization of sleep rhythms in multi-site thalamic and cortical recordings. *Soc Neurosci Abstr* 1993;19.

Steriade M, Contreras D, Curró Dossi R, Nuñez A. The slow (<1 Hz) oscillation in reticular thalamic and thalamocortical neurons: scenario of sleep rhythm generation in interacting thalamic and neocortical networks. *J Neurosci* 1993b;13:3284–3299.

Steriade M, Curró Dossi R, Contreras D. Electrophysiological properties of intralaminar thalamocortical cells discharging rhythmic ($\approx$40 Hz) spike-bursts at $\approx$1000 Hz during waking and rapid eye movement sleep. *Neuroscience* 1993c;56:1–9.

Steriade M, Curró Dossi R, Nuñez A. Network modulation of a slow intrinsic oscillation of cat thalamocortical neurons implicated in sleep delta waves: cortically-induced synchronization and brainstem cholinergic suppression. *J Neurosci* 1991a;11:3200–3217.

Steriade M, Curró Dossi R, Paré D, Oakson G (1991b). Fast oscillations (20–40 Hz) in thalamocortical systems and their potentiation by mesopontine cholinergic nuclei. *Proc Natl Acad Sci USA* 1991b; 88:4396–4400.

Steriade M, Datta S, Paré D, Oakson G, Curró Dossi R. Neuronal activities in brainstem cholinergic nucleir related to tonic activation processes in thalamocortical systems. *J Neurosci* 1990a;10:2541–2559.

Steriade M, Deschênes M. The thalamus as a neuronal oscillator. *Brain Res Rev* 1984;8:1–63.

Steriade M, Deschênes M, Domich L, Mulle C. Abolition of spindle oscillations in thalamic neurons disconnected from nucleus reticularis thalami. *J Neurophysiol* 1985;54:1473–1497.

Steriade M, Domich L, Oakson G, Deschênes M. The deafferented reticular thalamic nucleus generates spindle rhythmicity. *J Neurophysiol* 1987;57:260–273.

Steriade M, Glenn LL. Neocortical and caudate projections of intralaminar thalamic neurons and their synaptic excitation from midbrain reticular core. *J Neurophysiol* 1982;48:352–371.

Steriade M, Jones EG, Llinás RR. *Thalamic oscillations and signaling.* New York: Wiley-Interscience, 1990b.

Steriade M, McCarley RW. *Brainstem control of wakefulness and sleep.* New York: Plenum Press, 1990.

Steriade M, Nuñez A, Amzica F. A novel slow (<1 Hz) oscillation of neocortical neurons *in vivo*: depolarizing and hyperpolarizing components. *J Neurosci* 1993d;13:3252–3265.

Steriade M, Nuñez A, Amzica F. Intracellular analysis of relations between the slow (<1 Hz) neocortical oscillation and other sleep rhythms of the electroencephalogram *J Neurosci* 1993e;13:3266–3283.

Steriade M, Oakson G, Ropert N. Firing rates and patterns of midbrain reticular neurons during steady and transitional states of sleep-waking cycle. *Exp Brain Res* 1982;46:37–51.

Steriade M, Parent A, Hada J. Thalamic projections of nucleus reticularis thalami of cat: a study using retrograde transport of horseradish peroxidase and double fluorescent tracers. *J Comp Neurol* 1984a; 229:531–547.

Steriade M, Sakai K, Jouvet M. Bulbo-thalamic neurons related to thalamocortical activation processes during paradoxical sleep. *Exp Brain Res* 1984b;54:463–475.

Traub RD. Repetitive firing of Renshaw spinal interneurons. *Biol Cybernet* 1977;27:71–76.

Pain and the Brain: From
Nociception to Cognition,
edited by Burkhart Bromm and
John E. Desmedt, Advances in Pain
Research and Therapy Vol. 22.
Raven Press, Ltd., New York © 1995.

9

Thalamic Processing of Visceral Pain

*Christiane Vahle-Hinz, †Johannes Brüggemann, and
‡Klaus-D. Kniffki

*Institute of Physiology, University Hospital Eppendorf, D-20246 Hamburg; †Neurosurgery
Research Laboratory, State University of New York, Syracuse, New York 13210, USA and
‡Institute of Physiology, University of Würzburg, D-97070 Würzburg, Germany

SUMMARY

Visceral pain is distinct from somatic pain in a number of characteristics, including referral to skin areas and a usually diffuse localization. The neuronal mechanisms underlying these properties of visceral pain are poorly understood because there is little knowledge about processes of visceroception at higher stages of the central nervous system (CNS). Even the peripheral mechanisms underlying visceral pain are not yet resolved; it is, for instance, still a matter of debate whether specific visceral nociceptors exist similar to those of the skin.

In this chapter we review the results of animal studies on the receptors in visceral organs, the ascending pathways, and the thalamic areas involved in visceroception, and compare them to those of the somatic nociceptive system. Our focus is thereby on viscera of the lower abdominal space, with results from experiments which we undertook to study the thalamic processes of visceroception in the cat. These included: (a) a systematic mapping of the lateral thalamus for responses to electrical stimulation of the pelvic nerve, which innervates visceral organs of the lower abdominal space (urinary bladder, distal colon, reproductive organs); (b) a study of the responses of lateral thalamic neurons to natural stimulation of the urinary bladder; and (c) a neuroanatomic demonstration of the thalamic projections of the nucleus of the solitary tract (NTS), a major relay center for visceral pathways in the brain stem. All approaches showed a concentration of visceral inputs in a region surrounding the caudal to middle part of the ventral posterolateral (VPL) nucleus, i.e., to the periphery of the VPL (VPL_p) and the adjoining part of the posterior complex (PO). Most neurons with input from visceral receptors also had somatic receptive fields (RFs), which were of the low-threshold type. For two-thirds of the neurons, these RFs were located in areas on the lower back, the thigh, the tail, and/ or the heel, i.e., including dermatomes to which pain is referred from the visceral organs of the lower abdominal space. The responses of the thalamic neurons to distension of the urinary bladder with noxious intensities were excitatory or "inhibitory." The results of these studies suggest that the VPL_p and the adjoining PO in the lateral thalamus of the cat are involved in the encoding, localization, and referral of visceral pain.

INTRODUCTION

Visceral Versus Somatic Pain

Visceral pain has several characteristics distinct from somatic pain. First, results from actual or potential tissue damage which usually does not induce pain from internal organs a stimulus considered noxious and eliciting somatic pain. Visceral pain is, however, elicited when internal organs are distended beyond their normal physiological range or when inflamed organs contract or distend during their normal functions. Second, specific nociceptors have been identified as the peripheral sensors of noxious events in skin, muscles, and joints (for a review, see Willis 1985; see also Chapter 1), whereas it is still a matter of debate whether these nociceptors also exist in the viscera or whether visceral pain is signaled by a variation in intensity in the same population of afferent fibers that also submit nonpainful sensations and visceral reflexes (Jänig and Morrison 1986; Cervero 1988; Cervero and Jänig 1992). Such "intensity-encoding" primary afferent fibers are in fact abundant in many visceral organs; for example, Aδ- and C-fibers innervating the urinary bladder have been shown to respond in a graded fashion to passive distension and isovolumetric contraction at intravesical pressures of 10 to 70 mmHg, a range covering stimuli of innocuous and noxious intensity (Bahns et al. 1986, 1987). Apart from these, Häbler et al. (1990) have reported a small population (2.4%) of unmyelinated bladder afferents that could be activated only with high, presumably noxious pressure (30–50 mmHg). In addition, receptors with very high response thresholds have been described (9.5%; Häbler et al. 1990) that were unexcitable in the normal bladder but responded vigorously to contractions and distensions after an acute inflammation had been induced, closely resembling the behavior of the "silent" nociceptors first discovered in inflamed joints (Schaible and Schmidt 1988). The coexistence of different categories of visceral receptors (i.e., purely low-threshold, intensity-encoding, and high-threshold) has also been demonstrated in studies of the innervation of the esophagus (Sengupta et al. 1989, 1990).

In a recently proposed hypothesis, Cervero and Jänig (1992) suggested that the different categories of visceral receptors in varying combinations of activation subserve the different mechanisms underlying the various forms of visceral sensations and regulatory reflexes. In their view, low-threshold receptors, including the intensity-encoding receptors, are active during normal visceral function and may elicit nonpainful sensations. The intensity-encoding afferents also project to somatic nociceptive neurons; under normal circumstances, however, this input remains subliminal. Noxious visceral stimulation induces an increased input from the intensity-encoding afferents and additional activity in the high-threshold afferents, resulting in acute, brief visceral pain. Continuing irritation of the internal organ (e.g., by inflammation) leads to the sensitization of silent nociceptors, providing a third type of input to the nociceptive neurons. In this way, central neurons may be sensitized and normal visceral activity becomes painful.

In contrast to somatic pain, visceral pain can only be poorly localized, and pain from the viscera is often referred to areas of the skin. Since few dichotomizing afferent fibers innervating both skin and viscera have so far been demonstrated (e.g., only <0.5% of the unmyelinated fibers innervating the pelvic viscera send collaterals to the skin [Häbler et al. 1988a]), the main mechanism of pain referral appears to be the convergent projection of visceral primary afferent fibers onto somatic spinal-cord neurons (for a review, see Ness and Gebhart 1990). In fact, visceroceptive-specific neurons may occur, if at all, only rarely in the spinal cord. The convergent projection of visceral afferents is associated with a high degree of divergence, since these afferents make up only 2 to 7% of all primary afferents entering the spinal cord, but innervate up to 75% of the somatic neurons within their areas of termination (Cervero and Tattersall 1985, 1987; Jänig and Morrison 1986).

Ascending Visceroceptive Pathways

Primary afferent fibers innervating visceral organs of the lower abdominal space (urinary bladder, distal colon, and reproductive organs) project via the pelvic and hypogastric nerves to the sacral and lumbar spinal cord. Pelvic afferents, like those of other visceral nerves, terminate mainly in laminae I, II_0, and V to VIII of the spinal cord (de Groat 1986), sharing these laminae with the somatic afferents, which, however, also terminate in laminae II to IV. The somatic response characteristics of viscerosomatic neurons may be of the low-threshold, nociceptive-specific (NS) (i.e., high-threshold), or wide-dynamic-range (WDR) type depending on the viscus involved, the spinal-cord laminae and the species studied. Somatic NS neurons are mainly located in lamina I and WDR neurons in lamina V of the spinal cord. About half of the visceroceptive neurons in the cat and more than two-thirds in the monkey exhibit WDR-type somatic responses; the remaining neurons exhibit similar proportions of low- and high-threshold somatic responses in both species (Ammons et al. 1984a,b, 1985; Cervero and Tattersall 1985, 1987; Brennan et al. 1989).

In accordance with the wide divergence of visceral primary afferent fibers within the spinal cord, information from internal organs travels in a multitude of ascending pathways toward higher levels of the CNS. These include the spinothalamic tract (STT), which is the major pathway of the somatic nociceptive system, as demonstrated by electrical stimulation of visceral nerves (Hancock et al. 1975; Foreman et al. 1981; Rucker and Holloway 1982; Ammons et al. 1984b; Rucker et al. 1984) or natural activation of visceral organs (Milne et al. 1981; Ammons et al. 1984a). Others are the spinomesencephalic (Yezierski and Broton 1991), spinoreticular

(Foreman et al. 1984; Hobbs et al. 1990), and the dorsal column tracts (Rigamonti and Hancock 1978; Hubscher and Berkley 1992). Major visceroceptive relay nuclei in the brain stem are the nucleus of the solitary tract (NTS) and the parabrachial nucleus (PB), which receives part of its input from the NTS. Both nuclei also receive projections from nociceptive regions of the spinal cord (mainly lamina I; Menetrey and Basbaum 1987).

Thalamic Nociceptive Regions

The terminations of the ascending nociceptive pathways are distributed over a range of nuclei of the dorsal thalamus; these are commonly grouped into a medial thalamic region associated with the motivational–affective aspects of pain and a lateral region associated with its sensory–discriminative aspects. The medial region encompasses the mediodorsal nucleus (MD), the nucleus submedius (SM), and some of the intralaminar nuclei, mainly the central lateral nucleus (CL) and the parafascicular (Pf) and subparafascicular (SPf) nuclei. Nociceptive neurons in these nuclei usually exhibit large, often bilateral receptive fields (RFs), and their activity is highly influenced by anesthesia or the sleep/waking cycle (Casey 1966; Dostrovsky and Guilbaud 1988). Stimulation of medial thalamic nuclei in humans elicits diffuse pain sensations with strong affective components (Hassler 1976; Sano 1977).

The lateral thalamic nociceptive region encompasses the posterior complex (PO) and the ventrobasal complex (VB) or its peripheral area (VB_p). The PO is a large area whose anterior extensions envelop the VB at its mediodorsal (POm), dorsal (POd; as defined by Kniffki and Craig 1985), and lateral (PO1) aspects. The PO has long been regarded as the relay center for the sensory–discriminative aspect of somatic pain. Most of its nociceptive neurons have large RFs, in some cases extending over the entire body, and responses in these neurons are elicited by innocuous and noxious stimuli over a wide range of intensities without, however, encoding for these (Curry 1972; Guilbaud et al. 1977a). Representation of the parameters and sites of stimulation for the neuronal responses, as well as their somatotopic organization, are, however, generally the characteristics of CNS relay stations of sensory systems. A more likely candidate for this function in the nociceptive system is therefore the VB or VB_p. In the rat and monkey the lateral part of the VB, the ventral posterolateral (VPL) nucleus, which holds the representation of the low-threshold mechanoreceptors of the postcranial body, in addition to containing the terminations of projections from the dorsal column nuclei, receives projections from the lateral cervical nucleus and the STT (Berkley 1980). The trigeminal part of VB, the ventral posteromedial (VPM) nucleus, receives projections from the corresponding principal and spinal trigeminal nuclei, respectively. Nociceptive neurons with cutaneous RFs are therefore found within VB next to low-threshold mechanosensitive neurons in the rat and monkey. In the cat, STT terminations avoid the VB and aggregate around its periphery (Berkley 1980; Burton and Craig 1983; Craig and

Burton 1985). Here nociceptive neurons with predominantly trigeminal somatic RFs are located medially, within the periphery of VPM (VPM_p), while those with RFs on the postcranial body are found laterally in VPL_p (Honda et al. 1983; Kniffki and Mizumura 1983; Kniffki and Craig 1985; Yokota et al. 1987, 1988); hence, a somatotopic organization is present. Neurons with small RFs and responses encoding the intensity of noxious stimuli also occur within VB_p.

Knowledge about the thalamic processes of visceroception is very limited. Visceral inputs to the medial and/or lateral thalamus have been demonstrated by electrical stimulation of the greater splanchnic, vagal, hypogastric, and pelvic nerves (for references see Brüggemann et al. 1993, 1994b), or by natural activation of visceral receptors (Rogers et al. 1979; Carstens and Yokota 1980; Davis and Dostrovsky 1988; Vahle-Hinz et al. 1989; Brüggemann et al. 1989b, 1993, 1994a; Zagami and Lambert 1990; Chandler et al. 1992). However, the functional role of medial versus lateral thalamic visceroceptive regions, a viscerotopic organization, the stimulus-coding properties of thalamic visceroceptive neurons, and the degree of the somatovisceral convergence at the level of the thalamus remain to be defined.

This chapter reviews the results from studies undertaken to: (a) map the lateral thalamus of the cat with respect to input from a peripheral nerve supplying viscera of the lower abdomen; (b) verify this projection by recording responses of the neurons to natural stimulation of a viscus; (c) determine the somatovisceral convergence present in thalamic neurons; and (d) demonstrate the thalamic projection of a major nucleus of the visceral afferent pathway, the NTS (Brüggemann et al. 1993, 1994b; Vahle-Hinz and Harder 1993).

RESULTS AND DISCUSSION

Visceroceptive Region of the Lateral Thalamus

Mapping of the neuronal activity in response to electrical stimulation of the pelvic nerve results in distributions as shown in Fig. 1. Five electrode penetrations were reconstructed from Nissl-stained frontal sections; the locations of 13 visceroceptive neurons (Fig. 1, filled circles) were determined relative to four electrolytic lesions (open circles) and to their distance to neurons with low-threshold mechanoreceptive fields on the surface of the animal's body. Neurons responding to pelvic nerve stimulation were located in the area around the dorsal, lateral, and ventral aspects of VPL, but not within VPL. Although in the course of the experiments 67 electrode tracks penetrated VPL, and the effect of pelvic nerve stimulation was tested systematically along these tracks, not a single VPL neuron was found to respond to this stimulus.

The visceroceptive area around VPL extends over its periphery (VPL_p) and the dorsal (POd), lateral (PO1), and medial (POm; not present in Fig. 1) parts of the posterior complex. In addition to cytoarchitectonic criteria, these different areas of the lateral thalamus were differentiated by determining the RFs of their neurons to

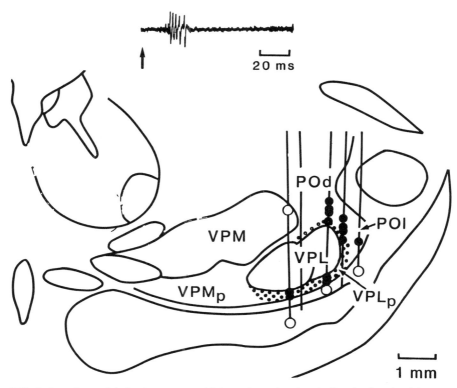

FIG. 1. Locations of thalamic neurons with input from the electrically stimulated pelvic nerve. Reconstruction of the electrode penetrations (*vertical lines*), the locations of recording sites of visceroceptive neurons (*filled circles*), and the locations of electrolytic lesions (*open circles*) made in a single frontal plane through the lateral thalamus of the cat. The nuclear borders were drawn from the Nissl-stained frontal section containing the four electrolytic lesions. The inset shows the registration of a response to electrical stimulation of the pelvic nerve (time marked by *arrow*) of one of the two neurons, which were located ventromedially in VPL_p. POd, POl, and in the dorsal and lateral part of the posterior complex, respectively. VPL = ventral posterolateral nucleus; VPL_p = periphery of the VPL (*stippled area*); VPM = ventral posteromedial nucleus; VPM_p = periphery of the VPM. (Modified from Brüggemann et al. 1994c).

innocuous mechanical stimulation of the body surface (Fig. 2; see also Fig. 5). Within VPL the well-known somatotopic representation of the contralateral half of the body is seen, standing upright with the forelimbs positioned medially and the hindlimbs laterally. The sizes of the RFs are small and decrease further from proximal to distal parts of the limbs. In contrast, the RFs of VPL_p neurons are larger or low-threshold mechanical RFs are absent. RFs of PO neurons are the largest; in 22% of the neurons within visceroceptive regions of PO, these RFs covered almost the entire contralateral side of the postcranial body, and in 8% of cases extended to the ipsilateral side. In a dorsoventral approach through POd, the neuronal RFs are

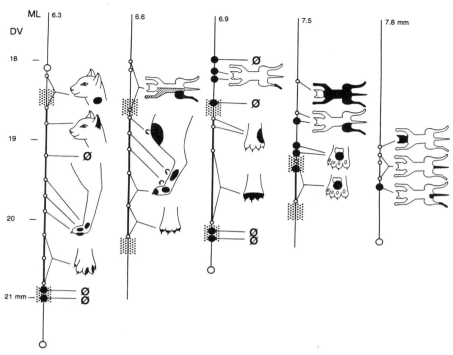

FIG. 2. Low-threshold cutaneous receptive fields (RFs) of neurons encountered in five electrode penetrations through stereotaxic plane A 9. The dorsoventral (DV) and mediolateral (ML) coordinates are given. The 200-μm-wide periphery of VPL (and VPM in the most medial track) above, below, and lateral to the nucleus is indicated by the *stippled areas* along the tracks. Large RFs covering the entire contralateral postcranial surface of the body with a focus on the hindlimb (*stippled* and *black areas* in the figurine, respectively) are shown for PO neurons and one VPL_p neuron (track at ML 6.6). The hindlimb RFs of VPL neurons in the track at ML 6.6 mm were located on the medial aspect of the limb, as indicated by the *curved arrows*. *Filled circles* = recording sites of neurons with input from the pelvic nerve; *large circles* = lesion sites; ∅ = no somatic RF found. Electrophysiologic map of the recording sites that were reconstructed histologically in Fig. 1. (Modified from Brüggemann et al. 1994b.)

seen to run from distal to proximal parts of the body. Thus, in POd there is another, although upside down, representation of the body surface in the lateral thalamus (Kniffki and Craig 1985). In addition, responses to noxious stimulation of cutaneous and subcutaneous tissues are found within VPL_p and PO, but again not within VPL in the case of the cat. Although VPL_p is only a small region (at the most 200 μm wide dorsoventrally), its neurons are not only distinct from those in PO with respect to RF size, but also in their ability to encode the parameters of noxious stimuli. Thus, VPL_p has been associated with processing of the discriminative aspects of nociception (Honda et al. 1983; Kniffki and Mizumura 1983).

Of all neurons with input from the pelvic nerve (n = 68), two-thirds were located

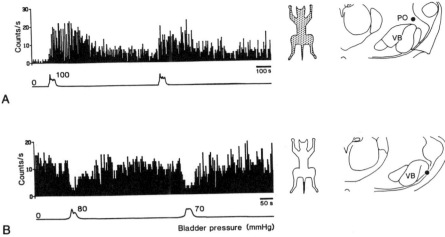

FIG. 3. Excitatory responses of a PO neuron **(A)** and inhibitory responses of a VPL$_p$ neuron **(B)** to bladder distension. Peristimulus-time histograms (bin width: 1 s) and intravesical pressure (lower traces), with baseline and peak values indicated, are shown on the left. The low-threshold cutaneous RFs of the respective neuron (**B**; *black area*) or of the background activity (**A**; *stippled area*) are delineated in the figurines. The locations of the recording sites within POd **(A)** or VPL$_p$ **(B)** are shown in the line drawings made from the histologic sections. (Modified from Brüggemann et al. 1993).

within VPL$_p$ and one-third in PO. When analyzing the rostrocaudal extension of this visceroceptive area, it was found to accompany the middle and caudal part of VPL (see Fig. 1 for a drawing of a frontal section through the caudal VPL), avoiding its rostral pole. Neurons responding to natural stimulation of a viscus (i.e., distension of the urinary bladder) were found in the same area (Fig. 3). In contrast to the neurons with pelvic nerve input, most of the neurons with input from the urinary bladder were located within regions of PO adjoining VPL$_p$. Only four of the 23 neurons responding to bladder stimulation were found in VPL$_p$. Apart from a possible sampling bias, these results may indicate that most VPL$_p$ neurons of this region receive inputs from pelvic viscera other than the urinary bladder. An alternative possibility would be that VPL$_p$ neurons receive a predominant input from a population of visceral afferent fibers that are normally unresponsive and are recruited only when inflammatory processes develop in the internal organs. A substantial proportion (9.5%) of unmyelinated afferent fibers innervating the urinary bladder has in fact been shown to exhibit these properties (Häbler et al. 1988b, 1990). An even larger proportion (54%) of spinal cord neurons with ascending projections had no detectable RF on a viscus, despite being activated by electrical stimulation of the pelvic, hypogastric, and/or lumbar colonic nerves (McMahon and Morrison 1982). These normally silent nociceptors may be sensitized by long-lasting visceral stimulation, and their activation may in turn lead to the sensitization of spinal cord and supraspinal neurons. VPL_p therefore might play a role in chronic aspects of visceral pain.

The distribution of visceroceptive neurons in the area of VPL_p and the adjoining PO was more dense (Figs. 1 and 2), by comparison with the scattered occurrence of visceroceptive neurons in nuclei of the medial thalamus, which included MD, the principal ventromedial nucleus (VMP), CL, center median nucleus (CM), and the paracentral nucleus (PAC) (Brüggemann et al. 1994a). Thus, for example, stimulation of the urinary bladder activated only few (8%) neurons in the medial thalamus of the cat (Vahle-Hinz et al. 1989; Brüggemann et al. 1989b, 1995), while more than twice as many (20%) were found in the lateral thalamus. In one study in monkey, visceroceptive STT neurons also had a preferential projection to the lateral thalamus (84%; Brennan et al. 1989), while another study reported a more even distribution (Ammons et al. 1985). In contrast to the involvement of several medial thalamic nuclei, the lateral visceroceptive region is concentrated in VPL (in the monkey) or PO and VPL_p (in the cat). The sparing of the cat's VPL from visceral inputs was also seen by Taguchi et al. (1987) and Asato and Yokota (1989) with electrical stimulation of visceral nerves. This difference between the cat and monkey, also present in the somatic nociceptive system, may partly be a reflection of the difference in the termination of the STT in the two species (Berkley 1980; Burton and Craig 1983), which underlines the importance of the STT for the transmission of visceroceptive signals.

Lateral as well as medial thalamic regions, however, receive other inputs that may contribute to thalamic visceroception. One of these was shown to originate from the nucleus of the solitary tract (NTS) of the brain stem by neuroanatomic tracing (Fig. 4; Vahle-Hinz and Harder 1993). Biotin-dextran was injected into the rostral part of the NTS on the left side of the brain stem and visualized by avidin-biotin immunohistochemistry using the method of Brandt and Apkarian (1992). The injection site was confined within the nuclear boundaries (Fig. 4A), and most of the tracer was taken up by neuronal somata and transported in an anterograde direction. Some retrogradely labeled neurons, however, were also seen, especially near the level of the injection. This labeling may have derived from *en passant* or cut fibers traversing the injection site. At the thalamic level, labeled fibers as well as terminals were seen, the latter being identified by bouton-like appendages. Terminal arbors were present bilaterally in medial thalamic nuclei, mainly in the mediodorsal nucleus (Fig. 4B), and in the intralaminar nuclei. In the lateral thalamus, terminals were found only contralaterally to the injection site, and were focused in the area dorsal and lateral of the VPL, i.e., within POd, PO1 and VPL_p (Fig. 4B and C). Labeled terminals also extended into the lamina between the medial and lateral subnuclei of VPL. These results show the direct projection of the NTS to the visceroceptive region of the lateral thalamus.

The NTS is viscerotopically organized, with general visceral inputs from the vagal nerve represented in its caudal part (Cechetto 1987; Person 1989). In addition, abdominal viscera project to this region of the NTS, as was shown for renal afferents (Simon and Schramm 1984). Somatovisceral convergence is abundant in

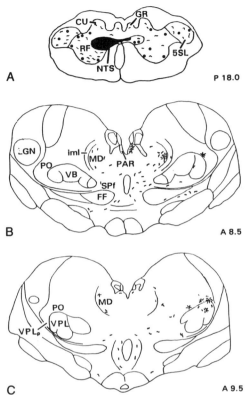

A   P 18.0

B   A 8.5

C   A 9.5

FIG. 4. Thalamic projection of neurons of the nucleus of the solitary tract (NTS). **A:** Injection site of the neuronal tracer biotin-dextran within the NTS in the brain stem (*black area*). *Dots* represent retrogradely labeled neuronal somata. **B, C:** Drawings of labeled terminals in the thalamus. The stereotaxic coordinates of the frontal planes are given on the right. CU = cuneate nucleus; FF = fields of Forel; GR = gracile nucleus; iml = internal medullary lamina; LGN = dorsal lateral geniculate nucleus; MD = mediodorsal nucleus; NTS = nucleus of the solitary tract; PAR = paraventricular nucleus; PO = posterior complex; RF = reticular formation; SPf = subparafascicular nucleus; VB = ventrobasal complex; VPL = ventral posterolateral nucleus; VPL$_p$ = periphery of VPL; 5SL = spinal trigeminal nucleus. (From Vahle-Hinz and Harder 1993).

NTS neurons deriving from direct projections of group I, II, and III afferent fibers, as well as from second-order afferents originating in several laminae of the spinal cord (Menetrey and Basbaum 1987; Person 1989). The major outflow from the NTS is to the parabrachial nucleus, which in turn also projects to the thalamus (Berkley and Scofield 1990). Among the other ascending pathway, the dorsal column medial lemniscal pathway has received more attention with regard to its role in visceroception since Hubscher and Berkley (1992), using natural stimulation of reproductive organs in the rat, showed the high degree of visceral convergence onto low-threshold somatic neurons of the dorsal column nuclei. Since most visceroceptive neurons had low-threshold somatic RFs and were located within VPL—the major target of the medial lemniscal pathway—Brüggemann et al. (1994a) discuss the possibility of this pathway being the major source of the viscerosomatic responses they found in the squirrel monkey's lateral thalamus. Whether the spinocervical tract is also involved in visceroception is still unresolved (Rigamonti and Michelle 1977; Cervero and Iggo 1978; McMahon and Morrison 1982). Fifty-nine percent of the neurons of the feline lateral cervical nucleus (LCN) have been shown to have somatic

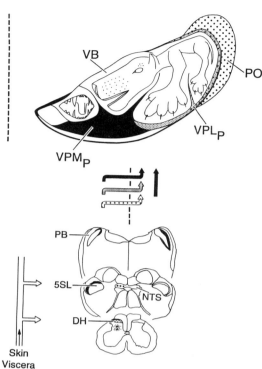

FIG. 5. Schematic overview of ascending inputs to the nociceptive and visceroceptive regions of the cat's lateral thalamus. The ventrobasal complex of the right side of the brain is shown, with its somatotopic map of the representation of the low-threshold mechanoreceptors on the body surface. DH = dorsal horn; NTS = nucleus of the solitary tract; PB = parabrachial nucleus; PO = posterior complex; VB = ventrobasal complex; VPM_p = periphery of the VPM; VPL_p = periphery of the VPL; 5SL = laminar part of the spinal trigeminal nucleus.

nociceptive response properties which, however, may be completely lost under anesthesia (Kajander and Giesler 1987); hence, visceroceptive properties may also be suppressed. Since the LCN projects to VPL_p and the adjoining region of PO, it may provide a source of the low-threshold somatic RFs seen in visceroceptive neurons of the anesthetized cat. Figure 5 gives a schematic overview over spinal cord and brain stem areas contributing to the input to the visceroceptive region in the lateral thalamus of the cat.

Response Properties of Visceroceptive Thalamic Neurons

In our study of the responses of thalamic neurons to natural visceral activation, distension of the urinary bladder was used, which rapidly increased the intravesical pressure to 50 to 70 mmHg. These stimuli were regarded as noxious on two grounds. First, these intensities and rates of distension are generally presumed to produce high-threshold activation of afferent fibers of the urinary bladder (for references see, e.g., Jänig and Morrison 1986; Bahns et al. 1986, 1987; Torrens and Morrison 1987). Second, rapid distension of the human urinary bladder within this pressure range causes severe pain (J. Brüggemann, A. V. Apkarian, and M. A. Turk, unpublished observations). Thalamic neurons in the cat were found to respond to noxious distention of the urinary bladder with increases (Fig. 3A) or decreases (Fig. 3B) in discharge rates. Whereas each of the two sequential excitatory responses of the POd neuron illustrated in Fig. 3A was followed by a long afterdischarge, other neurons more closely encoded the duration of the stimulus in their responses. The experimental stimuli sometimes elicited reflex bladder contractions, as occurred in this case, leading to short peaks in intravesical pressure of up to 100 mmHg. The "inhibitory" effects of urinary bladder distension were seen more often than was excitation in both VPL_p and PO neurons, but with similar reproducibility and short- or long-term changes in discharge. As shown for the VPL_p neuron in Fig. 3B, the relatively high ongoing activity decreased abruptly with the onset of stimulation and resumed shortly after the stimulation ended. There was no indication of a differential distribution within VPL_p or PO of neurons with different response properties to bladder stimulation. The response latencies measured after electrical stimulation of the pelvic nerve were for most thalamic neurons in the range of ≥ 10 to < 20 ms (inset, Fig. 1), indicating a transmission via small- and large-caliber myelinated nerve fibers.

Somatovisceral Convergence Present in Thalamic Neurons

The majority of the neurons in VPL_p and the adjoining PO with input from the pelvic nerve or urinary bladder also had somatic RFs when tested for convergent input from low-threshold somatic mechanoreceptors. Most of the neurons were excited by tap stimuli applied at a slow repetition rate, thus including inputs from cutaneous and "deep" structures. For two-thirds of the neurons with pelvic-nerve and urinary bladder input the RFs were confined to the contralateral part of the body and included the lower back, thigh, tail, and/or the heel, i.e., regions in the dermatomes of sacral and coccygeal spinal cord segments (Smith et al. 1991). RFs confined to the hindfoot, i.e., lower lumbar dermatomes, were present in one-fourth of the neurons with pelvic-nerve input. Large RFs extending over the entire contralateral side of the postcranial body were found more often in PO neurons than in VPL_p neurons; in these cases, however, RF foci were often located on the lower back and proximal hindlimb. Similar numbers of neurons with proximal-lower-body RFs were excited or inhibited by urinary bladder distension, whereas all neurons with large postcranial RFs were inhibited by this stimulus. Half of the neurons with pelvic nerve and bladder input were tested with noxious pinching of the skin in several places on all parts of the body. In particular, VPL_p neurons were tested with noxious somatic stimuli. Neither excitatory nor inhibitory responses were elicited by these stimuli.

These results show that the degree of somatovisceral convergence was very high for the thalamic visceroceptive neurons, and that all somatic inputs were of the low-threshold cutaneous or "deep" mechanosensitive type. This was a surprising finding, because the majority of visceroceptive spinal cord neurons, including those identified as projecting to the thalamus, have been shown to display WDR or multi-receptive somatic response properties in both the cat (Hancock et al. 1975; Guilbaud et al. 1977b; Rucker and Holloway 1982; Cervero 1983; Rucker et al. 1984; Honda 1985; Cervero and Tattersall 1985, 1987) and monkey (Foreman et al. 1981; Milne et al. 1981; Ammons et al. 1984a,b, 1985; Brennan et al. 1989). In addition, NS somatic input is present in a third of the visceroceptive neurons of the cat's dorsal horn (Cervero and Tattersall 1985, 1987) and in up to one-fourth of the visceroceptive STT neurons of the monkey (Foreman et al. 1981; Milne et al. 1981; Ammons et al. 1985; Brennan et al. 1989). Comparison of the results of studies at the spinal-cord level of the cat and monkey suggests species differences in the organization of the STT visceroceptive pathway. Among the three categories of somatic input to visceroceptive neurons, both the low-threshold and NS inputs occur about twice as often in the cat as in the monkey, in which about three-fourths of the neurons receive WDR inputs. It may be inferred, therefore, that somatic low-threshold and NS properties may also be more abundant in visceroceptive neurons at the thalamic level of the cat. The results of studies on visceroceptive thalamic neurons so far are conflicting. Whereas Chandler et al. (1992) reported values similar to those for STT neurons in the relative occurrence of WDR and NS as well as low-threshold/deep-somatic inputs to VPL neurons of the macaque monkey, the majority of visceroceptive VPL neurons in the squirrel monkey (Brüggemann et al. 1992, 1994a) and the rat (Berkley et al. 1993a) had low-threshold somatic RFs similar to our results in the thalamus of the cat. This may indicate a general shift in response properties of visceroceptive neurons recorded at the thalamic level as compared to those recorded in the spinal cord in all three species.

The finding that most of the lateral thalamic visceroceptive neurons exhibit convergent low-threshold somatic inputs is also consistent with neurosurgical reports. Electrical stimulation of the somatosensory thalamus generally elicits pure somatic, nonpainful sensations in awake humans who do not have a chronic pain syndrome (Dostrovsky et al. 1991; Lenz et al. 1993; see also Chapter 11). In a patient with chronic leg pain and angina pectoris, however, electrical stimulation in the lateral thalamus elicited both the perception of pain in the leg and the sensation of visceral pain. Reproduction of the visceral pain was unaccompanied by any of the pathologic processes that would normally accompany angina pectoris (Lenz and Dougherty, Chapter 11). This favors the idea that the strength of the synaptic connectivity of the somatosensory thalamus reorganizes during chronic pathologic processes.

Employing stimulation of several visceral organs, neither Berkley et al. (1993a) nor Brüggemann et al. (1994a) could detect a viscerotopic organization within the lateral thalamus. On the basis of their findings and reports by others, Brüggemann et al. (1994a) proposed that the same population of neurons used two different coding strategies for visceral and somatic inputs: a distributed population code for visceral inputs with highly overlapping RFs and a localized code for somatic inputs with only partially overlapping RFs, where only a small number of neurons is activated from a small RF. This interpretation led Brüggemann et al. (1994a) to a new model for referred pain. In brief, they propose that the highly distributed, seemingly nontopographic visceral input via the dorsal column pathway leads to poorly localizable visceral sensations. With repeated and intense visceral stimulation (e.g., during inflammation), the localized visceral inputs mediated by the STT, which are normally overridden by the somatic inputs from the dorsal column pathway, become potentiated and activate a local group of thalamic neurons. This localized activation results in a somatic perception (i.e., referred pain) superimposed on the dull visceral pain.

ACKNOWLEDGMENTS

Our experimental work described here was supported by grants from the Deutsche Forschungsgemeinschaft (Schwerpunktprogramm "Nociception und Schmerz").

REFERENCES

Ammons WS, Blair RW, Foreman RD. Responses of primate T_1-T_5 spinothalamic neurons to gallbladder distension. *Am J Physiol* 1984a;247:R995–R1002.

Ammons WS, Blair RW, Foreman RD. Greater splanchnic excitation of primate T_1-T_5 spinothalamic neurons. *J Neurophysiol* 1984b;51:592–603.

Ammons WS, Girardot M-N, Foreman RD. T_2-T_5 spinothalamic neurons projecting to medial thalamus with viscerosomatic input. *J Neurophysiol* 1985;54:73–89.

Asato F, Yokota T. Responses of neurons in nucleus ventralis posterolateralis of the cat thalamus to hypogastric inputs. *Brain Res* 1989;488:135–142.

Bahns E, Ernsberger U, Jänig W, Nelke A. Functional characteristics of lumbar visceral afferent fibers from urinary bladder and urethra in the cat. *Pflügers Arch* 1986;407:510–518.

Bahns E, Halsband U, Jänig W. Responses of sacral visceral afferents from the lower urinary tract, colon and anus to mechanical stimulation. *Pflügers Arch* 1987;410:296–303.

Berkley KJ. Spatial relationships between the terminations of somatic sensory and motor pathways in the rostral brainstem of cats and monkeys. I. Ascending somatic sensory inputs to lateral diencephalon. *J Comp Neurol* 1980;193:283–317.

Berkley KJ, Guilbaud G, Benoist JM, Gautron M. Responses of neurons in and near the thalamic ventrobasal complex of the rat to stimulation of uterus, cervix, vagina, colon, and skin. *J Neurophysiol* 1993a;69:557–568.

Berkley KJ, Hubscher CH, Wall PD. Neuronal responses to stimulation of the cervix, uterus, colon, and skin in the rat spinal cord. *J Neurophysiol* 1993b;69:545–556.

Berkley KJ, Scofield SL. Relays from the spinal cord and solitary nucleus through the parabrachial nucleus to the forebrain in the cat. *Brain Res* 1990;529:333–338.

Berman AL, Jones EG. *The thalamus and basal telencephalon of the cat. A cytoarchitectonic atlas with stereotaxic coordinates.* Madison, WI: University of Wisconsin Press, 1982.

Brandt HM, Apkarian AV. Biotin-dextran: a sensitive anterograde tracer for neuroanatomic studies in rat and monkey. *J Neurosci Methods* 1992;45:35–40.

Brennan TJ, Oh UT, Hobbs SF, Garrison DW, Foreman RD. Urinary bladder and hindlimb afferent input inhibits activity of primate T_2-T_5 spinothalamic tract neurons. *J Neurophysiol* 1989;61:573–588.

Brüggemann J, Apkarian AV, Cechetto DF, Mengel MKC, Vahle-Hinz C, Kniffki K-D. Splanchnic and vagal inputs to the medial region of the cat's thalamus. *Proc Int Union Physiol Sci* 1989a;17:97.

Brüggemann J, Apkarian AV, Cechetto DF, Mengel MKC, Vahle-Hinz C, Kniffki K-D. Viscero-somatic convergence in the medial region of the cat's thalamus. *Soc Neurosci Abstr* 1989b;15:1265.

Brüggemann J, Shi T, Apkarian AV. Squirrel monkey lateral thalamus: II. Viscero-somatic convergent representation of urinary bladder, colon and esophagus. *J Neurosci* 1994a;14:6796–6814.

Brüggemann J, Shi T, Stea RA, Stevens RT, Apkarian AV. Representation of bladder, colon and esophagus in the lateral thalamus of the squirrel monkey. *Soc Neurosci Abstr* 1992;18:495.

Brüggemann J, Vahle-Hinz C, Apkarian AV, Kniffki K-D. Somato-visceral convergence in thalamic regions of the cat. *J Neurophysiol* 1995;(*in press*).

Brüggemann J, Vahle-Hinz C, Kniffki K-D. Representation of the urinary bladder in the lateral thalamus of the cat. *J Neurophysiol* 1993;70:482–491.

Brüggemann J, Vahle-Hinz C, Kniffki K-D. Projections from the pelvic nerve to the periphery of the cat's thalamic ventral posterolateral nucleus and adjacent regions of the posterior complex. *J Neurophysiol* 1994b;72:2237–2245.

Burton H, Craig AD. Spinothalamic projections in cat, raccoon and monkey: A study based on anterograde transport of horseradish peroxidase. In: Macchi G, Rustioni A, Spreafico R, eds. *Somatosensory integration in the thalamus*. New York: Elsevier, 1983;17–41.

Carstens E, Yokota T. Viscerosomatic convergence and responses to intestinal distension of neurons at the junction of midbrain and posterior thalamus in the cat. *Exp Neurol* 1980;70:392–402.

Casey KL. Unit analysis of nociceptive mechanisms in the thalamus of the awake squirrel monkey. *J Neurophysiol* 1966;29:727–750.

Cechetto D. Central representation of visceral function. *Fed Proc* 1987;46:17–23.

Cervero F. Somatic and visceral inputs to the thoracic spinal cord of the cat: effects of noxious stimulation of the biliary system. *J Physiol (Lond)* 1983;337:51–67.

Cervero F. Visceral pain. In: Dubner R, Gebhart GF, Bond MR, eds. *Proceedings of the 5th world congress on pain: pain research and clinical management*, vol. 3. Amsterdam: Elsevier, 1988; 216–226.

Cervero F, Iggo A. Natural stimulation of urinary bladder afferents does not affect transmission through lumbosacral spinocervical tract neurones in the cat. *Brain Res* 1978;156:375–379.

Cervero F, Jänig W. Visceral nociceptors: a new world order? *Trends Neurosci* 1992;15:374–378.

Cervero F, Tattersall JEH. Cutaneous receptive fields of somatic and viscero-somatic neurons in the thoracic spinal cord of the cat. *J Comp Neurol* 1985;237:325–332.

Cervero F, Tattersall JEH. Somatic and visceral inputs to the thoracic spinal cord of the cat: marginal zone (lamina I) of the dorsal horn. *J Physiol (Lond)* 1987;388:383–395.

Chandler MJ, Hobbs SF, Fu Q-G, Kenshalo DR Jr, Blair RW, Foreman RD. Responses of neurons in ventroposterolateral nucleus of primate thalamus to urinary bladder distension. *Brain Res* 1992; 571:26–34.

Craig AD, Burton H. The distribution and topographical organization in the thalamus of anterogradely-transported horseradish peroxidase after spinal injections in cat and raccoon. *Exp Brain Res* 1985; 58:227–254.

Curry MJ. The exteroceptive properties of neurones in the somatic part of the posterior group (PO). *Brain Res* 1972;44:439–462.

Davis KD, Dostrovsky JO. Properties of feline thalamic neurons activated by stimulation of the middle meningeal artery and sagittal sinus. *Brain Res* 1988;446:401–406.

de Groat WC. Spinal cord projections and neuropeptides in visceral afferent neurons. In: Cervero F, Morrison JFV, eds. *Visceral sensation: progress in brain research*, vol. 67. Amsterdam: Elsevier, 1986;165–181.

Dostrovsky JO, Guilbaud G. Noxious stimuli excite neurons in nucleus submedius of the normal and arthritic rat. *Brain Res* 1988;460:269–280.

Dostrovsky JO, Wells FEB, Tasker RR. Pain evoked by stimulation in human thalamus. In: Sjigenaga Y, ed. *International Symposium on Processing Nociceptive Information*. Amsterdam: Elsevier, 1991.

Foreman RD, Blair RW, Weber RN. Viscerosomatic convergence onto T_2-T_4 spinoreticular, spinoreticular-spinothalamic, and spinothalamic tract neurons in the cat. *Exp Neurol* 1984;85:597–619.

Foreman RD, Hancock MB, Willis WD. Responses of spinothalamic tract cells in the thoracic spinal cord of the monkey to cutaneous and visceral inputs. *Pain* 1981;11:149–162.

Guilbaud G, Caille D, Besson JM, Benelli G. Single units activities in ventral posterior and posterior group thalamic nuclei during nociceptive and non-nociceptive stimulations in the cat. *Arch Ital Biol* 1977a;115:38–56.

Guilbaud G, Benelli G, Besson JM. Responses of thoracic dorsal horn interneurones to cutaneous stimulation and the administration of algogenic substances into the mesenteric artery in the spinal cat. *Brain Res* 1977b;124:437–448.

Häbler H-J, Jänig W, Koltzenburg M. Dichotomizing unmyelinated afferents supplying pelvic viscera and perineum are rare in the sacral segments of the cat. *Neurosci Lett* 1988a;94:119–124.

Häbler H-J, Jänig W, Koltzenburg M. A novel type of unmyelinated chemosensitive nociceptor in the acutely inflamed urinary bladder. *Agents Actions* 1988b;25:219–221.

Häbler H-J, Jänig W, Koltzenburg M. Activation of unmyelinated afferent fibers by mechanical stimuli and inflammation of the urinary bladder in the cat. *J Physiol* 1990;425:545–562.

Hancock MB, Rigamonti DD, Bryan RN. Convergence of visceral and cutaneous input onto spinothalamic tract cells in the thoracic spinal cord of the cat. *Exp Neurol* 1975;47:240–248.

Hassler R. Wechselwirkungen zwischen dem System der schnellen Schmerzempfindung und dem des langsamen, nachhaltigen Schmerzgefühls. *Langenbecks Arch Chir* 1976;342:47–61.

Hobbs SF, Oh UT, Brennan TJ, Chandler MJ, Kim KS, Foreman RD. Urinary bladder and hindlimb stimuli inhibit T_1-T_6 spinal and spinoreticular cells. *Am J Physiol* 1990;258:R10–R20.

Honda CN. Visceral and somatic afferent convergence onto neurons near the central canal in the sacral spinal cord of the cat. *J Neurophysiol* 1985;53:1059–1078.

Honda CN, Mense S, Perl ER. Neurons in the ventrobasal region of cat thalamus selectively responsive to noxious mechanical stimulation. *J Neurophysiol* 1983;49:662–673.

Hubscher CH, Berkley KJ. Neuronal responses to stimulation of uterus, cervix and vaginal canal in rat gracile nucleus. *Soc Neurosci Abstr* 1992;18:494.

Jänig W, Morrison JFB. Functional properties of spinal visceral afferents supplying abdominal and pelvic organs, with special emphasis on visceral nociception. In: Cervero F, Morrison JFB, eds. *Visceral sensation: progress in brain research* vol. 67. Amsterdam: Elsevier, 1986;87–114.

Kajander KC, Giesler GJ Jr. Responses of neurons in the lateral cervical nucleus of cat to noxious cutaneous stimulation. *J Neurophysiol* 1987;57:1686–1704.

Kniffki K-D, Craig AD. The distribution of nociceptive neurons in the cat's lateral thalamus: The dorsal and ventral periphery of VPL. In: Rowe M, Willis WD, eds. *Development, organization, and processing in somatosensory pathways*. New York: Alan R. Liss, 1985;375–382.

Kniffki K-D, Mizumura K. Responses of neurons in VPL and VPL-VL region of the cat to algesic stimulation of muscle and tendon. *J Neurophysiol* 1983;49:649–661.

Lenz FA, Seike M, Richardson RT, Lin YC, Baker FH, Khoja I, Jaeger CJ, Gracely RH. Thermal and pain sensations evoked by microstimulation in the area of human ventrocaudal nucleus. *J Neurophysiol* 1993;70:200–212.

McMahon SB, Morrison JFB. Spinal neurones with long projections activated from the abdominal viscera of the cat. *J Physiol* 1982;322:1–20.

Menetrey D, Basbaum AI. The distribution of substance P-, enkephalin- and dynorphin-immunoreactive neurons in the medulla of the rat and their contribution to bulbospinal pathways. *Neuroscience* 1987;23:173–187.

Milne, RJ, Foreman RD, Giesler GJ, Jr, Willis WD. Convergence of cutaneous and pelvic visceral nociceptive inputs onto primate spinothalamic neurons. *Pain* 1981;11:163–183.

Ness TJ, Gebhart GF. Visceral pain: a review of experimental studies. *Pain* 1990;41:167–234.

Person RJ. Somatic and vagal afferent convergence on solitary tract neurons in cat: electrophysiological characteristics. *Neuroscience* 1989;30:283–295.

Rigamonti DD, De Michelle D. Visceral afferent projection to the lateral cervical nucleus. In: Brooks, FP, Evans, PW, eds. *Nerves and the gut*. Thorofare, NJ: Charles B. Slack, 1977;327–333.

Rigamonti DD, Hancock MB. Viscerosomatic convergence in the dorsal column nuclei of the cat. *Exp Neurol* 1978;61:337–348.

Rogers RC, Novin D, Butcher LL. Hepatic sodium and osmoreceptors activate neurons in the ventrobasal thalamus. *Brain Res* 1979;168:398–403.

Rucker HK, Holloway JA. Viscerosomatic convergence onto spinothalamic tract neurons in the cat. *Brain Res* 1982;243:155–157.

Rucker HK, Holloway JA, Keyser GF. Response characteristics of cat spinothalamic tract neurons to splanchnic nerve stimulation. *Brain Res* 1984;291:383–387.

Sano K. Intralaminar thalamotomy (thalamolaminotomy) and postero-medial hypothalamotomy in the treatment of intractable pain. *Prog Neurol Surg* 1977;8:50–103.

Schaible H-G, Schmidt RF. Time course of mechanosensitivity changes in articular afferents during a developing experimental arthritis. *J Neurophysiol* 1988;60:2180–2195.

Sengupta JN, Kauvar D, Goyal RK. Characteristics of vagal esophageal tension-sensitive afferent fibers in the opossum. *J Neurophysiol* 1989;61:1001–1010.

Sengupta JN, Saha JK, Goyal RK. Stimulus-response function studies of esophageal mechanosensitive nociceptors in sympathetic afferents of opossum. *J Neurophysiol* 1990;64:796–812.

Simon OR, Schramm LP. The spinal course and medullary termination of myelinated renal afferents in the rat. *Brain Res* 1984;290:239–247.

Smith MV, Apkarian AV, Hodge CJ Jr. Somatosensory response properties of contralaterally projecting spinothalamic and nonspinothalamic neurons in the second cervical segment of the cat. *J Neurophysiol* 1991;66:83–102.

Taguchi H, Masuda T, Yokota T. Cardiac sympathetic afferent input onto neurons in nucleus ventralis posterolateralis in cat thalamus. *Brain Res* 1987;436:240–252.

Torrens M, Morrison JFB. *The physiology of the lower urinary tract*. Berlin: Springer, 1987; pp.

Vahle-Hinz C, Harder D. Thalamic projections of the nucleus tractus solitarii (NTS) in the cat. *Abstracts of the 7th world congress on pain*. Seattle: ASP Publications 1993;259.

Vahle-Hinz C, Apkarian AV, Brüggemann J, Kniffki K-D, Mengel MKC. Thalamic sites of autonomic regulation of orofacial nociception: Mediodorsal nucleus (MD) and periphery of the ventrobasal complex (VB$_p$). *Proc Finn Dent Soc* 1989;85:40.

Willis WD. *The pain system. The neural basis of nociceptive transmission in the mammalian nervous system*. Basel: Karger, 1985.

Yezierski RP, Broton JG. Functional properties of spinomesencephalic tract (SMT) cells in the upper cervical spinal cord of the cat. *Pain* 1991;45:187–196.

Yokota T, Asato F, Koyama N, Masuda T, Taguchi H. Nociceptive body representation in nucleus ventralis posterolateralis of cat thalamus. *J Neurophysiol* 1988;60:1714–1727.

Yokota T, Masuda T, Taguchi H, Koyama N. Viscerosomatic convergence onto nociceptive neurons in the shell region of nucleus ventralis posterolateralis. In: Schmidt RF, Schaible H-G, Vahle-Hinz C, eds. *Fine afferent nerve fibers and pain*. Weinheim: VCH Verlagsgesellschaft, 1987;427–437.

Zagami AS, Lambert GA. Stimulation of cranial vessels excites nociceptive neurones in several thalamic nuclei of the cat. *Exp Brain Res* 1990;81:552–566.

*Pain and the Brain: From
Nociception to Cognition,*
edited by Burkhart Bromm and
John E. Desmedt, Advances in Pain
Research and Therapy Vol. 22.
Raven Press, Ltd., New York © 1995.

10

The Use of Microelectrodes in the Human Brain

Ronald R. Tasker

*Division of Neurosurgery, The Toronto Hospital, Western Division,
Toronto, Ontario M5T 2S8, Canada*

SUMMARY

Microelectrode studies have been done in a variety of structures in the human brain in order to help the surgeon localize brain sites to be manipulated for the control of chronic pain, movement disorder, epilepsy, and psychiatric illness, particularly using stereotactic approaches. Such studies have not only accomplished their purposes but have also provided discrete information about the organization of normal brain structures, particularly somatosensory pathways. They have also cast light on pathologic brain function, such as mechanisms of tremor and chronic pain. Such "bench-to-bedside" applications of contemporary laboratory techniques offers hope of an increasingly better understanding of both disease and methods to control it.

INTRODUCTION

The now well-established technique of microelectrode recording of the activities of single cells in the laboratory is still recent enough that I can remember its beginning. The application of the technology to humans, on the one hand for physiologic localization during epilepsy and functional stereotactic surgery, and on the other for the study of normal and pathologic states of the nervous system, was slow in coming.

According to Redfern (1989), Wetzel and Snider (1958) were the first to use microelectrode recording in humans during pallidotomy. Various human applications soon followed, the technique being put into routine service in a number of centers by such investigators as Albe-Fessard and Guiot, Narabayashi and Ohye, Jasper and Bertrand, and, more recently, by ourselves. (Albe-Fessard 1973, 1974; Albe-Fessard et al. 1962, 1963a, 1963b, 1966a, 1966b, 1967; Arutjunov et al. 1970; Bates 1969, 1972; Bertrand et al. 1973; Bertrand and Jasper 1965; Bertrand et

TABLE 1. *Comparison of electrical stimulation and microelectrode recording for physiologic corroboration of target site during functional neurosurgery*

	Stimulation		Recording	
	Macroelectrode	Microelectrode	Low Impedance	High Impedance
Safety	Medium can deliver high output accidentally	High	High	High
Speed of exploration	Rapid	Medium	Medium	Slow
Sophistication of backup, potential for technical problems	Low	Medium	Medium	High
Ruggedness for repeated use	High	Medium	Medium	Lower
Possibility of recording and stimulating with same electrode	No	Yes	Yes	Yes
Need for patient cooperation	Yes	Yes	No	No
Variety of structures identified	High	High	Medium	Medium
Degree of functional compartmentalization	Low	Medium	Medium	High
Ability to detect somatotopography	Low	Medium	Medium	High
Chance of not obtaining a physiologic response on a given trajectory	Low	Medium	Medium	High
Spatial definition	± 2 mm	? <1 mm	<1 mm	Microns
Ability to detect pathologic processes	Low	Low	High	High

al. 1967, 1969; Carreras et al. 1967; Donaldson 1973; Fukamachi et al. 1973; Gaze et al. 1964; Gillingham 1966; Guiot et al. 1962, 1973; Hardy et al. 1979a, 1980b; Jasper 1966; Jasper and Bertrand 1963; Kelly et al. 1987; Ohye 1982; Tasker et al. 1986, 1987a,b, 1988)

Two types of microelectrodes have been employed in humans: semimicroelectrodes capable of recording the activity of multiple neurons and having the advantage of being rugged and largely insusceptible to electronic noise, and true microelectrodes capable of discriminating the action potentials of individual neurons.

The techniques used, which have been previously reported (see above), are similar to those used in the laboratory and will not be reiterated. Both types of electrode can be used alternately for recording and stimulation, thus increasing their value for physiologic localization.

This symposium is organized to explore the transition of pain from nociception to conscious awareness, and this chapter explores the use of microelectrode recordings in humans and their bearing on this issue. I will first summarize the findings made using microelectrodes in humans, including those concerned with somatosensory function and pain, and will then summarize the findings bearing on pain perception.

Microelectrode data consist of two bodies of information: that concerning the normal physiologic anatomy of the brain and that concerning pathologic processes.

Both have evolved from the use of microelectrode recordings for physiologic localization during functional, usually stereotactic, neurosurgery, either to verify that a probe has reached the intended target or to avoid damaging important neighborhood structures. In this capacity the use of microelectrodes competes with that of electrical stimulation; the use of both techniques together yields the best of both worlds. Table 1 compares the two techniques.

NORMAL PHYSIOLOGIC ANATOMY

Microelectrode recordings have been made in the cerebral cortex, mesencephalic tegmentum, cingulum, caudate, putamen, globus pallidus, optic tract, medial geniculate nucleus, pulvinar, and medial and lateral thalamus. Table 2 summarizes the responses recorded and, where known, the effects achieved by stimulation at the same site, as well as the application for that information. A summary of stimulation-induced responses can be found in the stereotactic atlas written by Schaltenbrand and Wahren (1977) and in Tasker et al. (1982).

Cerebral Neocortex

Recording in the cortex has been used fairly extensively for localization during epilepsy surgery. Comments relating to both normal and epileptic processes will be reviewed together. Li and Van Buren (1964, 1972; Li et al. 1965) studied cortical activity in epileptic patients, including four with continual epileptic discharges on electroencephalography (EEG) who showed trains of spike discharges with the absence of actual seizures. Rayport (1972) made a number of interesting observations in the neocortex and amygdala, hippocampus, and deep neocortex. During EEG alerting (desynchronization), he found that certain neurons ceased firing. Some neurons with what Rayport termed "pseudorhythmic" firing patterns became rhythmic in association with an EEG ictus. Using two cortical pipette electrodes simultaneously, he noted that neurons fired synchronously in response to EEG activation with pentylenetetrazol, and concluded that hypersynchronization was associated with an epileptic ictus. As an EEG spike occurred, different cortical neurons showed differing activities, consisting of the cessation of firing, increased firing, or no change.

Calvin (1972), in commenting on Rayport's paper, demonstrated neuronal burst activity associated with an EEG spike.

I will not further pursue the discussion of microelectrode studies of epileptic foci, since none of this work is known to impinge specifically on pain perception, and because pain induced by epileptic seizures is surprisingly rare.

Studies of normal cortical function have been pursued in great detail, particularly by Ojemann's group (Haglund et al. 1993; Ojemann 1990; Ojemann et al. 1992; Creutzfeld et al. 1989a,b,c). These investigators have been particularly interested in single-unit responses in temporal-lobe areas later to be resected. They have identi-

TABLE 2. *Results of electrical stimulation and recording in the brain*

Probable structure	Microelectrode recording	Stimulation-induced response	Application
Ventrocaudal nucleus	Tactile cells	Paresthesiae	DBS
Medial lemniscus	Nil	Paresthesiae	DBS
Sensory radiations	Nil	Paresthesiae	DBS
Ventral intermediate nucleus	Kinesthetic cells	Paresthesiae or a sense of movement, occasionally vertigo	Thalamotomy for dyskinesia
Posterior ventral oral nucleus	Voluntary cells	Movement at onset of stimulus train	Thalamotomy for dyskinesia
Spinothalamic tract including Vcpc	Rarely nociceptors	Warmth, coolness	Thalamotomy or tractotomy for pain
Cingulum	Rarely nociceptors	Various	Cingulotomy
Medial thalamus including thalamic lamina	Rarely nociceptors	Nil; sometimes burning in patients with neuropathic pain	Thalamotomy for pain
Internal capsule, peduncle, motor cranial nerves	Nil	Tetanization	Avoid these structures
Hypothalamus	Unidentified	Various autonomic, eye movements	Hypothalamotomy
Medial geniculate nucleus	Auditory cells	Buzzing, sometimes vertigo	Avoid structure
Lateral lemniscus	Nil	Buzzing, sometimes vertigo	Avoid structure
Optic tract, lateral geniculate	Light-sensitive neurons	Colored phosphenes	Avoid structure
Tectopulvinar tract	Unidentified	White phosphenes; obscuration of vision	Avoid structure
Central tegmental tract	Nil	Eye movements	Avoid structure
Medial longitudinal lemniscus	Nil	Eye movements	Avoid structure
Dorsomedian nucleus	Bursting cells	Nil	Localizing DBS for pain in PVG
PVG, parafascicular nucleus	Unidentified	Various: warmth, sense of satiety, pleasure, or nil	DBS
PAG	Unidentified	Various: sense of horror, discomfort, or nil	DBS
Cerebral cortex	Various	Various	Epilepsy and tumor surgery
Globus pallidus	Cells related to movement	Uncertain	Pallidotomy
Caudate	Cells related to movement	Uncertain	Pallidotomy; tissue implants
Putamen	Cells related to movement	Uncertain	Tissue implants
Reticular nucleus of thalamus	Cells related to movement	Uncertain	Probably avoid structure

fied specific areas related to particular components of speech, such as naming, as well as to functions such as face matching and the naming of objects and emotional expressions. For example, neurons in the superior temporal gyrus on both the dominant and nondominant side change their firing pattern, usually increasing their rate of firing, according to the phonetic but not the semantic aspects of spoken and heard speech; such responses are not seen in the middle or inferior temporal gyri. In polyphasic subjects, neurons were found that responded only to one language while neighboring cells responded to another. Such responses were peculiar to speech, and did not occur with other types of sound. All three gyri responded similarly to music.

Unusual somatosensory responses not seen in subcortical structures occurred in the neocortex, such as in neurons sensitive to skin stimulation in particular directions.

Although there appears to be a dearth of observations related to pain perception through nociceptive pathways in humans, it might well be profitable to use the technique of recording in association cortex to study pain perception in those rare patients with intractable pain who, for other reasons, undergo a wake craniotomy.

The Cingulum and Cingulate Cortex

Hutchison et al. (1993) and Davis et al. (1993) recorded neurons in the cingulate cortex with wide bilateral receptive fields (RFs) that responded to noxious stimuli during a cingulotomy done to relieve pain in a patient with a schizoaffective disorder. The authors noted that up to 3 months after bilateral cingulotomy the patient's rating of innocuous warm stimuli was diminished, while that of noxious heat and of cold was increased compared with these ratings in the preoperative assessment. Implication of the cingulum and cingulate cortex in pain perception is traditional in neurosurgery, and in conformity with the observations of Talbot et al. (1991), who showed that nociceptive stimuli caused activation of the parietal and cingulate cortex and thalamus as demonstrated by positron-emission tomography (PET).

Subcortical Structures

The Somatosensory System

Pain and Temperature Pathways

We have found the recording of pain and temperature neurons to be elusive.

Hitchcock and Lewin (1969) recorded increased cellular activity in the cuneate fasciculus, gracile fasciculus, caudal trigeminal nucleus, and spinothalamic tract (STT) in three patients in response to ipsilateral stimulation of the limbs and face, and (presumably contralateral) painful stimuli during percutaneous cordotomy.

Amano et al. (1978) have recorded neuronal activity with widespread bilateral

RFs responsive to nociceptive stimuli in the mesencephalic reticular formation (14.5 mm posterior to the middle of the anterior [AC] posterior [PC] commissure line, and 8 mm lateral to and 10 mm below the AC–PC line) in the course of a tractotomy for pain. The neurons were small and showed responses to pinprick with latencies in three ranges: <250, 400 to 800, and >1,000 msec. In our experience, stimulation at such sites usually elicits no conscious response, whereas stimulation in the nearby STT induces somatotopographically distributed feelings of warmth or coolness contralaterally.

Modesti and Waszac (1975) have recorded spontaneous activity in the medial thalamus. This was statistically significantly decreased by dorsal-column stimulation (DCS), although the temporal pattern and durations of the suppression with respect to the period of DCS varied. Four neurons showed a 1- to 3-sec increase in firing rate after the end of a bout of DCS. No neurons responded to electrical stimulation of the median nerve or to natural tactile or kinesthetic stimuli.

Sano and associates (Sano 1977; Sano et al. 1966; Ishijima et al. 1975) recorded a variety of neurons in the medial thalamus. None of 75 neurons in the dorsomedian nucleus (DM) or 35 neurons in the pretectal area responded to painful stimuli, but 20 of 80 neurons in the centromedian (CM) and parafascicular (Pf) nuclei responded to pinprick and two responded to heat. The nociceptors were of two types. The first, or type "A," had responses of short latency (30–90 msec) and short duration (150–300 msec) and were located in the medial and basal Pf nuclei; the second, or type "B," had longer (100–500 msec), more variable latencies and fluctuating lengthy (1–2 sec) responses, and were located in the CM and dorsal Pf nuclei. The type A neurons seemed to involve pathways conducting at 16 to 20 msec and had higher thresholds than the type B cells. One type A and one type B cell responded to heat stimuli. They had extensive bilateral RFs, although their responses to ipsilateral stimuli were weaker. Contra- or ipsilateral stimulation, especially in the posterior Pf nucleus, tended to increase existing pain or to produce contralateral burning pain. With more rostral stimulation, unpleasant, nonlocalized responses were evoked.

Lenz and associates (Seike et al. 1991; Lenz et al. 1993) have recorded cells, apparently in Hassler's parvicellular ventrocaudal nucleus (Hassler 1972), which is thought to be a relay for STT, that responded to noxious heat stimuli at sites where thermal sensations and pain can readily be elicited by macro- and microstimulation (Tasker et al. 1982; Dostrovsky et al. 1992; Halliday and Logue 1972).

The Muscle Spindle and Lemniscal Pathways

It has so far been impossible to distinguish the spindle and kinesthetic lemniscal pathways from one another physiologically in the human brain, although the separation between tactile and kinesthetic pathways can readily be made.

Tactile Pathway

The best-recognized structure in human microelectrode recording is the lemniscal tactile pathway. (Bertrand et al. 1967; Hardy et al. 1979b,c, 1981; Lenz et al. 1988a; Ohye et al. 1972) In its relay nucleus in the ventrocaudal nucleus (Vc), large neurons can readily be recognized that fire in response to hair bending or light touching, with either phasically and tonically responding neurons intermingled. The responses of these cells show no habituation and faithfully follow rapidly repeated stimuli. Their RFs may be minute (a millimeter or two in diameter), particularly on the lips and radial manual digits, and they are exquisitely arranged in a medial-lateral somatotopographic homunculus whose major components are representations of the lips and manual digits (66% of the neurons). The intraoral and other facial sites occupy a tiny area about 10 to 11 mm from the midline, while the area for the lips extends from 11 to 13 mm, that for the manual digits from 13 to 15 mm, and that for the upper limbs, trunk, and lower limbs from 15 to 17 mm from the midline on the average. Because of their minor representation, and the limited number of trajectories that can be made in any one patient, it is difficult to determine accurately the somatotopic organization of parts of the head, trunk, and proximal limbs with respect to that of the face and hands.

Neurons representing a particular bodily structure are arranged in stacks of laterally convex lamellae, so that an imaginary electrode traveling parasagittally and anteroposteriorly or superoinferiorly would encounter a long series of neurons with similar RFs except that at the superior and inferior extremes, RFs in more medial portions of the homunculus would be found. Trajectories made in a lateral-to-medial direction would encounter continually changing RFs (Fig. 1).

Stimulation of the sites at which tactile neurons are identified elicits paresthesiae with projected fields (PFs) that are often identical to the neurons' RFs. However, RF-PF mismatch is also seen, and is difficult to explain unless it results from the stimulation of clusters of fibers passing near the neurons.

Recording in thalamic radiations of the medial lemniscus with electrodes of the tip size used in human work is usually unrewarding.

To my knowledge, there has never been a suitable postmortem examination of a patient carefully explored with microelectrodes, and the conclusion that tactile neurons occur in the inferior 5 mm of Vc is therefore conjectural. Tactile RFs are contralateral to their neurons, except for occasional bilateral responses in the lips.

Kinesthetic Pathway

The pathway for spindle afferents whose activity may enter consciousness (Goto et al. 1968), and that subserve deep pressure and joint and muscle sense, can be readily identified with microelectrode recording, but not with electrical stimulation, and has been extensively studied (Bertrand et al. 1969; Hardy et al. 1980a,b,c; Maeda 1989; Ohye 1978, 1982, 1985, 1988; Ohye and Narabayashi 1972, 1979;

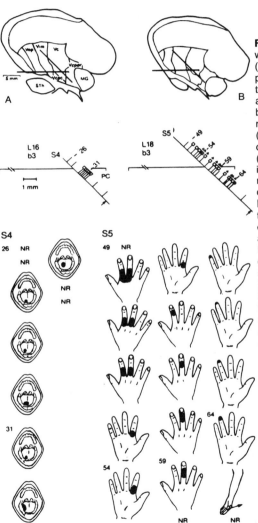

FIG. 1. RF mapping along two trajectories within parasagittal planes at 16 (A) and 18 mm (B) lateral to the midline. The stereotactically predicted course of each trajectory is drawn on the appropriate sagittal map of the thalamus, and the AC–PC line is indicated (top). Directly beneath these maps, the same trajectories are redrawn relative to the intercommissural line (AC–PC distance = 24.5 mm), with the position of the posterior commissure (PC) as indicated (middle). Lines at right angles to each trajectory indicate the positions at which single units were recorded. The response pattern of the cell is indicated by symbols at the end of these lines. Deep lemniscal (●) and cutaneous lemniscal touch (□) and pressure (■) responses are indicated. In some cases the cell had a slowly adapting (▲) or a rapidly adapting ( ) response. Lines with no squares or circles indicate the location of single units having no response to somatosensory stimulation. The most posterior location along the trajectory at which cells could be recorded is indicated (↑). Figurines depicting the size and location of RFs for each neuron encountered are displayed (bottom). NR indicates a neuron for which no RF was found. Figurines are numbered, and the cell corresponding to every fifth figurine is indicated by numbers along the trajectory. For deep cells responding to joint movement, the direction of the joint movement evoking a response is indicated (↑) on the corresponding figurine. Lettering to the upper left of the trajectory maps indicates the side (R or L), millimeters lateral to the midline, patient identification number (b3), and trajectory numbers (S4 and S5). MG = medial geniculate nucleus; Vop = ventralis oralis posterior; Vim = ventralis intermedius; Vc = ventrocaudal nucleus; Vcpc = ventrocaudal nucleus, pars parvocellularis; Vcpor = ventrocaudal portae; STh = subthalamic nucleus. (From Lenz et al. 1988, with permission.)

Ohye et al. 1972, 1975, 1977, 1982, 1985, 1989b) So-called deep cells, which respond to deep pressure but not muscle squeezing or joint bending, are especially noticeable in the fingertips, and appear to lie immediately rostral to tactile cells; however, Lenz et al. (1988a) were unable to show that this separation was statistically significant, even though the deep cells tended to be grouped together, distinct from tactile cells.

These deep neurons have fairly discrete RFs, especially in the hand, although not to the extent seen with tactile neurons, and have a medial-lateral homuncular arrangement like that of tactile cells. Along an anterosuperior-to-posteroinferior trajectory they are often found after muscle-tendon neurons and just before tactile neurons, usually with RFs similar to those of the ensuing tactile cells (Fig. 2).

Lying immediately rostral to tactile and deep neurons are kinesthetic neurons that, in the absence of any tactile response respond to two types of stimuli: contralateral muscle or tendon squeezing and joint bending. Lenz et al. (1988a) found that these cells tended to lie rostrodorsally to tactile cells, although they can also be found in small numbers caudally and, in my opinion, also inferiorly to tactile cells in a thin rim.

Typical responses of these neurons may be phasic or tonic; the effective stimuli consist of bending a particular contralateral joint in a particular direction or squeezing a particular contralateral muscle belly. Kinesthetic neurons related to the upper extremities are located rostrally to tactile upper-extremity neurons, and the same is true for other parts of the body.

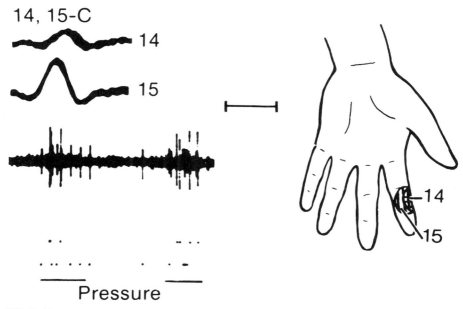

FIG. 2. Neuron sensitive to deep pressure but not joint bending. (Courtesy of F. A. Lenz, Department of Neurosurgery, Johns Hopkins University.)

Stimulation in the vicinity of kinesthetic neurons produces two types of response (Tasker et al. 1982). The most common are paresthesiae referred to larger areas of the body than the PFs in the tactile area, but usually in a similar body part to the one in which squeezing, deep pressure, or passive movement fired the neurons.

Rarely, stimulation elicits a different kind of response that is seemingly related to kinesthetic neurons, although activation of the more rostral dentatothalamic tract (see below) cannot be excluded. These responses imply that a movement is taking place, although none is witnessed, in a similar portion of the body to the origin of the RFs. Table 3 lists such responses obtained with macrostimulation, with which technique they seem to be more readily elicited than with microstimulation. The significance of inducing paresthesiae as opposed to the sensorimotor responses just described is unknown, although it is tempting to think that the former may arise in lemniscal and the latter in spindle afferent pathways.

The anatomic location of kinesthetic responses is controversial, with most authors stating that they arise in the ventral intermediate nucleus (Vim), although some relegate them to Vc.

TABLE 3. *Numbers of responses with motor connotations elicited by macrostimulation in the lateral thalamus rostral to Vc*

Response		No.
Wants to or has to move		10
Compression, pulsion		40
Pulling	10	
Drawing	5	
Pressure	5	
Tightening	9	
Grabbing	3	
Pinching	3	
Squeezing	1	
Pushing	1	
Choking	1	
Teeth close	2	
Rhythmic effects		18
Jaw pushing in and out	1	
Pulsation	6	
Jumping	3	
Flicking	2	
Eyelid twitching	2	
Throbbing	1	
Jerking	1	
Cheek sliding to and fro	1	
Tremor	1	
Part moving continuously		5
"Negative"		10
Weak	3	
Tired	3	
Heavy	3	
Loss of control	1	
Unspecified		1

The Pulvinar

Martin-Rodriguez et al. (1982) have recorded the spontaneous activity and sensorimotor effects in the pulvinar. Rhythmically firing units were not synchronous with any tremor, though five neurons that fired in relationship to the theta rhythm of the EEG were found. Thirteen units altered their firing in response to voluntary contralateral movements involving pressing and the release of pressing; nine neurons increased their firing rate after pressing (peak latency 100–400 msec), two increased their firing in relation to both pressing and release, while two decreased their firing with pressing. Another neuron increased its firing rate with pressing and release, decreased its firing with passive flexion, and increased its firing with thumb extension. Six units increased their firing in response to photic stimuli (70–140 msec latency), five of which also responded in relation to hand and jaw movements. One of three auditory units also responded to photic stimuli and voluntary movements. No tactile cells were found. Martin-Rodriguez et al. stressed the convergent relationships of pulvinar cells.

Periventricular Gray

The periventricular gray (PVG), probably medial Pf nucleus (Richardson and Akil 1977), is of interest as a target for chronic stimulation for the relief of intractable pain. Sometimes the target site in such cases can be recognized by electrical stimulation when a feeling of satiety, inebriation, pleasure, diffuse warmth, or pain relief is induced, but this is not a consistent finding.

In an attempt to improve the localization of electrode implantation, we have used microelectrode recordings and concluded that in an anterodorsal trajectory, the border between the dorsomedial (DM) and Pf nuclei can sometimes be discerned by the disappearance of burst-firing cells, so prevalent in DM, as the trajectory enters Pf. Young et al. (1990) seem to have made similar observations. Other evidence, however, suggests that this burst-firing activity arises in the centrolateral nucleus (CL) and is related to the presence of neuropathic pain (Jeanmonod et al. 1993).

The Visual System

The only structure in the visual system from which microelectrode recordings have been made appears to be the optic tract. This strategy is useful in pallidotomy, in which the optic tract is endangered by the ventroposterolateral lesion designed to relieve bradykinesia. Electrical stimulation of the optic tract elicits contralateral, usually white or bluish phosphenes, while recording reveals fibers whose action potentials respond somatotopographically to contralateral light stimuli.

The Auditory System

No organized study of the human auditory system has been done, but in recording during the course of thalamic exploration, auditory responses are found when the electrode wanders caudally and inferiorly, presumably in the medial geniculate nucleus. These responses are elicited by sounds delivered to the contralateral ear. Electrical stimulation induces low-pitched buzzing in the contralateral ear.

Motor Pathways

Voluntary Thalamic Cells

Moving rostrally in the ventrolateral thalamus from neurons that respond to passive movement reveals cells that change their firing in relationship to a contralateral voluntary movement. These have been observed by many groups (Crowell et al. 1968; Hongell et al. 1973; Jasper and Bertrand 1966; Lenz et al. 1990a; Li and van Buren 1972; Umbach and Ehrhardt 1965), perhaps most extensively by Raeva (1972, 1977, 1986; Raeva and Livanov 1975).

Umbach and Ehrhardt (1965) noted that 80% of neurons in the anterior and posterior ventral oral (Voa and Vop) nuclei altered their firing with voluntary movements, and recorded the changes that took place at: (a) the announcement that an order to move will be given; (b) the command to move; (c) the onset, during the course of; and (d) after the end of the actual movement. With (a), there was a decrease in frequency of spikes to 50 to 60% of their former levels for 150 to 200 msec, or a short inhibition followed by increased discharging; (b) produced a 100-msec inhibition followed by decreasing activity and, if tremor was present, tremor-synchronous activity; (c) led to various changes in activity with the blocking of neuronal spikes; and (d) was marked by possible inhibition followed by activation.

Raeva has divided voluntary cells into types A and B. In the thalamus she found 71% of voluntary-movement-related cells to be of type A, firing irregularly and spontaneously at 1 to 20 Hz and tending to be activated during voluntary acts. The remaining 29% of cells were of type B, with short, 3- to 5-Hz rhythmic discharges that tended to be inhibited during voluntary acts.

In the nucleus reticularis (NR) and neighboring structures Raeva found cells that responded with phasic activity or inhibition just after a verbal command to perform a voluntary movement. Phasic activation or inhibition occurred during preparation to carry out the movement; neither of these responses became habituated. Other NR neurons became activated just before or at the moment of onset of the electromyographic (EMG) activity of a voluntary task. No response to a verbal stimulus was seen unless it required a movement. Some NR cells fired rhythmically at 2 to 5 Hz, never in time with any tremor that might be present.

In the ventrolateral (VL) nucleus of the thalamus (Voa + Vop), on the other hand, neurons never responded to verbal commands unless they were close to NR, but fired in relation to a voluntary act. One type of cell fired 200 msec before the start of a movement and continued to do so throughout muscle contraction. A second type of cell either fired tonically or was tonically inhibited with maximal muscle contraction during a wide range of contralateral and, less often, ipsilateral movements. A third type of cell, which was nonrhythmic during spontaneous firing, fired rhythmically at the moment of initiation of a voluntary movement or just after completion of the movement. Sometimes a motor act had to be repeated to induce rhythmicity. This rhythmicity was unrelated to any tremor. A fourth type of cell which fired spontaneously and rhythmically at the frequency of, but not in phase with, any tremor had its rhythmicity suppressed during a voluntary movement. A final type of cell, located near NR, responded similarly to NR neurons.

In Vim Raeva found phasic and tonic units responding to specific passive movements (the kinesthetic cells discussed above) and to voluntary acts. These cells' rhythmicity was locked to that of any existing tremor.

Lenz et al. (1990a) identified voluntary neurons in the thalamus that also had RFs (combined cells; Fig. 3), usually in the form of a passive movement that opposed the voluntary act that triggered the response.

In our experience, thalamic voluntary cells were always related to specific contralateral voluntary acts and, being located rostrally to cells responding to passive movements and muscle perturbations, appear to be located in the dentatothalamic tract in Vop or rostral Vim, although Raeva reports finding them in Voa as well.

In our experience, stimulation at sites at which voluntary cells are recorded sometimes elicits a muscle contraction at the onset of a stimulus train; this habituates on repeated stimulation (Tasker et al. 1982). In a specific contralateral muscle group the response resembles those observed in the laboratory by Strick (1976), and appears to be derived from the transsynaptic activation of the motor cortex.

Basal Ganglia

Relatively few microelectrode studies in human basal ganglia have been reported, the first appearing to be that of Umbach and Ehrhardt (1965). However, renewed interest in pallidotomy to relieve parkinsonian bradykinesia (Laitinen et al. 1992) will undoubtedly lead to expanded interest in microelectrode recording in the globus pallidus (GP).

In GP, Umbach and Ehrhardt (1965) found voluntary units similar to those of VL; they were rhythmically synchronous, with 20-msec latencies, and their activity was suppressed on the order to move and at the termination of the movement.

Raeva (1972, 1977, 1986; Raeva and Livanov 1975) have studied GP, the caudate nucleus, and the putamen. In GP, spontaneous activity was usually "dense," of low voltage and high frequency (150 Hz), sometimes with silent intervals, and unaffected by voluntary movement. Thirty-five percent of GP neurons studied showed rhythmic firing at a rate near that of any tremor. Fifty percent of GP cells did not display high-frequency discharges but altered their firing rates over a 300- to

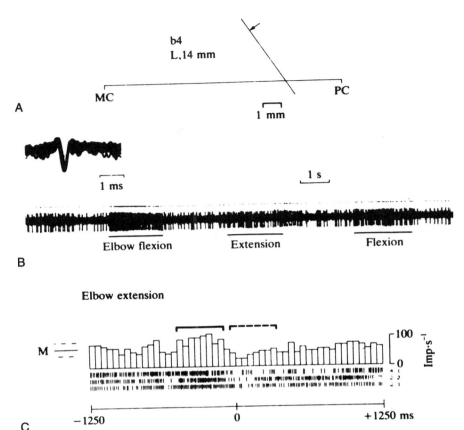

FIG. 3. Combined cell exhibiting activity related both to active movement and somatosensory stimulation. **A:** The location of the cell (*arrow*) in relation to the trajectory along which it was recorded (*oblique line*) and the intercommissural line, indicated by the posterior commissure (PC) and the midcommissural point (MC). The patient number (b4), parasagittal plane 14 mm to the left of midline (L, 14 mm), and scale are indicated in this panel. **B:** The response of the cell to passive elbow movement. The time scale is as indicated. Lines below the spike train in the lower panel of **B** indicate the approximate interval of elbow flexion and hold or extension and hold passive movements, as labeled. **C:** Raster and histogram for the activity of this cell during active elbow extension. (From Lenz et al. 1990, with permission.)

400-msec interval at the start or finish of a voluntary movement, some being excited, some inhibited, and others showed complex responses. GP neurons responded to both contralateral and ipsilateral voluntary movements, the activity sometimes being more pronounced with contralateral movements. Our findings are similar to these.

In the anteromedial putamen, Raeva found spontaneously active cells with low-voltage responses, discharging at 120 Hz or more, as well as cells that alternated between quiescence and grouped discharges, and others that fired rarely. Thirty percent of these cells had rhythmic discharges close to the frequency of any tremor. Putamenal cells fired briefly at the beginning and end of a contralateral and ipsilateral voluntary movement, by excitation, inhibition, or in a complex fashion. Caudate cells behave similarly. Any rhythmic activity was not synchronous with any tremor.

Miscellaneous Observations

Ohye et al. (1989a; see also Nakajima et al. 1978; Yoshida 1989) have used recording to delineate tumor margins through the abrupt electrical silence that occurs at these sites, while a number of workers (Fukamachi et al. 1977) have used the overall spontaneous "neural noise" recorded with a semimicroelectrode to differentiate one brain structure from another.

McClean et al. (1990) have recorded the patterns of thalamic somatosensory neurons firing in response to lip movements in speech.

Yamashiro et al. (1989) have correlated somatosensory evoked potentials (SEPs) recorded from the thalamus in response to median-nerve stimulation with single-unit recordings to confirm anatomic location, finding that continuous variations in SEPs occurred in all three directions through Vc. In caudal Vc the P15 peak showed the shortest and in anterior Vc the longest latency.

MICROELECTRODE RECORDINGS IN PATHOLOGIC STATES

This section will consider abnormalities in the firing patterns and arrangements of units in the brain.

Two types of abnormal unit activity have been recognized other than those associated with epilepsy, those associated with involuntary movement disorders and those associated with neurologic damage.

Neuronal Activity Associated with Dyskinesias

One of the most startling patterns of neuronal activity recorded in humans is that of "tremor cells," which are neurons that fire at the same rate as those of peripheral tremors. Originally reported in the thalamus by Albe-Fessard and colleagues (1962, 1963a,b, 1966a,b), these neurons have received considerable attention because of the interest in thalamotomy for Parkinson's disease (Bates 1969; Crowell et al. 1968; Hardy et al. 1964, 1979a; Lenz et al. 1984, 1985, 1987a,c, 1988d, 1990b; Lücking et al. 1972; Narabayashi 1982; Ohye and Albe-Fessard 1978; Ohye and Narabayashi 1972; Ohye et al. 1974; Schnider 1985; Schnider et al. 1989; Tasker et al. 1987b). Although extensively studied in Parkinson's disease, their occurrence in patients with other types of tremor, in which they appear to be less prominent, has been less well documented.

One of the problems in studying tremor cells is the inherent rhythmicity of the nervous system near the frequency of parkinsonian tremor but not actually synchronous with such tremor.

Tremor cells have been recorded in Vim and Vop, the zona incerta, GP, putamen, and caudate, and are of several types. Thalamic kinesthetic cells, by their nature, signal peripheral tremor because it "shakes" their receptors, passively activating them in time with the tremor; these cells therefore fire at tremor frequency only when tremor is present. A second group of cells appear to be candidates for tremor pacemaking. These are the subset of thalamic voluntary cells that discharge in advance of a particular contralateral voluntary movement and which also fire in time with tremor in patients with Parkinson's disease, even when peripheral tremor is absent. A third group of cells (no-response cells) fire in time with tremor but cannot be further identified. A fourth group fires near, but not at, tremor frequency.

Lenz and associates (Lenz et al. 1987a, 1988d, 1985, 1987c; Schnider 1985; Schnider et al. 1989; Tasker et al. 1987b) have studied the interrelationship between patterns of firing of thalamic tremor cells and peripheral tremor, examining the tightness of the linkage to and the concentration of neuronal activity at tremor frequency (Fig. 4). Lenz reasoned that the closer these relationships between neuronal firing and tremor frequency, the more likely it is that the neuron concerned is involved in the generation of tremor. Some voluntary cells both with and without RFs, as well as kinesthetic and no-response cells, demonstrated particularly tight

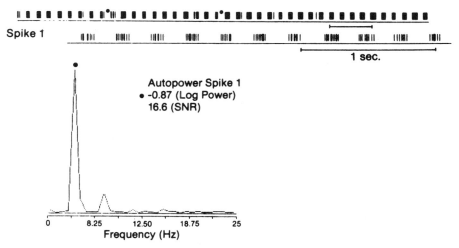

FIG. 4. Range of magnitudes of spike autopower peaks in the tremor-frequency band. Spike trains and corresponding spike autopower spectra are shown for a thalamic cell (spike 1). The spike train is shown on two different time scales so that the lower spike train corresponds to the interval in the upper spike train indicated by the dots. The dot above the spectrum indicates tremor frequency, as determined from the EMG autopower spectrum corresponding to that spike train. Numbers to the right of the spectrum indicate the $\log_{10}$ spike autopower and spike autopower signal to noise ratio (SNR) at tremor frequency. (From Lenz et al. 1988, with permission.)

linkages, especially in the case of voluntary cells with RFs and kinesthetic cells. He found a concentration of tightly linked neurons probably located in Vim or caudal Vop 3.5 mm above the intercommissural line and 2 mm rostral to the tactile relay in Vc.

Raeva and colleagues (Raeva 1972, 1977, 1986; Raeva and Livanov 1975) noted that thalamic tremor cells in Vop and Vim fired regularly and stably, with clear-cut burst and interburst intervals, constant numbers of spikes per burst, and silent inter-burst intervals. In GP, putamen, and caudate, however, rhythmic cells showed an unstable rhythm with variable burst and interburst intervals, the latter of which were not completely silent. However, some tremor cells in GP were found that behaved similarly to thalamic tremor cells.

Raeva also found differences between thalamic tremor cells and most tremor cells in the basal ganglion in their response to voluntary movement. The thalamic cells ceased firing during a voluntary movement, resuming their burst-firing pattern after a bout of enhanced firing when the movement was completed, a response that did not habituate. On the other hand, rhythmic cells in the basal ganglion showed dis-turbed rhythmicity and only partial inhibition at the beginning and end of a volun-tary act. During sustained motor acts, their neuronal firing accelerated and slowed alternately in periodic bursts. If I interpret Raeva's observations correctly, none of these tremor cells in the basal ganglion fired in time or phase with tremor frequency.

The firing of Voa and Vop neuron units whose firing became rhythmic during voluntary acts was independent of the presence or absence of peripheral tremor, but was in time with any existing tremor. In Raeva's experience, on the other hand, Vim units responded mainly to passive movements, but also to voluntary move-ments in a manner somatotopographically and contralaterally related. Most Vim cells were rhythmic, firing in correlation with tremor EMG.

Lücking et al. (1972) recorded tremor-synchronous activity in the prelemniscal radiations, where lesions effectively stopped tremor. They believed the cells re-sponsible for this activity to arise in cerebello-thalamorubral fibers.

Lenz et al. (1990b) have recognized in dystonia patients cells that fired in relation to the dystonia in much the same way as tremor cells do in relation to tremor.

Neuronal Responses Related to Neurologic Damage

Two types of abnormality can be found in patients who have suffered neurologic damage: burst-firing cells and somatotopographic reorganization of neurons.

Burst-firing Cells

Cells that fire in a spontaneous and rhythmic manner occur naturally in certain structures within the nervous system, as has already been mentioned. But these cells may appear at other sites in pathologic states, particularly in patients with damage to the nervous system. Their presence has been correlated with denervational neuronal hypersensitivity, often claimed to be a mechanism responsible for the steady component of neuropathic pain (Loeser et al. 1968). Such activity has been recorded frequently in the laboratory, but also in the spinal cord in a paraplegic patient with central pain (Loeser et al. 1968) and in the course of interruption of a dorsal-root entry zone (Jeanmonod et al. 1990) in a patient with neuropathic pain from a lesion of the cauda equina. The recordings in both cases were compared with the "normal" pattern seen in a spastic patient. We have recorded burst-firing cells in various sites including Vc, Vim, and Vop, usually in patients with neuropathic pain, and particularly but not exclusively in those with central pain of spinal or cerebral origin. With regard to identifying the pathogenesis of pain, such burst-firing cells are unfortunately also found in the thalamus of patients with multiple sclerosis who do not have pain but are undergoing surgery for tremor, those with stroke-induced dyskinesia who have no pain, and adjacent to previous thalamotomy lesions in patients with tremor who do not have pain. According to Gorecki et al. (1989), burst-firing cells appear to be markers of deafferentation rather than pain.

Lenz and colleagues (Lenz 1991; Lenz et al. 1987b, 1988c) studied the thalamus in a quadriplegic patient with central pain and in other patients with similar problems, noting several abnormalities that might be related to the presence of pain, including: (a) somatotopographic reorganization (discussed below); (b) unusual degrees of mismatch between RFs and PFs; (c) abnormal responses to electrical stimulation (burning instead of paresthesiae) in the thalamus near the junction of the normally innervated and deafferented parts; and (d) cells firing in bursts in the same area.

Lenz has observed that the burst-firing activity in the thalamus of patients with central pain resembles that of calcium spikes, and has supported this notion with further clinicopathologic studies (Lenz et al. 1989) (Fig. 5).

Yamashiro et al. (1991) also studied burst-firing cells, finding neurons firing regularly in groups of three to five trains of bursts at 4 to 5 Hz, resembling cells found in rats in the contralateral VP, zona incerta, and medial lemniscus at 1 to 3 months after section of C5 to T1 dorsal roots.

Hirayama et al. (1989) classified thalamic burst-firing cells into three groups: (a) those with regular burst and interburst intervals; (b) those with regular burst and irregular interburst intervals; and (c) those with irregular burst and interburst intervals. They suggested that the presence of cells of group (a) in Vc, and particularly those with RFs, correlated most closely with the presence of neuropathic pain (Fig. 6).

Somatotopographic Reorganization

In the course of mapping the human thalamus with microelectrode recording and microstimulation at the same site and with the same electrode, we have identified what appears to be somatotopographic reorganization in response to amputation, peripheral deafferentation, spinal-cord injury, and, especially, stroke. However,

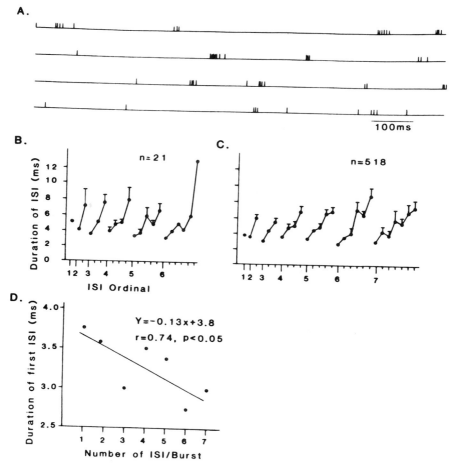

FIG. 5. Interstimulus interval (ISI) characteristics of bursts recorded in patients with pain. **A:** Digitized spike train of a cell recorded in a patient with central pain. Time scale as indicated. **B:** Plot of the average ISI duration (mean and SEM) as a function of the position of the ISI within a burst for 21 bursts recorded in that cell. For example, the three points joined by lines above and to the right of the number 3 show results for bursts composed of four action potentials or 31 ISIs. **C:** Same data as in **B** for 22 cells (518 bursts) recorded in two patients with spinal-cord transection. **D:** Plot of the mean duration of the first ISI in a burst as a function of the number of ISIs in the burst, for the data displayed in **C**. (From Lenz et al. 1989, with permission.)

like burst-firing cells, such reorganization is present in patients who have suffered deafferentation whether or not pain is present.

The reorganization may take several forms. In small thalamic strokes, silent "holes" may be found in Vc, with an apparent shift of tactile neurons representing a body part normally found in that "hole" to another site in the thalamus (Gorecki et al. 1989). At the junction in Vc between tactile neurons that normally represent

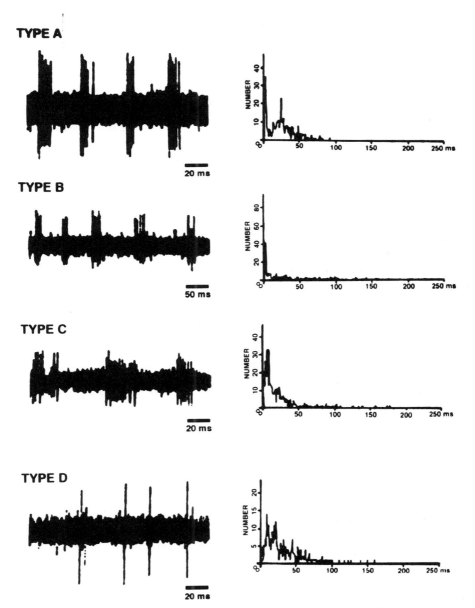

FIG. 6. Examples of the four types of burst-firing cells. For each cell type a photographic record of the activity is given on the left side of the figure, while on the right is the interspike-interval histogram (IH) constructed from the same cell from 10 sec of activity. Type A cells had an IH that was clearly bimodal, indicating that these cells tended to fire in bursts that occurred fairly regularly. Type B cells fired in bursts, as evidenced by short-latency peaks, but the bursts did not occur regularly, and thus there was no second peak in the IH. Type C cells were similar to type B except that the interspike intervals within the burst were not short or regular, thus resulting in a wider short-latency peak. Type D cells did not fire in bursts. (From Hirayama 1989, with permission.)

162

body parts above and below the level of spinal cord interruption, neurons with RFs below the level are, clearly, absent, but unusual numbers of neurons may be found representing parts of the body that normally have minimal representation in Vc (Lenz et al. 1987b). After loss of input from peripheral deafferentation to a portion of Vc, the lost RFs from the deafferented part may be replaced by RFs from body parts from which input is still intact. These abnormalities are one cause of mismatch between RFs and PFs; in the normal state, RFs and PFs induced by microstimulation are usually very similar, as in the stroke patient described in Fig. 7 (see also Fig. 8).

Ohye et al. (1985) also found evidence of thalamic reorganization when they compared patients who underwent surgery for movement disorders associated with Parkinson's disease and other conditions. Eight patients had stroke-induced tremor, two of the strokes being intrathalamic and six infrathalamic. In the stroke patients the proportions of kinesthetic cells were reduced, general cellular activity was reduced, tactile and kinesthetic cells were intermingled rather than distributed separately, and the percentage of facial tactile and kinesthetic neurons was increased at the expense of those representing hand and other body parts.

SUMMARY

As can be seen from the findings described in this chapter, studies of normal, individual neurons provide little information for the understanding of human pain. They have revealed something about the organization of hard-wired somatosensory pathways, but direct observations of pain pathways are elusive at all levels of the central nervous system (CNS). Studies elucidating the mechanism of pattern appreciation in the association cortex of the temporal lobe may prove helpful in understanding how we feel pain. Perhaps these studies will bear on findings related to the "time-on" theory that seems to demonstrate an ability for patients to detect a sensory stimulus without being consciously aware of it, as compared with conscious awareness of stimuli (Libet et al. 1991).

Abnormal neuronal firing (by burst-firing cells) and somatotopographic reorganization have been cited as possible mechanisms by which neuropathic pain may occur, but both phenomena occur in deafferented patients who do not have pain as well as in those who do; further refinements of technique will be required to determine when these features are algogenic and by what means.

OTHER STUDIES WITH MICROELECTRODES

Some indirect observations made with the microelectrode technique are of interest in understanding how we feel pain. Stereotactic procedures done in order to implant a chronically stimulating electrode (deep-brain stimulation; DBS) or to make a destructive lesion (medial thalamotomy, mesencephalic tractotomy) in an attempt to control intractable pain rely on the help of physiologic localization, with

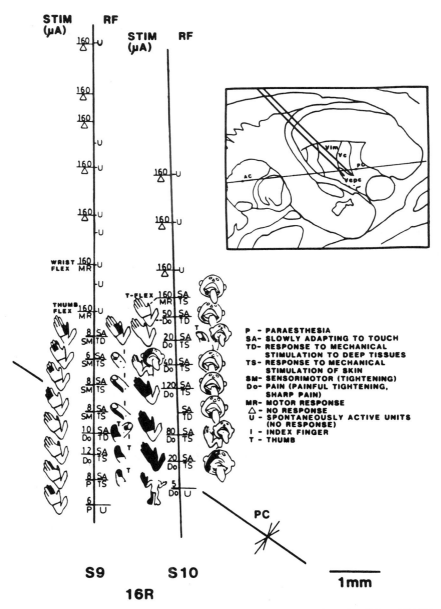

FIG. 7. Results of microstimulation and microrecording along two trajectories (S9 and S10) in a patient with pain secondary to supratentorial stroke. The two vertical lines are the trajectories, shown relative to the anterior commissure–posterior commissure line, with the posterior commissure (PC) as indicated. Figurines and letters to the right of each trajectory indicate the modality (TS or TD), response pattern (SA), and receptive field of cells recorded at the sites indicated along the trajectory. Letters, numbers, and figurines to the left of each trajectory respectively indicate the stimulation-evoked sensation (Do, P, or SM), stimulation threshold (in microam-

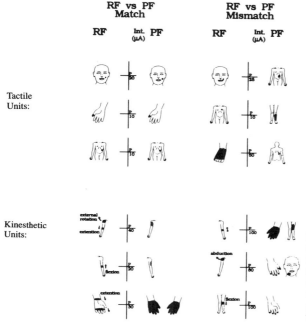

FIG. 8. Four figurine charts constructed from data collected in patients by microelectrode recording and microstimulation, showing on the left a high degree of RF–PF match for tactile (above) and kinesthetic (below) neurons, and on the right, RF–PF mismatch.

alternate recording and microstimulation done with the same electrode. In sensory structures, recording (studying RFs) is used to examine the integrity of the sensory system from receptor to thalamus, while stimulation (examining PFs) tests the integrity from thalamus to cortex, assuming that conscious awareness of sensation depends on the sensorimotor cortex.

This technique can be used both in patients with nociceptive pain, such as that caused by cancer, in whom somatosensory pathways may be intact, and in patients with neuropathic pain whose peripheral nervous system or CNS has been damaged. In patients with central pain caused by stroke, we have correlated the following in an attempt to better understand how these patients experience pain: (a) location and nature of pain; (b) location and size of the responsible lesion; (c) somatosensory loss; (d) thalamic RFs; (e) thalamic PFs; and (f) response of pain to surgery.

Twenty-nine patients with stroke-induced central pain were studied, all of whom had steady pain; 76% had allodynia and/or hyperpathia (evoked pain), and 14% had

---

FIG 7. *Continued.* peres), and area to which the sensation was referred in response to stimulation at the site indicated along the trajectory. The estimated location of nuclear boundaries in relation to these trajectories is indicated on the parasagittal map of the thalamus shown in the inset. Scale is as indicated. Abbreviations are as listed in the figure plus: Vc = ventrocaudal nucleus; Vcpc = ventrocaudal nucleus, pars parvocellularis; Vim = ventralis intermedius. This shows a good match between PFs and RFs, but also shows many sites in which pain (Do) was induced. (From Lenz 1988, with permission.)

neuralgic pain. The latter was too infrequent to study further. In most cases the lesion responsible for the pain was visualized with computed tomography (CT), but in four patients with infrathalamic lesions, the causative lesion was localized on clinical grounds; in two patients presumed to have supratentorial lesions, no appropriate lesion could be seen. Table 4 reviews the responsible lesions.

In each case a stereotactic procedure was done. Formerly, ventriculography but more recently and more often, CT was used to locate the AC–PC) line. Based on this information and with reference to an atlas, either a macroelectrode or, more usually, a microelectrode was directed toward the target through a twist-drill hole in the same sagittal plane as the target, in order to facilitate the analysis of physiologic data. Recording was done continuously, beginning about 10 mm above and extending 5 to 10 mm beyond the target, while microstimulation was done every millimeter. The collected data were displayed in figurine maps with PFs on one side and RFs on the other. Spinothalamic tract (6–9 mm from the midline) was located by first identifying the larger medial lemniscus (10–12 mm from the midline), where stimulation induced paresthetic contralateral PFs, and by then tracking dorsomedially until the quality of sensations induced in the contralateral PFs changed from paresthetic to warm, cold, hot, burning, or painful. Since medial thalamic nuclei such as Pf, thought to be associated with pain, were silent to electrical stimulation, their locations were extrapolated from that of the tactile relay in Vc, which was recognized by recording the RFs of tactile neurons or by producing paresthetic contralateral PFs by stimulation. PVG was usually located anatomically on the stereotactic CT scan at 2 mm lateral to the wall of the third ventricle, 5 mm above the AC–PC line, and 5 mm rostral to PC, although in some patients its stimulation induced a feeling of diffuse warmth, pleasure, satiety, and acute relief from pain. With microelectrode recording, the dorsal boundary of our PVG target (medial PF) may be recognized with microelectrode recording as the site at which spontaneous burst-firing cells in DM cease to be present.

On the basis of the physiologic data, either a DBS electrode was inserted for trial and eventually internalized if pain relief ensued, or a destructive lesion was made.

We first correlated the location and quality of pain with the size and location of the stroke lesion and with the somatosensory picture. The pain syndrome in these patients tended to be stereotyped, usually involving the hemibody, regardless of

TABLE 4. *Lesions in 29 patients with stroke-induced central pain*

Lesion	No. patients
None seen; presumed suprathalamic	2
Infrathalamic	4
Thalamic	6
Small suprathalamic	3
Large suprathalamic	8
Large thalmo-suprathalamic	3
Unknown	3

the extent of the lesion. The degree of sensory loss reflected the size and extent of the stroke, with similar pain syndromes marked by similar proportions of steady, neuralgic, and evoked pain occurring both in patients without clinically detectable sensory loss and in those with massive strokes. Burst-firing cells and somatotopographic reorganization were found in most patients and bore no recognizable relationship to their pain. Some patients displayed apparent migration of RFs from a damaged thalamic site into an adjacent intact one, and varying degrees of disorganization of the normal pattern of thalamic cells discussed earlier and of RF/PF mismatch were found. Table 5 reviews the possible patterns of abnormality that might be seen in the RFs and PFs of these patients.

In nine patients there was virtual absence (in three apparently complete) of RFs or PFs in the thalamus contralateral to the patient's pain (pattern 9 in Table 5). All of these patients had large lesions and extensive sensory loss or were suffering from steady and evoked pain (allodynia and/or hyperpathia), approaching the state seen in infantile hemiplegia or after hemispherectomy (Ralston 1962; Parrent et al. 1992a). If it is assumed that appreciation of pain depends on the cerebral cortex, such patients must experience pain ipsilaterally; otherwise, infrathalamic mechanisms of pain perception must be invoked. In one of these patients no physiologic responses were obtained with extensive exploration of the contralateral medial and lateral thalamus, but ipsilateral PVG stimulation at different loci evoked feelings of diffuse warmth, distress, and nausea, and relieved the patient's cold allodynia. In one further patient in whom both RFs and PFs were partially preserved contralateral to the pain, paresthesia-producing DBS contralateral to the pain was ineffective for pain relief. To our amazement, stimulation of the sensorimotor cortex (Tsubokawa et al. 1991) on the side ipsilateral to the pain (since the contralateral cortex had been largely destroyed by the stroke) induced paresthesiae ipsilateral to the stimulation in the patient's area of pain, and diminished its intensity, a result that continued for nearly a year of follow-up.

Other patients with constant and evoked pain showed varieties of alterations in RF/PF patterns, ranging from apparently normal (pattern 1) to severe damage to

TABLE 5. *Possible findings in Vc in patients with central pain from stroke*

Pattern no.	RFs	PFs
1	Intact	Intact
2	Intact	Deranged
3	Intact	Absent
4	Deranged	Intact
5	Deranged	Deranged
6	Deranged	Absent
7	Absent	Intact
8	Absent	Deranged
9	Absent	Absent

both systems. One would assume that in the apparently normal patients, stroke had produced minor damage undetectable by our methods but still capable of inducing pain, which was presumably mediated by contralateral pathways.

Between the two extremes, pain occurred in patients with reasonably intact RFs but PFs (thalamocortical structures) damaged to varying degrees, and vice versa (patterns 2–8). Although no example of absent RFs but intact PFs (pathway from receptor to thalamic neuron interrupted) (pattern 7) was found among the 29 stroke patients, one patient from whom an intramedullary cervical spinal-cord tumor had been removed, and who suffered from neuropathic pain and severe sensory loss in the right upper limb, showed this pattern. Thus, a deafferented thalamocortex, left "in neutral" and unresponsive to peripheral natural stimuli (no RFs), appeared capable of responding to artificial electrical stimulation, and therefore possibly also to intrinsic activation that might induce pain.

Some of the observations in our studies bear on structures that might be involved in the appreciation of central pain. If manipulation of a neurologic structure has an effect on a patient's pain, it is reasonable to suppose that that structure may be involved in pain signalling. This notion can be exploited either by observing the results of destroying structures or by modulating structures through acute or chronic stimulation. We have shown (Tasker et al. 1992) that in patients with central spinal cord pain, chronic stimulation is most effective for eliminating the steady element of the pain and destructive surgery for eliminating the evoked and intermittent elements. The same dichotomy seems to apply in brain central pain (Tasker and de Carvalho 1990), as shown in Table 6, with chronic stimulation of VC or the trigeminal nerve being more effective for relieving steady pain and thalamotomy or mesencephalic tractotomy being more effective for alleviating evoked pain; intermittent pain is too rare after stroke to permit significant conclusions to be drawn. We reasoned that if allodynia and hyperpathia were relieved by destructive surgery in pain pathways, they might also respond to PVG stimulation. In four of our 29 patients this strategy diminished evoked pain (Parrent et al. 1992b). Thus, allodynia and hyperpathia after stroke appear to depend on spinoreticulothalamic transmission but not steady pain.

Additional evidence for this conclusion comes from studies of acute stimulation. It has been pointed out by many (i.e., Tasker et al. 1982) how rarely electrical stimulation of the human brain evokes a feeling of pain except in patients with neuropathic pain. In these patients, and particularly those with stroke-induced pain

TABLE 6. *Response of different elements of stroke-induced central pain to surgery*

Pain type	% of patients improved	
	Destructive surgery	Chronic stimulation
Steady	30	50
Neuralgic	(100)	(0)
Evoked	60	25

that includes a hyperpathic or allodynic element (Gorecki et al. 1989; Davis et al. 1993) (see Fig. 7), acute stimulation of the spinoreticulothalamic pathways in the midbrain or medial and lateral thalamus elicited abnormal painful responses often similar to the patient's own pain. Thus, such sensations presumably arose in the reticulothalamic tract in the medial midbrain and thalamus, where no stimulation-induced responses normally occur, as well as in the spinothalamic tract, where they do. In the 29 patients in our study the same relationship seemed to exist.

Such painful responses to stimulation were also seen in the mesencephalon of patients in whom there appeared to be no preservation of thalamocortical structures implicating ipsilateral pathways. These observations suggest that allodynia and hyperpathia associated with central pain depend on pain pathways, just as does allodynia in neuropathic pain caused by peripheral nervous lesions, in which receptors that do not normally signal pain activate the pain pathway through perverted processing in the dorsal horn (Woolf 1992). Consequently, either contralateral or ipsilateral pathways may be involved in these two pathologic effects.

CONCLUSION

The use of microelectrodes offers a precise and objective method for physiologic localization in functional neurosurgery. It also offers an ideal application of the important principle of bringing "state-of-the-art, bench-to-bedside" expertise to bear on normal and abnormal brain function. It has not, however, unravelled the mysteries of the conscious processing of pain.

ACKNOWLEDGMENTS

The work described was partly supported by The Parkinson Foundation of Canada. The author wishes to thank Anne Chiacchieri for preparation of the manuscript.

REFERENCES

Albe-Fessard D. Electrophysiological methods for the identification of thalamic nuclei. *Z Neurol* 1973; 205:15–28.

Albe-Fessard D. Thalamic activity and Parkinson's disease. In: Umbach W, Koepchen HP, eds. *Central rhythm and regulation*. Stuttgart: Hyppokrates Verlag, 1974;353–362.

Albe-Fessard D, Arfel G, Guiot G, Hardy J, Vourch G, Hertzog E, Aleonard P, Derome P. Dérivations d'activités spontanées et évoquées dans les structures cérébrales profondes de l'homme. *Rev Neurol* 1962;106:89–105.

Albe-Fessard D, Arfel G, Guiot G. Activités électriques caractéristiques de quelques structures cérébrales chez l'homme. *Ann Chir* 1963a;17:1185–1214.

Albe-Fessard D, Guiot G, Hardy J. Electrophysiological localization and identification of subcortical structures in man by recording spontaneous and evoked activities. *EEG Clin Neurophysiol* 1963b;15: 1052–1053.

Albe-Fessard D, Arfel G, Guiot G, Derome P, Hertzog E, Vourch G, Brown H, Aleonard P, De la Herran J, Trigo JC. Electrophysiological studies of some deep cerebral structures in man. *J Neurol Sci* 1966a;13:37–51.

Albe-Fessard D, Guiot G, Lamarre J, Arfel G. Activation of thalamo-cortical projections related to tremorogenic processes. In: Purpura DP, Yahr MD, eds. *The thalamus*. New York: Columbia University Press, 1966b;237–253.

Albe-Fessard D, Arfel G, Derome P, Guilbaud G. Thalamic unit activity in man. *EEG Clin Neurophysiol* 1967;(Suppl 25):132–142.

Amano K, Tanikawa T, Iseki H, Kawabatake H, Notani M, Kawamura H, Kitamura K. Single neuron analysis of the human midbrain tegmentum. *Appl Neurophysiol* 1978;41:66–78.

Arutjunov A, Kadian A, Konovalov A, Raeva SN, Merschikova T, Seliverstov V. Experience of applying the microelectrode method in the neurosurgical clinic practice during single-stage stereotaxic operations for parkinsonism. *Vop Neirokhir* 1970;6:12.

Bates JAV. The significance of tremor phasic units in the human thalamus. In: Gillingham FJ, Donaldson IML, eds. *Third symposium on Parkinson's disease*.Edinburgh: Livingstone, 1969;118–124.

Bates JAV. Electrical recording from the thalamus in human subjects. In: Iggo A, ed. *Handbook of sensory physiology: somatosensory system*. Berlin: Springer Verlag, 1972;561–578.

Bertrand C, Martinez SN, Hardy J, Molina-Negro P, Velasco F. Stereotactic surgery for Parkinsonism: microelectrode recording, stimulation, and oriented sections with a leucotome. In: Krayenbühl H, Maspes PE, Sweet WH, eds. *Progress in neurological surgery*, vol. 5. Basel: Karger, 1973;79–112.

Bertrand G, Jasper H. Microelectrode recording of unit activity in the human thalamus. *Confin Neurol* 1965;26:205–208.

Bertrand G, Jasper H, Wong A. Microelectrode study of the human thalamus: organization in the ventrobasal complex. *Confin Neurol* 1967;29:81–86.

Bertrand G, Jasper H, Wong A, Matthews G. Microelectrode recording during stereotactic surgery. *Clin Neurosurg* 1969;16:328–355.

Calvin WH. Comments on human epileptic neurons. In: Somjen GG, ed. *Neurophysiology studied in man*. Amsterdam: Excerpta Medica, 1972;110–111.

Carreras M, Mancia D, Pagni C. Unit discharges recorded from the human thalamus with micro-electrodes. *Confin Neurol* 1967;29:87.

Creutzfeld O, Ojemann GA, Lettich E. Neuronal activity in the human lateral temporal lobe. I Repsonses to speech. *Exp Brain Res* 1989a;77:451–475.

Creutzfeld O, Ojemann GA, Lettich E. Neuronal activity in the human lateral temporal lobe. II Responses to the subjects' own voice. *Exp Brain Res* 1989b;77:476–489.

Creutzfeld O, Ojemann GA, Lettich E. Neuronal activity in the human lateral temporal lobe. III Activity changes during music. *Exp Brain Res* 1989c;77:490–498.

Crowell RM, Perret E, Siegfried J. "Movement units" and "tremor phasic units" in the human thalamus. *Brain Res* 1968;11:481–488.

Davis KD, Dostrovsky JO, Tasker RR, Kiss Z, Hutchison WD. Increased incidence of pain evoked by thalamic stimulation in post-stroke pain patients. *Soc Neurosci Abstr* 1993;19:1572.

Davis KD, Hutchison WD, Dostrovsky JO, Lozano AM. Altered pain and temperature perception following cingulotomy and capsulotomy in a patient with schizoaffective disorder. Presented at the International Association for the Study of Pain (IASP) Meeting, Paris, August 1993.

Donaldson IML. The properties of some human thalamus units. Some new observations and a critical review of the localization of thalamic nuclei. *Brain* 1973;96:419–440.

Dostrovsky JO, Wells FEB, Tasker RR. Pain sensations evoked by stimulation in human thalamus. In: Inoki R, Shigenaga Y, Yohyama M, eds. *Processing and inhibition of nociceptive information*. Amsterdam: Elsevier, 1992;115–120.

Fukamachi A, Ohye C, Narabayashi H. Delineation of the thalamic nuclei with a microelectrode in stereotaxic surgery for Parkinsonism and cerebral palsy. *J Neurosurg* 1973;39:214–225.

Fukamachi A, Ohye C, Saito Y, Narabayashi H. Estimation of the neural noise within the human thalamus. *Acta Neurochir* 1977;(Suppl 24):121–136.

Gaze RM, Gillingham FJ, Kalyanaraman S, Porter RW, Donaldson AA, Donaldson IML. Microelectrode recordings from the human thalamus. *Brain* 1964;87:691–706.

Gillingham FJ. Depth recording and stimulation. *J Neurosurg* 1966;(Suppl 2):382.

Gorecki J, Hirayama T, Dostrovsky JO, Tasker RR, Lenz FA. Thalamic stimulation and recording in patients with deafferentation and central pain. *Stereotact Funct Neurosurg* 1989;52:219–226.

Goto A, Kosaka K, Kubota K, Nakamura R, Narabayashi H. Thalamic potentials from muscle afferents in the human. *Arch Neurol* 1968;19:302–309.

Guiot G, Hardy J, Albe-Fessard D. Délimitation précise des structures souscorticales et identification des noyaux thalamiques chez l'homme par l'électrophysiologie stéréotaxique. *Neurochirurgica* 1962;5:1–18.

Guiot G, Derome P, Arfel G, Walter SG. Electrophysiological recordings in stereotaxic thalamotomy for Parkinsonism. In: Krayenbühl H, Maspes PE, Sweet WH, eds. *Progress in neurological surgery*, 5th ed. Basel: Karger, 1973;189–221.

Haglund MM, Ojemann GA, Lettich E, Bellugi U, Corina D. Dissociation of cortical and single unit activity in spoken and signed languages. *Brain Lang* 1993;44:19–27.

Halliday AM, Logue V. Painful sensations evoked by electrical stimulation in the thalamus. In: Somjen GG, ed. *Neurophysiology studied in man*. Amsterdam: Excerpta Medica, 1972;221–230.

Hardy J, Bertrand C, Martinez N. Activités cellulaires thalamiques liées au tremblement parkinsonien. *Neurochirurgie* 1964;10:449.

Hardy TL, Bertrand G, Thompson CJ. Position and organization of thalamic cellular activity during diencephalic recording. II Joint- and muscle-evoked activity. *Appl Neurophysiol* 1980a;43:28–36.

Hardy TL, Bertrand G, Thompson CJ. Thalamic recordings during stereotactic surgery. I Surgery topography of evoked and nonevoked rhythmic cellular activity. *Appl Neurophysiol* 1979a;42:185–197.

Hardy TL, Bertrand G, Thompson CJ. Thalamic recordings during stereotactic surgery. II Location of quick-adapting touch-evoked (novelty) cellular responses. *Appl Neurophysiol* 1979b;42:198–202.

Hardy TL, Bertrand G, Thompson CJ. Organization and topography of sensory responses in the internal capsule and nucleus ventralis caudalis found during stereotactic surgery. *Appl Neurophysiol* 1979c; 42:335–351.

Hardy TL, Bertrand G, Thompson CJ. Position and organization of thalamic cellular activity during diencephalic recording I. Pressure evoked activity. *Appl Neurophysiol* 1980b;43:18–27.

Hardy TL, Bertrand G, Thompson CJ. Topography of bilateral-movement-evoked thalamic cellular activity found during diencephalic recording. *Appl Neurophysiol* 1980c;43:67–74.

Hardy TL, Bertrand G, Thompson CJ. Touch-evoked thalamic cellular activity. The variable position of the anterior border of somesthetic S1 thalamus and somatotopography. *Appl Neurophysiol* 1981;44: 302–313.

Hassler R. The division of pain conduction into systems of pain sensation and pain awareness. In: Janzen R, Keidel WD, Herz A, Steichele C, eds. *Pain basic principles: Pharmacology, therapy*. Stuttgart: Thieme; Edinburgh: Livingstone, 1972;98–112.

Hirayama T, Dostrovsky JO, Gorecki J, Tasker RR, Lenz FA. Recordings of abnormal activity in patients with deafferentation and central pain. *Stereotact Funct Neurosurg* 1989;52:120–126.

Hitchcock E, Lewin M. Stereotactic recording from the spinal cord of man. *Br Med J* 1969;4(5074): 44–45.

Hongell A, Wallin G, Hagbarth KE. Unit activity connected with movement initiation and arousal situations recorded from the ventrolateral nucleus of the human thalamus. *Acta Neurol Scand* 1973;49:681–698.

Hutchison WD, Davis KD, Lozano AM, Dostrovsky JO. Single unit recording and macrostimulation in cingulate cortex of an awake patient. Presented at the IASP Meeting, Paris, August, 1993.

Ishijima B, Yoshimasu N, Fukushima T, Hori T, Sekino H, Sano K. Nociceptive neurons in the human thalamus. *Confin Neurol* 1975;37:99–106.

Jasper HH. Recording from micro-electrodes in stereotaxic surgery for Parkinson's disease. *J Neurosurg* 1966;(Suppl 2):219.

Jasper HH, Bertrand G. Exploration of the human thalamus with micro-electrodes. *Physiologist* 1963; 7:167.

Jasper HH, Bertrand G. Thalamic units involved in somatic sensation and voluntary and involuntary movements in man. In: Purpura DP, Yahr MD, eds. *The thalamus*. New York: Columbia University Press, 1966;365–390.

Jeanmonod D, Sindou M, Mauguière F. Intraoperative electrophysiological recordings during microsurgical DREZ-tomies in man. *Stereotact Funct Neurosurg* 1990;54/55:80–85.

Jeanmonod D, Magnin M, Morel M. Thalamus and neurogenic pain: physiological, anatomical and clinical data. *Neurol Rep* 1993;4:475–478.

Kelly PJ, Ahlskog JE, Goerss SJ, Daube JR, Duffy JR, Kall BA. Computer-assisted stereotactic ventralis lateralis thalamotomy with microelectrode recording control in patients with Parkinson's disease. *Mayo Clin Proc* 1987;62:655–664.

Laitinen LV, Bergenheim AT, Hariz MI. Ventroposterolateral pallidotomy can abolish all parkinsonian symptoms. *Stereotact Funct Neurosurg* 1992;58:14–21.

Lenz FA. The thalamus and central pain syndromes: human and animal studies. In: Casey KL, ed. *The central pain syndromes*. New York: Raven Press, 1991;171–182.

Lenz FA, Dostrovsky JO, Tasker RR, Yamashiro K, Kwan HC, Murphy JT. Single-unit analysis in the human ventral thalamic nuclear group: somatosensory responses. *J Neurophysiol* 1988a;59:299–316.

Lenz FA, Dostrovsky JO, Kwan HC, Tasker RR, Yamashiro K, Murphy JT. Methods for microstimulation and recording of single neurons and evoked potentials in the human central nervous system. *J Neurosurg* 1988b;68:630–634.

Lenz FA, Kwan HC, Dostrovsky JO, Tasker RR. Characteristics of the bursting pattern of action potentials that occurs in the thalamus of patients with central pain. *Brain Res* 1989;496:357–360.

Lenz FA, Kwan HC, Dostrovsky JO, Tasker RR, Murphy JT, Lenz YE. Single unit analysis of the human ventral thalamic nuclear group. Activity correlated with movement. *Brain* 1990a;113:1795–1821.

Lenz FA, Martin R, Kwan HC, Tasker RR, Dostrovsky JO. Thalamic single-unit activity occurring in patients with hemidystonia. *Stereotact Funct Neurosurg* 1990b;54/55:159–162.

Lenz FA, Schnider S, Tasker RR, Kwong R, Kwan H, Dostrovsky JO, Murphy JT. The role of feedback in the tremor frequency activity of tremor cells in the ventral nuclear group of human thalamus. *Acta Neurochir* 1987a;(Suppl 39):54–56.

Lenz FA, Seike M, Richardson RT, Lin YC, Baker FH, Khoja I, Yeager CJ, Gracey RH. Thermal and pain sensation evoked by microstimulation in the area of human ventrocaudal nucleus. *J Neurophysiol* 1993;70:200–212.

Lenz FA, Tasker RR, Dostrovsky JO, Kwan HC, Gorecki J, Hirayama T, Murphy JT. Abnormal single-unit activity recorded in the somatosensory thalamus of a quadriplegic patient with central pain. *Pain* 1987b;31:225–236.

Lenz FA, Tasker RR, Dostrovsky JO, Kwan HC, Gorecki J, Hirayama T, Murphy JT. Abnormal single-unit activity and responses to stimulation in the presumed ventrocaudal nucleus of patients with central pain. In: Dubner R, Gebhart GF, Bond MR, eds. *Proceedings of the Vth World Congress on Pain.* Amsterdam: Elsevier, 1988c;158–164.

Lenz FA, Tasker RR, Kwan HC, Murphy JT, Nguyen-Huu HH. Techniques for the analysis of spike trains in the human central nervous system. *Acta Neurochir* 1984;(Suppl 33):57–61.

Lenz FA, Tasker RR, Kwan HC, Schnider S, Kwong R, Murayama Y, et al. Single unit analysis of the human ventral nuclear group: correlation of thalamic "tremor cells" with the 3–6 Hz component of Parkinsonian tremor. *J Neurosci* 1988d;8:754–764.

Lenz FA, Tasker RR, Kwan HC, Schnider S, Kwong R, Murphy JT. Cross-correlation analysis of thalamic neurons and EMG activity in Parkinsonian tremor. *Appl Neurophysiol* 1985;48:305–308.

Lenz FA, Tasker RR, Kwan HC, et al. Selection of the optimal lesion site for the relief of Parkinsonian tremor on the basis of spectral analysis of neuronal firing patterns. *Appl Neurophysiol* 1987c;50:338–343.

Li CL, Friauf W, Cohen G, Tew JM. A method of recording single cell discharges in the cerebral cortex of man. *EEG Clin Neurophysiol* 1965;18:187–190.

Li CL, van Buren JM. Reciprocal activation and inhibition of cortical neurons and voluntary movements in man: cortical cell activity and muscle movement. *Nature* 1964;203:264–265.

Li CL, van Buren JM. Micro-electrode recordings in the brain of man with particular reference to epilepsy and dyskinesia. In: Somjen GG, ed. *Neurophysiology studied in man.* Amsterdam: Excerpta Medica, 1972;49–63.

Libet B, Pearl DK, Morledge DE, Gleason CA, Hosobuchi Y, Barbaro NM. Control of the transition from sensory detection to sensory awareness in man by the duration of a thalamic stimulus. *Brain* 1991;114:1731–1757.

Loeser JD, Ward AA, White LE. Chronic deafferentation of human spinal cord neurons. *J Neurosurg* 1968;29:48–50.

Lücking CH, Struppler A, Erbel F, Reiss W. Stereotactic recording from human subthalamic structures. In: Somjen GG, ed. *Neurophysiology studied in man.* Amsterdam: Excerpta Medica, 1972;95–99.

Maeda T. Lateral coordinates of nucleus ventralis intermedius target for tremor alleviation. *Stereotact Funct Neurosurg* 1989;52:191–199.

Martin-Rodriguez J, Buño W, Garcia-Austt E. Human pulvinar units, spontaneous activity and sensorimotor influences. *EEG Clin Neurophysiol* 1982;54:388–398.

McClean MD, Dostrovsky JO, Lee L, Tasker RR. Somatosensory neurons in human thalamus respond to speech-induced orofacial movements. *Brain Res* 1990;513:343–347.

Modesti LM, Waszak M. Firing patterns of cells in human thalamus during dorsal column stimulation. *Appl Neurophysiol* 1975;38:251–258.

Nakajima H, Fukamachi A, Isobe I, Miyazaki M, Shibazaki T, Ohye C. Estimation of neural noise— Functional anatomy of the human thalamus. *Appl Neurophysiol* 1978;41:193–201.

Narabayashi H. Tremor mechanisms. In: Schaltenbrand G, Walker AE, eds. *Stereotaxy of the human brain.* Stuttgart: Thieme, 1982;510–514.

Ohye C. Anatomy and physiology of the thalamic nucleus ventralis intermedius. In: Ito M, et al., eds. *Integrative control functions of the brain*, vol. 1. Tokyo: Kodansha, 1978;152–163.

Ohye C. Depth microelectrode studies. In: Schaltenbrand G, Walker AE, eds. *Stereotaxy of the human brain. Anatomical, physiological, and clinical applications*. Stuttgart: Thieme, 1982;372–389.

Ohye C. Neurons of the thalamic ventralis intermedius nucleus—Their special reference to tremor. *Adv Neurol Sci* 1985;29:224–231.

Ohye C. Selective thalamotomy for movement disorders: microrecording stimulation techniques and results. In: Lunsford LD, ed. *Modern stereotactic surgery*. Boston: Martinus Nijhoff, 1988;315–331.

Ohye C, Albe-Fessard D. Rhythmic discharges related to tremor in humans and monkeys. In: Chalazonitis N, Boisson M, eds. *Abnormal neuronal discharges*. New York: Raven Press, 1978;37–48.

Ohye C, Fukamachi A, Miyazaki M, Isobe I, Nakajima H, Shibazaki T. Physiologically controlled selective thalamotomy for the treatment of abnormal movement by Leksell's open system. *Acta Neurochir* 1977;37:93–104.

Ohye CH, Fukamachi A, Narabayashi H. Spontaneous and evoked activity of sensory neurons and their organization in the human thalamus. *Z Neurol* 1972;203:219–234.

Ohye C, Hirai T, Miyazaki M, Shibazaki T, Nakajima H. Vim thalamotomy for the treatment of various kinds of tremor. *Appl Neurophysiol* 1982;45:245–250.

Ohye C, Nakamura R, Fukamachi A, Narabayashi H. Recording and stimulation of the ventralis intermedius nucleus of the human thalamus. *Confin Neurol* 1975;37:258.

Ohye CH, Narabayashi H. Activity of thalamic neurons and their receptive fields in different functional states in man. In: Somjen GG, ed. *Neurophysiology studied in man*. Amsterdam: Excerpta Medica, 1972;79–84.

Ohye CH, Narabayashi H. Physiological study of presumed ventralis intermedius neurons in the human thalamus. *J Neurosurg* 1979;50:290–297.

Ohye CH, Saito Y, Fukamachi A, Narabayashi H. An analysis of the spontaneous rhythmic and non-rhythmic burst discharges in human thalamus. *J Neurol Sci* 1974;22:245–259.

Ohye C, Shibazaki T, Hirai T, Kawashima Y, Hirato M, Matsumura M. Plastic change of the thalamic organization in the cases with tremor after stroke. *Appl Neurophysiol* 1985;48:288–292.

Ohye C, Shibazaki T, Hirai T, Matsumura M, Kawashima Y, Hirato M. Microrecording for the study of thalamic organization for tumour biopsy and removal. *Stereotact Funct Neurosurg* 1989a;52:136–144.

Ohye C, Shibazaki T, Hirai T, Wada H, Hirato M, Kawashura Y. Further physiological observations on the ventralis intermedius neurons in the human thalamus. *J Neurophysiol* 1989b;61:488–500.

Ojemann GA. Organization of language cortex derived from investigations during neurosurgery. *Semin Neurosci* 1990;2:297–305.

Ojemann JG, Ojemann GA, Lettich E. Neuronal activity related to faces and matching in human right nondominant temporal cortex. *Brain* 1992;115:1–13.

Parrent AG, Lozano AM, Dostrovsky JO, Tasker RR. Central pain in the absence of functional sensory thalamus. *Stereotact Funct Neurosurg* 1992a;59:9–14.

Parrent AG, Lozano AM, Tasker RR, Dostrovsky JO. PVG stimulation suppresses allodynia and hyperpathia in man. *Stereotact Funct Neurosurg* 1992b;59:82.

Raeva SN. Unit activity of some deep nuclear structures of the human brain during voluntary movement. In: Somjen GG, ed. *Neurophysiology studied in man*. Amsterdam: Excerpta Medica, 1972;64–78.

Raeva SN. Role of neurons of the neostriatum and non-specific thalamus in the organization of goal-directed activity. *Hum Physiol* 1977;3:972–984.

Raeva SN. Localization in human thalamus of units triggered during "verbal commands," voluntary movements and tremor. *EEG Clin Neurophysiol* 1986;63:160–173.

Raeva SN, Livanov MN. Microelectrode study of neuronal mechanisms of human voluntary mnesic activity. *Hum Physiol* 1975;1:27–34.

Ralston BL. Hemispherectomy and hemithalamectomy in man. *J Neurosurg* 1962;19:909–912.

Rayport M. Single neuron studies in human epilepsy. In: Somjen GG, ed. *Neurophysiology studied in man*. Amsterdam: Excerpta Medica, 1972;100–109.

Redfern RM. History of stereotactic surgery for Parkinson's disease. *Br J Neurosurg* 1989;3:271–304.

Richardson DE, Akil H. Pain reduction by electrical brain stimulation in man. I: Acute administration in periaqueductal and periventricular sites. *J Neurosurg* 1977;47:178–183.

Sano K. Intralaminar thalamotomy (thalamo-laminotomy) and posteromedial hypothalamotomy in the treatment of intractable pain. In: Krayenbühl H, Maspes PE, Sweet WH, eds. *Progress in neurological surgery, vol. 8: Pain—Its neurosurgical management. Part II: Central procedures*. Basel: Karger, 1977;50–103.

Sano K, Yoshioka M, Ogashiwa M, Ishijima B, Ohye C. Thalamolaminotomy. A new operation for relief of intractable pain. *Confin Neurol* 1966;27:63–66.

Schaltenbrand G, Wahren W. *Atlas for stereotaxy of the human brain.* Stuttgart: Thieme, 1977.

Schnider SM. Detection of feedback in the central nervous system of parkinsonian patients using system identification techniques. M.S. Thesis, Department of Electrical Engineering, University of Toronto, July 1985.

Schnider SM, Kwong RH, Lenz FA, Kwan HC. Detection of feedback in the central nervous system using system identification techniques. *Biol Cybernet* 1989;60:203–212.

Seike M, Lenz FA, Lin YC, Baker FH, Gracely RH, Richardson R. Neurons in human Vc respond to noxious heat stimuli. *Soc Neurosci Abstr* 1991;17:294.

Strick PL. Activity of ventrolateral thalamic neurons during arm movement. *J Neurophysiol* 1976;39: 1032–1044.

Talbot JD, Marrett S, Evans AC, Meyer E, Bushnell C, Duncan GH. Multiple representations of pain in human cerebral cortex. *Science* 1991;251:1355–1358.

Tasker RR, de Carvalho GTC, Dolan EJ. Intractable pain of spinal cord origin: clinical features and implications for surgery. *J Neurosurg* 1992;77:373–378.

Tasker RR, de Carvalho GTC. Pain in thalamic stroke. *Proceedings of the 13th Annual Meeting of the Inter-Urban Stroke Academic Association,* Queen Elizabeth Hospital, Toronto, 1990;1–25.

Tasker RR, Dostrovsky JO, Yamashiro K, Chodakiewitz J, Albe-Fessard DG. The physiological basis of VIM thalamotomy for involuntary movement disorders. In: Struppler A, Weindl A, eds. *Clinical aspects of sensory motor integration.* Berlin: Springer-Verglag, 1987a;265–276.

Tasker RR, Dostrovsky JO, Yamashiro K, Lenz FA, Chodakiewitz J. Effets sensitifs et moteurs de la stimulation thalamique chez l'homme. Applications cliniques. *Rev Neurol* 1986;142:316–326.

Tasker RR, Organ LW, Hawrylyshyn PA. *The thalamus and midbrain of man.* Springfield, IL: Charles C Thomas, 1982.

Tasker RR, Lenz FA, Yamashiro K, Gorecki J, Hirayama T, Dostrovsky JO. Microelectrode techniques in localization of stereotactic targets. *Neurol Res* 1987b;9:105–112.

Tasker RR, Yamashiro K, Lenz FA, Dostrovsky JO. Thalamotomy in Parkinson's disease: micro-electrode techniques. In: Lunsford D, ed. *Modern stereotactic surgery.* Norwell, UK: Academic Press, 1988;297–313.

Tsubokawa T, Katayama Y, Yamamoto T, Hirayama T, Koyama S. Treatment of thalamic pain by chronic motor cortex stimulation. *Pace* 1991;14:131–134.

Umbach W, Ehrhardt K. Microelectrode recording in the basal ganglia during stereotaxic operations. *Confin Neurol* 1965;26:315–317.

Wetzel N, Snider RS. Neurophysiological correlates in human stereotaxis. *Q Bull Northwestern University Medical School* 1958;32:386–392.

Woolf CJ. Excitability changes in central neurons following peripheral damage: role of central sensitization in the pathogenesis of pain. In: Wilkins W, ed. *Hyperalgesia and allodynia.* New York: Raven Press, 1992;221–243.

Yamashiro K, Iwayama K, Kurihara M, Mori K, Niwa M, Tasker RR, Albe-Fessard D. Neurons with epileptiform discharge in the central nervous system and chronic pain. *Acta Neurochir* 1991;(Suppl 52):130–132.

Yamashiro K, Tasker RR, Iwayama K, Mori K, Albe-Fessard D, Dostrovsky JO, Chodakiewitz JW. Evoked potentials from the human thalamus: correlation with microstimulation and single unit recording. *Stereotact Funct Neurosurg* 1989;52:127–135.

Yoshida M. Electrophysiological characterization of human subcortical structures by frequency spectrum analysis of neural noise (field potential) obtained during stereotactic surgery. Preliminary presentation of frequency power spectrum of various subcortical structures. *Stereotact Funct Neurosurg* 1989; 52:157–163.

Young RF, Rinaldi P, Albe-Fessard D, Chodakiewitz J, Bloomfield S. Spontaneous neuronal activity in the intralaminar nuclei of patients with deafferentation pain. Presented at the 58th Meeting of the AANS, Nashville, April 28–May 3, 1990.

*Pain and the Brain: From
Nociception to Cognition,*
edited by Burkhart Bromm and
John E. Desmedt, Advances in Pain
Research and Therapy Vol. 22.
Raven Press, Ltd., New York © 1995.

11

Pain Processing in the Ventrocaudal Nucleus of the Human Thalamus

Frederick A. Lenz and Patrick M. Dougherty

Department of Neurosurgery, Johns Hopkins University, Baltimore, Maryland 21287-7713

SUMMARY

Studies in humans have demonstrated that neurons responsive to painful stimuli are located at the posterior border of the core area of the Vc, and in the posteroinferior area. Stimulation in these areas evoke somatic or visceral pain at the sites of receptive fields of neurons that respond to noxious stimuli. The spinothalamic tract (STT) terminates in the area where cells responding to painful stimuli are recorded. Reorganization of Vc occurs after major deafferentation. Abnormal burst firing is observed in the deafferented areas of thalamus and is probably related to loss of spinothalamic inputs. These findings suggest that the region of Vc signals acute and chronic pain in humans.

INTRODUCTION

The ventrocaudal nucleus (Vc), the principal somatosensory nucleus of the human thalamus, is widely recognized as a site at which innocuous somatosensory information is processed and transmitted to cortex. Recent studies suggest that somatosensory information concerning noxious stimuli is also processed in Vc. In this chapter we will briefly review the organization of innocuous mechanoreceptive inputs to Vc and then consider recent findings concerning the role of Vc in the processing of noxious somatosensory information.

ORGANIZATION OF INNOCUOUS MECHANORECEPTIVE INPUTS TO VC

The region of Vc is divided into two areas on the basis of physiologic criteria. The core area is the area in which the majority of cells respond to innocuous cutaneous stimulation (Perl and Boivie 1975; Loe et al. 1977; Kaas et al. 1984; Jones 1985; Lenz et al. 1988). Below and behind the core is a less cellular area arbitrarily termed the posteroinferior area (Lenz et al. 1993a,b, 1994a). The locations of receptive fields (RFs) for the cells in Vc remain unchanged over distances of several millimeters in the anteroposterior and dorsoventral directions, but change markedly over similar distances in the mediolateral direction. From medial to lateral the sequence of neuronal cutaneous RFs progresses from intraoral through the face, thumb, fingers (radial to ulnar), and arm to leg (Lenz et al. 1988). This mediolateral somatotopy (Lenz et al. 1988) is consistent with some (Cohen and Grundfest 1953; Albe-Fessard et al. 1963; McComas et al. 1920; Bates 1972; Guiot et al. 1973) but not all studies of human thalamus (Ohye 1982).

Cells with deep receptive fields are usually located anteriorly and dorsally in the core of Vc, but are sometimes posterior to those with cutaneous RFs (Jasper and Bertrand 1966; Bertrand et al. 1967; Fukamachi et al. 1973; Hardy et al. 1980; Kelly et al. 1987). Cutaneous cells are often found clustered according to their types of responses into zones showing rapidly or slowly adapting responses or showing responses to pressure versus touch stimuli (Lenz et al. 1988). This clustering was found to be significant, and was consistent with recent reports of the detailed organization of the principal sensory nucleus in nonhuman primates (Jones and Friedman 1982; Kaas et al. 1984).

CELLS IN THE REGION OF VC RESPONSIVE TO PAINFUL THERMAL STIMULI

Cells responding to noxious heat have been located close to the posterior inferior aspect of the core area of Vc or in the posteroinferior area, while cells responding to innocuous cooling have been located only within the posterior inferior aspect of the core. A significantly greater response to painful heat than to innocuous mechanical and thermal stimuli was observed for 6% of cells studied in the core of Vc (Lenz et al. 1993b). Half of the cells responding to noxious stimuli also exhibited significant phasic responses to cold stimuli. Responses to noxious heat were significantly greater than control for 5% of cells studied in the posteroinferior area. None of the cells in the posteroinferior area responded to innocuous stimuli.

The production of pain by threshold microstimulation was significantly correlated with the location of neurons that responded to noxious heat stimuli. Cells responsive to noxious heat were recorded at a significantly greater proportion of sites at which microstimulation evoked pain (66%) than at sites where sensations other than pain were evoked (1.5%). Innocuous thermal sensations were not evoked by microstimulation at any of the sites at which cells responsive to noxious heat were recorded. These results demonstrate that cells responsive to noxious stimuli probably signal pain and are located in the posterior inferior aspect of the core of Vc, and in the posteroinferior area. The location of these cells is consistent with the conclusion that they receive input from the spinothalamic tract (STT). Anatomic studies at autopsy of patients who have had anterolateral cordotomy show that the human STT terminates in Vc (Mehler et al. 1960; Mehler 1962, 1966) as irregular clusters that may be concentrated posteroinferiorly in the dorsal Vc parvocellularis (Mehler 1966) or the caudal portion of Vc (Mehler 1962). Terminations are also observed posterior to Vc in the limitans and Vc portae nuclei (Mehler 1966).

SENSATIONS EVOKED BY MICROSTIMULATION IN THE REGION OF VC

Microstimulation studies suggest a partitioning of thermal/pain sensations at different locations in the region of Vc. Thermal/pain sensations were evoked by stimulation over a relatively large area extending up to 4 mm posterior to the core and up to 4 mm below the anterior commissure–posterior commissure (AC–PC) line. Within the core of Vc, sites at which stimulation evoked thermal/pain sensations were located near the border with the posteroinferior area. Thermal/pain sensations were evoked at a significantly greater percentage of all sites located in the posteroinferior area (30%) than at sites in the core area of Vc (5%). The threshold current for evoking sensation did not vary with the location of the stimulation site (core/posteroinferior) or quality of the sensation (paresthesia or thermal/pain). Therefore the difference between the proportion of sites in the core and posteroinferior areas at which thermal/pain and paresthesia sensations were evoked is not explained by differences in thresholds.

There is also anatomic organization based on the nature of thermal/pain sensations. For example, the sensation of warmth was evoked by stimulation at sites located significantly posteriorly to sites at which pain or cool sensations were evoked. Stimulation sites at which thermal/pain sensations are evoked were located at the medial aspect of the cutaneous core of Vc, between the representation of cutaneous structures on the face and hand.

Properties of the projected fields (PFs) also vary with the thalamic location of the stimulation site. Thus, the sensation of paresthesia was more likely to be evoked in a large PF by stimulation in the posteroinferior area (11%) than in the core (3%). Differences in the size of the PFs were related to descriptor quality within the thermal/pain category. The sensation of cool was usually evoked in small PFs located on the lips. The sensation of warmth or pain occurred in PFs that were larger than those in which cool sensations were evoked on the same part of the body (Lenz et al. 1993a). The locations of PFs in terms of depth relative to the skin also varied relative to the location of the stimulation site. Evoked sensations were more likely to be referred to deep than to superficial structures at stimulation sites in the posteroinferior (56%) than in the core area (28%).

In summary, microstimulation in the posteroinferior area of Vc evokes thermal sensations or pain often referred to large RFs and subcutaneous structures. A population of cells in the posterior aspect of the core and in the posteroinferior area respond to noxious heat. Sites at which pain is evoked by stimulation are significantly correlated with sites at which cells respond to noxious stimuli. These results demonstrate that the posterior part of the core area and the posteroinferior area of Vc are involved in signalling acute pain.

VISCERAL PAIN EVOKED BY MICROSTIMULATION IN THE AREA OF Vc

Visceral pain can be evoked by stimulation in the area of Vc (Lenz et al. 1994a). The sensation of angina was evoked in a patient undergoing implantation of a deep-brain-stimulating electrode for treatment of pain secondary to arachnoiditis. She had a past history of unstable angina that had become stable following coronary balloon angioplasty. At and posterior to the location of cells with cutaneous RFs on the left chest wall, stimulation coincided precisely with the sensation of angina (stimulation-associated angina). The pain was described with a standard pain questionnaire having forty-five descriptors (Lenz et al. 1994a). The descriptors chosen for the stimulation-associated angina were identical to those chosen for the patient's usual angina. However, stimulation-associated angina began and stopped instantaneously with stimulation, which is typical of sensations evoked by thalamic microstimulation (Lenz et al. 1993a) but quite unlike the patient's usual angina, which lasted for minutes and began and ended gradually (Roughgarden 1966; Matthews 1985). Sensations in the arm but not the leg have been described in angina of cardiac origin (Matthews 1985; Braunwald 1988; Pasternak et al. 1992). In contrast, the stimulation-associated angina was coincident with a tingling sensation in the leg. Microstimulation at sites located posterior and inferior to Vc frequently evokes sensations simultaneously in more than one part of the body (Lenz et al. 1993a). Finally, clinical, hemodynamic, electrophysiologic, and biochemical measures of cardiac function showed no evidence of myocardial strain or injury related to the patient's stimulation-associated angina. For example, no tachycardia or ST-segment changes such as those often observed with angina of cardiac origin (Roughgarden 1966; Friesinger and Robertson 1985; Hauser et al. 1985) were observed in this patient. Furthermore, the absence of angina over a period of two months around the time of the implantation procedure argues strongly against the possibility of the evoked sensations having been due to unstable angina (Rutherford and Braunwald 1992). In summary, the characteristics of stimulation-associated angina strongly suggest that its sensation in this case was related to the thalamic stimulation.

In contrast to the results in this patient, stimulation during explorations in 50 patients without a history of angina never produced stimulation-associated angina. In these 50 patients sensations were evoked on the chest wall by stimulation at 19 sites. A sample of 19 sites at which microstimulation evoked sensations on the chest wall, three of which were on the left chest wall, may be too small to reliably demonstrate stimulation-associated angina. If more patients were studied, examples of stimulation-associated angina might be found in patients without a history of angina. On the other hand, production of stimulation-associated angina in a patient with a history of angina may be an example of the increased incidence of micro-stimulation-evoked pain that occurs in patients with chronic pain (Lenz et al. 1993a). Alterations in the sensations evoked by thalamic microstimulation in patients with chronic pain might be related to an activity-dependent plasticity of nociceptive systems resembling that demonstrated in the spinal cord (Dubner 1991; Woolf 1991).

STT cells in the upper thoracic spinal cord that project to the monkey nucleus equivalent to Vc (ventral posterior thalamus) respond to coronary artery occlusion (Blair et al. 1984) and intracardiac injection of bradykinin (Blair et al. 1982; Meller and Gebhart 1992). Additionally, cells at the posterior aspect of the nucleus equivalent to Vc in the cat respond to intracardiac injections of bradykinin (Horie and Yokota 1990) and stimulation of cardiac sympathetic nerves (Taguchi et al. 1987). Neurons in the thalamic principal sensory nucleus also encode visceral inputs from gastrointestinal and genitourinary systems in rats and monkeys (Brüggemann et al. 1992; Berkley et al. 1993). Therefore, experimental studies suggest that cells in the thalamic principal sensory nucleus encode noxious visceral and cardiac stimuli. In combination with these experimental results, the human report described above (Lenz et al. 1994a) argues forcefully that the region of the human Vc signals angina and perhaps other visceral sensations.

ALTERATIONS IN PHYSIOLOGY OF Vc IN PATIENTS WITH CHRONIC PAIN

Mapping of the region of Vc was done in patients with chronic pain secondary to spinal-cord transection (spinal patients). Neurons with RFs adjacent to the area of sensory loss in these patients occupied more of the thalamic homunculus than did neuronal RFs for the same body part in patients with movement disorders (Lenz et al. 1994b). For example, in a patient with spinal-cord transection at the eighth thoracic level, the representation of the trunk occupied 1.2 mm of a trajectory through the part of the thalamus in which leg is often represented (Lenz et al. 1988; 1994b). In a patient with spinal transection at the sixth cervical level, the representation of the neck and occiput occupied 1.5 mm of a trajectory through the forearm representation (Fig. 2 in Lenz et al. 1987). In patients with movement disorders, the neck and trunk are usually represented over trajectory lengths of 0.1 to 0.3 mm. The discrepancy between representation of this area in spinal patients and patients with movement disorders suggests that the representation of the border area is increased in spinal patients.

Somatotopic reorganization is also strongly suggested by the presence of an RF/PF mismatch (Lenz et al. 1994b). In patients with movement disorders, the PF is usually located in the same part of the body as the RF of cells recorded at the stimulation site (Lee et al. 1989; Lenz et al. 1994), as expected. In the thalamic area representing the border of the anesthetic part of the body of patients with spinal-cord transections, there was a significant increase in the number of sites with an absolute mismatch, so that the RF did not overlap the PF (Lenz et al. 1994b). The phenome-non of mismatch predicts that somatosensory stimulation at the border of the area of sensory loss might be mislocalized to the anesthetic part of the body. In fact, mis-localization of sensations to the anesthetic part of the body is a sensory symptom occurring in patients with pain following injuries to the nervous system (Leijon et al. 1989).

In the area of Vc that would normally represent the leg, which is the anesthetic part of the body in cases of spinal transection, neurons often had no RFs (Lenz et al. 1994b). Neurons without RFs were often recorded at sites where stimulation evoked sensations in PFs on the leg. This latter finding suggests that a central representation of the anesthetic part of the body exists years after interruption of input from that part of the body. The area of thalamus representing the border zone and the anes-thetic area is termed the border-zone/anesthetic area throughout this chapter. The persistence of the central representation of anesthetic areas may be the physiologic basis for phantom sensations in these areas after neural injuries or amputation (Jen-sen and Rasmussen 1989). Changes in the central representation that occur in the absence of sensory input may be responsible for alterations in the size and shape of phantoms (Jensen and Rasmussen 1989).

SPONTANEOUS ACTIVITY IN THE REGION OF
Vc IN SPINAL PATIENTS

Significant abnormalities have also been observed in the spontaneous activity in Vc recorded in patients with central pain secondary to spinal-cord transection (Lenz et al. 1989, 1994b). In Vc of patients without somatosensory abnormality, cells fire regularly at a rate of approximately 10 spikes per second, and two-thirds of the spike trains can be described by a Poisson distribution (Lenz et al. 1994b). Analysis of higher-order interspike interval histograms showed that few spike trains exhibit high-frequency burst firing. In contrast, cells recorded in border-zone/anesthetic areas showed a significantly higher likelihood of a having burst-firing pattern. In-dices of burst firing activity were orders of magnitude greater for cells in the border-zone/anesthetic area that lacked RFs than they were for control cells.

Cells in the border-zone/anesthetic area without RFs also showed differences in their activity between bursts, as measured by the pre-burst interval and the primary-event rate. The pre-burst interval measures the period of silence before a burst. The primary-event rate includes independent action potentials, but only the first action potential in any burst, and so is an indicator of action potentials occurring outside bursts. Cells in the border-zone/anesthetic area that lacked RFs had longer pre-burst intervals and lower primary-event rates than others. Moreover, the pre-burst in-tervals of cells in this area were inversely correlated with primary-event rates, sug-gesting that the latter determine the former and that these cells have a tonically decreased firing rate between bursts.

The most intense burst-firing is found in cells that appear to be located in the posterior aspect of the core of Vc and in the posteroinferior area (Lenz et al. 1994b). It is in these areas that spinothalamic terminations are most dense (Mehler et al. 1960; Mehler 1962; Mehler 1966). This type of burst firing is also found in other spinothalamic terminal zones (e.g., the intralaminar nuclei) in patients with pain following injuries to the nervous system (Rinaldi et al. 1991). These results suggest that burst firing occurs preferentially in cells that normally receive inputs from the STT.

Recent studies in animals may provide insight into the mechanisms that underlie the increase in burst firing associated with loss of spinothalamic input to Vc. The pattern of burst-firing activity observed in spinal patients is very similar (Lenz et al. 1989) to that occurring in the thalamic oscillatory mode in cats (McCarley et al. 1983; Domich et al. 1986). This pattern has been found in different animal preparations to be characteristic of bursts associated with the occurrence of a calcium spike (Deschenes et al. 1984; Jahnsen and Llinas 1984b; Domich et al. 1986). It is also associated with sleep in both cats (McCarley et al. 1983) and humans (Lenz et al. 1993c). Experimental studies have clarified the conductances underlying this burst-firing or oscillatory mode (for reviews see Steriade and Deschenes 1984; Steriade and Llinas 1988; Steriade et al. 1990; see also chapter 8). The oscillatory mode occurs when the cell is hyperpolarized with respect to its normal resting membrane potential. In this state, inhibitory postsynaptic potentials (IPSPs) are prolonged by the activation of a fast transient potassium conductance: the A current. The gradual return toward resting membrane potential de-inactivates a low-threshold, rapidly inactivating calcium current. During this calcium spike, the cell fires a series of action potentials at high frequency in what is termed a calcium-spike associated burst (Jahnsen and Llinas 1984a; Roy et al. 1984). Calcium-spike-associated bursts are characterized by specific patterns of interspike intervals (Domich et al. 1986).

The other main mode of thalamic activity is the relay mode. The relay mode is facilitated when the membrane is kept at a depolarized potential with respect to the resting membrane potential. At depolarized membrane potentials, small depolarizations activate a slowly inactivating sodium conductance that provides a small, continuous depolarizing current. This depolarizing current produces a sodium action potential that is followed by an afterhyperpolarization caused by both calcium-independent and calcium-dependent potassium conductances. The afterhyperpolarization produces a refractory period that generates the constant firing rate characteristic of the relay mode.

The rate of primary events for cells in the border-zone/anesthetic area that lack RFs seems to be decreased as the result of a diminished tonic excitatory level rather than from isolated inhibitory events occurring at a normal resting membrane potential (Steriade and Glenn 1982). This suggests that deafferented cells in the border-zone/anesthetic area are fundamentally different from those in control areas, perhaps because of the interruption of afferent input and tonic facilitation to the border-zone/anesthetic area. The loss of excitatory input could be related to interruption of the STT, the only spinal pathway directly afferent to the thalamus that was interrupted in the spinal patients in the studies described here. Spinothalamic inputs seem to be transmitted via excitatory amino acids. Anatomic studies have found glutamate-like immunoreactivity at higher concentrations in spinothalamic terminals than in other neural elements in the submedius of the cat (Ericson et al. 1992) and posterior nucleus of the monkey (Ericson et al. 1993).

Recent studies in anesthetized rats have shown that responses to different types of somatic stimulation were blocked selectively by different excitatory amino-acid antagonists/blockers (Eaton and Salt 1990). Responses to noxious stimuli, presumably transmitted through the STT, may be mediated through an NMDA (N-methyl-D-aspartate) receptor (Eaton and Salt 1990). Cells in the primate STT fire tonically at a rate of approximately 10/sec (Surmeier et al. 1989). If primate spinothalamic input is mediated by excitatory amino acids acting at an NMDA receptor, the loss of this potent excitatory drive might lead to hyperpolarization and increased burst firing in the postsynaptic neurons.

Interruption of sensory input can also affect inhibitory processes in the thalamus. Following complete interruption of afferent input from the arm by dorsal rhizotomy, decreased labelling for γ-aminobutyrate$_A$ receptors, but not decreased numbers of γ-aminobutyrate-positive cells, have been reported in the monkey nucleus equivalent to Vc (Rausell et al. 1992). Consequently, the balance of excitatory and inhibitory inputs leading to calcium-spike associated burst firing is unclear. Regional changes in this balance presumably vary by area in the region of Vc, and by the presence or absence of an RF.

Whatever the mechanism for its occurrence, the burst-firing activity in the posteroinferior area of Vc may be related to the sensation of pain experienced by spinal patients in the anesthetic part of the body. Several lines of evidence have related the posteroinferior area to the sensory aspect of pain in humans. The STT terminates in this area (see above). Neurons in this area respond preferentially to pain-producing stimuli (Lenz et al. 1993b). Stimulation evokes the sensation of pain more often in this area than in the core of Vc (Hassler and Riechert 1959; Hassler 1970; Halliday and Logue 1972; Dostrovsky et al. 1991; Lenz et al. 1993a). Application of a local anesthetic agent in the monkey nucleus equivalent to Vc markedly decreases the animal's ability to discriminate temperature in the noxious range (Duncan et al. 1993). These findings suggest that the posteroinferior area of Vc is involved in signaling acute pain, and that burst-firing activity at and posterior to the posterior border of Vc may be appreciated as pain.

ACKNOWLEDGMENTS

Some of the studies described in this review were supported by grants to F.A.L. from the Eli Lilly Corporation, and by grants NS28598, P01-HS32386-01 and K08 NS01384 from the National Institutes of Health.

REFERENCES

Albe-Fessard DG, Arfel G, Guiot G. Activites electriques characteristiques de quelques structures cerebrales chez l'homme. *Ann Chir* 1963;17:1185–1214.

Bates JAV. Electrical recording from the thalamus in human subjects. In: Iggo A, ed. *Handbook of sensory physiology: somatosensory system*. Berlin: Springer Verlag, 1972;561–578.

Berkley KJ, Guilbaud G, Benoist J-M, Gautron M. Responses of neurons in and near the thalamic ventrobasal complex of the rat to stimulation of the uterus, cervix, vagina, colon and skin. *J Neurophysiol* 1993;69:557–568.

Bertrand G, Jasper H, Wong A. Microelectrode study of the human thalamus: functional organization in the ventrobasal complex. *Confin Neurol* 1967;29:81–86.

Blair RW, Ammons WS, Foreman RD. Responses of thoracic spinothalamic and spinoreticular cells to coronary artery occlusion. *J Neurophysiol* 1984;51:636–648.

Blair RW, Weber N, Foreman RD. Responses of thoracic spinothalamic neurons to intracardiac injection of bradykinin in the monkey. *Circ Res* 1982;51:83–94.

Braunwald E. The history. In: Braunwald E, ed. *Heart disease: A textbook of cardiovascular medicine*. Philadelphia: W. B. Saunders, 1988;1–12.

Brüggemann J, Shi T, Stea RA, Stevens RT, Apkarian AV. Representation of bladder, colon and esophagus in the lateral thalamus of the squirrel monkey. *Soc Neurosci Abstr* 1992;18:495.

Cohen SM, Grundfest H. Thalamic loci of electrical activity initiated by afferent impulses in the cat. *J Neurophysiol* 1953;17:193–207.

Deschenes M, Paradis M, Roy JP, Steriade M. Electrophysiology of neurons of lateral thalamic nuclei in cat: resting properties and burst discharges. *J Neurophysiol* 1984;51:1196–1219.

Domich L, Oakson G, Steriade M. Thalamic burst patterns in the naturally sleeping cat: a comparison between cortically-projecting and reticularis neurones. *J Physiol (Lond)*, 1986;379:429–449.

Dostrovsky JO, Wells FEB, Tasker RR. Pain evoked by stimulation in human thalamus. In: Sjigenaga Y, ed. *International symposium on processing nociceptive information*. Amsterdam: Elsevier, 1991.

Dubner R. Neuronal plasticity and pain following peripheral tissue inflammation or nerve injury. In: Dubner R, Gebhart GF and Bond MR, eds. *Proceedings of the VIth World Congress on Pain*. Amsterdam: Elsevier 1991; 263–276.

Duncan GH, Bushnell MC, Oliveras JL, Bastrash N, Tremblay N. Thalamic VPM nucleus in the behaving monkey. III. Effects of reversible inactivation by lidocaine on thermal and mechanical discrimination. *J Neurophysiol* 1993;70:2086–2096.

Eaton SA, Salt TE. Thalamic NMDA receptors and nociceptive sensory synaptic transmission. *Neurosci Lett* 1990;110:297–302.

Ericson A-C, Broman J, Blomqvist A. Glutamate-like immunoreactivity in primate spinothalamic tract terminals. *Soc Neurosci Abstr* 1993;19:1571.

Ericson AC, Blomqvist A, Craig AD, Ottersen OP, Broman J. Enrichment of glutamate-like immunoreactivity in spinothalamic tract terminals in the nucleus submedius of cat. *Soc Neurosci Abstr* 1992; 18:832.

Friesinger GC, Robertson RMS. Haemodynamics in stable angina pectoris. In: Julian DG, ed. *Angina Pectoris*, Edinburgh: Churchill Livingstone, 1985;25–37.

Fukamachi A, Ohye C, Narabayashi H. Delineation of the thalamic nuclei with a microelectrode in stereotaxic surgery for parkinsonism and cerebral palsy. *J Neurosurg* 1973;39:214–225.

Guiot G, Derome P, Arfel G, Walter SG. Electrophysiological recordings in stereotaxic thalamotomy for parkinsonism. In: Krayenbuehl H, Maspes PE, and Sweet WH, eds. *Progress in neurological surgery*. Basel: Karger, 1973; 189–221.

Halliday AM, Logue V. Painful sensations evoked by electrical stimulation in the thalamus. In: Somjen GG, ed. *Neurophysiology studied in man*. Amsterdam: Excerpta Medica, 1972;221–230.

Hardy TL, Bertrand G, Thompson CJ. Position and organization of thalamic cellular activity during diencephalic recording. II: Joint and muscle evoked activity. *Appl Neurophysiol* 1980;43:28–36.

Hassler R. Dichotomy of facial pain conduction in the diencephalon. In: Hassler R and Walker AE, eds. *Trigeminal neuralgia. Pathogenesis and pathophysiology*. Stuttgart: Thieme, 1970;123–138.

Hassler R, Riechert T. Klinische und anatomische Befunde bei stereotaktischen Schmerzoperationen im Thalamus. *Arch Psychiat Nervenkr* 1959;200:93–122.

Hauser AM, Vellappillil G, Ramos RG, Gordon S, Timmis GC, Dudlets P. Sequence of mechanical, electrocardiographic and clinical effects of repeated coronary artery occlusion in human beings: echocardiographic observations during coronary angioplasty. *J Am Coll Cardiol* 1985;5:193–197.

Horie H, Yokota T. Responses of nociceptive VPL neurons to intracardiac injection of bradykinin in the cat. *Brain Res* 1990;516:161–164.

Jahnsen H, Llinas R. Ionic basis for the electroresponsiveness and oscillatory properties of guinea-pig thalamic neurones in vitro. *J Physiol (Lond)* 1984a;349:247–349.

Jahnsen H, Llinas R. Electrophysiological properties of guinea-pig thalamic neurones: an in vitro study. *J Physiol (Lond)* 1984b;349:205–226.

Jasper HH, and Bertrand G. Thalamic units involved in somatic sensation and voluntary and involuntary movements in man. In: Purpura DP, and Yahr MO. eds. *The thalamus*. Columbia University Press, New York: 1966;365–390.

Jensen TS, Rasmussen P. Phantom pain and related phenomena after amputation. In: Wall PD and Melzack R, eds. *Textbook of pain*, Edinburgh, London, Melbourne, New York: Churchill Livingstone, 1989;508–521.

Jones EG. *The thalamus*. New York: Plenum, 1985.

Jones EG, Friedman DP. Projection pattern of functional components of thalamic ventrobasal complex on monkey somatosensory cortex. *J Neurophysiol* 1982;48:521–544.

Kaas JH, Nelson RJ, Sur M, Dykes RW, Merzenich MM. The somatotopic organization of the ventroposterior thalamus of the squirrel monkey, Saimiri Sciureus. *J Comp Neurol* 1984;226:111–140.

Kelly PJ, Ahlskog JE, Goerss SJ, Daube JR, Duffy JR, Kall BA. Computer-assisted stereotactic ventralis lateralis thalamotomy with microelectrode recording control in patients with Parkinson's disease. *Mayo Clin Proc* 1987;62:655–664.

Lee L, Dostrovsky JO, Tasker, RR, Lenz FA. Relationship of thalamic neuronal responses and microstimulation evoked sensations elicited at the same sites in man. *Soc Neurosci Abstr* 1989;15:384.

Leijon G, Boivie JJG, Johansson I. Central post-stroke pain-neurological symptoms and pain characteristics. *Pain* 1989;36:13–25.

Lenz FA, Dostrovsky JO, Tasker RR, Yamashiro K, Kwan HC, Murphy JT. Single-unit analysis of the human ventral thalamic nuclear group: somatosensory responses. *J Neurophysiol* 1988;59:299–316.

Lenz FA, Gracely RH, Hope EJ, Baker FH, Rowland LH, Dougherty PM, Richardson RT. The sensation of angina can be evoked by stimulation of the human thalamus. *Pain* 1994A;59:119–125.

Lenz FA, Kwan HC, Dostrovsky JO, Tasker RR. Characteristics of the bursting pattern of action potentials that occur in the thalamus of patients with central pain. *Brain Res* 1989;496:357–360.

Lenz FA, Kwan HC, Martin R, Tasker RR, Richardson RT, Dostrovsky JO. Characteristics of somatotopic organization and spontaneous neuronal activity in the region of the thalamic principal sensory nucleus in patients with spinal cord transection. *J Neurophysiol* 1994b;72:1570–1587.

Lenz FA, Seike M, Lin YC, Baker FH, Richardson RT, Gracely RH. Thermal and pain sensations evoked by microstimulation in the area of the human ventrocaudal nucleus (Vc). *J Neurophysiol* 1993a;70:200–212.

Lenz FA, Seike M, Lin YC, Baker FH, Rowland LH, Gracely RH, Richardson RT. Neurons in the area of human thalamic nucleus ventralis caudalis respond to painful heat stimuli. *Brain Res* 1993b;623: 235–240.

Lenz FA, Tasker RR, Dostrovsky JO, Kwan HC, Gorecki J, Hirayama T, Murphy JT. Abnormal single-unit activity recorded in the somatosensory thalamus of a quadriplegic patient with central pain. *Pain* 1987;31:225–236.

Lenz FA, Vitek JL, DeLong MR. Role of the thalamus in parkinsonian tremor: evidence from studies in patients and primate models. *Stereotact Funct Neurosurg* 1993c;60:94–103.

Loe PR, Whitsel BL, Dreyer DA, Metz CB. Body representation of ventrobasal thalamus of macaque: a single unit analysis. *J Neurophysiol* 1977;40:1339–1355.

Matthews MB. Clinical diagnosis. In: Julian DG, ed. *Angina pectoris*. Edinburgh, London, Melbourne, New York: Churchill Livingstone, 1985;62–83.

McCarley RW, Benoit O, Barrionuevo G. Lateral geniculate nucleus unitary discharge in sleep and waking: state and rate specific aspects. *J Neurophysiol* 1983;50:798–818.

McComas AJ, Wilson P, Martin-Rodriguez J, Wallace C, Hankinson J. Properties of somatosensory neurons in the human thalamus. *J Neurol Neurosurg Psychiatry* 1970;33:716–717.

Mehler WR. The anatomy of the so-called "pain tract" in man: an analysis of the course and distribution of the ascending fibers of the fasciculus anterolateralis. In: French JD and Porter R, eds. *Basic research in paraplegia*. Springfield, IL: Charles C. Thomas, 1962;26–55.

Mehler WR. The posterior thalamic region in man. *Confin Neurol* 1966;27:18–29.

Mehler WR, Feferman ME, Nauta WHJ. Ascending axon degeneration following anterolateral cordotomy. An experimental study in the monkey. *Brain* 1960;83:718–750.

Meller ST, Gebhart GF. A critical review of the afferent pathways and the potential chemical mediators involved in cardiac pain. *Neuroscience* 1992;48:501–524.

Ohye C. Depth microelectrode recordings. In: Schaltenbrand G and Walker AE, eds. *Stereotaxy of the Human Brain*. Stuttgart: Thieme, 1982;372–389.

Pasternak RC, Braunwald E, Sobel BE. Acute myocardial infarction. In: Braunwald E, ed. *Cardiac disease*. Philadelphia: W. B. Saunders, 1992;1200–1291.

Perl ER, Boivie JJG. Neural substrates of somatic sensation. In: Hunt CC, ed. *MTP international review of science. Physiology series 1. Neurophysiology*. Baltimore: University Park Press, 1975;303–411.

Rausell E, Cusick CG, Taub E, Jones EG. Chronic deafferentation in monkeys differentially affects nociceptive and non-nociceptive pathway distinguished by specific calcium-binding proteins and down-regulates gamma-aminobutyric acid type A receptors at thalamic levels. *Proc Natl Acad Sci USA* 1992;89:2571–2575.

Rinaldi PC, Young RF, Albe-Fessard DG, Chodakiewitz J. Spontaneous neuronal hyperactivity in the medial and intralaminar thalamic nuclei in patients with deafferentation pain. *J Neurosurg* 1991;74:415–421.

Roughgarden JW. Circulatory changes associated with spontaneous angina pectoris. *Am J Med* 1966;41:947–961.

Roy JP, Clercq M, Steriade M, Deschenes M. Electrophysiology of neurons of lateral thalamic nuclei in cat: mechanisms of long-lasting hyperpolarizations. *J Neurophysiol* 1984;51:1220–1235.

Rutherford JD, Braunwald E. Chronic ischemic heart disease. In: Braunwald E, ed. *Cardiac disease*. Philadelphia: W. B. Saunders, 1992;1292–1363.

Steriade M, Deschenes M. The thalamus as a neuronal oscillator. *Brain Res Rev* 1984;8:1–63.

Steriade M, Glenn LL. Neocortical and caudate projections of intralaminar thalamic neurons and their synaptic excitation from midbrain reticular core. *J Neurophysiol* 1982;48:352–371.

Steriade M, Jones EG, Llinas RR. *Thalamic oscillations and signaling*. New York: John Wiley & Sons, 1990;431.

Steriade M, Llinas RR. The functional states of the thalamus and the associated neuronal interplay. *Physiol Rev* 1988;68:649–742.

Surmeier DJ, Honda CN, Willis WD. Patterns of spontaneous discharge of primate spinothalamic neurons. *J Neurophysiol* 1989;61:106–115.

Taguchi H, Masuda T, Yokota T. Cardiac sympathetic afferent input onto neurons in nucleus ventralis posterolateralis in cat thalamus. *Brain Res* 1987;436:240–252.

Woolf CJ. Central mechanisms of acute pain. In: Dubner R, Gebhart GF and Bond MR, eds. *Proceedings of the 6th world congress on pain*. Amsterdam: Elsevier, 1991;25–34.

Pain and the Brain: From Nociception to Cognition, edited by Burkhart Bromm and John E. Desmedt, Advances in Pain Research and Therapy Vol. 22. Raven Press, Ltd., New York © 1995.

12

Subcortical Stimulation in Humans and Pain

*Jan Gybels and †Ron Kupers

Departments of Neurosurgery and †Brain and Behaviour Research, University of Leuven, B-3000 Leuven, Belgium

SUMMARY

Electrical stimulation of the brain in conscious patients is one of the few techniques that has permitted direct insight into the living human brain. It is well established now that subcortical stimulation can both provoke and suppress pain in humans. This chapter discusses the results of thalamic microstimulation studies, done during therapeutic stereotaxic interventions. These studies have shown that different responses are induced in patients with deafferentation pain and patients with movement disorders or somatic pain. In patients without abnormalities of the somatosensory system, electrical stimulation of the ventrocaudal (Vc) and intralaminar nuclei of the thalamus rarely provokes pain. In contrast, stimulation in patients with deafferentation pain more readily evokes pain sensations. These results suggest that injury to the nervous system causes functional alterations in the somatosensory and medial thalamus. Subcortical electrical stimulation can also suppress pain. In current clinical practice, the two classic targets stimulated for the relief of chronic pain are the somatosensory thalamic nuclei and the periventricular (PVG) and periaqueductal (PAG) gray matter. Whereas somatosensory thalamic stimulation is almost exclusively used for treating deafferentation pain, stimulation of the PVG and PAG is mainly used for treating nociceptive pain. Brain stimulation for the treatment of persistent pain is not an established method. It is done largely by those neurosurgeons who have a major interest in pain and its pathophysiology, and in their hands it is a safe method. Knowledge of how electrical stimulation may suppress persistent pain remains fragmentary, and in explaining it one is on less firm ground than was initially thought.

INTRODUCTION

Before functional positron-emission tomographic (PET) scanning became available, electrical stimulation of the brain in conscious patients, done primarily for diagnostic purposes, was one of the few methods that permitted direct insight into the living human brain. Although sensory physiologic studies in humans are plagued with many difficulties, they have the unique advantage of permitting the awake subject to provide a verbal description of the sensory event. It should be kept in mind that the value of the information obtained with this technique depends heavily on the experimental skills used to stimulate the brain and assess the patient's behavioral and verbal reactions to the stimuli. In almost five decades during which stereotactic operations have been performed, it has become clear that stimulation of subcortical structures can both provoke and suppress pain, and that the responses are different in subjects with and without pain.

STIMULATION THAT PROVOKES PAIN

In humans, pain can be elicited by stimulating many subcortical structures (Gybels and Sweet 1989), such as the peripheral nerve (Ochoa and Torebjörk 1989), spinal cord (Tasker et al. 1991), brain stem (Nashold et al. 1969), thalamus, and subcortical white matter (Talairach et al. 1960). We limit our review to the diencephalon because it is the structure that has been frequently stimulated in pain-free patients (e.g., those with Parkinson's disease) as well as in patients with different types (nociceptive and neurogenic) of persistent pain. Our leitmotiv will be to examine whether thalamic stimulation leads to different (pain) experiences in patients with and without a pain syndrome.

Stimulation in the Ventrobasal Complex (VPL-VPM) (Vce-Vci-Vcpc)

In 1959, Hassler and Riechert stimulated the parvocellular portion of the ventrocaudal nucleus (Vcpc), which lies posteriorly and inferiorly in the ventral posterolateral–ventral posteromedial (VPL–VPM) complex, in patients in whom a thalamotomy was performed for the treatment of pain. Stimulation of the Vcpc provoked sensations not of paresthesiae, but of cramplike, burning pain. Halliday and Logue (1972), while stimulating a small area at the lower end of the VPL–VPM nuclei, provoked sensations of sharp pain, ache, or burning in five pain-free patients undergoing stereotactic thalamotomy for parkinsonism. The responses were produced with low current strengths of 0.01 to 0.03 mA, and the same stimulus evoked only a sensation of "tingling, electricity or pins and needles" without a painful quality when the electrode was moved a few millimeters away. These observations are important because the general belief had previously been that thalamic stimulation could induce painful paresthesiae only in patients who are already complaining of pain, and that even in such cases pain was encountered only with the use of strong suprathreshold stimuli. According to Hassler and Riechert (1959), the Vcpc receives afferents from the neospinothalamic tract. This agrees well with observations in the primate, in which spinothalamic tract (STT) terminations are most dense in the ventral caudal aspect of the ventrobasal complex (VB) (Berkley 1980).

Tasker and collaborators (Tasker and Organ 1972; Tasker et al. 1972, 1977; Emmers and Tasker 1975) reported a dual representation in the human somatosensory thalamus. According to these authors, stimulation of the anterior portion of the ventrocaudal nucleus (Vc), and of what can be considered the lemniscal relay of the posterior columns of the spinal cord, elicits sensations such as tingling, vibration, and electric shock. These strictly contralateral discrete responses are somatotopically organized from medial to lateral; the lemniscal area for the mouth lies about 8 mm from the midline against the centrum medianum and that for the foot about 18 mm from the midline against the internal capsule. In sharp contrast, stimulation of the more posterior portions of the ventrocaudal complex and the posterior adjacent structures (as far caudally as the anterior portion of the medial geniculate body) elicits a sensation of warm or cool and sometimes of burning pain, chiefly but not exclusively in the contralateral half of the body. The orientation of this second bilaterally represented homunculus is more or less vertical, standing (the term used by Tasker) as it were in the posterior thalamus between about 12 and 16 mm from the midline, and immediately posterior to the contralateral, horizontally oriented lemniscal homunculus, with its feet in the medial geniculate body. It occupies the posterior and ventral portion of the VB complex and part of the posterior group of nuclei (Tasker 1969).

What are the effects of stimulation of Vc in patients with central pain? This has been studied in great detail by Lenz and co-workers (1988). By means of microelectrodes, the Vc was stimulated at multiple sites (30 sites in two patients with thalamic pain, 35 sites in three patients following spinal-cord injury, and 75 sites in four patients with parkinsonian tremor). The effect of stimulation of Vc in the parkinsonian group was very different from the effect in patients with "central" pain. Pain responses were not observed in any of the control (parkinsonian) patients, whereas numerous pain responses were evoked by stimulation in the Vc of patients with thalamic pain. However, among patients with pain secondary to spinal-cord injury, only one patient reported the sensation of pain in response to electrical stimulation. In a more recent study (Lenz et al. 1993), these authors investigated the effect of threshold microstimulation (TMS) in patients with movement disorders and patients with pain due to lesions of the peripheral nervous system. In contrast to their 1988 study, Lenz and colleagues included no patients with central pain in this study. They distinguished between the responses obtained in the core region and in the posteroinferior zone of Vc. Thermal/pain sensations were evoked at a greater percentage of the stimulation sites in the posteroinferior region (30%) than in the core region (5%), suggesting that both regions are functionally distinct. Pain was evoked at 17% of all stimulation sites in the core and posteroinferior regions of the thalamus representing parts of the body in which the chronic-pain patients in the earlier study experienced chronic pain. In the same patients, TMS produced pain in only 2% of the investigated areas of the thalamus representing parts of the body in which the chronic-pain patients did not experience chronic pain. This is not different from the 3% of such sites found in patients with movement disorders. Table 1 summarizes these different observations.

TABLE 1. *Results of stimulation in the ventrobasal complex (VPL–VPM) (Vce-Vci-Vcpc) in patients with and without pain*

Author, year	Patients	Stimulation site	Stimulation-evoked responses
Hassler et al. 1959	Central pain	Vcpc	Cramplike, burning pain
Halliday et al. 1972	Parkinson's disease	VPL–VPM ventral-caudal	Sharp, ache or burning pain
Tasker et al. 1972, 1975, 1977	Movement disorder	VPL–VPM (anterior lemniscal)	Tingling, vibration
		VPL–VPM (posterior)	Warm, cool, sometimes burning pain
Lenz et al. 1988	Movement disorder	Vc	No pain
	Central pain	Vc	Pain
Lenz et al. 1993	Movement disorder	Vc core region	Mainly paresthesiae
		Vc posteroinferior	Paresthesiae, thermal sensations, sometimes pain (3%)
	Peripheral Deafferentation pain	Vc representing painful zone	Pain in 17% of the stimulation sites
		Vc representing nonpainful zones	Pain in only 2% of the stimulation sites

Stimulation of the Intralaminar Nuclei

Results of stimulation of the intralaminar nuclei are summarized in Table 2. According to certain authors (Richardson 1974; Tasker 1982), intralaminar stimulation does not evoke sensations within the range of parameters that excite other sensory structures. When responses do occur, the high intensity of the stimulation current suggests conduction to the adjacent Vc and medial lemniscus. Others have reported a variety of responses, usually unpleasant sensations in the contralateral half of the body together with an aggravation of existing pain ipsilateral and contralateral to the stimulation site (Cassinari et al. 1963; Mark and Ervin 1965; Sano et al. 1966; Sano 1977). Other described effects are dizziness and dyspnea (Richardson and Akil 1977), motor and paresthetic effects (Adams and Rutkin 1965), and pain, heat, and motor effects (Hassler and Riechert 1959; Hassler 1972). Sano and co-workers (Sano et al. 1970; Sano 1977) observed that stimulation in the anterior part of the intralaminar nuclei produced an "unpleasant" sensation that could not be localized anywhere in the body. In contrast, stimulation in the posterior part of the internal medullary lamina (in an area ranging from about 4 to 14 mm posterior to the midpoint of the intercommissural line) gave rise to a diffuse burning pain in the contralateral half of the body. It was commonly observed that irrespective of the site of stimulation, the threshold for aggravating the spontaneously existing pain was lower than the threshold for eliciting a diffuse burning pain. Still, according to the same authors, the parafascicular nucleus (Pf), the parvocellular portion of the centrum medianum (CM), and the nucleus limitans are especially sensitive to electrical stimulation. Tasker and colleagues (1983) performed a careful quantitative analysis of the effect of intralaminar stimulation in a large group of patients. They pointed out

TABLE 2. Results of stimulation in the intralaminar nuclei in patients with and without pain

Structure	Without pain	With pain	Authors
Intralaminar		Pain ↑	Tasker 1982 Richardson 1974 Cassinari et al. 1963 Mark et al. 1965
Anterior intralaminar	Unpleasant sensation		Sano et al., 1966 Sano et al. 1970, 1977
Posterior intralaminar Intralaminar	Diffuse burning	Burning ↑ Central allodynia ↑	Tasker et al. 1983
	Dizziness Dyspnea Movement		Several authors

that patients with deafferentation pain show a peculiar sensitivity to electrical stimulation of the medial mesencephalic tegmentum and medial thalamus. Such stimulation induces no "natural" sensations, but instead a contralateral, poorly localized burning pain that frequently resembles the pain from which the patient suffers. It further appeared that the effect of stimulation was dependent on the presence of allodynia or hyperpathia: stimulation induced pain in 62% of patients with allodynia or hyperpathia and in only 8% of patients without these sensory abnormalities. In Tasker's words (Tasker 1990): "The induction of pain by CNS stimulation may be a central marker for hyperpathia and allodynia—a central allodynia, as it were, mediated by the spinothalamic tract, VB complex and probably the reticulo-thalamic system. The converse does not appear to be true: the presence of hyperpathia and allodynia does not necessarily imply that central allodynia is present."

Burning sensations elicited by electrical stimulation are most prominently found in the medial thalamus. They are not always clearly referable to the deafferented areas, but instead refer nonsomatotopographically to large areas of the contralateral body. This is in contrast with stimulation of VB, where burning sensations are referred topographically to the deafferented area (Tasker 1990).

STIMULATION THAT SUPPRESSES PAIN

Animal experiments provide ample evidence that stimulation of certain cerebral structures can suppress acute experimentally induced pain (Oliveras and Besson 1988). In addition, there is some evidence that the same holds true for experimentally induced persistent pain (Kupers et al. 1988; Kupers and Gybels 1993). In humans, the picture is the opposite: there is much evidence that pathologic persistent pain can be suppressed by stimulation of subcortical structures such as the PAG–PVG and VPL–VPM area, the Kölliker–Fuse nucleus, the septal area, and

Structure	Number of cases	Number of stim. (100 csec, 1 msec, 10 sec; 0.5 - 2 mA)	$s_2 < s_1$	$s_2 = s_1$	$s_2 > s_1$
Frontal cortex (area 9 ?)	9	160	24	102	34
Parietal cortex (area 19 ? - 39 ?)	12	119	39	50	30
Nucleus caudatus and Fundus striati	4	31	1	28	2
VPL and Vcpc	$\left.\begin{matrix}17\\2\end{matrix}\right]$ 19	$\left.\begin{matrix}290\\16\end{matrix}\right]$ 306	$\left.\begin{matrix}141\\12\end{matrix}\right]$ 153	$\left.\begin{matrix}112\\2\end{matrix}\right]$ 114	$\left.\begin{matrix}37\\2\end{matrix}\right]$ 39
CM - Pf	3	23	2	19	2
VL	10	79	20	52	7

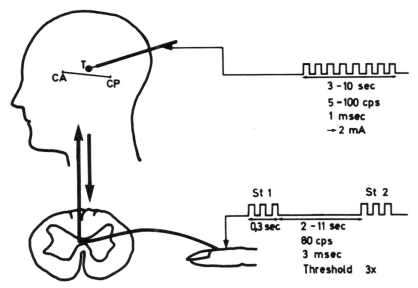

FIG. 1. Results of brain stimulation in 26 patients who underwent stereotactic surgery for a variety of diseases, mainly parkinsonism. The subject had to make comparisons of the subjective intensity of two equally noxious electrical skin stimuli, St1 and St2. A brain structure was stimulated during the second noxious stimulus. Three categories of judgment were permitted: the sensation (S2) provoked by the second stimulus is equal to (S2 = S1), greater than (S2>S1), or smaller than (S2<S1) the sensation (S1) provoked by the first stimulus. The figure shows that VPL–VPM stimulation suppresses acute pain sensation in humans. (From Gybels et al. 1976, with permission.)

the hypothalamus (Gybels and Sweet 1989). However, there is less convincing evidence for a suppressive effect of such stimulation on acute pain (Duncan et al. 1991), although there are some indications that VPL–VPM stimulation can mask the sensation of acute pain in humans (Gybels et al. 1976; see Fig. 1).

In the following discussion we will examine whether stimulation of different thalamic targets suppresses different types and different characteristics of persistent pain in humans. It should be stressed that an objective evaluation of the clinical efficacy of deep brain stimulation (DBS) is obscured by the lack of well-controlled studies (Duncan et al. 1991). The majority of the clinical reports on DBS are case histories, and the outcome measures are often too rough or incomprehensive, which makes a rigorous statistical analysis of the findings extremely difficult. In only a small number of studies was an attempt made to assess the effect on pain as well as on other outcome measures, such as consumption of analgesics, physical activities, and life-style. Moreover, practically no double-blind or placebo-controlled studies have been conducted, and only rarely has the therapeutic outcome been assessed by a disinterested third party.

General Results

We reviewed the literature on DBS up to 1993. As shown in Table 3, this survey comprised 37 reports with a total of 1,843 patients (for references see Gybels and Sweet 1989).

In these cases, where the same authors reviewed their clinical data more than once, only the results of the latest of their reviews were considered. Since the way of quantifying the results differed among the authors, the following scoring system was adopted: pain relief scores of 50% or more and verbal ratings of excellent to good were considered as successes. Patients in whom no electrode or stimulator was internalized because of the lack of a favorable response to trial stimulation were considered therapeutic failures. However, not all the authors reported these early treatment failures, and hence the following results overestimate the real therapeutic efficacy of DBS. Among the 1,843 patients, DBS was considered successful in 51% (934). When the data obtained for neuropathic and nociceptive pain are analyzed separately, it appears that 47% of the 866 patients suffering neuropathic pain and 51% of the 469 patients suffering nociceptive pain benefited from brain stimulation. This seems to signify that brain stimulation is more or less equally effective in both categories of pain. In 637 of the 1,843 cases, a distinction was made between the initial results (i.e., at trial stimulation) and the long-term results. In these patients, a significant decrease was observed in therapeutic effectiveness with the passage of time, from an initial success rate of 71% to a success rate at long-term follow-up of 49%. This means that in about 70% of the patients the response to trial stimulation was judged sufficient for internalization, and that 70% of these showed good results at long-term follow-up. This decrease in success rate occurred in patients with PAG–PVG stimulation (from 77% to 57%) and in patients with stimulation of the VPL–VPM (from 66% to 42%).

A large variability exists in the therapeutic outcome reported by the different authors. It is not very likely that this variability can be explained by differences in pain pathology, since: (a) in the larger studies, the major pain syndromes are all approximately equally well represented; and (b) even when the results obtained in a particular diagnostic category are compared, the same variability between the au-

TABLE 3. *Results of clinical studies on brain stimulation*

Author, year	N_t	Target	Pain type	% Success
Richardson and Akil 1977	30	PVG	N, S	70
Gybels 1979	7	PAG–PVG	S	16
Lazorthes 1979	226	PVG	N (107)	40
			S (36)	47
		VPM–IC	N (83)	28
Mazars et al. 1979	205	VPL–VPM	N (99)	84
			S (22)	0
		PAG–PVG	N (84)	18
Hosobuchi 1980	62	VPL–VPM	N	84
			S	0
		PAG–PVG	S	15
Mundinger and Salomao 1980	32	LM	N	53
Schvarcz 1980	6	PAG–PVG	N	100
Turnbull et al. 1980	18	VPL–VPM	N	57
Dieckmann and Witzman 1982	52	VPL–VPM or PVG	esp. N	28
Boivie and Meyerson 1982	5	PVG	S	80
Groth et al. 1982	339	VPL–VPM PAG–PVG	N, S	57 (74)
Plotkin 1982	60	VPL–VPM PAG	N	79
Shulman et al. 1982	24	VPL–VPM	N	67
Lazorthes et al. 1983	8	PVG	S	87
Meyerson 1983	41	VPL–VPM	N (13)	17
		PVG	N (11)	0
			S (18)	50
Siegfried 1983	61	VPL–VPM	N	78
Broggi et al. 1984	9	VPL–VPM	N	44 (67)
Broseta et al. 1984	7	VPM	N	0 (86)
Hood and Siegfried, 1984	8	VPL–VPM	N	50
Tsubokawa et al. 1984	14	VPL–IC	N, S	64
Young et al. 1984	29	VPL–VPM PAG–PVG	N, S	45
Kumar and Wyant, 1985	18	esp. PVG	N, S	78
Namba et al. 1985	11	VPL–VPM IC–LM	N	55
Schvarcz, 1985	10	septal area	N	60
Young et al. 1985	48	PAG–PVG VPL–VPM	N, S	73
Baskin et al. 1986	9	PAG–PVG	S	89
Hosobuchi, 1986	122	PAG–PVG	S	77 (82)
		VPL–VPM	N	58 (68)
Young and Brechner, 1986	17	PAG–PVG VPL–VPM	N, S	59 (94)
Levy et al. 1987	141	VPL–IC	N	30 (61)
		PAG–PVG	S, N	32 (56)
Young and Chambi, 1987	52	PAG–PVG	S, N	56 (87)
		VPL–VPM	N	55
Gybels and Kupers, 1990	36	VPL–VPM	N	31 (61)
Kumar et al. 1990	48	VPL–VPM	esp. N	10 (20)
		PAG–PVG		63 (74)
Siegfried, 1991	168	VPL–VPM	N	48 (71)
Tsubokawa et al. 1991	12	motor cortex	N	75 (83)
Meyerson et al. 1992	12	motor cortex	N	41
Tasker et al. 1992	13	VPL–VPM	N	31
Young et al. 1992	6	Kölliker-Fuse	N	50 (83)

Nt = total number of patients; N = neuropathic pain; S = somatogenic or nociceptive pain. The numbers between parentheses in the % success column refer to the initial success rates. Adapted from Gybels and Sweet (1).

thors remains (see further). In general, the larger and older series reported much more favorable results than did the smaller and more recent series. For instance, the cooperative American study (339 patients), with a mean follow-up of 17 months, obtained a success rate of 57% (Groth et al. 1982). Mazars (205 patients) and Siegfried (168 patients) respectively reported 84% and 48% successes in neuropathic pain (Mazars et al. 1979; Siegfried 1991). Hosobuchi (122 patients) obtained a success rate of 77% for PAG–PVG stimulation and 58% for VPL–VPM stimulation (Hosobuchi 1986). In sharp contrast, in the study by Levy et al. (1987), only 30% of the 84 patients suffering neuropathic pain and 32% of the 57 patients suffering nociceptive pain responded favorably to DBS. Tasker's results and our own are in the same range: only about 30% of the patients were considered as therapeutic success (Gybels and Kupers 1990; Tasker et al. 1992). Let us again emphasize that in these evaluations, patients who did not respond favorably to trial stimulation, and in whom no stimulator was therefore internalized, were also considered as treatment failures.

Results of Thalamic Stimulation in Specific Pain Conditions

With respect to the question of whether certain pain syndromes respond better to brain stimulation than others, we analyzed the data in the studies described above according to diagnostic category. Since we were afraid that the mean percentages for success might too strongly reflect the (usually much better) results obtained in the larger series, instead of giving a view of what was found among the different investigators, we also calculated median success scores. Thereto, we selected the studies in which a certain diagnostic category appeared at least four times. After this we transformed all of the results into a percent success score. In this way the results of the smaller series carried the same impact as the results of the larger studies. After this we calculated the median value of these transformed scores. Table 4 shows the results of this survey.

TABLE 4. *Results of DBS per diagnostic category and stimulation target*

Effect	No. of patients	Success range (min.–max.)	Median success score
VPL–VPM stimulation			
Phantom/stump pain	84	20–98%	49%
Brachial plexus pain	49	20–85%	43%
Post-herpetic pain	50	0–72%	40%
Post-cordotomy pain	26	40–100%	85%
Spinal cord lesion	63	0–100%	25%
Peripheral nerve lesion	33	50–100%	74%
Anesthesia dolorosa	103	0–86%	33%
Thalamic pain	100	0–63%	30%
PAG–PVG stimulation			
Cancer pain	125	20–100%	64%
Low back pain	299	32–83%	76%

VPL–VPM Stimulation

Despite the large variability in the reported success rates for each of the diagnostic categories, some tentative conclusions can be drawn. Pain due to peripheral nerve lesions and postcordotomy pain seem to respond best to somatosensory thalamic stimulation. The poorest results are obtained in the category of pain from spinal-cord lesions, thalamic pain, and anesthesia dolorosa. It is tempting to conclude that in those cases in which there is atrophy at the level of the dorsal horn and somatosensory thalamus, thalamic stimulation will result in a poor outcome. There is some clinical evidence that in these cases it might be worthwhile to try motor-cortex stimulation (Tsubokawa et al. 1991; Meyerson et al. 1992).

PAG–PVG Stimulation

According to the results of the studies of DBS summarized in Table 4, low-back pain seems to respond well to PAG–PVG stimulation. Unfortunately, in this syndrome the question of whether PAG–PVG stimulation preferentially affects the nociceptive component of low-back pain has not been addressed. In view of the positive results of DBS in cancer pain, PAG–PVG stimulation has an indication in those patients in whom there is a moderate expectancy of long life (more than 6 months) and in whom opioids provide insufficient pain relief or produce unmanageable side effects.

The indication for VPL–VPM stimulation is usually neuropathic pain, while that for PAG–PVG stimulation is mainly cancer pain or low-back pain. Table 3 shows that most authors, following the lead taken by Hosobuchi (1986), do in fact use PAG–PVG stimulation sites for nociceptive pain and VPL–VPM sites for neuropathic pain. However, a certain number of reports have shown that nociceptive pain can also be suppressed by VPL–VPM stimulation (Mazars 1975; Tsubokawa et al. 1985) and that neuropathic pain may sometimes be abolished by PVG stimulation (Richardson and Akil 1977).

It should also be pointed out that the different clinical features of pain may respond in different ways to VPL–VPM stimulation. Tasker and colleagues (1992) showed that in patients with intractable pain of spinal cord origin, neurostimulation (both DBS and spinal cord stimulation) suppressed steady pain in 36% of cases, but reduced intermittent pain only in 16%, and did not affect evoked pain at all.

The "Time-On" Theory of Conscious and Unconscious Mental Functions and Thalamic Stimulation

As we have seen, subcortical electrical stimulation in patients has permitted us to trace some nociceptive pathways. In addition, it has shown that changes in these and other pathways occur in patients suffering from persistent neurogenic pain. Stimulation in the diencephalon, and more particularly the PVG and VPL–VPM, can also suppress persistent pain in some patients. However, this is by no means the case in all patients, and it is unclear why this is so. These data teach us something about how the brain deals with nociceptive inputs and denervation, but do not show us much about the transduction of neuronal activity into conscious experience. In this respect, the work of Libet and co-workers (1991) has to be mentioned. They proposed a "time-on" theory to explain the cerebral distinction between conscious and unconscious mental functions. This theory states that a substantial minimum duration of appropriate neuronal activation, lasting up to about 0.5 sec, is required to elicit a conscious sensory experience, but that activation of durations distinctly below this minimum can mediate sensory detection without awareness. This theory has been tested directly in patients with persistent pain, using electrodes implanted in the thalamus. Stimuli (72 pulses/sec) above and below such minimum train durations (0–750 msec) were delivered to the VB thalamus via electrodes implanted chronically for the control of intractable pain. Detection was measured by the subject's forced choice as to stimulus delivery in one of two intervals, regardless of any presence or absence of sensory awareness. Subjects also indicated their awareness level of any stimulus-induced sensation in every trial. The results showed that: (a) detection (correct in more than 50% of cases) occurs even with stimulus durations too brief to elicit awareness; and (b) to move from mere detection to even an uncertain and often questionable sensory awareness requires a significantly longer additional duration of pulses. Thus, simply increasing the duration ("time-on") of the same repetitive input to the cerebral cortex can convert an unconscious cognitive function (detection without awareness) into a conscious one (detection with awareness; see Libet 1993 for a discussion).

In conclusion, the results of thalamic stimulation in patients with and without pain, and the observation described above about the cerebral time-on factor in sensory awareness, clearly show that stimulation methodologies in conscious patients have a potentiality that goes beyond localization. They offer the possibility of probing into the physiologic mechanisms that generate complex somatosensory experiences.

REFERENCES

Adams JE, Rutkin BB. Lesions of the centrum medianum in the treatment of movement disorders. *Confin Neurol* 1965;26:231–236.

Berkley KJ. Spatial relationships between the terminations of somatic sensory and motor pathways in the rostral brainstem of cats and monkeys. I. Ascending somatic inputs to lateral diencephalon. *J Comp Neurol* 1980;193:283–317.

Cassinari V, Infuso L, Pagni CA. Some experiences with stereotactic surgery of pain. *Excerpta Medica International Congress Series* 1963;60:121–123.

Duncan GH, Bushnell MC, Marchand S. Deep brain stimulation: a review of basic research and clinical studies. *Pain* 1991;45:49–59.

Emmers R, Tasker RR, eds. *The human somesthetic thalamus.* New York: Raven Press, 1975.

Groth K, Adams J, Richardson D, Hosobuchi Y, Ray C, Turnbull I, Long D. *Deep brain stimulation for chronic intractable pain.* Minneapolis: Medtronic Inc., 1982.

Gybels JM, Kupers R. Deep brain stimulation in the treatment of chronic pain in man: where and why? *Neurophysiol Clin* 1990;20:389–398.

Gybels JM, Sweet WH. *Neurosurgical treatment of persistent pain*. Basel: Karger, 1989.

Gybels JM, Van Hees J, Peluso F. Modulation of experimentally produced pain in man by electrical stimulation of some cortical, thalamic, and basal ganglia structures. *Adv Pain Res Ther* 1976;1:475–478.

Halliday AM, Logue V. Painful sensations evoked by electrical stimulation in the thalamus. In: Somjen GC, ed. *Neurophysiology studied in man*. Amsterdam: Excerpta Medica 1972;221–230.

Hassler R, Riechert T. Klinische und anatomische Befunde bei stereotaktischen Schmerzoperationen im Thalamus. *Arch Psychiatr Z Ges Neurol* 1959;200:93–122.

Hassler R. The division of pain conduction into systems of pain sensation and pain awareness. In: Janzen R, Keidel WD, Herz A, Steichele C, eds. *Pain: basic principles, pharmacology, therapy*. Stuttgart: Thieme, 1972;98–112.

Hosobuchi Y. Subcortical electrical stimulation for control of intractable pain in humans. Report of 122 cases (1970–1984). *J Neurosurg* 1986;64:543–553.

Kupers RC, Gybels JM. Electrical stimulation of the ventroposterolateral thalamic nucleus (VPL) reduces mechanical allodynia in a rat model of neuropathic pain. *Neurosci Lett* 1993;150:95–98.

Kupers RC, Vos BPJ, Gybels JM. Stimulation of the nucleus paraventricularis thalamic suppresses scratching and biting behaviour of arthritic rats and exerts a powerful effect on tests for acute pain. *Pain* 1988;32:115–125.

Lenz FA, Seike M, Richardson RT, Lin YC, Baker FH, Khoja I, Jaeger CJ, Gracely RH. Thermal and pain sensations evoked by microstimulation in the area of human ventrocaudal nucleus. *J Neurophysiol* 1993;70:200–212.

Lenz FA, Tasker RR, Dostrovsky JO, Kwan HC, Gorecki J, Hirayama T, Murphy JT. Abnormal single-unit activity and responses to stimulation in the presumed ventrocaudal nucleus of patients with central pain. In: Dubner R, Gebhart GF, Bond MR, eds. *Proceedings of the Vth World Congress on Pain*. Amsterdam: Elsevier, 1988;157–164.

Levy RM, Lamb S, Adams JE. Treatment of chronic pain by deep brain stimulation: long term follow-up and review of the literature. *Neurosurgery* 1987;21:885–893.

Libet B. The neural time factor in conscious and unconscious events. In: *Experimental and theoretical studies of consciousness*. Ciba Foundation Symposium 174. Chichester, UK: John Wiley & Sons, 1993;123–146.

Libet B, Pearl DK, Morledge DE, Gleason CA, Hosobuchi Y, Barbaro NM. Control of the transition from sensory detection to sensory awareness in man by the duration of a thalamic stimulus. The cerebral "time-on" factor. *Brain* 1991;114:1731–1757.

Mark VH, Ervin FR. Role of thalamotomy in treatment of chronic severe pain. *Postgrad Med* 1965; 37:563–571.

Mazars GJ. Intermittent stimulation of nucleus ventralis posterolateralis for intractable pain. *Surg Neurol* 1975;4:93–95.

Mazars GJ, Mérienne L, Cioloca C. Comparative study of electrical stimulation of posterior thalamic nuclei, periaqueductal gray, and other midline mesencephalic structures in man. *Adv Pain Res Ther* 1979;3:541–546.

Meyerson BA, Lindblom U, Linderoth B, Lind G. Motor cortex stimulation as treatment of trigeminal neuropathic pain. *Acta Neurochir* 1992;117:89.

Nashold BS, Wilson WP, Slaughter DG. Sensations evoked by stimulation in the midbrain of man. *J Neurosurg* 1969;30:14–24.

Ochoa J, Torebjörk E. Sensations evoked by intraneural microstimulation of C nociceptor fibres in human skin nerves. *J Physiol (Lond)* 1989;415:583–599.

Oliveras J-L, Besson J-M. Stimulation-produced analgesia in animals: behavioural investigations. *Prog Brain Res* 1988;77:141–157.

Richardson DE. Thalamotomy for control of chronic pain. *Acta Neurochir* 1974;(Suppl 21):77–88.

Richardson DE, Akil H. Pain reduction by electrical brain stimulation in man. I. Acute administration in periaqueductal and periventricular sites. *J Neurosurg* 1977;47:178–183.

Sano K. Intralaminar thalamotomy (thalamolaminotomy) and postero-medial hypothalamotomy in the treatment of intractable pain. *Prog Neurol Surg* 1977;8:50–103.

Sano K, Yoshioka M, Ogashiwa M, Ishijima B, Ohye C. Thalamolaminotomy. A new operation for relief of intractable pain. *Confin Neurol* 1966;27:63–66.

Sano K, Yoshioka M, Sekino H, Mayanagi Y, Yoshimasu N, Tsukamoto Y. Functional organization of the internal medullary lamina in man. *Confin Neurol* 1970;32:374–380.

Siegfried J. Therapeutical neurostimulation—indications reconsidered. *Acta Neurochir* 1991;(Suppl 52): 112–117.

Talairach J, Tournoux P, Bancaud J. Chirurgie pariétale de la douleur. *Acta Neurochir* 1960; 8:153–250.

Tasker RR. Thalamotomy for pain: lesion localization by detailed thalamic mapping. *Can J Surg* 1969; 12:62–74.

Tasker RR. Thalamic stereotaxic procedures. In: Schaltenbrand G and Walker AE, eds. *Stereotaxy of the human brain*, 2nd ed. Stuttgart: Thieme-Stratton 1982;484–497.

Tasker RR. Management of nociceptive, deafferentation and central pain by surgical intervention. In: Fields HL, ed. *Pain syndromes in neurology*. London: Butterworths, 1990;143–200.

Tasker RR, de Carvalho GTC, Dolan EJ. Intractable pain of spinal cord origin: clinical features and implications for surgery. *J Neurosurg* 1992;77:373–378.

Tasker RR, de Carvalho GTC, Dostrovsky O. The history of central pain syndromes, with observations concerning pathophysiology and treatment. In: Casey KL, ed. *Pain and central nervous system disease: The central pain syndromes*. New York: Raven Press, 1991;31–58.

Tasker RR, Organ LW. Mapping of the somatosensory and auditory pathways in the upper midbrain and thalamus in man. In: Somjen GC, ed. *Neurophysiology studied in man*. Amsterdam: Excerpta Medica 1972;169–187.

Tasker RR, Organ LW, Hawrylyshyn P. The sensory organization of the human thalamus. *Appl Neurophysiol* 1977;39:137–154.

Tasker RR, Richardson P, Newcastle B, Emmers R. Anatomical correlation of detailed sensory mapping of the human thalamus. *Confin Neurol* 1972;34:184–196.

Tasker RR, Tsuda T, Hawrylyshyn P. Clinical neurophysiological investigation of deafferentation pain. *Adv Pain Res Ther* 1983;5:713–738.

Tsubokawa T, Katayama Y, Yamamoto T, Hirayama T. Deafferentation pain and stimulation of the thalamic sensory relay nucleus: clinical and experimental study. *Appl Neurophysiol* 1985;48:582–591.

Tsubokawa T, Katayama Y, Yamamoto T, Hirayama T, Koyama S. Chronic motor cortex stimulation for the treatment of central pain. *Acta Neurochir* 1991;(Suppl 52):137–139.

Pain and the Brain: From Nociception to Cognition, edited by Burkhart Bromm and John E. Desmedt, Advances in Pain Research and Therapy Vol. 22. Raven Press, Ltd., New York © 1995.

13

Imaging the Brain in Pain: Potentials, Limitations, and Implications

*Kenneth L. Casey, †Satoshi Minoshima, ‡Thomas J. Morrow, §Robert A. Koeppe, and ¶Kirk A. Frey

¶*Internal Medicine (Division of Nuclear Medicine), *‡Veteran's Affairs Medical Center, University of Michigan Medical Center, Ann Arbor, Michigan*

SUMMARY

The recent development of methods for imaging the functional activity of the waking human brain has added a highly important dimension to neuroscience in general and to the study of pain mechanisms in particular. Tomographic images of changes in regional cerebral blood flow (rCBF) can now be constructed, using freely diffusible radiotracers such as $H_2{}^{15}O$, with a half-life of 2 min. Image resolution is now on the order of 3 to 5 ml in volume, and stereotaxic reconstruction methods allow the identification of changes in rCBF within cerebral cortical and subcortical structures, including those within the posterior fossa. Subtracting images obtained during control conditions from those obtained during test or experimental conditions produces images that can reveal increases in cerebral blood flow that are associated uniquely with the test condition. There is substantial evidence that these increases in rCBF are generated by metabolic by-products of synaptic activity, probably including nitric oxide (NO). Positron-emission tomographic (PET) images of rCBF have been made of the brains of normal subjects receiving repetitive heat stimulation of one arm. Subtraction images were made from scans taken during stimulation with innocuous (<45°C) as compared with noxious (>45°C) heat. Taken together, the data obtained from three different PET facilities, including our own, show a pattern of rCBF activation that includes structures that may be assumed, on the basis of other evidence, to mediate different components of pain and pain modulation. Thus, rCBF activation of the contralateral ventral thalamus and primary (S1) cortex probably represents the sensory–discriminative component of pain, while the activation of structures associated with autonomic and limbic-system functions, such as the insula and anterior cingulate cortex, may reflect the affective aspect of the pain experience. The activation of pain-modulatory and premotor systems may be represented by the increased rCBF in the dorsomedial midbrain and midline cerebellum, respectively. However, the function subserved by each of the components of this pain-related rCBF activation pattern can be determined only by further experiments directed toward an analysis of this inter-regional network.

INTRODUCTION

The development of brain imaging is an example of how technical advances can determine the direction of scientific inquiry. Before the mid-1970s, imaging the human brain was unknown to most of us in the neurologic branches of medicine and in neuroscience. The implementation of computerized tomography (CT) and, subsequently, magnetic resonance imaging (MRI) gave us the opportunity to correlate disease-related anatomic changes in brain structure with changes in neurologic function. This opportunity continues to improve as the spatial resolution of the brain images improves, and we are only beginning to take advantage of it. There are many questions that can be answered by the proper application of tests of neurologic function to subjects with well-identified lesions of the nervous system. Most of these questions could not have been addressed before CT and MRI became available, and, because scarcely a decade has passed since then, most have yet to be asked.

The development of positron-emission tomography (PET) in the 1980s added another technical advance that further expanded the opportunities for research on the function of the human brain (Raichle 1987; Walker 1984). It then became possible to examine changes in regional metabolic function, such as glucose utilization and neurotransmitter receptor binding, that were produced by changes in brain function due to disease or induced by specific sensory or motor events. Improvements in spatial resolution, image-analysis methods, and the use of radiolabelled water (Ter-Pogossian et al. 1969) now make it possible to identify small, transient, statistically significant changes in rCBF in brain regions only 3 to 5 ml in volume. This now allows us to address more refined and specific questions about human brain function. In this chapter we discuss the use of current rCBF studies done with PET in the analysis of pain mechanisms.

TECHNICAL ASPECTS OF PET rCBF STUDIES

In PET, rCBF is computed from the counts of gamma rays emitted by the annihilation of positrons from a radioactive compound in the blood and electrons within the surrounding media. In current studies, water (as $H_2{}^{15}O$) is injected intravenously or carbon dioxide (as $C{}^{15}O_2$) is inhaled and converted in the lungs to $H_2{}^{15}O$. The ^{15}O has a half-life of 122 sec. This is sufficient for rCBF measurements because at the rCBF levels being measured in human studies, a bolus injection (e.g., 66 mCi) of $H_2{}^{15}O$ is nearly completely diffused into brain tissue on the first arterial pass (Ter-Pogossian et al. 1969). The counts of emissions from a given volume of brain tissue therefore provide a good estimate of the amount of blood within that brain region during the counting period. The difference in the number of counts between sequential counting periods provides an estimate of rCBF within the specified volume of brain tissue. The location of that volume (a voxel) within the brain is computed from the difference in time required for the gamma-ray emission from the volume to activate a pair of detectors directly opposite one another.

The volume within which counts are made is the voxel. With current technology, voxels are typically 15.6μl in volume. With the analytical methods used in our facility, there are approximately 95,000 voxels in the gray matter of the average human brain. However, the spatial resolution of PET is limited by the ability of the radiation detectors used in the technique to differentiate the radiation emitted from two separate point sources. Because the radioemissions spread outward from each point source, there is a spatial limitation on the detectable distance between them. For PET, this distance is the width of the distribution of radioactivity at one-half the maximum counting rate, called the "full width at half maximum" (FWHM). The FWHM defines the spatial resolution for PET scanners; for a typical scanner today, this is between 10 to 15 mm. However, the spatial resolution can be increased considerably (to less than half the FWHM) by measuring sequential changes in the spatial distribution of radioactivity.

To determine whether a task or a stimulus has produced an increase in rCBF, the rCBF computed during a control condition is subtracted from that computed during the test condition. Areas of significant changes in rCBF and the locations of volumes of interest (VOI) are determined stereotaxically. This requires a stereotaxic alignment of rCBF images based on the intercommissural line, so that the differences in rCBF are compared within the same brain regions (Minoshima et al. 1992, 1993). The resulting subtraction image then shows those brain regions with differences in rCBF between the two conditions.

The next problem is to determine which differences are statistically significant (Friston et al. 1991). This is done in two ways. In an independent statistical summation analysis, the average change in rCBF is computed over all 95,000 voxels in the gray matter of the brain, and those voxels or groups of voxels with rCBF changes that deviate from the mean are identified. Because of the small variance produced by the large number of voxels, the level of significance must be corrected (Adler and Hasofer 1976). After this correction, significant changes in rCBF are typically between 3 and 4.5 standard deviations (SD) from the mean change in global CBF, and are associated with changes of 3 to 5% in rCBF. The reliable detection of such small changes usually requires a summation of the subtraction images from several subjects. In a second method of analysis, VOIs are selected on the basis of *a priori* hypotheses. The average rCBF increase (or decrease) is computed across these VOIs and regional deviations from this mean are identified. In this case, the t statistic, corrected for multiple comparisons among the number of VOIs selected, is used to determine the statistical significance of rCBF changes.

THE INTERPRETATION OF CHANGES IN rCBF

There is substantial evidence that rCBF is highly positively coupled to synaptic activity (Sokoloff 1978), although the degree of this coupling shows some regional variation (Raichle 1987). A major factor controlling rCBF is the local production of nitric oxide (NO) (Iadecola 1993; Dirnagl et al. 1993). This NO is produced in neurons by calcium–calmodulin-activated NO synthase (Vincent and Hope 1992). Because calcium influx is the triggering event for presynaptic neurotransmitter release, NO production predominantly reflects the activity within the synaptic neuropil. However, NO synthase is not evenly distributed among neurons (Vincent and Hope 1992), and the absence of an increase in rCBF may therefore not signify synaptic inactivity. Recently, evidence has been presented that NO may not be the link between neuronal activity and rCBF in the rat somatosensory system (Wang et al. 1993). Nonetheless, on the basis of other studies, including those cited below, it is reasonable to assume that regional increases in CBF are produced by regional increases in synaptic activity, and that a significant component of this vascular response is mediated by NO production (Fox et al. 1987; Northington et al. 1992; Lindauer et al. 1993).

No method currently exists for distinguishing between increased inhibitory and excitatory synaptic activity with PET studies of rCBF. Because increases in local metabolism are seen during increased inhibitory synaptic activity (Ackerman et al. 1984), increases in rCBF would be expected during the activity of either excitatory or inhibitory synapses. The neurophysiologic significance of decreases in rCBF is less clear; presumably, this could reflect a decrease in synaptic activity induced by active synaptic inhibition elsewhere, but this has not been established in PET rCBF studies.

PET rCBF STUDIES OF PAIN

There have been three PET rCBF studies of heat-induced pain in normal humans. In each study, heat stimuli were delivered to the skin with a contact thermal probe. Innocuous heat was used as the control state and noxious heat as the test state. The subjects rated the intensity of the stimulation in each study, assuring that a salient difference between the conditions was the painful nature of the most intense stimulus. Talbot et al. (1991) showed that painful, repetitively applied cutaneous heat produced increased rCBF in the contralateral S1, S2, and anterior cingulate cortices (Broadmann's area 24). In subsequent studies, these investigators have shown that painful cutaneous heat is also associated with activity in the contralateral thalamus (Coghill et al. 1992). Jones et al. (1991b), using similar methods, also showed heat-pain-associated activation of the contralateral thalamus and anterior cingulate cortices, but did not find increased rCBF in the S1 or S2 cortices. Differences in stimulation procedures and methods of analysis may account for these differences.

In our study (Casey et al. 1994), data acquisition encompassed a broader axial span and included structures within the posterior fossa. Painful repetitive cutaneous heat was shown to differentially activate the contralateral S1, S2, and anterior cingulate cortices as well as the medial dorsal midbrain (in the region of PAG) and cerebellar vermis. Significant increases in rCBF were also found in the ipsilateral thalamus and contralateral insular and ipsilateral S2 cortices (Fig. 1, see Colorplate 1). To assure that this cerebral blood-flow activation pattern (CBFAP) was associated with perception of the stimulus as painful, we tested additional subjects and applied heat stimuli with similar differences in intensity to the same site after bilaterally reducing the baseline skin temperature. The stimuli raised the skin temperature by 10 or 20°C, as before; they were easily discriminated in intensity, but were not perceived as noxious. Under these conditions, no significant increases in rCBF were found. Thus, our study confirmed the metabolic activation found in the earlier studies, and added ipsilateral and subthalamic structures to the CBFAP for repetitive cutaneous heat pain.

The results are consistent with the interpretation that the structures showing significant increases in rCBF are components of the neural mechanisms mediating the sensory, affective, and premotor components of the acute pain produced by repetitive heat stimuli. With the exception of the cerebellar vermis, all of the structures showing pain-related increases in rCBF in this study have been considered important components of the pain-sensory mechanism or the autonomic response to nociceptive stimulation. There is nociceptive input to the cerebellum (Jie and Pei-Xi 1990; Ekerot et al. 1991a; 1991b), but it is likely that the cerebellar activation produced in our study is related to some aspect of motor preparation or suppression that accompanies nociceptive stimulation in the setting of these experiments. The PAG and adjacent midbrain reticular formation are known to participate in the transmission and modulation of nociceptive information (Gebhart 1982; Sjolund and Bjorklund 1982; Yaksh and Hammond 1982; Basbaum and Fields, 1984; Willis 1985). The role of the VP thalamus in pain is well established (Albe-Fessard et al. 1985). The increased rCBF seen in the ipsilateral thalamus in our experiments may have been related to nociceptive inputs from ipsilateral projections of the spinothalamic tract (STT) or from spinoreticulothalamic pathways (Willis and Coggeshall 1978; Willis 1985). The S1 cortex probably mediates the spatial and temporal components of pain (Kenshalo and Willis 1991). The somatosensory cortex within the lateral sulcus has been implicated in pain mechanisms on the basis of human clinical (Davison and Schick 1935; Biemond 1956; Berthier et al. 1988; Greenspan and Winfield 1992) and animal (Jones and Burton 1974; Burton and Jones 1976; Chudler et al. 1986; Dong et al. 1989) studies. As a defining structure of the limbic system, the anterior cingulate gyrus may mediate hedonic aspects of pain (Melzack and Casey 1968). This region receives somatic input from parietal cortical areas 5 and 7 (Jones and Powell 1970), spinothalamically responsive medial and intralaminar thalamic nuclei (Finch et al. 1984; Vogt et al. 1987; Zeng and Stuesse 1991; Sikes and Vogt 1993), and, in the cat, from VP thalamic neurons (Yasui et al. 1988).

Three PET studies of patients with chronic pain have been reported. Decreased blood flow was observed in the hemithalamus of morphine-treated patients contralateral to pain caused by cancer; the blood flow was restored following pain-relieving anterolateral chordotomy (Di Piero et al. 1991). In another report (Jones et al. 1991c), cancer pain in one patient was associated with increased rCBF in the prefrontal and ipsilateral temporal cortices, the caudate and putamen, and the insula and anterior cingulate gyrus. Morphine increased the rCBF in these same areas. In a PET study of opioid receptor binding, Jones et al. (1991a) found evidence for reduced binding potential in the thalamus and anterior cingulate gyrus of two rheumatoid arthritis patients during a painful exacerbation of their disease.

In addition to these PET studies of rCBF, single-photon emission computed tomography (SPECT) has been applied to the study of chronic pain in patients and tonic experimental pain in normal subjects. Cesaro et al. (1991) found thalamic hyperactivity in two patients with pain due to lesions of the central nervous system (central pain). Canavero et al. (1993) found evidence for reduced rCBF in the parietal lobe contralateral to the location of pain in some patients with central pain. Apkarian et al. (1992) found reduced rCBF in the somatosensory cortex contralateral to the site of tonic heat pain in normal subjects. The data acquisition and analysis procedures in SPECT are quite different from those in PET, and there is less spatial resolution with SPECT. Nonetheless, the results of both PET and SPECT studies in chronic clinical pain and tonic experimental pain strongly suggest the possibility of different CBFAPs for different types of pain.

THE LIMITATIONS OF PET STUDIES OF rCBF AND OTHER IMAGING STUDIES OF PAIN

The primary limitation of the PET and SPECT studies discussed above and of related studies is that they reveal, albeit quantitatively, some by-product of neuronal synaptic activity, such as blood flow or the presence of a metabolite; the valence of the activity, whether excitatory or inhibitory, cannot be determined with currently available methods. Perhaps the future will bring the possibility of quantitative imaging of changes in the local concentration of specific neurotransmitters with known synaptic actions. Until then, it will be necessary to supplement PET and other imaging studies with information obtained from electrophysiologic studies.

Another obvious limitation of PET and SPECT studies is the temporal resolution of the sample of activity. With present technology, changes in synaptic activity must be sampled for approximately one minute to achieve reliable results. This means that brief, transient changes or frequent fluctuations in neuronal activity cannot be detected, although they may be a critical component of the brain process under investigation. The newly developed technique of functional MRI may help alleviate this problem (Ogawa et al. 1993). This method uses endogenous deoxyhemoglobin, which has iron with unpaired electrons, as a paramagnetic contrast agent. Because synaptic activity can increase rCBF beyond that required to meet the demands of oxygen consumption (Fox and Raichle 1986), the excess oxyhemoglobin results in a decrease in the capillary and venous deoxyhemoglobin concentration, which can be detected with appropriate MR pulse sequences (Ogawa et al. 1990). With this method, functional images with voxels of nearly 5μ have been obtained with acquisition times on the order of 10 sec. The location of the MR signal, however, may be some distance from the site of synaptic activity (Menon et al. 1993), and, as with PET, the valence of the synaptic activity must be determined by other methods. Moreover, in contrast to PET, MR activation studies are not quantitative.

The spatial resolution of PET will continue to undergo improvement as data-acquisition and analysis methods are refined. With present technology, the boundaries of even the larger thalamic nuclei cannot be delineated. Currently, this same limitation also applies to functional MR studies. Spatial resolution at this level of analysis will be necessary, however, if imaging studies are to advance our understanding of the functional circuitry of pain.

Finally, a perhaps less obvious limitation of all imaging studies is that they are only as good as the specificity of the function they are intended to study. In the case of pain studies, every effort must be made to assure that the difference between the control and the test image is limited to pain or to some chosen component of pain, such as the physical nature of the stimulus, the location of the pain, or differences in perceived intensity or affect (Price 1988).

INTERPRETING RESULTS TO DATE

Given the foregoing limitations, what can be said of the current imaging studies of pain? What new information have they presented? And what is its significance?

Taking the PET studies of rCBF collectively, there appears to be a predictable CBFAP associated with the perception of acute, repetitive, cutaneous heat pain. This CBFAP includes the contralateral S1, S2, insular, and anterior cingulate cortices and the contralateral thalamus. These structures have shown pain-related activation in two or more PET studies of rCBF in normal subjects. Although each of these areas has been identified with pain mechanisms based on other clinical and experimental evidence (Casey 1978; Sweet 1982; Willis 1985; Fields 1987; Bonica 1990), it is probably true that this particular pattern of activity would not have been predicted by all—or perhaps even by most—neuroscientists and neurologic clinicians. This is because of important uncertainties and apparent contradictions in the total body of evidence implicating each of these structures in various aspects of pain. The CBFAP presented by the PET rCBF studies focuses our attention on each of its components—and on the CBFAP itself—in large part because it represents a specific function of the conscious human brain and thus avoids the uncertainties associated with species differences, anesthetics, and whether pain or unconscious nociception is present. This leads to new questions about the function of each of the components of the CBFAP and their functional interrelationships. It seems unlikely that such questions would arise so obviously in the absence of the current PET results.

The existence of a pain-related CBFAP emphasizes the point that pain is not due to neuronal activity in a single "center" or structure, but involves the participation of several functionally distinct but interactive and interrelated brain areas. The activation of some areas may be positively correlated, suggesting common or closely related functions. Regions that participate primarily in the inhibitory modulation of nociceptive transmission may, under specific experimental or clinical conditions, be distinguished from CBFAP elements mediating other aspects of the pain experience or response. The task of understanding pain mechanisms involves analyzing the complex dynamics of the constellation of structures participating in the CBFAP.

The data available from other imaging studies of chronic clinical pain and tonic experimental pain suggest that there may be significant CBFAP differences between types of pain, depending on how they are elicited and how they are perceived. How great these differences may be remains to be determined. It seems reasonable to anticipate that all pains would share some common CBFAP elements but would also show significant differences in accord with how differently they are perceived. Indeed, it would be surprising if this were not the case.

THE FUTURE, AND SOME PHILOSOPHICAL IMPLICATIONS

Given the pace of progress in the imaging and electrophysiologic and chemical analysis of the human brain, it is easily conceivable that we will eventually be able to specify, simultaneously at the regional and molecular levels, the physiologic state of the brain that is associated uniquely with a specific experience, such as a particular type of pain. This means, for example, that one of our descendants will be able to view a composite, probably dynamic, moving image, displaying the detailed spatial distribution of the neurochemical and electrophysiologic events taking place in a brain, and that he or she will be able to say, with a high degree of certainty: "This young woman is experiencing a moderately severe, cramping pain in her left ovarian region, but she doesn't seem much concerned about it." Or "This patient with central pain in the left leg would benefit from an increased dose of gamma calcium channel and NMDA3-alpha suppressor to reduce that thalamic burst-firing."

In addition to the practical implications of such potential developments, there are philosophical implications, which should be recognized in keeping with the spirit of this symposium. If we can predict experience from images of the brain, where does this leave the mind-body problem (Puccetti and Dykes 1978; Fodor 1981)? Will we have "solved" it? Will we know when we have solved it? Or, if there is no solution, is there a problem? We must leave the answers to these questions to the professional philosophers.

ACKNOWLEDGMENTS

The authors gratefully acknowledge the support, advice, and encouragement of David E. Kuhl, M.D. The expert technical assistance of Jill Rothley, Todd Hauser,

Paul Kison, Edward McKenna, Andrew Weeden, and Laura Pastoriza was essential for the conduct of this study, and is greatly appreciated.

REFERENCES

Ackerman RF, Finch DM, Babb TL, Engel J Jr. Increased glucose metabolism during long-duration recurrent inhibition of hippocampal pyramidal cells. *J Neurosci* 1984;4:251–264.

Adler RJ, Hasofer AM. Level crossings for random fields. *Ann Probabil* 1976;4:1–12.

Albe-Fessard D, Berkley KJ, Kruger L, Ralston HJ III, Willis WD Jr. Diencephalic mechanisms of pain sensation. *Brain Res Rev* 1985;9:217–296.

Apkarian AV, Stea RA, Manglos SH, Szeverenyi NM, King RB, Thomas FD. Persistent pain inhibits contralateral somatosensory cortical activity in humans. *Neurosci Lett* 1992;140:141–147.

Basbaum AI, Fields HL. Endogenous pain control systems: brainstem spinal pathways and endorphin circuitry. *Annu Rev Neurosci* 1984;7:309–338.

Berthier M, Starkstein S, Leiguarda R. Asymobolia for pain: A sensory-limbic disconnection syndrome. *Ann Neurol* 1988;24:41–49.

Biemond A. The conduction of pain above the level of thalamus opticus. *Arch Neurol Psychiatry* 1956; 75:231–244.

Bonica JJ. *The management of pain*. Philadelphia: Lea and Febiger, 1990.

Burton H, Jones EG. The posterior thalamic region and its cortical projection in new world and old world monkeys. *J Comp Neurol* 1976;168:249–302.

Canavero S, Pagni CA, Castellano G, Bonicalzi V, Bello' M, Duca S, Podio V. The role of cortex in central pain syndromes: Preliminary results of a long-term technetium-99 hexamethylpropyleneamine-oxime single photon emission computed tomography study. *Neurosurgery* 1993;32:185–191.

Casey KL. Neural mechanisms of pain. In: Carterette EC, Friedman MP, eds., *Handbook of perception, Vol VIB, Feeling and Hurting*. New York: Academic Press, 1978;183–230.

Casey KL, Minoshima S, Berger KL, Koeppe RA, Morrow TJ, Frey KA. Positron emission tomographic analysis of cerebral structures activated specifically by repetitive noxious heat stimuli. *J Neurophysiol* 1994;71:802–807.

Cesaro P, Mann MW, Moretti JL, Defer G, Roualdès B, Nguyen JP, Degos JD. Central pain and thalamic hyperactivity: A single photon emission computerized tomographic study. *Pain* 1991;47: 329–336.

Chudler EH, Dong WK, Kawakami Y. Cortical nociceptive responses and behavioral correlates in the monkey. *Brain Res* 1986;397:47–60.

Coghill RC, Talbot J, Evans A, Gjedde A, Meyer E, Duncan GH, Bushnell MC. Human cerebral processing of noxious and innocuous stimuli. *Soc Neurosci Abstr* 1992;18:386.

Davison C, Schick W. Spontaneous pain and other subjective sensory disturbances. *Arch Neurol Psychiatry* 1935;34:1204–1237.

Di Piero V, Jones AKP, Iannotti F, Powell M, Perani D, Lenzi GL, Frackowiak RSJ. Chronic pain: A PET study of the central effects of percutaneous high cervical cordotomy. *Pain* 1991;46:9–12.

Dirnagl U, Lindauer U, Villringer A. Role of nitric oxide in the coupling of cerebral blood flow to neuronal activation in rats. *Neurosci Lett* 1993;149:43–46.

Dong WK, Salonen LD, Kawakami Y, Shiwaku T, Kaukoranta EM, Martin RF. Nociceptive responses of trigeminal neurons in SII-7b cortex of awake monkeys. *Brain Res* 1989;484:314–324.

Ekerot CF, Garwicz M, Schouenborg J. Topography and nociceptive receptive fields of climbing fibres projecting to the cerebellar anterior lobe in the cat. *J Physiol (Lond)* 1991a;441:257–274.

Ekerot CF, Garwicz M, Schouenborg J. The postsynaptic dorsal column pathway mediates cutaneous nociceptive information to cerebellar climbing fibres in the cat. *J Physiol* (Lond) 1991b;441:275–284.

Fields HL. *Pain*. New York: McGraw-Hill, 1987.

Finch DM, Derian EL, Babb TL. Afferent fibers to rat cingulate cortex. *Exp Neurol* 1984;83:468–485.

Fodor JA. The mind-body problem. *Sci Am* 1981; 244:114–123.

Fox PT, Burton H, Raichle ME. Mapping human somatosensory cortex with positron emission tomography. *J Neurosurg* 1987;67:34–43.

Fox PT, Raichle ME. Physiological uncoupling of cerebral blood flow and oxidative metabolism during somatosensory stimulation in human subjects. *Proc Natl Acad Sci USA* 1986;83:1140–1144.

Friston KJ, Frith CD, Liddle PF, Frackowiak RSJ. Comparing functional (PET) images: the assessment of significant change. *J Cereb Blood Flow Metab* 1991;11:690–699.

Gebhart GF. Opiate and opioid peptide effects on brainstem neurons: relevance to nociception and antinociceptive mechanisms. *Pain* 1982;12:93–140.

Greenspan JD, Winfield JA. Reversible pain and tactile deficits associated with a cerebral tumor compressing the posterior insula and parietal operculum. *Pain* 1992;50:29–39.

Iadecola C. Regulation of the cerebral microcirculation during neural activity: is nitric oxide the missing link? *Trends Neurosci* 1993;16:206–214.

Jie W, Pei-Xi C. Cerebellar evoked potential elicited by stimulation of C-fiber in saphenous nerve of cat. *Brain Res* 1990;552:144–146.

Jones AK, Liyi Q, Cunningham VV, Brown DW, Ha-Kawa S, Fujiwara T, Friston KF, Silva S, Luthra SK, Jones T. Endogenous opiate response to pain in rheumatoid arthritis and cortical and subcortical response to pain in normal volunteers using positron emission tomography. *Int J Clin Pharmacol Res* 1991a;11:261–266.

Jones AKP, Brown WD, Friston KJ, Qi LY, Frackowiak RSJ. Cortical and subcortical localization of response to pain in man using positron emission tomography. *Proc R Soc Lond* [B] 1991b;244: 39–44.

Jones AKP, Friston KJ, Qi LY, Harris M, Cunningham VJ, Jones T, Feinman C, Frackowiak RSJ. Sites of action of morphine in the brain. *Lancet* 1991c; 338:825.

Jones EG, Burton H. Cytoarchitecture and somatic sensory connectivity of thalamic nuclei other than the ventrobasal complex. *J Comp Neurol* 1974;154:395–432.

Jones EG, Powell TPS. An anatomical study of converging sensory pathways within the cerebral cortex of the monkey. *Brain* 1970;93:793–820.

Kenshalo DR Jr, Willis WD Jr. The role of the Cerebral Cortex in Pain Sensation. In: Peters A, Jones EG, eds. *Cerebral cortex*, New York: Plenum Press, 1991;153–212.

Lindauer U, Villringer A, Dirnagl U. Characterization of CBF response to somatosensory stimulation. Model and influence of anesthetics. *Am J Physiol (Heart Circ Physiol)* 1993;264:H1223–H1228.

Melzack R, Casey KL. Sensory, Motivational, and Central Control Determinants of Pain. In: Kenshalo DR Jr., ed. *The skin senses*, Springfield, IL: Charles C. Thomas, 1968;423–439.

Menon RS, Ogawa S, Tank DW, Ugurbil K. Tesla gradient recalled echo characteristics of photic stimulation-induced signal changes in the human primary visual cortex. *Magn Reson Med* 1993;30:380–392.

Minoshima S, Berger KL, Lee KS, Mintun MA. An automated method for rotational correction and centering of three-dimensional functional brain images. *J Nucl Med* 1992;33:1579–1585.

Minoshima S, Koeppe RA, Mintun MA, Berger KL, Taylor SF, Frey KA, Kuhl DE. Automated detection of the intercommissural line for stereotactic localization of functional brain images. *J Nucl Med* 1993;34:322–329.

Northington FJ, Matherne GP, Berne RM. Competitive inhibition of nitric oxide synthase prevents the cortical hyperemia associated with peripheral nerve stimulation. *Proc Natl Acad Sci USA* 1992;89: 6649–6652.

Ogawa S, Lee TM, Kay AR, Tank D. Brain magnetic resonance imaging with contrast dependent on blood oxygenation. *Proc Natl Acad Sci USA* 1990;87:9868–9872.

Ogawa S, Lee TM, Barrere B. The sensitivity of magnetic resonance image signals of a rat brain to changes in the cerebral venous blood oxygenation. *Magn Reson Med* 1993;29:205–210.

Price DD. *Psychological and neural mechanisms of pain.* New York: Raven Press, 1988.

Puccetti R, Dykes RW. Sensory cortex and the mind-brain problem. *Behav Brain Sci* 1978;3:337–375.

Raichle ME. Circulatory and metabolic correlates of brain function in normal humans. In: Plum F, ed. *Handbook of physiology, section 1: The nervous system*, vol. 5. *Higher functions of the brain, Part 2*, Bethesda, MD: American Physiological Society, 1987;643–674.

Sikes RW, Vogt BA. Nociceptive neurons in area 24 of rabbit cingulate cortex. *J Neurophysiol* 1993; 68:1720–1732.

Sjolund B, Bjorklund A. *Brain stem control of spinal mechanisms.* Amsterdam: Elsevier, 1982.

Sokoloff L. Relationship between functional activity and energy metabolism in the nervous system: Whether, where and why? In: Lassen NA, Ingvar DH, Raichle ME and Friberg L eds. *Brain Work and Mental Activity*, Copenhagen: Munksgaard, 1991;52–64.

Sweet WH. Cerebral localization of pain. In: Thompson RA, Green JR, eds. *New perspectives in cerebral localization*, New York: Raven Press, 1982;205–242.

Talbot JD, Marrett S, Evans AC, Meyer E, Bushnell MC, Duncan GH. Multiple representations of pain in human cerebral cortex. *Science* 1991;251:1355–1358.

Ter-Pogossian MM, Eichling JO, Davis DO. The determination of regional cerebral blood flow by means of water labeled with radioactive oxygen. *Radiology* 1969;93:31–40.

Vincent SR, Hope BT. Neurons that say NO. *Trends Neurosci* 1992;15:108–113.

Vogt BA, Pandya DN, Rosene DL. Cingulate cortex of the rhesus monkey: I. Cytoarchitecture and thalamic afferents. *J Comp Neurol* 1987;262:256–270.

Walker MD, ed. Research issues in positron emission tomography. *Ann Neurol* 1984;15(Suppl.):S1–S204.

Wang Q, Kjaer T, Jorgensen MB, Paulson OB, Lassen NA, Diemer NH, Lou HC. Nitric oxide does not act as a mediator coupling cerebral blood flow to neural activity following somatosensory stimuli in rats. *Neurol Res* 1993;15:33–36.

Willis WD. *The pain system: The neural basis of nociceptive transmission in the mammalian nervous system*. Basel: Karger, 1985.

Willis WD, Coggeshall RE. *Sensory mechanisms of the spinal cord*. New York: Plenum Press, 1978.

Yaksh TL, Hammond DL. Peripheral and central substrates involved in the rostral transmission of nociceptive information. *Pain* 1982;13:1–86.

Yasui Y, Itoh K, Kamiya H, Ino T, Mizuno N. Cingulate gyrus of the cat receives projection fibers from the thalamic region ventral to the ventral border of the ventrobasal complex. *J Comp Neurol* 1988; 274:91–100.

Zeng D, Stuesse SL. Morphological heterogeneity within the cingulate cortex in rat: a horseradish peroxidase transport study. *Brain Res* 1991;565:290–300.

Pain and the Brain: From Nociception to Cognition, edited by Burkhart Bromm and John E. Desmedt, Advances in Pain Research and Therapy Vol. 22. Raven Press, Ltd., New York © 1995.

14

PET Imaging of Pain-Related Somatosensory Cortical Activity

Anthony K.P. Jones and Stuart W.G. Derbyshire

Rheumatic Diseases Center, Hope Hospital, University of Manchester Salford, M6 8HD, England

SUMMARY

Positron-emission tomography (PET) provides the facility to make multiple serial measurements of changes in regional cerebral blood flow (rCBF) in response to painful and nonpainful stimuli. In this context, rCBF is used as an indirect index of neuronal activity (Raichle 1987). Intermittent thermal stimuli applied to the skin have been used as a source of either painful or nonpainful heat. Serial measurements of rCBF response to either stimulus are made in groups of individuals. If the two types of stimuli are matched in their spatial and temporal components, the effects of the "suffering" component of the stimulus, in contrast to the sensory–discriminatory components, can be analyzed by subtracting the effects of nonpainful from painful heat. This is the basis of maps generated by PET of the human brain's response to acute and tonic pain. The somatosensory cortex is most likely to be involved in the spatial localization of pain. It is unlikely to be involved in the affective–motivational or cognitive–evaluative components of pain. However, attention to one or another component of a painful stimulus may be important in determining the nature of the response of the cortical projections of the medial and lateral pain systems. The potential for mutual inhibition between these two systems requires further exploration. In particular, if the somatosensory cortex is not primarily concerned with processing the "suffering" component of pain, we require an explanation of why a lesion of its thalamocortical projections can lead to severe, intractable pain. Reciprocal inhibition between these two systems would provide one possible mechanism for this, but the relevant inhibitory pathways have yet to be described.

INTRODUCTION

Although there is clear evidence for nociceptive inputs into the somatosensory cortex, the precise physiologic role of this cortex in the experience of pain remains uncertain. This chapter delineates what is known about the types of inputs concerned with the processing of sensory information, in the context of nociceptive inputs into the somatosensory cortex and what has been observed in functional imaging studies of the brain. Prior to discussion of the possible role of the somatosensory cortex in the processing of nociceptive stimuli, some of the more robust aspects of anatomy and sensory physiology are considered.

ANATOMY AND PHYSIOLOGY OF THE SOMATOSENSORY CORTEX

The primary somatosensory cortex (S1) is generally considered to include Broadman's areas, 1, 2, and 3 (3a and 3b) in monkeys, apes, and humans. Each of these architectonic strips contains separate representations of the body surface. Complete somatotopic representations of the body surface exist in areas 1 and 3b and probably in area 2 of the somatosensory cortex (Kaas et al. 1981). Area 3b is the closest homolog to S1 in nonprimates and prosimians, in that it has a complete representation of the body surface and is responsive throughout to light touch. In addition to the densely packed small cells in layer IV, area 3b has a substantial input from the ventroposterior nucleus of the thalamus in common with S1 in nonprimates. Projections from area 3b are to other regions of area 3b, S2, and area 1. The superficial and deep layers are rapidly adapting, whereas the intermediate layers are slowly adapting. The relationship between these two types of cells and the input from rapidly and slowly adapting receptors in the skin is not yet clear. However, these observations suggest that processing modules in the somatosensory cortex may be more bandlike than columnar. There is also a clear delineation of levels of integration between the different somatosensory cortical strips. Area 3a is activated predominantly by muscle-spindle receptors, with adjacent mapping of cutaneous input to area 3b. Area 2 is activated both by cutaneous receptors and deep tissue receptors in muscles, joints, and tendons, and therefore appears to represent a higher level of integration (Kaas 1987). It receives information from deep receptors via the ventroposterior complex of the thalamus and possibly the anterior pulvinar, whereas cutaneous information is relayed via areas 3b and 1, and the ventroposterior nucleus of the thalamus.

The secondary sensory cortex (S2), on the lateral fissure, responds to cutaneous stimuli and receives input from areas 3b, 1, and 2, and thalamic inputs from the ventroposterior inferior nucleus (VPI) and ventroposterior nucleus (VP) of the thalamus. S2 is thought to be an important link with the limbic cortex, and has important connections with the anterior cingulate cortex.

The somatosensory cortex is therefore well equipped not only to represent a constantly changing profile of events at the body surface, but also to represent these events in relation to sensory events in some of the underlying structures.

The Somatosensory Cortex in Pain Processing

Against this background, there is good evidence for second-order projection of nociceptive inputs to the somatosensory cortex, mainly via the lateral and ventral components of the spinothalamic tracts (STT). Over 90% of the neurons of these components of the STT encode cutaneous nociceptive stimuli in the primate (Willis and Coggeshall 1991), and their terminations are therefore useful markers of areas of the thalamus likely to be processing nociceptive stimuli. These inputs have been well documented for some time, and have provided substantial evidence for the involvement at some level of the somatosensory cortex in the processing of pain.

Both the dorsal and ventral components of the STT have extensive projections to both the medial and lateral thalamic nuclei (Bowsher 1957; Apkarian and Hodge 1989). The medial thalamic nuclei have major projections to the anterior cingulate cortex and prefrontal cortex (Vogt et al. 1985). Area 24 of the anterior cingulate cortex has been strongly implicated as an area involved in nociception (Sikes and Vogt 1992, Vogt et al. 1993) and avoidance learning (Gabriel et al. 1991a, b). Nociceptive responses in area 24 are nonsomatotopic and can be blocked by blocking medial thalamic activity in rabbits (Sikes and Vogt 1992). Behavioral measures of pain responses in rats after formalin injection into the forepaw can be blocked by lidocaine injections into the cingulum bundle (Vaccarino and Melzack 1989). Nociceptive responses have also been recorded in the prefrontal cortex (Tsubokawa et al. 1981). Double labeling experiments in monkeys suggest that the spinothalamic projections to the thalamus are relayed to S1 via the ventral posterolateral (VPL), ventral posteroinferior (VPI), and centrolateral nuclei (CL) (Gingold et al. 1991). Similar experiments suggest that the VPI, VPL, posterior nuclear complex (PO_a), and CL nuclei relay spinothalamic information to S2 (Stevens et al. in press). The VPL_c (caudal division) is one of the main relay nuclei of the STT to S1. Despite this, some distinguished workers have found it difficult to identify neurons responding specifically to nociceptive stimuli in this nucleus in unanesthetized monkeys (Poggio and Mountcastle 1963), although pain could be elicited in patients undergoing craniotomy by stimulation of the more caudal neurons of the thalamus (Hassler 1972). Stimulation of VPL_c has even been used to relieve certain types of intractable pain (Hosobuchi 1986). A further apparent paradox is that lesions anywhere along the spinothalamic projection, from the brain stem to S1, may cause intractable pain (Boivie and Leijon 1991).

Apkarian and Hodge (1989) have pointed out that "nociception does not seem to be a sensory modality that is prominently represented in either the first or the second somatic sensory area of the parietal cortex. Since the terminals of the DSTT and the VSTT (ventral and lateral spinothalamic tracts in the thalamus) are scattered in small patches, since the cortical projections from the VPL_c are restricted to small areas, since VPL_c cells in a given somatotopic area project to multiple cortical zones and not all VPL_c cells project to the cortex, the precise cortical destinations of VPL_c cells are still unknown."

Ablation of S1 in patients is not associated with any change in the threshold for pain, although the discriminative components of the sensation may be reduced (Head 1920). Ablation of S1 in patients with intractable pain is rarely successful in the relief of pain (Gybels and Sweet 1989). Seizures involving S1 or S2 rarely cause pain (Penfield and Jasper 1954; Angelergue and Hecaen 1958; Young and Blume 1983; Young et al. 1986).

The role of the somatosensory cortex in pain processing has also been questioned on the basis of Penfield's observation that pain was difficult to elicit by stimulating the cortical surface (Penfield and Boldrey 1937). This is in sharp contrast to other types of sensations, which might be classified as primary sensations, and which may be elicited by stimulating specific areas of the cortical surface. Penfield paid particular attention to the primary somatosensory cortical strip, and was able to elicit a sensation approaching pain in only 11 of 800 stimulations in awake patients undergoing craniotomy. These early studies obviously did not include the whole of the cortex, in particular the deep cortical surface of the insula, cingulate cortex, and medial frontal cortex. However, these observations did lead Penfield and Boldrey (1937) to state that "pain (probably) has little, if any true cortical representation." However, pain is not a primary sensation. It is an integrated emotional response to potential or actual tissue damage. It is therefore perhaps not surprising that stimulation of a single area of S1 does not elicit pain.

Guilbaud and colleagues have recorded responses to the movement of a joint in S1, and have observed expansion of the receptive field during inflammation (Guilbaud 1985). It has been assumed that these very interesting observations represent the expansion of a nociceptive receptive field, rather than of a receptive field relating to joint-position sense. The lack of response to simple pressure over the inflamed joint in S1 raises the possibility of the latter interpretation (personal communication). Kenshalo and Isense (1983) have conclusively demonstrated units in the somatosensory cortex of monkeys that respond to noxious stimulation to a greater extent than to nonnoxious stimulation. However, the level of response to mechanical stimuli of increasing intensity showed a fairly gradual increase, with no evidence of a sharp increase at nociceptive levels of intensity. It therefore seems likely that the somatosensory cortex is equipped to localize and encode the intensity of stimulation in the noxious range. What is not clear is what these responses represent in terms of sensory experience. Whether they represent the differential localization of intense stimulation or whether they represent first pain is not clear. The question therefore becomes: To what extent is the somatosensory cortex involved in the processing of pain and contribution to pain experience, and how might it interact with other areas of the cortex such as the insula, prefrontal and anterior cingulate cortices, which are now also strongly implicated in the human pain response?

METHODOLOGIC ASPECTS OF MEASUREMENT OF METABOLIC AND VASCULAR RESPONSES FOR THE IMAGING OF CEREBRAL RESPONSES TO SENSORY STIMULATION

General Aspects

Positron-emission tomography (PET) is a technique for accurately measuring, in time and space, very small concentrations of radioactivity in living tissue (Lucignani et al. 1989). Cyclotron-generated short- and longer-lived positron-emitting isotopes (e.g., ^{11}C, ^{18}F, ^{15}O) have been incorporated into a range of molecules to provide tracers capable of providing information about specific biologic processes after inhalation (e.g., $C^{15}O_2$ for blood flow) or i.v. injection (e.g. H_2 ^{15}O for blood flow, ^{18}FDG for deoxyglucose metabolism, ^{11}C-RO15 for benzodiazepine binding, ^{11}C-diprenorphine for opiate-receptor binding) without interfering with those processes.

At present, PET and single-photon emission computed tomography (SPECT) are the only means by which integrated (whole brain) cerebral metabolic and pharmacological responses to pain can be studied in humans. The relative contributions of tomographic imaging techniques and electrophysiologic methods have recently been extensively reviewed (Chen 1993 a,b), and will not be further examined here. The discussion will be mainly limited to PET methodology. However, it is our view that each of these techniques has its own complementary contribution to make. The combined use of functional imaging and electrophysiologic techniques is likely to be particularly productive in interpreting some of the changes in regional cerebral blood flow (rCBF) detected by PET, particularly in relation to attention and variability of psychological state during PET studies (Itoh et al. 1993). The recently developed means to accurately coregister functional PET images with structural magnetic resonance (MR) images of the brain has considerably enhanced the effective (but not actual) spatial resolution of PET (Woods et al. 1992). The development of functional magnetic resonance imaging (FMRI) to measure a combination of changes in blood flow, volume, and deoxyhemoglobin, although at an early stage in terms of quantitation, is likely to provide a powerful tool for resolving certain issues of brain function at a higher resolution than does PET. These exciting techniques have been pioneered by Belliveau and colleagues and have been recently reviewed elsewhere (Belliveau et al. 1991).

PET Scanning

The reasons for the sensitivity and localizing capacity of PET are intrinsic to the nature of positron emission. Shortly after the release of a positron (a positively charged electron), it is annihilated by collision with an electron, resulting in the emission of two photons traveling at almost 180° to each other. PET utilizes this property by recording the simultaneous arrival of two such photons at a cylindrical bank of detectors around the source. Simultaneous arrivals of positrons of the appropriate energy (511 keV) are electronically recorded as coincidence events. This allows the physical collimation used in SPECT to be replaced by electronic collimation. The recording of several such events at different angles from a single source allows the source of radioactivity to be computed. The recording of multiple coincidence events by a ring of detectors facilitates the construction of a two-dimensional image of radioactivity. However, emission scans require correction for variable attenuation of the photon energy within tissues of different densities. This is achieved by doing a transmission scan with an external source of positrons.

Through the use of this transmission scan, the emission scan is reconstructed to produce parametric images, in multiple time-frames, of the distribution of radioactivity.

Only tissue concentrations of radioactivity can be measured. The biologic specificity of the measurements will therefore depend on the specificity of the tracer used and the ability to quantitate the kinetic parameters relating to its dynamic distribution in different tissue compartments.

Simultaneous dynamic measurement of regional cerebral radioactivity in multiple slices is now routinely acquired through PET. Simultaneous continuous arterial sampling of radioactivity is usually required to provide a continuous arterial input function for the absolute quantitation of tissue kinetics. After the reconstruction of each emission scan, a series of dynamic scans of regional tracer distribution is obtained in multiple brain slices. Appropriate models for the *in vivo* behavior of the particular tracer being used are applied to these whole-brain and arterial-dynamic data sets to generate parameters for binding (Jones et al. 1993) to receptor/reuptake sites or for flow and metabolism (Lammertsma et al. 1990). Data collection with a multiringed scanner allows whole-brain data sets to be collected simultaneously and continuously with a temporal resolution of 1 sec and spatial resolution of 6.5 mm at full-width half-maximum (FWHM), which is the physical resolution capacity of the system. However, the high chemical resolution provided by PET makes it possible to visualize smaller volumes of tissue if the contrast with the surrounding tissue is high and the appropriate ligand is used (e.g., periaqueductal grey [PAG] in the brain stem can be visualized with flow activation [Fig. 1, see Colorplate 2] and [^{11}C]diprenorphine for opiate receptor binding).

Scanning in Three-Dimensional Mode

Until recently, individual detector rings were separated by lead septa in order to reduce background counts from scatter and random coincidences. This results in a hybrid of electronic and physical (septa) collimation. Systems having such rings make maximum use of the coincidence events in the plane of each detector ring, but make poor use of the total photon emission from the tissue being scanned. The recent introduction of commercial scanners with the capacity to retract their septa has resulted in full electronic collimation. This results in a threefold increase in sensitivity across the whole brain (Bailey et al. 1991a), with a fivefold increase in sensitivity at the center of the field of view. The greater resulting scatter is corrected through use of a dual-energy window-scatter correction (Grootoonk et al. 1991). The increase in noise is compensated for by the more efficient use of the administered radioactivity (Townsend et al. 1991). The greater resulting sensitivity of scanning in the three-dimensional mode has resulted in a commensurate improvement in signal-to-noise (S/N) ratios (improvement in noise equivalent counts of three in the center of the field), and a consequent substantial improvement in the quality of radioligand and metabolic studies. Specifically, the point-source sensitivity is six to seven times greater than with the standard CTI 931 scanner recording with the septa in place (Bailey et al. 1991a), while in practice there is a threefold increase in useful counts over the whole brain, with a fivefold increase at the center of the field of view. Thus, individual subjects can be studied alone by reducing the radiation dose to increase the number of scans per individual.

Another consequence of the development of retractable septa is that in the case of flow activation studies, more measurements of flow can be made in single subjects using less radioactivity per measurement. This has meant that significant results can now be obtained in single subjects whereas the pooling of results from several subjects had previously been necessary.

Principles of PET Activation Studies

Acute changes in neuronal function are usually accompanied by changes in cerebral blood flow (CBF) (Raichle 1987). Changes in cerebral function can therefore be detected by measuring regional changes in cerebral blood flow (rCBF), provided that a correction is made for the variability of global blood flow. The recent development of statistical methods for analyzing whole brain data sets (Fox and Mintum 1989) has led to a proliferation of information about the functional anatomy of the brain over the last 4 years.

In order to localize different aspects of cerebral function within the brain, experiments using PET scanning must be carefully designed to provide specific answers to specific questions. Repeated measures of rCBF are made in response to a sensory, psychological, cognitive, or motor challenge. The subtraction of the irrelevant components of the stimulus or task is an integral component of studies of this type. Because there is likely to be variability in the subject's psychological state during a study, in addition to variation in the attention given to a task, most studies so far have concentrated on pooling data from repeated measure on groups of six to 12 subjects (Fig. 1). The methods for pooling these group data and making the appropriate subtractions have been greatly advanced by Friston and colleagues (Friston 1990, 1991). Their approach requires that each data set be placed into a standardized stereotactic space in relation to the atlas of Talairach (Talairach and Tournoux 1988). Corrections are made for variations in global flow. Each individual data set is then pooled to create a single data set in order to subtract the effects of one condition from the other. This approach permits subtraction of the effects of different conditions on rCBF within a group or comparisons of effects between groups of subjects.

PAIN ACTIVATION STUDIES

The aim of our studies was to identify the principal areas of pain processing in the human brain and to subsequently examine the differences in patterns of response in patients with different types of chronic pain. The latter will not be described here, but have been reviewed elsewhere (Jones and Derbyshire, in press). In this section we will concentrate on the methodology used in our pain-activation studies and give some examples of recent results in groups of normal volunteers as an illustration of some of the issues rather than as an exhaustive catalogue of results. A more complete discussion of our results in the context of those obtained by other investigators will follow.

The principle of most of these studies was that somatosensory discriminatory components of a thermal stimulus (its spatial and temporal localization) were subtracted from the acute thermal pain component of the stimulus, with the result that only the emotional, motivational, cognitive, and evaluative components of the pain responses were examined. Obviously a major component of these responses is the "suffering" component of pain. The thermal stimulus used in our studies at the Hammersmith Hospital, was intermittent and highly reproducible. It was applied to the back of the hand in one position only and at the same frequency, in order to control for the temporal and spatial components of the stimulus. Other centers have moved the location of stimulus around the hand between measurement in order to avoid habituation.

Data Acquisition

Subjects

Six right-handed male volunteers, aged 28 to 50 years (mean age 35 years), and six right-handed female volunteers, aged 47 to 69 years (mean age 54.2 years) took part in the study. A further male volunteer received a series of 12 scans as an individual study. Permission to carry out these studies was obtained from the AR-SAC-UK (Administration of Radioactive Substances Advisory Committee, UK) and the Research Ethics Committee of Hammersmith Hospital.

Procedure

The heat stimulus, used for both hot and painfully hot stimulations, was obtained with a Marstock thermal threshold stimulator (Somedic: Thermotest Type 1; Fruhstorfer et al. 1976), which delivers reproducible, intermittent ramps of increasing heat via a water-cooled probe. Scans were obtained from our volunteer groups with a PET scanner (CTI model 931-08/12 Knoxville, TN) (Spinks et al. 1988). Data were obtained for single subject analysis with another PET scanner (CTI model 953B Knoxville, TN) in three-dimensional mode. Prior to the scan, temperatures that were reproducibly experienced as nonpainfully hot or painfully hot on the back of the right hand were carefully established for each subject, using the thermal threshold stimulator.

Each subject was positioned in the scanner in such a way that the axis of the scanner was approximately parallel to the glabellar–inion line, which is in turn parallel to the line between the anterior and posterior commissures (AC–PC line). A transmission scan was performed prior to the emission scans. Each subject underwent six or 12 sequential scans over the course of a single 2- or 3-hour session. Each scan provided a single measurement of relative rCBF. In each subject rCBF was measured by recording the distribution of cerebral radioactivity following inhalation of the freely diffusible, positron-emitting, ^{15}O-labeled tracer carbon dioxide $C^{15}O_2$ (931 scanner) or $H_2^{15}O$ (953B scanner). Any increase in rCBF entails an increase in the amount of radioactivity recorded from the same region (Mazziotta et al. 1985; Fox and Mintum 1989). Each thermal stimulus was begun 5 sec prior to the start of the scan. Subjects were warned before the start of each stimulation but were not told whether the painful or nonpainful temperature was to be applied. The two stimuli were alternated from scan to scan, in order to avoid any possible order effects; the series commenced with a nonpainfully hot stimulus in half the subjects and a painfully hot stimulus in the other half. Each scan lasted 2 min, during which time an intermittent and precisely reproducible ramp of increasing heat was applied to the back of the right hand every 15 sec. After each measurement of rCBF, retrospective verbal confirmation was obtained that the subject had experienced the stimulus appropriately as nonpainfully hot or painfully hot. No other measurement was made during the time of stimulation, in order to avoid altering the sensory input.

Data Analysis

Groups

The object of the analysis of these studies was first to make statistical comparisons of changes in blood flow between the different stimulation conditions in such a way that the effect of increasing heat intensity without pain could be compared with the effect of painful thermal stimulation. The second objective was to make statistical comparisons of changes in blood flow between the two groups such that the effect of pain on a female group could be compared with the effect of pain on a male group. To make these comparisons, the following procedures were done. Correction for head movement between scans was done by aligning all of the scan images with the first image using automated image registration (AIR) software specifically developed for this purpose (Woods et al. 1992). Each realigned set of scans from every patient was reoriented into a standardized stereotactic anatomic space. A correction was made for global changes in blood flow between scans. These two procedures allow flow values for each stimulus condition to be pooled across subjects. Finally a statistical comparison of blood flow distributions between conditions and groups was performed to identify sites of significantly changed regional flow (Friston et al. 1991).

The AC–PC line was identified directly from the PET image, and the data were transformed into a standard stereotactic space according to the stereotactic atlas of Talairach and Tournoux (1988). In order to increase the signal-to-noise ratio and accommodate variability in functional anatomy, each image was smoothed in the x, y, and z dimensions with a Gaussian filter of 20 mm (FWHM). Differences in global activity were removed following a pixel-by-pixel analysis of covariance (Friston et al 1990). The differences between one condition and another were assessed with the appropriate contrast (weighting of the six condition means) using the t statistic (Friston et al 1991). This analysis is performed for each pixel, and the resulting set of t values constitutes the t-statistical parametric map (SPM $\{t\}$) of the area of interest. The significance of this SPM was assessed by comparing the observed and expected pixels above a specific criterion ($p<0.001$). The resulting 0.001 significance pertains to this suprathreshold subset, or profile of pixels. The threshold limit of $p<0.001$ was chosen because empirical studies with phantoms have shown that this threshold protects against false positives (Bailey et al 1991b). Note that because the significance relates to the profile of rCBF changes, individual foci are reported for descriptive purposes only.

Two sorts of statistical comparison were performed: (a) A comparison to assess the differences in the neurophysiologic responses to pain between the two groups; and (b) a comparison to determine the effects of pain in both groups. The interaction term was assessed with the appropriate contrast to define the t statistic. This contrast effectively tests for a difference in rCBF increases due to pain, these differences being assessed between the two groups (males and females). The error variance used to compute the t statistic was the average error variance for each pixel based on the one way analyses of variance (ANOVAs) described above. In analyzing simple effects of pain for both groups combined, the nonpainfully hot conditions (increasing heat, anticipation of pain) were subtracted from the painfully hot conditions (increasing heat, anticipation of pain, pain) for all 12 subjects combined. The resulting SPM $\{t\}$ highlighted brain regions that responded to pain by increasing their rCBF.

Throughout the data analysis we used one-tailed tests of significance, looking for: (a) increases in the pain-induced rCBF response in the female subjects over and above those seen in the male subjects for the interaction SPM$\{t\}$, and (b) increases in rCBF due to pain.

Single Study

A procedure similar to the one described above was used for analyzing the pattern of rCBF change in individual subjects. Each image was smoothed in the x, y, and z dimensions with a Gaussian filter of 20 mm (FWHM), while the SPM$\{t\}$ was smoothed with a secondary filter of 4 mm FWHM.

The search for areas of significance was conducted in the same manner as above except with an omnibus threshold of $p = 0.01$ to interrogate the whole brain for significant change in response to pain with a chi-square protection against false positives.

PET–MRI coregistration

For the individual subject, an MRI was obtained using a 1-Tesla Picker HPQ Vista system with an RF spoiled volume acquisition that is relatively T1 weighted to give good grey/white contrast and anatomic resolution. After reconstruction the MR images were also aligned parallel with the intercommissural line and interpolated to yield a cubic voxel size of $0.977 \times 0.977 \times 0.977$ mm^3, which permitted co-registration with PET images.

For the coregistration of SPM and MR images obtained from single three-dimensional activation, the steps of image realignment to the intercommissural line and anatomic standardization were omitted. Also, the filtering was considerably reduced with a primary filter of 10 mm FWHM and no secondary filter. The ANOVA and the generation of a thresholded SPM{t} were identical. The SPM{t} was then coregistered with the subject's own MRI scan. Such superimposition allowed us to determine the position of the region of maximal change in rCBF in relation to the gyral and sulcal pattern of the subject's brain.

Results

In the comparison of rCBF increases in the males with increases in the females, no between-group analysis revealed any significant differences between the groups. The results for both of these groups were therefore pooled and reanalyzed.

Table 1 shows the areas of significant increases ($p<0.001$) in rCBF from the comparison of painful heat with nonpainful heat for all 12 of the subjects combined. The results of a single pain activation study on a normal volunteer acquired in three-dimensional mode, are demonstrated in Fig. 1 (see Colorplate 2). The details in Table 1 are reproduced in Fig. 2 (see Colorplate 3), which shows these focal activ-

TABLE 1. *Areas of significant change in rCBF in response to pain (thermal painful phasic heat to the right hand versus nonpainful heat) pooled from a group of 12 male and female normal volunteers. Within-group comparison for the pooled control group*

Region	Side	Coordinates (mm)			Associated z-value
		x	y	z	
1. PAG	(M)	2	−50	−20	3.113
2. Thalamus/insula/lentiform nucleus	(L)	−24	−10	8	3.887
3. Thalamus/lentiform nucleus	(R)	22	6	8	3.843
4. Prefrontal cortex (BA 44)/insula cortex	(R)	42	10	16	3.401
5. Prefrontal cortex (BA 10)	(R)	22	34	24	3.099
6. Inferior parietal/temporal cortex	(R)	56	−42	28	3.380
7. Anterior cingulate (BA 24)	(L)	−8	−10	40	3.818

All values shown are significant at $p < 0.001$. The x, y, and z coordinates refer to the standard 3D coordinates described in the atlas of Talairach and Tournoux (1988).

ities as SPMs at the appropriate levels in the brain. The main areas showing significant activation are thalamus, insula, and anterior cingulate cortex (area 24) contralateral to the thermal stimulus and the putamen/thalamus, prefrontal cortex (area
10), and inferior parietal/temporal cortex (areas 39 and 40), in addition to an area of
activation in the brain stem corresponding to the PAG. The increase at the center of
all of these areas was significant at $p < 0.001$.

REVIEW OF CORTICAL RESPONSES TO PAIN

Three PET centers have now published results of thermal pain stimulation in
normal volunteers (Jones et al. 1991a, b; Talbot et al. 1991; Minoshima et al. 1993).
All three groups used some form of acute intermittent thermal heat pain applied
either to the back of the right hand or the forearm of right-handed normal male
volunteers, and subtracted the effects of nonpainful heat from painful heat. The
Hammersmith group kept the thermal probe in the same place during each measurement of rCBF in each subject in order to minimize attention to position, whereas the
Montreal and Ann Arbor groups moved the stimulus around the forearm in order to
minimize habituation.

There is both agreement and disagreement over the areas of the brain that showed
significant increases in blood flow. There is now agreement between the groups on
contralateral (to stimulus) thalamic and anterior cingulate increases in blood flow.
Both the Ann Arbor and Hammersmith groups have shown significant increases in
the cortex of the contralateral insula, lentiform nucleus, and PAG. The latter became significant only with a larger experimental group in the Hammersmith series
(12 normal volunteers), for which there was a sufficient spread of scans that included the brain stem in the field of view. In addition the Hammersmith group has
shown significant activation of the prefrontal cortex (area 10), which was not demonstrated by the two other groups.

The main area of divergence has had and still has to do with the responses recorded in the somatosensory cortex. Both the Montreal and Ann Arbor groups have
reported significant increases in blood flow in the somatosensory cortex on the side
contralateral to the stimulation, although subsignificant ipsilateral increases in flow
were also apparent in the Montreal group's results. The Hammersmith group was
unable to demonstrate consistent responses in the somatosensory cortex initially in a
group of six normal volunteers (Jones et al. 1991a) and subsequently in a group of
12 normal volunteers (Derbyshire et al. 1993, Derbyshire et al. submitted). One
possible explanation for this discrepancy is that there was greater attention to position for the two research groups that varied the position of stimulation within each
experiment (Jones et al. 1991b). Another potential explanation for the discrepancies
in the various groups' findings is that with each painful heat stimulation there is a
variable ramp of nonpainful stimulation leading up to the sensation of pain. In fact it
is only the upper pinnacle of the stimulus that is actually painful. Apart from the
increasing heat there is therefore a considerable and variable sensory–discrimina-

tive component to the stimulus. Each subject was given an intermittent painful heat stimulus at a level above the pain threshold which they judged would be tolerable during the experiment. It is therefore possible that once localization of a painful stimulus has taken place (the effect of which the design of our experiments was designed to minimize), the main determinants of changes in flow (either increased or decreased) are more dependent on the sensory–discriminative component of the stimulus and attention to the spatial components of the stimulus. That is not to say that the "suffering" components of ongoing pain are not processed at all in the somatosensory cortex, but rather that quantitatively, they are not the main determinants of the significant changes in flow. Apkarian and colleagues (1994) found that tonic pain inhibits touch discrimination and have documented decreases in rCBF in the somatosensory cortex contralateral to tonic thermal pain, using SPECT in normal volunteers. This raises the issue of temporally dependent reversal of flow in the somatosensory cortex in response to pain. The significance and consistency of such responses require further study. First, however, there is a need to study the variability of response in the somatosensory cortex with single, three-dimensional, normal pain-activation studies. Preliminary PET studies by the Hammersmith group along these lines suggest highly variable changes in flow in this area of the cortex. We would therefore suggest that the presence of pain *per se* is unlikely to be the principal determinant of changes in flow in the somatosensory cortex. Moreover, PET lacks the spatial resolution to distinguish between S1, S2, and the cortex of the insula. We would therefore suggest that careful repeated individual functional magnetic resonance imaging (fMRI) studies, which permit control of the attentional and sensory–discriminative components of pain from one experiment to another, are likely to be the best way to resolve these issues.

REFERENCES

Angelergue R, Hecaen H. La douleur au cours des lesions des hemispheres cerebraux. *J Psychol Norm Pathol* 1958;55:42–69.

Apkarian AV, Hodge CJ. Primate spinothalamic pathways: 1. A quantitative study of the cells of origin of the spinothalamic pathway. *J Comp Neurol* 1989;288:447–473.

Apkarian AV, Stea R, Bolanowski SJ. Supression of a sense of touch by pain: A touch gate. Submitted.

Apkarian AV, Stea RA, Manglos SH, Szevernyi NM, King RB, Thomas FD. Persistent pain inhibits contralateral somatosensory cortical activity in humans. *Neurosci Lett* 1992;140:141–147.

Bailey DL, Jones T, Spinks TJ, Gilardi MC, Townsend DW. Noise equivalent count measurements in neuro-PET scanner with retractable septa. *IEEE Trans Med Imaging* 1991a;10:256–260.

Bailey DL, Jones T, Spinks TJ. A method for measuring the absolute sensitivity of positron emission tomography scanners. *Eur J Nucl Med* 1991b;18:374–379.

Belliveau JW, Kennedy DN, McKinstry RC, Buchbinder BR, Weisskoff RW, Cohen MS, Vevea JM, Brady TJ, Rosen BR. Functional mapping of the human visual cortex by magnetic resonance imaging. *Science* 1991;254:716–719.

Boivie J, Leijon G. Clinical findings in patients with central post-stroke pain. In Casey KL, ed. *Pain and central nervous system disease: the central pain syndromes*. New York: Raven Press, 1991;65–75.

Bowsher D. Termination of the central pain pathway in man: the conscious appreciation of pain. *Brain* 1957;80:606–624.

Chen ACN. Human brain measures of clinical pain: a review I. Tomographic mappings. *Pain* 1993a; 54:115–132.

Chen ACN. Human brain measures of clinical pain: a review II. Tomographic imagings. *Pain* 1993b; 54:133–144.

Derbyshire SWG, Jones AKP, Devani P, Friston KJ, Feinman C, Harris M, Pearce S, Frackowiak RSJ. Cerebral responses to pain in patients with atypical facial pain. *J Cereb Blood Flow Metab* 1993; 13:S799.

Derbyshire SWG, Jones AKP, Devani P, Friston KJ, Brown WD, Watson J, Pearce S. Cortical and subcortical responses to pain in male and female volunteers measured by positron emission tomography. *Eur J Neurosci*.

Fox PT, Mintum MA. Noninvasive functional brain mapping by change-distribution analysis of averaged PET images of $H_2{}^{15}O$ tissue activity. *J Nucl Med* 1989;30:141–149.

Friston KJ, Frith CD, Liddle PF, Lammertsma AA, Dolan DD, Frackowiak RSJ. The relationship between local and global changes in PET scans. *J Cereb Blood Flow Metab* 1990;10:458–466.

Friston KJ, Frith CD, Liddle PF, Frackowiak RSJ. Comparing functional (PET) images: The assessment of significant change. *J Cereb Blood Flow Metab* 1991;11:690–699.

Fruhstorfer H, Lindblom U, Schmidt WG. Method for quantitative estimation of thermal thresholds in patients. *J Neurol Psychiatry* 1976;39:1071–1075.

Gabriel M, Kubota Y, Sparenborg S, Straube K, Vogt BA. Effects of cingulate cortical lesions on avoidance learning and training-induced unit activity in rabbits. *Exp Brain Res* 1991a;86:585–600.

Gabriel M, Vogt BA, Kubota Y, Poremba A, Kang E. Training-stage related neuronal plasticity in limbic thalamus and cingulate cortex during learning: a key to mnemonic retrieval. *Behav Brain Res* 1991b;46:175–185.

Gingold SI, Greenspan JD, Apkarian AV. Anatomic evidence of nociceptive inputs to primary somatosensory cortex: relationship between spinothalamic terminal and thalamocortical cells in squirrel monkeys. *J Comp Neurol* 1991;308:467–491.

Grootoonk S, Spinks T, Jones T. Correction for scatter using a dual energy window technique with a tomograph operated without septa. *Conference Record of the IEEE Medical Imaging Conference* 1991;3:1569–1573.

Guilbaud G. Thalamic nociceptive systems. In: Iggo A, Iverson LL, Cervero F, eds. Nociception and pain, *Phil Trans R Soc Lond [B]* 1985;308:299–310.

Gybels JM, Sweet WH. Pre- and postcentral gyrectomy. In: Gybels JM, Sweet WH, eds. *Neurosurgical treatment of persistent pain*. Basel, Munich, Paris, London, New York: Karger, 1989;254–256.

Hassler R. The division of pain conduction into systems of pain sensation and pain awareness. In: Jansen R, Keidel WD, Hertz A, Steichele C, eds. *Pain*. London: Churchill Livingstone, 1972;98–112.

Head H. Sensation and the cerberal cortex. In: Head H, Rivers WHR, Sherren J, eds. *Studies in neurology* (II). London: Hodder and Stoughton, 1920;639–810.

Hosobuchi Y. Subcortical electrical stimulation for the control of intractable pain in humans. Report of 122 cases (1970–1984). *J Neurosurg* 1986;64:543–553.

Itoh M, Jeong M, Fujiwara T, Watabe H, Okamura N, Seo S, Watanuki S, Fukuda H, Ido T. Instability of subject's psychological state during PET activation study monitored by EEG. In: Uemura K, Jones T, Lassen NA, Kanno I, eds. *Quantitation of brain function: tracer kinetics and image analysis in brain PET*. Amsterdam, London, New York, Tokyo: Excerpta Medica, 1993;627–633.

Jones AKP, Derbyshire SWG. Positron emission tomography as a tool for understanding the cerebral processing of pain. In: Boivie J, Hansson P, Lindblom U, eds. *Touch, temperature and pain in health and disease. Progress in pain research and management*. Seattle: IASP Press, vol. 3. (*in press*).

Jones AKP, Cunningham VJ, Ha-Kawa S, Fujiwara T, Qi L, Luthra SK, Ashburner J, Osman S, Jones T. Quantitation of ${}^{11}C$-diprenorphine cerebral kinetics in man acquired by PET using presaturation, pulse-chase and tracer alone protocols. *J Neurosci Methods* 1993;51:123–134.

Jones AKP, Friston KJ, Brown D, Qi L, Frackowiak RSJ. Cortical and subcortical localisation of response to pain in man using positron emission tomography. *Proc Soc Lond [B]* 1991a;244:39–44.

Jones AKP, Friston K, Frackowiak RSJ. Cerebral localisation of responses to pain in man using positron emission tomography. *Science* 1991b;255:215–216.

Kaas JH. Somatosensory cortex. In: Adelman G, ed. *Encyclopaedia of neuroscience*. Boston, Basel, Stuttgart: Birkhäuser, 1987;1113–1117.

Kaas JH, Nelson RJ, Sur M, Merzenich MM. Organization of somatosensory cortex in primates. In: Schmitt FO, Worden FG, Adelman G, Dennis SG, eds. *The organisation of the cerebral cortex*. Cambridge, MA: MIT Press, 1981;237–261.

Kenshalo DR, Jr., Isense O. Responses of the primate SI cortical neurons to noxious stimuli. *J Neurophysiol* 1983;50:1479–1496.

Lammertsma AA, Cunningham VJ, Deiber MP, Heather JD, Bloomfield PM, Nutt JG, Frackowiak RSJ, Jones T. Combination of dynamic and integral methods for generating reproducible functional CBF images. *J Cereb Blood Flow Metab* 1990;10:675–686.

Lucignani G, Moresca RM, Fazio F. PET-based neuropharmacology: state of the art. *Cerebrovasc Brain Metab Rev* 1989;1:271–287.

Mazziotta JC, Huang SC, Phelps ME, Carson RE, Macdonald NS, Mahoney K. A non-invasive positron computed tomography technique using oxygene-15 labeled water for the evaluation of the neuro-behavioural task batteries. *J Cereb Blood Flow Metab* 1985;5:70–78.

Minoshima S, Frey KA, Koeppe RA, Berger KL, Fessler JA, Kuhl DE, Casey KL. PET localisation of response to thermal stimuli in human. *J Cereb Blood Flow Metab* 1993;13:S260.

Penfield W, Boldrey E. Somatic motor and sensory representation in the cerebral cortex of man as studied by electrical stimulation. *Brain* 1937;60:389–443.

Penfield W, Jasper H. Sensory seizures—auras. In: *Epilepsy and the functional anatomy of the human brain.* London: J. & A. Churchill Ltd., 1954;389–411.

Poggio GF, Mountcastle VB. The functional properties of ventro-basal thalamic neurons studied in anaesthetised monkeys. *J Neurophysiol* 1963;26:775–806.

Raichle ME. Circulatory and metabolic correlates of brain function in normal humans. In: Plum F, ed. *American Physiological Society handbook of physiology.* Section 1. *The nervous system*, vol. V, part 2, Washington, DC: American Physiological Society 1987;643–674.

Sikes RW, Vogt BA. Nociceptive neurons in area 24 of rabbit cingulate cortex. *J Neurophysiol* 1992; 68:1720–1732.

Spinks TJ, Jones T, Gilardi MC, Heather JD. Performance characteristics of a whole body positron tomograph. *IEEE Trans Nucl Sci* 1988;35:721–725.

Stevens RT, London SM, Apkarian AV. Spinothalamic projections to the secondary somatosensory cortex (SII) in squirrel monkey. *Brain Res (in press).*

Talairach J, Tournoux P. Co-planar stereotaxic atlas of the human brain. Stuttgart, New York: Georg Thieme Verlag, 1988.

Talbot JD, Marrett S, Evans AC, Meyer E, Bushnell MC, Duncan GH. Multiple representations of pain in the human cerebral cortex. *Science* 1991;251:1355–1358.

Townsend DW, Geissbuhler A, Defrise. Fully 3D reconstruction for a PET camera with retractable septa. *IEEE Trans Med Imaging* 1991;10:S5–S12.

Tsubokawa T, Katayama Y, Ueno Y, Morijasu N. Evidence for involvement of the frontal cortex in pain-related cerebral events in cats: increase in local cerebral blood flow by noxious stimuli. *Brain Res* 1981;217:179–185.

Vaccarino AL, Melzack R. Analgesia produced by injection of lidocaine into the anterior cingulum bundle of the rat. *Pain* 1989;39:213–219.

Vogt BA. The cingulate cortex. In: Jones EG, Peters A, eds. *The cerebral cortex.* New York, London: Plenum Press, 1985;89–149.

Vogt B, Sikes RW, Vogt LJ. Anterior cingulate cortex and the medial pain system. In: Vogt BA, Gabriel M, eds. *Neurobiology of cingulate cortex and limbic thalamus: a comprehensive handbook.* Boston, Basel, Berlin: Birkhäuser, 1993;313–344.

Willis WD, Coggeshall RE. Sensory pathways in the dorsal funiculus. In: Willis WD, Coggeshall RE, eds. *Sensory mechanisms of the spinal cord.* New York: Plenum Press, 1991;245–306.

Young GD, Blume WT. Painful epileptic seizures. *Brain* 1983;106:537–554.

Young GD, Barr HWK, Blume WT. Painful epileptic seizures involving the second sensory area. *Ann Neurol* 1986;106:412.

Pain and the Brain: From
Nociception to Cognition,
edited by Burkhart Bromm and
John E. Desmedt, Advances in Pain
Research and Therapy Vol. 22.
Raven Press, Ltd., New York © 1995.

15

Anatomical and Functional Neuro-imaging in Headache

Nabih M. Ramadan and Panayiotis Mitsias

Ambulatory Department of Neurology, Headache Center, Henry Ford Hospital and Health Sciences Center, Detroit, Michigan 48202, USA

SUMMARY

The introduction of computerized tomography (CT) and magnetic resonance imaging (MRI) to the practice of medicine has allowed the determination of the structural cause of headache in various neurologic conditions including: (a) cerebral neoplasm; (b) intracranial hemorrhage (subdural, subarachnoid, intraparenchymal, intraventricular); (c) cerebrovascular malformations; (d) venous and arterial cerebral infarction; (e) hydrocephalus (obstructive, communicating); (f) infections of the central nervous system (CNS) (e.g., herpes simplex, toxoplasmosis); and (g) congenital malformations of the cranium or craniocervical junction. The use of these anatomical neuroimaging techniques in patients with clinical histories suggestive of a primary headache such as migraine, cluster headache, or tension-type headache should be restricted to the occasional instance in which abnormal neurologic findings are made or when the headache features are atypical. For example, positional head pain in a patient with papilledema and characteristics of migraine headache should be investigated with an MRI or CT scan to rule out a space-occupying lesion causing increased intracranial pressure. Also, confusion or altered mental status accompanying a migraine-like headache is not typical of migraine, and an imaging study is indicated to rule out conditions such as a subdural hematoma. Cranial MRI is superior to CT in identifying structural lesions, particularly in the posterior cerebral fossa; however, the cost and limited availability of MRI prohibit its routine use in the evaluation of an acute severe headache. Furthermore, cerebral hemorrhage is better visualized with CT than with MRI when the blood is fresh (i.e., less than 24 hours old). Functional neuroimaging studies, such as magnetic resonance spectroscopy (MRS), single-photon emission computed tomography (SPECT), [133]xenon cerebral blood flow (CBF) methods, or positron-emission tomography (PET) are important research tools useful for investigating the mechanisms of headache and its accompanying cerebral metabolic and hemorrheologic changes. So far, however, these techniques have not resolved the controversy over a primary ischemic versus a neuronal origin of the neurologic symptoms of migraine; MRS seems promising for making the distinction. Transcranial Doppler ultrasonography is a noninvasive technique that helps us to identify cerebral aneurysms or arteriovenous malformations causing headache. When combined with CBF measurements, transcranial Doppler ultrasonography identifies hemodynamic changes associated with headache. Whether these changes are the direct cause of the headache or the result of it remains to be determined.

INTRODUCTION

Headache is one of the most common complaints of patients seeking medical advice. A complete history of the frequency, severity, onset, duration, and location of the headache; its precipitating, aggravating, and relieving factors; a history of symptoms accompanying the headache, such as nausea, photophobia, neck rigidity, and focal sensorimotor complaints; and a comprehensive family history are the essentials in formulating a differential diagnosis of the conditions that can cause headache. A general physical and detailed neurologic examination help us to make the diagnosis of the ailment in the majority of patients. Rarely, the physician performs laboratory and/or neuroimaging studies to rule in or rule out a provisional diagnosis made during the patient's interview. In this chapter we will describe the role of cranial CT and MRI in evaluating patients with headache. The value of cerebral blood flow (CBF) techniques [transcranial Doppler (TCD); single-photon emission computed tomography (SPECT); ^{133}xenon-CBF studies], and metabolic and functional imaging [magnetic resonance spectroscopy (MRS); positron-emission tomography (PET)] in understanding the pathogenesis of headache will be outlined. It is to be emphasized that CBF techniques and functional and metabolic imaging are not essential to make the diagnosis of the medical condition causing headache; rather, they shed light on the mechanisms and physiologic sequelae of head pain, and can therefore be of future therapeutic value.

ANATOMIC IMAGING

Cranial CT Scanning

Cranial CT scanning is indicated in the evaluation of headache when the following diagnoses are entertained: (a) a cerebral mass (e.g., brain abscess, tumor, subdural hematoma); (b) venous or arterial cerebral infarction; (c) vascular malformation of the brain (e.g., cerebral aneurysm, arteriovenous malformation); and (d) subarachnoid (SAH), subdural (SDH), epidural, or intraparenchymal hemorrhage (ICH). In addition to these indications, the decision to order a CT scan is influenced by nonmedical factors. Among these are: (a) the physician's type of practice (physicians who practice in a litiginous environment order CT scans more often than those who do not practice in such an environment); (b) the type of medical facility to which the patient presents (patients who are seen in emergency departments and specialty clinics are more likely to have a CT scan than patients seen in family practice clinics); and (c) the reaction of the patient to the physician's explanation of the headache cause(s); "It is unlikely that your headache is related to a tumor or stroke" is reassuring to some patients, but others may believe that they fall into the small percentage of people who do have a neoplasm or a stroke; patients in the latter group will not be reassured until they find a physician who will order the imaging study, preferably an MRI scan.

Many recent reports have suggested that cranial CT is overused in conditions associated with headache. Mitchell et al. (1993) used cranial CT to prospectively evaluate 350 consecutive patients complaining of headache; only 2% had "significant" radiologic findings. These same patients had abnormal physical or neurologic examinations. Incidental CT findings (e.g., atrophy, basal ganglia calcification) were detected in another 25% (Mitchell et al. 1993). In a primary-care setting, about 350 CT scans were ordered in 19 months in order to investigate subjects with headache (Becker et al. 1993). The most common reasons for obtaining the radiologic study were: (a) suspected intracranial mass (48%); (b) patient's request or medicolegal (17%); and (c) suspected SAH (9%). Of 293 scans reviewed, 14 (5%) positively identified the cause of the headache and 44 (15%) demonstrated incidental findings. The authors concluded that "physicians must exercise good clinical judgment in their attempt to identify treatable disease in a cost-effective way." In another report from two university medical centers providing primary and specialized referral services (Kahn et al. 1993), a retrospective analysis of the indications for cranial CT in subjects with acute nontraumatic headache indicated that an intracranial process was present in 10.8% of 1,111 studies performed (cerebral infarction [4%]; neoplasm [2.7%]; SAH [1.3%]; SDH [1.1%]; and others [1.8%]). Subjects with migraine-like symptoms and those with "other headaches" had similar proportions of acute intracranial findings. Interestingly, the likelihood of a positive scan was highest when the subject was an inpatient (21.2%), as opposed to an outpatient (11.7%) or an emergency-room subject (6.9%). In contrast, Fodden et al. (1989) found that 16% of a total of 106 CT scans performed in the emergency room for the evaluation of subjects with headache demonstrated "serious neurological pathology" such as intracranial hemorrhage or neoplasm.

Migraine is diagnosed clinically according to the criteria of the International Headache Society (IHS) (Olesen 1988). Sometimes, patients complain of headaches that mimic migraine ("migraine mimic") (Welch and Levine 1990); a cranial CT scan may be indicated in such instances. A partial list of conditions that can mimic migraine, and clues to their diagnoses, is represented in Table 1. Cranial CT scanning shows evidence of subarachnoid blood in over 90% of cases of subarachnoid hemorrhage (Scotti et al. 1977; Fontanarosa 1989). Exceptions are: (a) patients who are severely anemic; (b) small hemorrhages in the brain-stem region; and (c) SAH older than 2 weeks (Prager and Mikulis 1991). Arteriovenous malformations can be demonstrated on contrast-enhanced CT scans as serpiginous areas of enhancement,

TABLE 1. *Conditions mimicking migraine*

Condition	Clues to diagnosis
Subarachnoid hemorrhage	Explosive headache; symptoms and signs of meningeal irritation; altered mental status
Arteriovenous malformation	Heachache usually develops before neurologic symptoms; seizure history in some patients; cranial bruits
Ischemic stroke	Focal neurologic symptoms and signs much more emphasized than the headache
Arterial dissection	Neck pain; Horner's syndrome; cerebral ischemic symptoms
Benign intracranial hypertension	Characteristically positional headache; papilledema
Subdural hematoma	Confusion; history of head trauma; positional headache; papilledema
Cerebral venous/sinus thrombosis	Positional headache; seizures; peripartum; hematologic predisposition (e.g., protein C deficiency)
CNS neoplasm	Positional headache; papilledema

usually in the cerebral convexities. The value of CT in cervicocephalic arterial dissection is to demonstrate areas of cerebral infarction. Increased density in the distal carotid artery can sometimes be visualized and suggests the presence of an intraluminal clot (Fig. 1). A common CT finding in patients with benign intracranial hypertension (BIH) is slit ventricles, probably related to interstitial edema (Weisberg 1985). In cerebral venous and sinus thrombosis (CVT), the enhanced CT scan can show an empty delta sign (Fig. 2); a cord sign and hemorrhagic infarction can also be demonstrated (Lefkowitz 1989). Space-occupying lesions such as tumors of

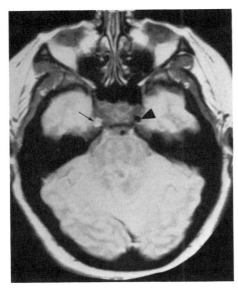

FIG. 1. Cranial MRI (TR = 2,900 msec, TE = 30 msec). The patient presented with a right frontotemporal headache preceded by positive visual phenomena in the right eye. Compare the normal flow void phenomenon in the left cavernous internal carotid artery (*arrowhead*) and its absence (occlusion) on the right side (*small arrow*). Right internal carotid artery dissection was angiographically confirmed.

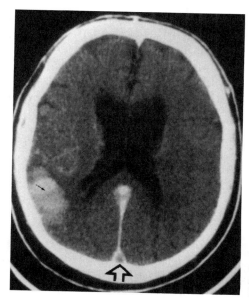

FIG. 2. Cranial CT scan with contrast infusion. The patient presented with acute headache and confusion. Note the "empty delta" sign (*open arrow*) and the right parietotemporal hemorrhagic infarction (*small arrow*).

the central nervous system (CNS) are seen on cranial CT scan as areas of hypodensity that enhance with intravenous contrast medium. Variable degrees of cerebral edema and mass effect are also observed. A subdural hematoma goes into various pathologic stages, which on CT are reflected as: (a) hyperdensity surrounded by cerebral edema; (b) isodensity with or without cerebral edema and a surrounding enhancing rim with contrast injection; and (c) hypodensity when the blood has resolved and has been replaced by cerebrospinal fluid (i.e., subdural hygroma).

Cluster headache is also diagnosed clinically according to the IHS criteria (Olesen 1988). As in the case of migraine, conditions mimicking cluster headache (Table 2) must be looked for and, when suspected, the pertinent laboratory and/or imaging studies should be performed.

TABLE 2. *Conditions mimicking cluster headache*

Condition	Clues to diagnosis
Herpetic infections	Oral/facial blisters; facial hyperpathia
Aseptic meningitis	Fever; symptoms and signs of meningeal irritation
Arteriovenous malformation	Long duration of headache; cranial bruit; accompanying focal neurologic symptoms and/or signs
Cerebral aneurysm	Poorly localized hemicephalic pain; strong family history of cerebral aneurysms
CNS neoplasm (primary or metastatic)	Age >50 years; no or short-duration remissions; endocrinologic abnormalities; focal neurologic signs/symptoms (visual field loss, cranial nerve palsy, etc.)

The majority of patients who present with symptoms of daily, dull, bilateral, and mild to moderate headache are correctly diagnosed as having tension-type headache (Weingarten et al. 1992). Rarely, type I Chiari malformation (Stovner 1993) and BIH without papilledema (Ramadan 1993) can present similarly. A cranial CT, or more appropriately an MRI, will demonstrate the tonsillar herniation of a type I Chiari malformation and slit ventricles may be demonstrated on cranial CT in cases of BIH.

Cranial MRI

In the early 1980s, the introduction of clinical cranial MRI revolutionized the field of diagnostic imaging in neurologic disorders. Ever since, cranial MRI has been increasingly used, and maybe overused, to diagnose ailments causing headache. MRI is clearly more sensitive than CT in identifying cerebral neoplasms and abscesses, but is not as sensitive in detecting hyperacute (<24 hours) hemorrhage (SAH or ICH) (Bradley 1993). Patients with acute headache who are suspected of having cerebral hemorrhage or obstructive hydrocephalus are best evaluated with CT. Cranial MRI is helpful in diagnosing occult vascular malformations that cause headaches but which are not readily delineated on cerebral angiography (Ramadan et al. 1989a). Areas of hemorrhage are occasionally observed around these lesions. Some neurosurgeons choose to excise such malformations when hemorrhage is demonstrated because of the potential risk of rebleeding. Cranial MRI is also indicated for diagnosing the rare patient with headache and Chiari malformation (Stovner 1993). Another role for cranial MRI and MR venography is in the evaluation of the patient with headache and suspected cerebral venous thrombosis (CVT) (Tietjen and Mitsias 1993). Finally, when investigating a "migraine-like" complaint, an MRI is ordered in preference to a CT scan with contrast-dye injection because of the anecdotally reported increased risk of dye-related complications in migraineurs.

Several authors recently have reported that patients with migraine have T_2-weighted hyperintensities on MRI, suggestive of subclinical cerebral ischemia. Kaplan et al. (1987) reviewed the MRI studies of nine patients with headache [migraine (6-one migraine aura without headache); cluster (1); tension-type (2)] and found hyperintense T_2 signals in three (two migraine and one tension-type). These lesions were not present on cranial CT. Soges et al. (1988) reported that 46% of 24 migraineurs had hyperintense white-matter signals on T_2-weighted MRI. Similarly, Igarashi et al. (1991) reported T_2-weighted MRI abnormalities in 29.4% of migraineurs younger than 40 years and in 11.2% of controls. Prager et al. (1991) found that 27 of 58 (47%) patients with migraine without aura and eight of 19 (42%) patients with migraine plus aura had white-matter abnormalities on T_2-weighted MRI. These studies are open to significant criticism because of one or more of the following: (a) small number of cases; (b) retrospective nature of the analysis; (c) investigator not blinded to headache diagnosis; (d) lack of controls; and (e) use of historical controls. Furthermore, the results of the studies have not repro-

TABLE 3. *Indications for neuroimaging studies in headache*

1. Explosive headache
2. Headache and neurologic signs and/or symptoms
3. Changing character of headache (e.g., intensity, quality) in a patient with a history of a primary headache (migraine, tension-type, cluster)
4. Headache induced or exacerbated by cough or other Valsalva maneuvers
5. Migraine or clusterlike headache occurring for the first time after the age of 40 years
6. Headache in a patient with human immunodeficiency virus (HIV) infection
7. Headache in immunocompromised patients

duced in a prospective controlled study of MRI changes in subjects with migraine plus aura (Ziegler et al. 1991). The controversy about white-matter changes and their significance in migraineurs cannot be resolved without a large, prospective, case-controlled study comparing the incidence, location, and distribution of MRI abnormalities in the general population to those in subjects with primary headaches (migraine and tension-type).

Conclusion

In this era of cost-effective medical practice, expensive neuroradiologic studies such as MRI or CT should be ordered only when clinically indicated. In 1982, the U.S. National Institutes of Health recommended the use of CT when a patient presents with a headache that is "severe, constant, unusual, or associated with abnormal neurological signs" (NIH Consensus Development Panel 1982). More recently, Edmeads (1990) felt that a neuroimaging study was indicated to evaluate a subject with headache when: (a) it is the worst headache the subject has experienced; (b) its onset occurs with exertion; (c) the neck is not supple; (d) the neurologic examination is abnormal; or (e) the patient's condition worsens under observation. Another expert in the field of headache felt that the use of MRI or CT "all depends on the circumstances" (Campbell 1993). We recommend obtaining a cranial CT or MRI when any of the conditions mentioned in Table 3 exist. These indications are, however, only general guidelines. The ultimate decision to order a CT scan should be made on a case-by-case basis, as suggested by Edmeads (1990) and Campbell (1993).

FUNCTIONAL IMAGING

Cerebral Blood Flow (CBF)

Cerebral circulatory disturbances have long been considered an important feature in the pathophysiology of migraine. Wolff and co-workers (1963) suggested that focal cerebral vasospasm leading to focal ischemia is responsible for the prodromal neurologic deficits in migraine with aura, while the headache results from cerebral vasodilation. Well-known laboratories working in CBF research have obtained contradictory data, probably for a number of methodologic reasons.

CBF during the Aura of Migraine (Classic Migraine)

Early studies uniformly revealed hypoperfusion during the aura phase of migraine (Skinhoj and Paulson 1969; Simard and Paulson 1973; Norris et al. 1975; Mathew et al. 1976; Edmeads 1977; Hachinski et al. 1977). More recently, Olesen et al. (1981a) used the intracarotid injection of [133]Xenon-CBF with 254 collimated detectors covering a single hemisphere and observed what they termed *spreading oligemia (SO)*: a spreading moderate reduction in CBF, starting at the occipital pole and gradually moving forward at a calculated rate of $\cong 3$ mm/min (Lauritzen et al. 1983a). In some patients, SO was preceded by a short-lived focal and perifocal hyperemia. The SO finally either involved the entire hemisphere or remained confined to the occipital region, where it localized to areas corresponding to the neurologic deficit. Occasionally the oligemia persisted well into the headache phase of migraine, indicating that the headache is not the result of cerebral vasodilation. In addition, reduced CBF was sometimes seen in the frontal lobe, independent of the posterior site at which SO began, indicating that the SO did not cross the central or lateral sulcus. The progression rate of the SO and its dependence on the major cortical structural features indicate a relation to Leao's *spreading depression (SD)* (Leao 1944; Leao and Morrison 1945). Thus, SO could be an epiphenomenon accompanying SD, and focal symptoms of migraine might result from the prolonged inhibition of cortical neurons after SD. Of note is that the regional CBF (rCBF) in the oligemic areas varied between 34 and 67 ml/100 mg/min, values well above the ischemic range. Olsen et al. (1987, 1989) challenged these findings, arguing that the blood flows would be within the ischemic range after correcting for the 40% rCBF overestimation caused by Compton scatter. They also added that the so-called *dissociated vasomotor paralysis*, which is marked by normal autoregulation but reduced responsiveness to changes in arterial pCO_2, can be explained by Compton scatter, while Lauritzen et al. (1983b) stated that dissociated vasomotor paralysis and the impaired blood-flow response in the oligemic areas during physiologic activation procedures support the hypothesis of a local metabolic disturbance—the SD of Leao—that is responsible for the blood-flow reduction during the aura of migraine. Recently, Friberg et al. (1987) measured rCBF in hemiplegic migraine and demonstrated hypoperfusion originating in the frontal lobe and spreading posteriorly, with mean rCBF values below the ischemic threshold, supporting Olsen's hypothesis that ischemia is the cause of the neurologic deficits in migraine, and that the instability of cerebrovascular tone in the hypoperfused areas, which have a fluctuating size, gives the impression of a spreading pattern.

CBF During the Headache Phase of Migraine With Aura

Skinhoj and Paulson (1969) described increased rCBF in the headache phase of classic migraine. In 1973, Skinhoj confirmed this finding which, together with the increase in cerebrospinal fluid lactate levels, led him to speculate that the hyperperfusion was secondary to intracerebral acidosis (Skinhoj 1973). Norris et al. (1975) found that the initially reduced CBF (during the aura phase) became normalized within 1 hour and increased 20 min later. Increased rCBF persisting up to 48 hours after resolution of the headache (Sakai and Meyer 1978), diffusely increased rCBF and regional cerebral blood volume during the headache phase (Mathew et al. 1976), and bilateral hyperemia (Edmeads 1977) were subsequently reported.

Olesen et al. (1981a) observed severe headache in four of eight patients at a time when global or focal reduction in rCBF was the regional flow abnormality in the absence of signs of nonhomogeneous brain perfusion. He suggested that intracerebral vasodilatation could not have caused the headache. Lauritzen et al. (1983a) reported that five of nine patients developed headache at the time of rCBF investigation, four at a time of global oligemia and one when experiencing parietal hyperemia and frontal oligemia. In a subsequent report, Olesen et al. (1990) showed that in the early headache phase, rCBF was focally reduced in 34 of 56 patients, was normal in seven, and was increased in two. At later stages of the attack, hyperperfusion and headache coexisted in several patients, and hyperperfusion frequently outlasted the headache. Anderson et al. (1988), using ^{133}Xe inhalation SPECT, demonstrated delayed hyperemia from 3 to 8 hours after the onset of the attack. All patients developed headache while focal posterior hypoperfusion, confined to the tomographic representation of the cortex and occasionally spreading to the underlying white matter, was still present. Usually the shift from hypoperfusion to hyperemia occurred at the time when patients described their headaches as regressing and changing from "throbbing" to "pressure-like." During the phase of hyperemia, a reversed side-to-side asymmetry was seen and the hyperemia was focal and localized to the areas previously hypoperfused. The delayed, long-lasting hyperemia is likely due to reactive hyperemia after ischemia. These results suggest that it is unlikely that the headache is triggered by the hyperemia, and that a state of arteriolar vasoconstriction, leading to transient focal cerebral ischemia, is present. In a large study, Juge (1988) found either hyperemia or oligemia in the first 48 hours after the onset of headache in patients with "Sylvian expression" (symptoms of anterior cerebral circulation dysfunction), while patients with posterior cerebral symptoms more frequently had oligemia. The abnormalities normalized within 10 to 21 days. Using high-resolution color-coded images of local cerebral blood flow, Kobari et al. (1990) reported increased rCBF values in cortical and subcortical grey matter during the headache, which were more pronounced in patients with classic than with common migraine. Bilateral hemispheric hyperperfusion was seen independent of laterality of the headache.

CBF During the Headache Phase of Migraine Without Aura (Common Migraine)

It has always been difficult to encompass the entity of migraine without aura within the classic migraine theory of Wolff (1963). Earlier studies showed increased CBF and a reduced pCO_2 response during fully developed attacks and for up to 48 hours after the attacks (Mathew et al. 1976; Sakai and Meyer 1978). More recently, Juge (1988) demonstrated increased mean hemispheric fast flows, as compared to controls, during the first 48 hours of attacks of migraine without aura. The hyperemia was distributed in all regions, dominating anteriorly and bilaterally, even when the headache was lateralized. Similarly, Kobari et al. (1990) found symmetric and bilateral local increases in CBF in the cortical and subcortical grey matter during the headache, and not correlating with the preponderant side of the headache. In contrast, Olesen et al. (1981b) observed an absence of changes in CBF during attacks of migraine without aura. They also could not demonstrate any alterations in CBF just before attacks induced by red wine or foodstuffs. Lauritzen and Olesen (1984), using the ^{133}Xe inhalation rCBF method, studied 12 patients at 3 to 20 hours after the onset of the headache, and found normal and symmetric mean hemispheric, basal ganglionic, and cortical blood flows both ipsi- and contralateral to the pain.

CBF in Interictal Migraine Studies

Mathew et al. (1976) found no significant interictal differences in CBF in migraineurs and controls, while Sakai and Meyer (1978) showed that the diffuse hyperemia accompanying the headache phase outlasted the migraine by an average of 2 days. Using the ^{133}Xe inhalation method, Levine et al. (1987) reported no significant difference in mean CBF between migraineurs and controls. However, asymmetric probe pairs, more evident posteriorly, were found more frequently in migraineurs, independent of migraine type, which may be relevant to the spreading oligemia generally thought to proceed from the occipital lobes forward. Robertson et al. (1989) found that migraineurs studied interictally have lower rCBF and more frequent rCBF asymmetries than controls, suggesting differences in the cerebrovascular resistance tone in migraine patients that may contribute to the threshold for a migraine attack. Between attacks of classic migraine, Lauritzen et al. (1983b, 1984) found normal baseline CBF, preserved autoregulation, normal responsiveness to pCO_2, and normal physiologic activation of rCBF. Finally, Schlake et al. (1989), using ^{123}I-iodoamphetamine SPECT, showed a regional reduction of tracer uptake in patients with migraine with aura, suggesting that migraine attacks occur in connection with exacerbations of preexisting changes in cerebral autoregulation.

Conclusion

The studies of rCBF in migraine have yielded conflicting results. If the spreading reduction in rCBF truly exists, it remains to be determined whether it is purely secondary to decreased neuronal function (metabolic depression of CBF) or whether constriction of cortical arterioles (arteriolar spasm-ischemia) plays a primary role in the regional flow reduction. To definitely resolve the controversy, it will be necessary to conduct either PET studies with measurements of the oxygen extraction fraction or ^{31}P-nuclear magnetic resonance (^{31}P-NMR) spectroscopy with measurements of cerebral metabolism.

TRANSCRANIAL DOPPLER ULTRASONOGRAPHY

The role of transcranial Doppler ultrasonography (TCD) in headache and migraine is still investigational. The technique allows the measurement of blood flow velocities (BFV) in the major cerebral arteries of the circle of Willis, such as the middle cerebral (MCA) or anterior cerebral artery (ACA). Thus, constriction or dilatation of these vessels can be observed and monitored. Indirectly, the state of cerebral perfusion can also be assessed.

TCD in Interictal Migraine Studies

In a review of the literature until 1992, Young and Silberstein (1992) summarized the TCD findings in migraine and cluster headache. In migraineurs (with or without aura), BFVs and CO_2 reactivity were increased, suggesting an increased tone of the cerebral conductance vessels. Changes in pulsatility indices (PI) have not been consistent, however. Thie et al. (1990a) reported that PIs are low in migraineurs interictally, indicating dilatation of the resistance vessels either primarily or secondarily to the stenosis of the conductance arteries. In contrast, Totaro et al. (1992) reported high PIs in migraineurs with aura as compared to controls.

TCD in Ictal Migraine Studies

As compared to controls, both increased and decreased BFVs in migraineurs have been reported (Young and Silberstein 1992; Thie et al. 1990b; Totaro et al. 1992). The timing of the TCD study as being done during the hyperemic or during the oligemic phase could have been different in these reports. This would certainly affect BFV measurements, hence yielding conflicting results. Combining TCD studies with cerebral perfusion measurements such as ^{133}Xe inhalation CBF (Friberg et al. 1991) would, at least partially, solve the controversy and provide further insight into the vascular accompaniments of migraine attacks. Moreover, TCD can be used to study the effect, if any, of anti-migraine drugs on the cerebral circulation.

Studies in Selected Nonmigraine Headaches

Wallash (1992a, 1993) reported increased interictal BFVs in episodic tension-type headache and in migraine as compared to controls, suggesting that migraine and tension-type headache share a similar pathogenesis. Patients with chronic tension-type headache had no changes in BFV (Wallash 1992b). During the remission period of cluster headache, Dahl et al. (1990) reported that the BFVs ipsilateral to the side of the headache were greater than those in the contralateral MCA. Shen (1993) found that the BFVs of the ipsilateral ACA, rather than MCA were greater on the symptomatic than on the asymptomatic side. Micieli et al. (1993) reported normal and Ertsey et al. (1993) found lower interictal BFVs ipsilateral to the side of cluster headache, than on the asymptomatic side. These findings are too conflicting to provide any conclusion. Similarly, the results of the ictal studies have been contradictory. Finally, Shen (1993) reported a statistically insignificant lower vasomotor reactivity in three patients with chronic paroxysmal hemicrania than in nine controls.

POSITRON-EMISSION TOMOGRAPHY (PET)

PET During the Aura of Migraine

Measurements of cerebral metabolism have never been made during a typical migraine aura. During an episode of severe hemiplegia lasting 3 weeks without evidence of cerebral infarction on CT scan, Baron and Bousser (1985) found an increase in CBF and decrease in O_2 extraction, with relatively preserved O_2 utilization in the other hemisphere, at 1 week after the onset of the neurologic deficit. These findings could be consistent with the so-called "luxury perfusion" without evidence of cerebral ischemia. The examination was normal a year later. On the other hand, Herold et al. (1985) reported decreased CBF and an increased O_2 extraction fraction, without variation in local O_2 consumption, in a woman studied 90 min after the onset of a left hemiparesis associated with homolateral hemicrania. These findings correspond to the so-called "misery perfusion" which, in this case, suggested simple oligemia. The examination was normal 3 weeks later. CBF, oxygen consumption, and the O_2 extraction fraction were normal in another patient 8 hours after the onset of migraine with aura (Chabriat 1992).

PET During the Headache

Using ^{15}O PET, Herold et al. (1985) found no abnormality in O_2 consumption after the onset of headache in two patients with migraine without aura. These results were insufficient for Herold and colleagues to conclude that the metabolic activity is normal during the headache phase of migraine, and would not imply an absence of other disturbances in cellular energy, as suggested by the NMR spectroscopy studies done on the two patients. Sachs et al. (1986), using PET to test the hypothesis that a decrease in the rate of cerebral glucose metabolism (CMR-Glu) occurs at an early stage in a migraine attack and to determine whether this condition accompanies the headache phase, found that migraine subjects exhibited a marked decline in their global CMR-Glu during the early phase of the attack, and that a regional decline in CMR-Glu corresponded to the headache site, while none of the subjects displayed focal neurologic deficits. In contrast, normal controls showed a global increase in CMR-Glu.

PET in the Study of Serotonin Receptors Outside Migraine Attacks

Although still in its infancy, the study of serotonin receptors by PET could represent an interesting arena of research that will shed light on the pathophysiology and pharmacology of migraine, and also on the effects of the 5-hydroxytryptamine (5-HT) system on the regulation of CBF. Brain 5-HT_2 receptors have been implicated in the pathogenesis of migraine because they appear to be related to cortical neuronal activity and to the endogenous pain-control system, and could influence cerebral circulation. In addition, 5-HT_2 antagonists are of proven benefit in migraine prophylaxis. Using PET and ^{18}F-setoperone, a 5-HT_2-specific radioligand, Chabriat et al. (1993) studied the regional cortical volumes of distribution of 5-HT_2 receptors in nine migraineurs (six with and without aura and three without aura) and 12 normal controls. They found inconsistent regional or global modifications in ^{18}F-setoperone binding in the cortex of migraineurs, despite a significant effect of aging alone. These results suggest that cortical 5-HT_2 receptors are unaltered between attacks of migraine.

Conclusion

Overall, PET has shown only hemodynamic disturbances in migraineurs. These observations are preliminary, and studies combining CBF and metabolism will be necessary to better understand the origin of neurologic manifestations accompanying or preceding migraine.

MAGNETIC RESONANCE SPECTROSCOPY (MRS)

The precise mechanisms responsible for head pain during an attack of migraine are unknown. A popular but overly simplistic and unproven theory implies that brain acidosis caused by prodromal vasospasm-induced ischemia subsequently leads to an increase in CBF and hence to throbbing headache (Skinhoj 1973). Measurements of CBF during attacks of migraine have yielded controversial data that have been interpreted as showing spreading oligemia, spreading depression, or even focal ischemia. *In vivo* ^{31}P-MRS may be useful in resolving this controversy.

In one study, Welch et al. (1989) reported a lower mean phosphocreatine-to-inorganic phosphate ratio (PCr/Pi) in patients studied during a migraine attack. Patients with migraine with aura exhibited a significantly lower mean PCr/Pi and mean PCr/TP (total phosphate) ratio than did normal controls, while in patients with migraine without aura these values were lower than in controls, but not significantly so. In addition, there was an increase, albeit not statistically significant, in the Pi/TP ratio in both groups. Cerebral pH did not change, which does not support the earlier consideration that migraine headache is caused by brain acidosis. Overall, these results are consistent with an alteration in high-energy phosphate metabolism in the cerebral cortex of migraineurs during an attack. A low PCr/Pi ratio may indicate cerebral ischemia during an attack, but the absence of pH shifts argues against this possibility. Barbiroli et al. (1992) showed reduced PCr/Pi and PCr/ATP ratios in the brain (occipital lobes) and muscle of patients with migraine with aura, and an elevated intracellular pH. The slope of the initial PCr/Pi recovery in muscle after exercise was markedly reduced. These results suggest mitochondrial dysfunction in migraine.

Also using ^{31}P-MRS, Ramadan et al. (1989b) reported elevated pMg and therefore low free Mg levels in patients studied during attacks of migraine. The authors concluded that these results should be interpreted cautiously because of the small number of subjects studied and because the same subjects were not tested both during and between attacks.

We suggest that an inherited mitochondrial defect in the turnover of high-energy phosphates, coupled with an environmentally modifiable magnesium deficiency, makes the brain hyperexcitable and therefore susceptible to migraine. This attractive theory needs further testing using MRS.

REFERENCES

Anderson AR, Friberg L, Olsen TS, Olesen J. Delayed hyperemia following hypoperfusion in classic migraine. *Arch Neurol* 1988;45:154–159.

Barbiroli B, Montagna P, Cortelli P, Funicello R, Iotti S, Monari, L, Pierangeli G, Zaniol P, Lugaresi E. Abnormal brain and muscle energy metabolism shown by ^{31}P magnetic resonance spectroscopy in patients affected by migraine with aura. *Neurology* 1992;42:1209–1214.

Baron JC, Bousser MG. Circulation et métabolisme du cerveau au cours de la migraine. In: Meyer P, Albi H, Jaillo P, Lhoste F, eds. *Les antimigraineux*. Paris: Masson, 1985;36–45.

Becker LA, Green LA, Beaufait D, Kirk J, Froom J, Freeman WL. Use of CT scans for the investigation of headache. A report from ASPN, part I. *J Fam Pract* 1993;37:129–134.

Bradley WG. MR appearance of hemorrhage in the brain. *Radiology* 1993;189:15–26.

Campbell JK. CT or not CT?- That is the question. *Headache* 1993;33:52.

Chabriat H. Positron emission tomography and migraine. *Pathol Biol* 1992;40:344–348.

Chabriat H, Tehindrazanarinelo A, Samson Y, Boullais N, Bousser MG. PET study of cortical 5HT2 serotoninergic specific binding in migraine. *Cephalalgia* 1993;13(Suppl 13):19.

Dahl A, Russel D, Nyberg-Hansen R, Rootwelt K. Cluster headache: transcranial doppler ultrasound and rCBF studies. *Cephalalgia* 1990;10:87–89.

Edmeads J. Cerebral blood flow in migraine. *Headache* 1977;17:148–152.

Edmeads J. Challenges in the diagnosis of acute headache. *Headache* 1990;30(Suppl 2):537–540.

Ertsey C, Áfra J, Jelencsik I, Csanda E, Dabasi G, Pánczél G. SPECT and TCD studies in cluster headache patients. *Cephalalgia* 1993;13(Suppl 13):198.

Fodden DI, Peatfield RC, Milsom PL. Beware the patient with a headache in the accident and emergency department. *Arch Emerg Med* 1989;6:7–12.

Fontanarosa PB. Recognition of subarachnoid hemorrhage. *Ann Emerg Med* 1989;18:1199–1205.

Friberg L, Olsen TS, Roland PE, Lassen NA. Focal ischaemia caused by instability of cerebrovascular tone during attacks of hemiplegic migraine. *Brain* 1987;110:917–934.

Friberg L, Olesen J, Iversen HK, Sperling B. Migraine pain associated with middle cerebral artery dilatation: reversal by sumatriptan. *Lancet* 1991;338:13–17.

Hachinski VC, Olesen J, Norris JW, Larsen B, Enevoldsen B, Lassen NA. Cerebral hemodynamics in migraine. *Can J Neurol Sci* 1977;4:245–359.

Herold S, Gibbs JM, Jones AKP, Brooks DJ, Frackowiak RSJ, Legg NJ. Oxygen metabolism in classical migraine. *J Cereb Blood Flow Metab* 1985;5(Suppl 5):445–446.

Igarashi H, Sakai F, Kan S, Okada J, Tazaki Y. Magnetic resonance imaging of the brain in patients with migraine. *Cephalalgia* 1991;11:69–74.

Juge O. Regional cerebral blood flow in the different clinical types of migraine. *Headache* 1988;28: 537–549.

Kahn CE, Sanders GD, Lyons EA, Kostelic JK, MacEwan DW, Gordon WL. Computed tomography for nontraumatic headache: current utilization and cost-effectiveness. *Can Assoc Radiol J* 1993;44: 189–193.

Kaplan RD, Solomon GD, Diamond S, Freitag FG. The role of MRI in the evaluation of a migraine population: preliminary data. *Headache* 1987;27:315–318.

Kobari M, Meyer JS, Ichijo M, Kawamura J. Cortical and subcortical hyperperfusion during migraine and cluster headache measured by Xe CT-CBF. *Neuroradiology* 1990;32:4–11.

Lauritzen M, Olsen TS, Lassen A, Paulson OB. Changes in regional cerebral blood flow during the course of classic migraine attacks. *Ann Neurol* 1983a;13:633–641.

Lauritzen M, Olsen TS, Lassen A, Paulson OB. Regulation of regional cerebral blood flow during and between migraine attacks. *Ann Neurol* 1983b;14:569–572.

Lauritzen M, Olesen J. Regional cerebral blood flow during migraine attacks by xenon-133 inhalation and amazon tomography. *Brain* 1984;107:447–461.

Leao AAP. Spreading depression of activity in cerebral cortex. *J Neurophysiol* 1944;7:359–390.

Leao AAP, Morrison RS. Propagation of spreading cortical depression. *J Neurophysiol* 1945;8:33–45.

Lefkowitz D. Cortical thrombophlebitis and sinovenous disease. In: Vinken PJ, Bruyn GW, Klawans HL, eds; Toole JP, co-ed. *Handbook of clinical neurology*, vol. 54, revised series 10: *Vascular diseases*, part II. Amsterdam: Elsevier 1989;395–423.

Levine SR, Welch KMA, Ewing JR, Joseph R, D'Andrea G. Cerebral blood flow asymmetries in headache-free migraineurs. *Stroke* 1987;18:1164–1165.

Mathew NT, Hrastnik F, Meyer JS. Regional cerebral blood flow in the diagnosis of vascular headache. *Headache* 1976;16:252–260.

Micieli G, Bosone D, Cavallini A, Tassorelli C, Nappi G. Cerebral blood velocity changes in cluster headache: evidence for a bilateral asymmetrical impairment. *Cephalalgia* 1993;13(Suppl 13):197.

Mitchell CS, Osborn RE, Grosskreutz SR. Computed tomography in the headache patient: is routine evaluation really necessary? *Headache* 1993;33:82–86.

National Institutes of Health Consensus Development Panel. Computed tomographic scanning of the brain. *JAMA* 1982;247:1955–1958.

Norris JW, Hachinski VC, Cooper PW. Changes in cerebral blood flow during a migraine attack. *Br Med J* 1975;3:676–677.

Olesen J. (Chairman, Headache Classification Committee of the International Headache Society). Classification and diagnostic criteria for headache, cranial neuralgias and facial pain. *Cephalalgia* 1988; 8(Suppl 7):1–96.

Olesen J, Larsen B, Lauritzen M. Focal hyperemia followed by spreading oligemia and impaired activation of rCBF in classic migraine. *Ann Neurol* 1981a;9:344–352.

Olesen J, Tfelt-Hansen P, Henriksen L, Larsen B. The common migraine attack may not be initiated by cerebral ischemia. *Lancet* 1981b;2:438–440.

Olesen J, Friberg L, Olsen TS, Iversen HK, Lassen NA, Andersen AR, Karle A. Timing and topography of cerebral blood flow, aura, and headache during migraine attacks. *Ann Neurol* 1990;28:791–798.

Olsen TS, Friberg L, Lassen A. Ischemia may be the primary cause of the neurologic deficits in classic migraine. *Arch Neurol* 1987;44:156–161.

Olsen TS, Lassen NA. Blood flow and vascular reactivity during attacks of classic migraine limitations of the Xe-133 intraarterial technique. *Headache* 1989;29:15–20.

Prager JM, Mikulis DJ. The radiology of headache. *Med Clin North Am* 1991;75:525–544.

Prager JM, Rosenblum J, Mikulis DJ, Diamond S, Freitag FG. Evaluation of headache patients by MRI. *Headache Q* 1991;2:192–196.

Ramadan NM. Intracranial hypertension and migraine. *Cephalalgia* 1993;13:210–211.

Ramadan NM, Deveshwar R, Levine SR. Magnetic resonance and clinical cerebrovascular disease: An update. *Stroke* 1989a;20:1279–1283.

Ramadan NM, Halvorson H, Vande-Linde A, Levine SR, Helpern JA, Welch KMA. Low brain magnesium in migraine. *Headache* 1989b;29:590–593.

Robertson WM, Welch KMA, Levine SR, Schultz LR. The effects of aging on cerebral blood flow in migraine. *Neurology* 1989;39:947–951.

Sachs H, Wolf A, Russell AG, Christma DR. Effect of reserpine on regional cerebral glucose metabolism in control and migraine subjects. *Arch Neurol* 1986;43:1117–1123.

Sakai F, Meyer JS. Regional cerebral hemodynamics during migraine and cluster headaches measured by the ^{133}Xe inhalation method. *Headache* 1978;18:122–132.

Schlake HP, Bottger IG, Grotmeyer KH, Husstedt IW. Brain imaging with ^{123}I-IMP-SPECT in migraine between attacks. *Headache* 1989;29:344–349.

Scotti G, Ethier R, Melançon D, Terbrugge K, Tchang S. Computed tomography in the evaluation of intracranial aneurysms and subarachnoid hemorrhage. *Radiology* 1977;123:85–90.

Shen JM. Transcranial doppler sonography in chronic paroxysmal hemicrania. *Headache* 1993;33:493–496.

Simard D, Paulson OB. Cerebral vasomotor paralysis during migraine attack. *Arch Neurol* 1973;29:207–209.

Skinhoj E. Hemodynamic studies within the brain during migraine. *Arch Neurol* 1973;25:95–98.

Skinhoj E, Paulson OB. Regional cerebral blood flow in internal carotid distribution during migraine attack. *Br Med J* 1969;3:569–570.

Soges LJ, Cacayorin ED, Petro GR, Ramachadran TS. Migraine: evaluation by MRI. *AJNR* 1988;9:425–429.

Stovner LJ. Headache associated with the Chiari type I malformation. *Headache* 1993;33:175–181.

Thie A, Fuhlendorf A, Spitzer K, Kunze K. Transcranial doppler evaluation of common and classic migraine. Part I. Ultrasonic features during the headache free period. *Headache* 1990a;30:201–208.

Thie A, Fuhlendorf A, Spitzer K, Kunze K. Transcranial doppler evaluation of common and classic migraine. Part II. Ultrasonic features during attacks. *Headache* 1990b;30:209–215.

Tietjen GE, Mitsias P. Cerebral venous thrombosis. *Heart Dis Stroke* 1993;2:19–25.

Totaro R, De Matteis G, Marini C, Prencipe M. Cerebral blood flow in migraine with aura: a transcranial doppler sonography study. *Headache* 1992;32:446–451.

Wallash TM. Transcranial doppler ultrasonic features in episodic tension-type headache. *Cephalalgia* 1992a;12:293–296.

Wallash TM. Transcranial doppler ultrasonic features in episodic tension-type headache. *Cephalalgia* 1992b;12:385–386.

Wallash TM. Middle cerebral artery flow velocities in primary headaches. *Cephalalgia* 1993;13(Suppl 13):71.

Weingarten S, Kleinman M, Elperin L, Larson EB. The effectiveness of cerebral imaging in the diagnosis of chronic headache. *Arch Intern Med* 1992;152:2457–2462.

Weisberg LA. Computed tomography in benign intracranial hypertension. *Neurology* 1985;35:1075–1088.

Welch KMA, Levine SR. Migraine-related stroke in the context of the International Headache Society classification of head pain. *Arch Neurol* 1990;47:458–462.

Welch KMA, Levine SR, D'Andrea G, Schultz LR, Helpern JA. Preliminary observations on brain energy metabolism in migraine studied by in vivo phosphorus ^{31}P NMR spectroscopy. *Neurology* 1989;39:538–541.

Wolff HG. *Headache and other head pain*, 2nd ed. New York: Oxford University Press, 1963.

Young WB, Silberstein SD. Transcranial doppler: technique and application to headache. *Headache* 1992;32:136–142.

Ziegler DW, Batnisky S, Barter R, McMillan JH. Magnetic resonance image abnormality in migraine with aura. *Cephalalgia* 1991;11:147–150.

*Pain and the Brain: From
Nociception to Cognition,*
edited by Burkhart Bromm and
John E. Desmedt, Advances in Pain
Research and Therapy Vol. 22.
Raven Press, Ltd., New York © 1995.

16

Pain-Related Generators of Laser-Evoked Brain Potentials: Brain Mapping and Dipole Modelling

*Andrew C. N. Chen and †Burkhart Bromm

*Rhematic Diseases Center, Hope Hospital, University of Manchester, Salford M6 8HD
UK; and †Institute of Physiology, University Hospital Eppendorf,
D-20246 Hamburg, Germany*

SUMMARY

This contribution reviews brain-potential mapping and electrical source analysis in an attempt to identify cortical generators involved in the processing of experimentally induced pain. Brief (2 msec) radiant heat pulses emitted by a novel infrared thulium laser stimulator were applied to the right temple of 10 healthy male volunteers (20–25 years), activating nociceptive afferents of the upper branch of the trigeminal nerve. For investigation of the reliability of data and calculations derived from the procedure, the 10 subjects had to participate in three identical sessions, 1 week apart, in which the same four blocks of stimuli (interblock intervals of 20 min) were repeatedly applied. The electroencephalogram (EEG) was recorded at 31 scalp sites following the international 10/20 system, and laser-evoked brain potentials (LEPs) were built by averaging the 500-msec poststimulus segments in all recordings over the 40 stimuli per stimulus block. Data were subjected to brain electrical source analysis (BESA; Scherg 1990); results with the single-moving-dipole (SMD) approximation were compared with those obtained with multiple dipoles of varying strengths and orientations (multiple spatio-temporal dipoles; MSTD). The grand mean LEP as averaged over the 10 subjects, three sessions, and four blocks of stimuli (N = 120) indicates three major components of poststimulus segments of 300 msec, at about 100, 150, and 230 msec, dependent on scalp site. The SMD technique approximates the potential distributions over the scalp at a given time from a single dipole with calculated site, orientation, and strength. This dipole normally moves from one sample point to another. Its pathway (trajectory) through the brain began in all 10 subjects at the contralateral (left) somatosensory cortex area at 80 msec, moved forward to the frontal head (at about 130 msec), and then moved backward into the right hemisphere (at about 180 msec) and into the midline posterior central region (at about 210 msec), disappearing at the end of the analysis period (300 msec) in deep central structures under the vertex. MSTD modelling revealed four clearly identifiable generators: dipole I, with a maximum negativity at 106 msec in the contralateral trigeminal secondary somatosensory cortical area (19.0 mm beneath the cortex); dipole II, with a maximum negativity at 6 msec later in the corresponding ipsilateral area (13.6 mm near the surface of the cortex); dipole III, with a maximum positivity at 130 msec in the frontal cortex of the head (35 mm beneath the cortical surface); and dipole IV, describing both the late vertex negativity at 150 msec and the consecutive positivity at 220 msec under the vertex in deep (33.1 mm) brain structures. In the generalized spheric head model of BESA dipole IV was projected into the rostral part of the anterior cingulate gyrus.

These late brain potentials, however, were bilaterally symmetrical, with a maximum at the vertex, and had a distribution that is considerably larger in a lateral than in a longitudinal direction. It might therefore be possible to approximate these potential distributions with two parallel dipoles that are laterally shifted into the right and left deep hemispheres.

INTRODUCTION

The "decade of the brain" provided research with a series of more or less noninvasive methods for monitoring normal and disturbed cerebral function, including computed tomography (CT), magnetic resonance imaging (MRI), positron-emission topography (PET), radioimmunocytochemistry, single-photon emission computed tomography (SPECT), microangiography, autoradiography, Doppler sonography, microthermography, multilead electroencephalography (EEG), and multichannel magnetoencephalography (MEG) (for a review, see AAAS, 1993). The role of these techniques in pain research has recently been reviewed by one of us (Chen 1993a, b), and new results with promising techniques are described in several chapters of this book.

The oldest of these techniques is brain potential mapping. In this technique, an EEG is continuously recorded with up to 124 electrodes (Gevins et al. 1990), and interpolated potential distributions are displayed at each site of the scalp and at each time point measured. In this way cortical areas responsible for spike and wave generation in epileptic seizures, for example, can be specified. Another approach in research with functional EEG mapping is the multilead measurement of brain potentials evoked by all kinds of stimuli, including noxious stimulation [e.g., in the comparison of potential distributions in response to selective Aδ- or C-fiber stimulation (see Chapter 3 for details)]. Very impressive are the maps made during different states of a voluntary movement with spatially different cortical activity in its intention, performance, and suppression phases, particularly in patients with a loss in sensorimotor function. An immense amount of data on EEG mapping was gathered in EEG laboratories all over the world, and the question rose of how to best display and manage all of these clinical findings in order to avoid false conclusions.

Even modern comprehensive books about functional brain-potential mapping and data evaluation (Duffy 1986; Pfurtscheller and Lopes da Silva 1988) do not provide a mathematical identification of sources relevant for the measured potential distribution, even in terms of data reduction, with the exception of some graphic estimations. One reason for this may be that most researchers in this field agree with the statement of Helmholtz (1853) that the "inverse" problem, of the unique determination of sources responsible for measured and evaluated potential distributions, is not solvable, whereas the "forward" calculation of potential distributions from a source in a given conductor is easy. This doubt was given additional support by the fact that the electrical and geometric properties of the manifold tissues in the head are not sufficiently well known for such calculations. In our opinion, a major merit of initial biomagnetic research (see Chapter 17) was its stimulation of the development of source-localization procedures in the evaluation of signal distributions spread over the scalp, using additional physiologic and neuroanatomic data. Biomagnetometry normally involves no ferromagnetic substances that might disturb the magnetic fields in the body, and there was therefore an immediate impetus to estimate current dipoles from magnetic fields measured over the body by magnetocardiography, for example (Baule and McFee 1965; for a review see Stroink, 1992) or over the scalp by magnetoelectrography (MEG) (Cohen 1968; see also Cuffin and Cohen 1977; Cuffin et al. 1991).

One of the first approaches to estimating brain sources from EEG recordings by applying the electrical-field theory and numerical iteration procedures was reported by Henderson et al. (1975). In 1984 Scherg reported a computerized procedure, brain electrical source analysis (BESA), which was subsequently completed (e.g., Scherg and coworkers 1984, 1986, 1989, 1990, 1991, 1992, 1993) and which allows the calculation of a series of simultaneously active generators from measured scalp-potential distributions if well-defined physiologic constraints are established. For example, the "inverse" problem is solvable if the site of the generator is given and only its orientation and strength are allowed to vary. BESA can be used in the single-moving-dipole mode, which assumes that the potential distributions over the scalp at each sampled time point are generated by only a single dipole that moves in time. This single-dipole approximation is often used in source-localization procedures (e.g., Lehmann 1989), particularly in analyses of stimulus-evoked magnetic-field maps recorded by MEG (e.g., Wood et al. 1985; Sutherling et al. 1988; Hari et al. 1990; see Chapter 17). However, the main feature of BESA is its multiple spatiotemporal dipole analysis, which is based on the assumption that brain potentials are generated by multiple, simultaneously active cortical regions that produce electrical fields which overlap in time and space.

BESA has been applied to brain potentials evoked by different sensory modalities [e.g. the visual (Simpson et al. 1990; Plendl et al. 1993) and auditory systems

(Scherg 1984, 1993; Ponton et al. 1993)]. However, little research has so far been published on generators of somatosensory evoked potentials (SEP). Recently, Franssen et al. (1992) described the generators of short-latency potentials in response to electrical stimulation of the median nerve. The main result was that the generators identified by BESA fit well with the primary sensory (S1) cortical areas known so far: N20 and P22 were respectively modelled by a tangentially and a radially oriented dipole in the region of the contralateral cortical hand area; a third dipole, with a maximum activity at 14 msec, was located in the brain stem. In patients with a somatosensory deficit, the two generators in the corresponding cortical areas were found to be distorted or even missing.

Most knowledge about brain generators responsible for the long-latency somatosensory potentials evoked at the vertex has been gathered through invasive techniques in animals or during surgery in humans, leading to a wide variety of hypotheses about their localizations, which have included primary sensory cortical areas, the frontal association cortex, areas in the mesial cortex, areas in the corpus callosum, diencephalic regions, sensorimotor areas, and the cingulate gyrus (for a review, see e.g., Allison 1992).

This chapter reports results with BESA applied to a large set of multilead EEG data obtained through repeated measurements on the same subjects with a thulium laser stimulus administered to the left temple of healthy subjects, thus activating the upper branch of the trigeminal nerve. We used BESA for both the single-moving-dipole and the multiple spatiotemporal-dipole approximations, and compared the results of these two modelling methods for understanding the pain-related neural generators of laser-evoked potentials (LEP). The subjects had to participate in three identical sessions (exactly 1 week apart), with four identical experiments exactly 30 min apart, done at each session in order to test the reliability of the results of measurement and source analysis.

METHODOLOGIC DETAILS

Data Collection

Pain-Inducing Stimuli

Brief (2-msec) laser-emitted heat stimuli (thulium YAG crystal, 1.8 μm wavelength) were delivered to the right temple by means of a flexible light conductor (the stimulated body area was 20 mm^2); the subjects had to wear protective eyeglasses. Four intensities of 310, 340, 370, and 400 mJ were used for all subjects and sessions; these intensities were clearly within the painful range (mean pain threshold intensity: 280 mJ). The intensities were varied randomly in blocks of 40 stimulus applications; the interstimulus intervals varied between 10 and 20 sec. Each laser stimulus was followed, with a delay of 3 sec, by a tone (500 Hz; 20-msec duration;

65 dB SPL) that prompted the subject to rate the magnitude of the pain created by the stimulus on a visual analogue scale.

Subject and Study Design

Ten healthy male medical students (20–25 years) were comfortably seated in a noise-free chamber with a regulated room temperature (22–24°C). In preceding adaptation sessions, the subjects were familiarized with the entire experimental procedure. Subjects were paid to participate and provided informed consent in accordance with the Helsinki Declaration. The study was approved by the institute's Human Subject Committee. The first of the four experimental sessions was only for familiarization with the experimental surroundings. In each session, five blocks of stimuli were applied, each lasting for 20 min, with interblock intervals of 30 min (the first stimulus block was repeated for adaptation). For each subject, 12 potential sets (three sessions with four blocks of stimuli) were evaluated. The experiments have been described in detail elsewhere (Kazarians et al. 1995).

EEG Recording and Data Management

EEG was recorded with Ag/AgCl electrodes (bandpass: 0.5–250 Hz), using a 32-channel Nicolet amplifier, with linked earlobes as the reference. The standard international 10/20 system was chosen for the 31 EEG recording sites, with an additional 10 interpolated locations in both precentral and postcentral sites, following the American EEG Society guideline (Fig. 1). Two channels were used to measure the vertical electrooculogram (EOG) from supra- and infraorbital electrodes for the control of artifacts in each EEG segment; the 32nd channel monitored stimulus parameters. The interelectrode impedances were below 5 kΩ. For each laser stimulus, the peristimulus EEG segment of 1.1-sec duration (400 msec before and 700 msec after stimulus onset) was digitized (CED 1401; 300-Hz sampling rate) and stored on a magneto-optical disc. The poststimulus EEG segments were averaged with a micro-VAX II computer over the 40 stimuli of each block (block LEP), over all blocks for each session (session LEP: four blocks), over all sessions for each subject (subject LEP: four blocks × three sessions), and over the total sample (grand mean LEP: four blocks × three sessions × 10 subjects). LEP components with latencies between 75 and 300 msec—the typical interval of pain-related potentials (see Chapter 3)—were evaluated.

Topographic Mapping

For the analysis of topography, the LEPs recorded from the 31 EEG channels were fed into a mapping program (a modified version of the program developed by

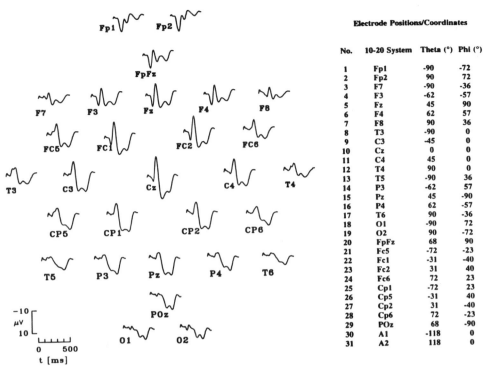

FIG. 1. Locations of recording electrodes in BESA coordinates. Brain potentials in response to brief laser heat pulses applied to the right temple are recorded simultaneously at the scalp sites and averaged over blocks of 40 stimuli (laser-evoked potentials, LEPs). Grand mean LEPs are the averages over the four stimulus blocks per session, three repeated sessions, and 10 subjects in the study (altogether, 120 LEPs). Electrode positions follow the international 10/20 system and are shown at right, in BESA coordinates. The head is approximated by a hemisphere with a scalp radius of 85 mm. The origin is defined by the intersection point between the lines T3–T4 (x-axis) and Oz–Fpz (y-axis); the z-axis runs through Cz; positions on the scale are described by spherical coordinates with the angles phi (x–y plane) and theta (x–z plane). (From Bromm and Chen 1995, with permission.)

Coppola et al. 1982) to compute estimated amplitudes for the whole scalp with a spatial resolution of 3 mm. The value of a given pixel was computed by calculating the weighted mean of the values from the four closest electrodes, with each electrode value weighted by the inverse of its distance from the examined pixel. In order to allow for a small variability in peak latency at different lead positions, mean amplitudes over 10 msec (three sampling points) were taken. The resulting instantaneous potential maps were displayed on a graphics screen. For the analysis of the isopotential contours and peak maxima at each instaneous latency point, a mapping program for the micro-VAX-II was employed. Each brain electrical activity map was sequentially displayed for every 6 msec in the latency range analyzed.

Brain Electrical Source Analysis (BESA)

Principles of BESA

We used the commercially available BESA program provided by Scherg (BESA manual 1992, version 1.9; Scherg and Berg 1992). It allows the calculation of sources from measured potential maps under certain assumptions adapted from neurophysiologic and anatomic knowledge. Basically, the program calculates potential distributions over the scalp from preset voltage dipoles within the brain; the sites, orientations, and strengths of these dipoles are repeatedly varied until an optimal agreement between the measured and calculated maps is achieved. The solutions, of course, are not unique, and depend on the starting conditions in terms of the numbers and sites of the dipoles and assumptions about head geometry and other factors. In the single-moving-dipole (SMD) mode, only a single generator was assumed for each measured time point; the initial parameters can be chosen with few constraints. By iteration of the site, orientation, and strength of this dipole, residual variance was minimized. Consequently, with the application of this method for each sampled time point (the evaluation lasting between 80 and 250 msec), another generator appears; the footpoints of these generators build the pathway of the "moving" dipole, called the trajectory.

In the multiple spatiotemporal-dipole (MSTD) mode, the cerebral dipoles were present in certain brain areas on the basis of the findings in the potential maps (see below, Fig. 2, see Colorplate 4); the number of dipoles was estimated by principal-component analysis. The sites, orientations, and strengths of the dipoles were then improved by iteration, comparing the measured and calculated maps. Once these characteristics were determined, the dipoles remained at the same sites while varying in orientation and activity throughout the entire epoch range. In detail, this procedure involved the following steps: (a) siting the dipole at the approximate brain location; (b) selecting the latency times of local maxima; (c) fitting the parameters of each dipole for location, orientation, and strength to achieve a maximum stability in LEP topographic prediction (i.e., minimizing residual variances); and (d) repeating the fit for all dipoles together, with fixed sites, but varying dipole strengths and orientations.

BESA Coordinates and Head Geometry

In BESA, the human head is approximated by a standard sphere (outer radius 85 mm) consisting of three layers: the scalp (thickness 7 mm), skull (thickness 8 mm), and cortex (surface radius 70 mm). The center of the concentric spheres is the intersection point of the cartesian coordinates x, y, and z. The x-axis is defined by the line through T3 and T4, the y-axis by the line through Oz and Fpz, and the z-axis runs through Cz. In the case of a particular head, these axes do not necessarily intersect and are not necessarily rectangular (for more discussion see Towle et al. 1993). In this study, however, we followed the original BESA methodology.

Each calculated dipole was determined from six parameters: three for location, two for orientation, and one for strength. The location was described in the x, y, z system (in millimeters). In addition, the cortex depth of the dipoles was given, on the basis of the radius from the corresponding point of the cortical surface to the center. The orientation was described in angles (°); ϕ was the horizontal angle in the xy-plane, measured counterclockwise from the nearest point on the x-axis (positive or negative x), and θ was the vertical angle, measured from the z-axis, with values between 0 and 180° being positive for the right hemisphere. The strength was given in μVeff, scaled such that a horizontal $\phi = 0°$, $\theta = 90°$) dipole of 1.0 μVeff amplitude located below Cz at $y = 50$ mm (60% of the total radius; cortex depth 20 mm) produced a voltage difference of 0.5 μVeff between C3 and C4. In Fig. 1 the electrode sites employed on the scalp (international 10/20 system) are given in BESA coordinates.

Statistical Analyses

Consistency of the results in repeated experiments during each session and across weeks was given by standard deviations within (SDw) and between subjects (SDb). To compare the dipole parameters across sessions, a two-way repeated-measures analysis of variance (ANOVA) was conducted, with one main factor for session and the other for dipole number. In comparing the differences of means, *post hoc* analysis at alpha = 0.05 was performed with Fisher's least significant difference (LSD) test.

LEP MAPS EVOKED BY PAINFUL TRIGEMINAL
NERVE STIMULATION

Series of topographic maps over the entire latency interval measured (700 msec) were constructed to depict the spatiotemporal distributions of LEPs in response to pain-inducing stimulation of the upper trigeminal nerve. The grand-mean map, averaged over the 10 subjects, three sessions, and four blocks of 40 stimuli, is given in Fig. 2 (see Colorplate 4). The figure clearly demonstrates that: (a) no LEP was consistently obtained at 70 msec; (b) a frontal positivity and contralateral temporal negativity with focal extrema were present at 90 msec; (c) a correponding ipsilateral focal negativity emerged at 100 msec; (d) the contralateral negativity reached its maximum at 106 msec; (e) convergence of bilateral negativity at the vertex was seen at 130 msec; (f) vertex negativity reached its peak intensity at 150 msec; (g) this vertex negativity shifted toward the ipsilateral right frontal cortex at 180 msec; (h) a sharp reversal of vertex negativity to vertex positivity was evident at 220 msec; (i) the vertex positivity exhibited posterior spreading between 250 and 350 msec with the probable activation of P300; and (j) the vertex negativity returned by 450 msec and lasted to the end of the analysis at 700 msec, probably representing the contingent negative variation.

In pain research, the late LEP components, at up to 250 msec, are usually regarded as reflecting Aδ-fiber activity (see Chapter 3). Pain-related brain responses to activation of C-fibers with conduction velocities of 1 msec or less are expected to appear later. In the case of trigeminal-nerve stimulation, the neuronal conduction distance amounts to approximately 10 cm, so that cognitive potentials with latencies of more than 300 msec may be contaminated by C-fiber responses. We therefore stopped BESA analysis within 300 msec poststimulus EEG segments and focused on Aδ-fiber responses only. The data for the maps in Fig. 2 provided estimates of the "starting values" for dipole localization.

SINGLE MOVING-DIPOLE ANALYSIS OF GRAND-MEAN LEP MAPS

As mentioned above, the moving-dipole analysis identifies a single generator at each time point; connecting the sites of this dipole at different times results in a trajectory through the brain. We evaluated the poststimulus epoch between 80 and 300 msec in time steps of 10 msec, which resulted in 23 dipole sites. These are, for some time periods, very similar, whereas in other time periods large distances were covered. Fig. 3 illustrates the course of the trajectory obtained from the evaluation of the grand-mean LEP maps given in Fig. 2. The main plot gives a three-dimensional perspective; the small panels show both coronal and horizontal two-dimensional planes of the same trajectory, with x directed to the right ear, y to the front, and z to the vertex. The dipole starts at 80 msec in contralateral cortical areas in the left hemisphere, moves slowly frontally and upward during the period between 110 and 150 msec, then moves backward, where it finally dives at the midline in the center of the brain, with latencies above 230 msec.

Trajectories like that given in Fig. 3, however, are misleading, since they do not discriminate between dipoles with high energy and a large total variance and those that obviously reflect only "noise." More interesting, therefore, are analyses of the time intervals in which the dipoles do not move, in which the same neuronal areas remain active. For example, dipoles 6, 7, and 8, with latencies between 130 and 150 msec, seem to describe a constant area in the frontal brain, whereas for other time intervals there was a rapid change in location coordinates (e.g., for dipoles 11, 12, and 13). Moreover, the total variance (fit precision) explained by the respective dipoles varied remarkably for different time periods. In certain stable periods it was as large as 98%, while at other time points, especially those marked by a rapid transition to new sites, it was less than 60%.

Table 1 lists the source parameters of these single dipoles in detail from 80 to 300 msec, in 10-msec steps. Twenty-three dipoles are given, one for each time point. The parameters of these dipoles are sometimes rather similar to those of neighboring dipoles and sometimes very different. Quantitative determination of the identity and interdependency of these dipoles is difficult on the basis of source parameters, since no indices are elaborated to cluster similar dipoles, and a rule for selecting meaningful criteria for this purpose is still not known.

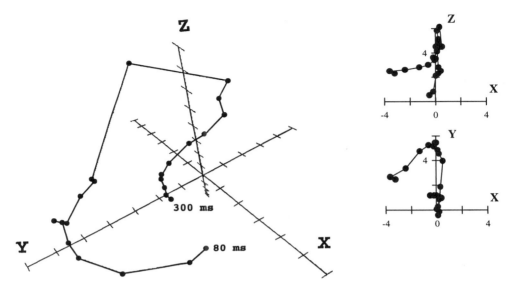

FIG. 3. Pathway of the single-moving dipole calculated from grand-mean LEP maps. From the maps given in Fig. 2 the site, strength, and orientation of the dipole was calculated at each sampled time point [which explains] a maximum of the measured EEG potential distributions. The illustration shows the line through the sites of all succeeding dipoles, calculated in the latency range of 80 to 300 msec in steps of 10 msec, which results in 23 points. According to the BESA coordinates, x points to the right ear, y to the front, and z to the vertex; distances are given in centimeters. The main figure shows a three-dimensional perspective; the small panels show both coronal and horizontal two-dimensional planes of the same trajectory. The trajectory starts in the contralateral cortex in the left hemisphere (80 msec), slowly moves to the frontal cortex at the period of 120 to 160 msec, then swings backward and down into the center of the brain at latencies above 210 msec.

For the source localization of the major pain-related late N150 and P220 components, we can focus on two particular dipole clusters in Table 1 that might show comparable coordinates, strengths, and percentages of variance explained. These are the dipoles 5 to 8 at about 140 msec and the dipoles around 16 at 230 msec. These two dipole clusters differed distinctly in site, with dipole 7 being 48 mm anterior to the vertex and dipole 6 about 4 mm posterior to the vertex, both being approximately in the midline of the brain. Furthermore, dipole 7 and its neighbors were 13 to 15 mm beneath the frontal cortex, while the dipoles around dipole 16 were 25 to 30 mm beneath the central cortex near the vertex. The strength of the two dipoles was rather similar, but their orientations differed. These results indicate that the two waveform components of LEPs usually regarded in pain research could stem from brain generators with clearly different spatial locations. The fit precision of the identified dipoles ranged from 88–90% around dipole 7, and from 93 to 98% around dipole 16. Between these two dipoles was a region with low stimulus-

TABLE 1. *Source parameters of the single-moving dipoles*

Dipoles	Time (msec)	Location (mm)			Orientation (°)		Strength (μV_{eff})	Cortex depth (mm)	Fit precision (%)
		x	y	z	θ	φ			
1	80	−35	24	28	67	46	1.4	19.4	91
2	90	−37	30	29	64	46	2.1	14.0	92
3	100	−27	45	20	62	58	3.5	13.6	86
4	110	−13	52	15	72	74	4.2	14.4	81
5	120	−7	48	18	92	78	4.8	15.6	87
6	130	−4	47	28	115	78	5.4	15.5	90
7	140	−4	48	32	136	74	5.7	14.6	89
8	150	−7	46	32	146	71	5.8	14.1	88
9	160	4	38	31	165	55	5.5	21.4	77
10	170	14	32	14	−178	54	4.6	32.1	78
11	180	23	34	3	−169	20	3.6	28.7	80
12	190	13	6	66	126	28	1.2	2.6	55
13	200	3	−14	51	162	−27	3.2	17.4	88
14	210	3	−11	44	166	−35	4.3	24.4	96
15	220	2	−12	35	169	−46	5.8	33.1	98
16	230	1	−4	30	174	−2	6.6	39.5	95
17	240	1	2	29	172	46	6.8	41.5	96
18	250	−1	11	26	163	76	7.0	41.9	97
19	260	−2	15	22	155	80	7.1	43.1	94
20	270	−3	16	21	152	81	7.0	43.1	93
21	280	−5	17	17	147	81	6.8	45.6	95
22	290	−7	18	14	145	81	6.7	46.2	96
23	300	−8	18	12	145	82	6.7	47.5	95

induced EEG activity in which fit precision was extremely low. The lowest variance, of only 55%, was found for dipoles around dipole 12, at 190 msec. In this region the transition occurred in polarity from vertex negativity to positivity, explaining this small variance. Inspection of the entire data set of scalp-potential distributions, as given in Fig. 2, however, provides evidence that several dipoles seem to be active at the same times. In such cases, the single dipole approximation will localize its solution somewhere between the sites of the coactive generators. For example, the frontal generator is obviously still active when the vertex negativity arises. Similarly, at least two additional separate dipoles are required to explain the observed negativity between 106 and 112 msec, one in the frontal brain and the other on the ipsilateral side. On the other hand, the bilaterally symmetrical vertex potential distribution of N150 seems to be similar to that of P230, which indicates comparable brain sites for both generators. Thus, the given values of fit precision still have to be called low; they cannot be used as crucial criteria in deciding modelling validity. In the following section we show that the results obtained here with the single-dipole approximation contrast with those produced if several generators are assumed to act simultaneously.

MULTIPLE SPATIOTEMPORAL-DIPOLE ANALYSIS OF
GRAND-MEAN LEP MAPS

Multiple spatiotemporal-dipole (MSTD) modelling usually begins with a principal-component analysis (PCA) to estimate the number of dipoles underlying the potential distributions. In our data set, five principal components (PCs) were sufficient to explain 93.7% of variances in the grand-mean LEPs and, on the average, 91.5% of these variances if PCA was applied in the 10 subject LEPs, as described by Bromm and Chen (1995). To avoid confusion, it should be mentioned that PCA is a purely statistical analysis; components resulting from it are orthogonal, that is, they are statistically independent of one another. The numbers and waveforms of the PCs are naturally different from the biophysical or physiologic dipoles identified from the brain-potential distributions produced by different mathematical procedures. Nevertheless, the number of PCs often yields a good approximation of the number of dipoles in source analysis.

Accordingly, we began MSTD modelling with five dipoles, which were roughly preset as follows: dipoles I and II in the contra- and ipsilateral somatosensory cortices, dipole III in the midline frontal cortex, and dipoles 4 and 5 in frontocentral and centroparietal sites in the deep midline brain. An interesting result was that the latter two dipoles could be located at the same site without losing considerable accuracy of approximation (Bromm and Chen 1994). For these reasons, we combined dipoles 4 and 5 into a single dipole IV, the maximum activities of which described both the vertex negativity N150 and vertex positivity P220, and performed the further grand-mean LEP analysis with only four dipoles.

Fig. 4 demonstrates the locations, orientations, and maximum strengths of the resulting four dipoles for the coronal, axial, and lateral views shown in the three columns at the right of the figure. Their maximum activities exhibited different latencies: dipole I in the contralateral somatosensory cortex showed a maximum activity at 106 msec, dipole II in the ipsilateral somatosensory cortex a maximum activity at 112 msec, dipole III in the frontal cortex a maximum activity at 130 msec, and dipole IV a maximum activity at 150 msec and, with reversed polarity, at 220 msec. Dipole source potentials (strengths) as a function of time are seen in the left column of the figure. All dipoles were active during the entire period of analysis, and contributed to the grand-mean potential maps to varying degrees that depended on the respective latencies (for details see Bromm and Chen 1995). Dipoles I and II showed very similar waveforms; the ipsilateral dipole II exhibited a delay in peak amplitude of about 5 msec against the contralateral dipole I. The frontal dipole III of the grand-mean LEPs was located in the middle frontal area, with an anterior-posterior orientation, although the activity of this dipole did not end within the analyzed poststimulus EEG periods. The greatest activity was seen for dipole IV, describing the two consecutive components beneath the vertex.

In Table 2 the final locations of the four dipoles are listed in BESA coordinates. The locations of dipoles I and II were at nearly homologous sites in each hemisphere (note the different sign of x); their orientations were mirror images of each other for

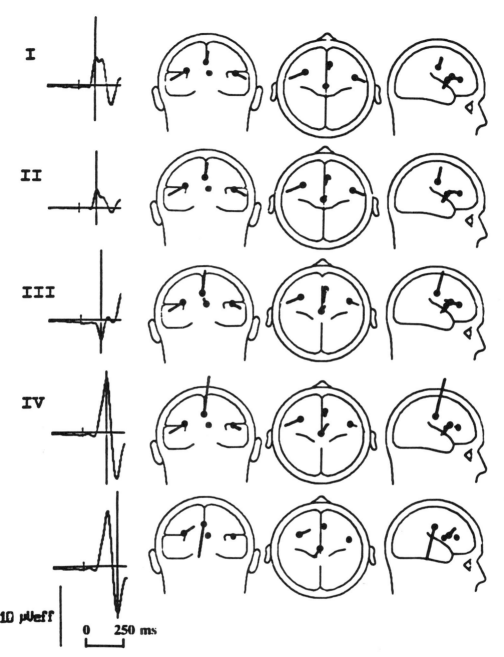

FIG. 4. Multiple dipoles calculated from the grand-mean LEP maps. Four dipoles account for more than 93% of the total variance of LEP maps, with peak maxima at 106 msec (dipole I, left somatosensory cortex), 112 msec (dipole II, ipsilateral), 130 msec (dipole III, frontal), 150 msec, and 220 msec (dipole IV, central). The locations of the dipoles fixed in time, orientation, and strength are given at respective peak latencies. In the lefthand column is shown the dipole source potential, DSP, for the four dipoles, as a function of time. (From Bromm and Chen 1995, with permission.)

TABLE 2. *Dipole coordinates of grand-mean LEPs[a]*

Dipole	I	II	III	IV
Site	Contralateral	Ipsilateral	Frontal	Vertex
Latency (msec)	106.3	112.1	130.4	150.6/220.5
Location (mm)				
Lateral, x	−36.7	50.2	6.4	−1.4
Frontal, y	28.1	20.6	42.5	3.2
Vertical, z	21.5	15.2	16.2	36.7
Orientation (°)				
ϕ	24.8	−21.5	82.7	59.0/59.0
θ	−119.4	117.3	106.3	16.1/−164.2
Strength (μV_{eff})	5.3	1.8	1.7	8.7/7.6
Cortex depth (mm)	19.0	13.6	24.1	33.1

[a]Site parameters are given in cartesian coordinates (x, y, z), orientation in spherical coordinates ($\phi = xy$ plane and $\theta = xz$ plane). Strength is the mean power averaged over the 70- to 250-msec analysis period.

both the angles ϕ and θ (for a definition of these angles see the section on brain electrical source analysis). Obviously the strength of the contralateral dipole was greater. Dipole III was clearly frontal (note the high value of y); its direction was downward ($\theta > 90°$) looking toward the forehead ($\phi \approx 90°$). The antiparallel orientations of dipole IV at the two latencies describe both the N110 and P230 components (note the complementary values of θ and the identical values of ϕ). Although the z-value was greatest for dipole IV, this dipole was nevertheless localized in the deepest cortex, at 33.1 mm measured from the cortical surface to the center.

The maps in Fig. 5 illustrate the contribution made by each of the identified dipoles to the scalp distribution of the grand-mean LEPs at the dipoles' respective peak-activity latencies. At 107 msec, dipole I reached its peak intensity on the contralateral site, but dipoles II and IV were also active; dipole III was relatively quiet. These simultaneous activities resulted in the modelled compound potential map, which is contrasted with the measured grand-mean LEP map in the lower third of the figure. At 112 msec, dipole II reached its peak maximum at the ipsilateral site, while dipoles I, III, and IV were also active. Again, the topographic model composed from the activities of the four dipoles closely resembled the recorded topography. The same was true for the 130-msec time point, at which dipole III exhibited its maximum activity at the frontal site while the three other generators were also considerably activated. At 150 msec, dipole IV generated its maximum negativity at the vertex site, while dipole I was still active, and dipoles II and III became quiet. Dipole IV then reversed its polarity and exhibited a positive maximum at 220 msec at the vertex. At this time, dipole I at the contralateral site also showed a reversed polarity, from negativity to positivity on the scalp, while dipoles II and III remained quiet. To sum up, the topographic model closely resembled the recorded topography for all time points analyzed.

With the four dipoles obtained by MSTD modelling, a precision of fit (see above)

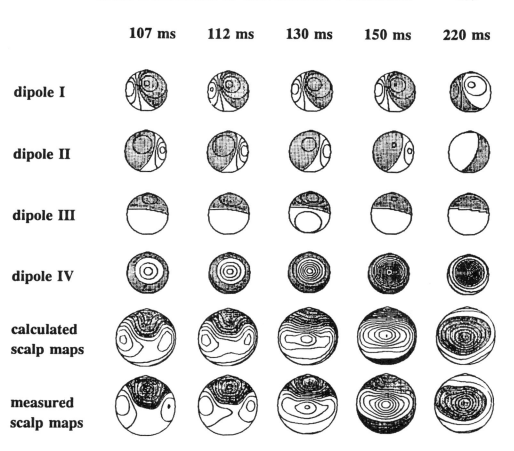

| | **107 ms** | **112 ms** | **130 ms** | **150 ms** | **220 ms** |

dipole I

dipole II

dipole III

dipole IV

calculated scalp maps

measured scalp maps

spacing between field lines 1 μV

FIG. 5. Comparison of measured and predicted grand-mean LEP maps. The potential maps calculated from each dipole at its respective maximum activity, as well as the resulting total LEP map, are compared with the measured map (+ = dark, − − = white). At all times all generators contribute to the brain-potential distributions, though with variable strengths. (From Bromm and Chen 1995, with permission.)

between 97.2 and 98.8% was obtained in those time intervals in which the dipoles were maximally active. When we averaged the fit precisions over the entire post-stimulus interval analyzed (between 80 amd 300 ms), a mean value of 93.5% was obtained. Although this accuracy amounts to only about 5% more than that obtained with the single-dipole approximation (mean value over the 23 dipoles, 88.4%), this increase in precision is decisive in brain-source analysis.

DIPOLE CONSISTENCY IN REPEATED MEASUREMENTS AND IN DIFFERENT INDIVIDUALS

In a manner similar to that described above, MSTD analysis was applied to all individual LEP distributions for each of the 10 subjects and for each of the three study sessions. The LEPs of the four blocks of stimuli per session were combined to reduce the signal-to-noise ratio (session LEPs are averages over the four blocks per session); this was possible because a preliminary study showed an extremely high intrasession reliability of vertex LEPs in response to upper trigeminal-nerve stimulation (Kazarians et al. 1995). For all subjects, dipole IV provided sufficient information for calculating the potential distributions of the N150 and P230 components: beginning with two separate dipoles having different sites and opposite polarities repeated iterations yielded a single resulting dipole in the deep brain beneath the vertex.

To document the differences between individuals and sessions, the source parameters of the individual LEPs were averaged across all subjects and sessions. The mean parameters of the four dipoles as the average of the 30 BESA analyses (10 subjects, three sessions; for details see Bromm and Chen 1995) were largely the same as those of the grand-mean LEP (all individual maps were pooled and BESA was applied once, Table 2). The mean precision of fit was again 93.5% if averaged over the 10 subjects, ranging from 92.9% to 98.1% for individuals. For the individual group LEP map evaluations, standard deviations (SDs) within and between subjects were calculated (Table 3). Within the same subjects, a high reliability of dipole coordinates was found, with a mean redetection accuracy of sites of better than 5 mm. This is very near the theoretical limit for errors in brain-source identification (Mosher et al. 1993). Only the frontal dipole III showed a considerable variability in its coordinates in repeated sessions (mean SD = 5 mm), as will be described below.

TABLE 3. *Intra- and interindividual variability of dipole parameters*[a]

Dipole	I Contralateral SDw/SDb	II Ipsilateral SDw/SDb	III Frontal SDw/SDb	IV Vertex SDw/SDb
Latency (msec)	1.7/7.4	1.7/7.2	1.0/10.6	0.4/4.9
Location (mm)				
x	0.9/13.5	2.7/6.6	5.0/10.9	2.0/7.1
y	1.3/13.7	4.6/12.9	4.5/19.7	6.2/14.7
z	2.6/12.7	1.7/14.8	5.0/23.9	2.8/11.1
Orientation (°)				
ϕ	3.0/31.0	8.1/19.2	15.6/48.7	16.2/46.8
θ	11.7/22.5	0.7/65.8	31.6/70.3	10.9/47.1
Strength (μV_{eff})	0.8/3.0	0.7/1.8	0.6/2.1	0.5/4.2

[a]BESA was applied to each measured LEP map per session (10 subjects × 3 sessions = 30 maps). The individual solutions were compared with the corresponding mean values. Standard deviations of each dipole parameter were calculated for repeated sessions within the same subject (SDw) and for the same session between different subjects (SDb).
Within-subject variability: less than 5 mm (mean SDw for *x*, *y*, *z*).
Between-subject variability: less than 15 mm (mean SDb for *x*, *y*, *z*).

There was also high variability in the frontal coordinate (y) of the central dipole IV, which may in part be due to the variability of the frontal generator. In other words, if the same subject participates at weekly intervals in different sessions of an experiment of constant design, similar potential maps and thus highly reliable generators will result from the BESA procedure. This is an important finding, for example, if these methods are to be applied to test pharmacologic treatments that alter pain perception or pain-relevant brain potentials. It is also important for clinical applications, such as in comparing disturbed pain sensitivity with that in the healthy body area of a particular patient.

Interindividually, the SD of dipole coordinates was found to be much larger (mean SDb = 15 mm) than it was within a given patient. The variability for the frontal dipole III was again large, with a site variability of up to 25 mm: each subject produced an individual frontal generator in response to painful trigeminal simulation. This generator may be involved in eye movements or in task performance, or may be initiated by voluntary motor responses that were suppressed in our study. The main reason for the large interindividual variability in dipole identification is that a single uniform head model (a sphere with a constant radius) has been used for BESA of different subjects. As reflected by the high variability of dipole III, however, there are obviously additional individual differences in generator sites (see the conclusion of this chapter).

In a final analysis of variances with repeated measures, neither a "session" effect on the dipole parameters x, y, z, depth, θ, ϕ, and strength (F-values between 0.16 and 0.97, $p > 0.05$), nor a "session by dipole" interaction (F-values between 0.21 and 0.49, $p > 0.05$) was found, indicating that the dipole parameters did not vary systematically with session repetitions. In contrast, the differences between corresponding coordinates of the four dipoles were large (F-values between 30.79 and 1,129.50, $p < 0.0001$). To examine the significance of coordinate differences, *post hoc* comparisons of mean values were performed, with the result that dipole I and dipole II showed a significant difference in cortical depth (19.0 versus 13.6 mm), in the frontal coordinate (28.1 versus 20.6 mm), and in strength (5.3 versus 1.8 μVeff). Dipole III was widely distributed and exhibited significant differences in all of its coordinates as compared to those of the other dipoles. Dipole IV showed significant differences in location, orientation (except in phi), and strength as compared with those of both dipoles I and II.

In summary, MSTD modelling of LEPs in response to painful upper-trigeminal-nerve stimulation resulted in four major brain dipoles, with locations in contralateral and ipsilateral secondary somatosensory cortical areas, in the frontal area, and in the deep midline cortex. The topographic maps predicted from these generators fitted well with the recorded scalp-potential distributions in time and space.

CONCLUSIONS

Most brain-source analysis from multilead recordings is still based on the single-moving-dipole approximation, assuming a single dipole to be responsible for a measured brain-signal distribution at a series of sampled time points. This is especially true for the analysis of magnetic fields in MEG (for a review, see e.g., Cuffin et al. 1991; Sato et al. 1991). Only recently have powerful programs become available for calculating multiple dipoles in morphologically defined layers of the head, such as certain cortical areas (Fuchs et al. 1994). However, many investigators of electrical brain maps prefer the single moving-dipole approximation (e.g., from simple determinations of maxima and minima in global-field power maps [e.g., Lehmann 1989]). This "two-extreme description" is based on the observation that many maps give the impression of a simple "mountain-valley landscape" of potentials. In any case, the single-dipole approximation of momentary maps, measured with up to 124 electrodes (Gevins et al. 1990), means a reduction of data to only the six parameters needed to describe one dipole. This may often be sufficient, especially if a series of similar experiments is performed on the same subjects (e.g. to investigate the action of psychotropic substances). The physiologic meaning of the resulting data, however, is poor, since functioning of the brain is typically based on multiple processing of the information received in different cortical and subcortical structures.

In any case, the single moving-dipole approximation is inadequate if the map to be evaluated already indicates several centers of brain activity. For detecting the number of independent sources, multivariate statistical analysis may be helpful. This was the case in the LEP distributions measured in response to painful trigeminal activation with brief infrared radiant heat pulses in our study. In the latency range between 80 msec and 300 msec, the brain potential maps we derived indicated the existence of several sources for all time points sampled. For this reason, a single source of activity provided by single-moving-dipole approximations was localized somewhere between the simultaneously active brain areas. Interestingly, during those time periods in which several dipoles are obviously active (e.g., between 80 and 150 msec), the precision of fit with the single-dipole mode still reached values between 81% and 90%. In other words, a congruence between measured and calculated potential distributions of up to 90% is insufficient for a neurophysiologically relevant identification of brain generators responsible for measured distributions of potentials (or fields). Within those time periods in which the map clearly indicates only a single extremum (e.g., between 220 and 250 msec) the single-dipole solution had a precision of fit of 97% or better. Averaged over the entire latency period evaluated (80–300 msec), the single-moving-dipole approximation yielded an overall precision of fit of only 88% in our LEP data.

On the other hand, as more simultaneously active dipoles are admitted in the analysis of brain-potential maps, more information is needed to preset the initial parameters of sites, strengths, and orientations. The major finding in our study of the need for four dipoles for an optimal approximation of measured potential distributions, in fact means that $4 \times 6 = 24$ parameters are needed to describe a map at each time point. Once determined, the sites of these generators are fixed, and for the remainder of the analysis period, only three parameters (two for orientation, one for strength) need to vary. This reminds us of a sentence ascribed to the German mathematician David Hilbert (1862–1943): "Give me a differential equation system with 4 parameters, and I promise you to build an elephant; give me an additional 5th parameter and he will even be able to move his trunk!" Nevertheless, the multiple spatial-temporal-dipole mode yielded plausible sources for the measured maps. If the parameters are determined with additional information from neuroanatomic imaging, such as MRI, SPECT, or PET scans (see the preceding chapters), approximations with multiple-dipole data result in brain sources that fit our neurophysiologic data much more closely than those obtained with the simpler single-dipole model. In our data we found a mean precision of 93% averaged over the entire latency range analyzed. In single time periods in which only a single dipole is obviously active (e.g., between 220 and 250 msec), the precision reached the 97% level obtained with the single moving-dipole mode.

We found that the fits of maps at around 110 msec could be markedly improved by adding a second dipole (II) in the corresponding ipsilateral cortex, the activity of which was smaller than that for dipole I. The small shift in peak latencies (106 msec versus 112 msec) indicates that both dipoles may be activated in parallel by discrete thalamocortical projection systems rather than by cortico-cortical association tracks. Hari et al. (1990), by means of MEG measurements of SEPs in response to electrical finger stimulation, also found a similar ipsilateral dipole with a peak latency of 110 msec that was shifted by 5 msec against the contralateral generator at 105 msec.

The neurons in the secondary somatosensory cortex (SII; area 7) and in the retroinsular cortex of the primate receive thalamic input from the inferior nucleus of the ventroposterior (VP) complex, but the involvement of this complex in nociception is still in dispute. Burton (1986) described a respone of the majority of neurons in SII to innocuous mechanical stimuli, but of only a few neurons (<3%) in SII to noxious stimuli. Kenshalo and Willis (1991) concluded that these neurons in SII and area 7 are probably not involved in pain perception, but may participate in learning and attention to events that produce pain. In contrast, recent human studies have implicated the involvement of SII in processing experimental pain. These studies include the MEG source localization of painful trigeminal tooth stimulation (Hari et al. 1984) and the increased metabolism found with PET in radiant noxious heat stimulation (Jones et al. 1991). Whether SII is involved in nociception and/or nonpainful somatosensory activation (Allison et al. 1992) and attention requires further clarification.

Dipole III identified in our study was localized in the frontal cortex. Whereas all of the other dipoles showed a very constant behavior over repeated sessions and within different subjects, dipole III exhibited marked interindividual variability. It is difficult to distinguish the frontal activity reflected in dipole III from artifacts due to eye movements or blinks, although all of the EEG segments that showed motor contamination were eliminated from further analysis. But even if no eye movements are detected, voluntary suppression of reaction to the stimulus may induce signals in the EEG that fall within the latency range of dipole III. On the other hand, it is clinically known that the frontal cortex is strongly involved in pain experience (for a review, see Levin et al. 1991). Another aspect of frontal activity is related to mechanisms of attention and arousal, and to other nonspecific reactions in the ascending reticular activation system (Guilbaud et al. 1984).

Interestingly, a single central dipole (IV) could explain the potential distribution of the two most prominent late components considered in pain research. Both the late vertex negativity at 150 msec and the positivity at 220 msec contain components that vary significantly with the painfulness of a stimulus as felt and indicated by the subject (for details see Chapter 3). As a consequence, the potency of analgesic or anesthetic agents is often documented by their ability to attenuate these late components, and these components are considerably modulated in patients with disturbed pain sensitivity (for a review, see Bromm 1989). In our study the site of dipole IV was constant, and localized under the vertex at a cortical depth of 33 mm, perhaps in the cingulate gyrus (Talairach and Tournoux 1988). This locus is part of the limbic cortex and is probably involved in the affective processing of painful information, as suggested in several human and animal studies (e.g., Sweet 1982; see also Chapters 1, 2, 11). In our study, activity of dipole IV began 90 msec after stimulation, achieved a first maximum at 150 msec, and then changed in polarity, explaining the P220 potential distribution.

The scalp potential distribution of the large vertex negativity, however, shows a very broad lateral extension, reaching from T3 to T4, whereas the longitudinal distribution was much smaller. This finding was reinforced by global-field power analysis, which indicated the existence of two dipoles with similar activities, localized symmetrically in the left and right hemispheres. The potentials resulting from such parallel dipoles with identical activity are, of course, maximal at the vertex, as described in all electrical mapping studies so far. The existence of two parallel dipoles is also strongly supported by investigations with MEG. The source localization of pain-induced potentials by mapping with the single-moving-dipole approximation has located the dipole eccentrically in areas of SII (Hari et al. 1984; Huttunen et al. 1986; Laudahn and Bromm 1993; see also Chapter 7). In fact, as has been shown by Scherg et al. (1989), bilaterally eccentric sources can produce fairly symmetrical topographic evoked-potential maps. The same was found in multicenter study testing BESA with simulated data (Miltner et al. 1994). Nevertheless, with BESA applied to the potential distributions described in this chapter, a single deep generator was sufficient to describe all of the components of pain-related potentials with high accuracy. Future anatomic and functional brain-imaging studies, such as with MRI, PET, or MEG, are needed to characterize this dipole in greater detail.

ACKNOWLEDGMENTS

We wish to thank Heiko Kazarians and Kriemhild Saha for collecting the experimental data evaluated here. This research was supported by a German grant (DFG-Br 310/20-1).

REFERENCES

AAAS Science innovation: Biomedicine in the age of imaging. Science 1993;261:554–561.
Allison T, McCarthy G, Wood CC. The relationship between human long-latency somatosensory evoked

potentials recorded from the cortical surface and from the scalp. *Electroencephalogr Clin Neurophysiol* 1992;84:301–314.

Baule GM, McFee R. Theory of magnetic detection of the heart's electrical activity. *J Appl Phys* 1965;36:2066–2073.

Bromm B. Laboratory animal and human volunteers in the assessment of analgesic efficacy. In: Chapman RC, Loeser H, eds. *Issues in pain measurement. Advances in pain research and therapy,* vol. 8. New York: Raven Press, 1989;117–143.

Bromm B, Chen ACN. Brain electrical source analysis of laser-evoked potentials in response to painful trigeminal nerve stimulation. *Electroencephalogr Clin Neurophysiol* 1995;95:in press.

Burton H. Second somatosensory cortex and related areas. In: Jones EG, Peters A, eds. *Cerebral cortex,* vol. 5, New York: Plenum Press, 1986;31–98.

Chen ACN. Human brain measures of clinical pain: a review. I. Topographic mappings. *Pain* 1993a; 54:115–132.

Chen ACN. Human brain measures of clinical pain: a review. II. Tomographic imagings. *Pain* 1993b; 54:133–144.

Cohen D. Magnetoencephalography: evidence of magnetic fields produced by alpha rhythm currents. *Science* 1968;161:784–786.

Coppola R, Buchsbaum MS, Rigal F. Computer generation of surface distribution maps of measures of brain activity. *Comput Biol Med* 1982;12:191–199.

Cuffin BN, Cohen D. Dipole calculation from biomagnetic fields. *IEEE Trans Biomed Eng* 1977; 24:372–379.

Cuffin BN, Cohen D, Yunokuchi K, Maniewski R, Purcell C, Cosgrove GR, Ives J, Kennedy J, Schomer D. Tests of EEG localization accuracy using implanted sources in the human brain. *Ann Neurol* 1991;29:132–138.

Duffy RH. *Topographic mapping of brain electrical activity.* Boston: Butterworths, 1986.

Franssen H, Stegeman, DF, Moleman J, Schoobaar RP. Dipole modelling of median nerve SEPs in normal subjects and patients with small subcortical infarcts. *Electroencephalogr Clin Neurophysiol* 1992;84:40–417.

Fuchs M, Wischmann HA, Wagner M, Krüger J. Coordinate system matching for neuromagnetic and morphological reconstruction overlay. *IEEE Trans Biomed Eng* 1995;in press.

Gevins A, Brickett P, Costales B, Le J, Reutter B. Beyond topographic mapping: towards functional-anatomical imaging with 124-channel EEGs and 3D- MRIs. *Brain Topogr* 1990;3:53–64.

Guilbaud G, Peschanski M, Bession JM. Experimental data related to nociception and pain at the supra-spinal level. In: Wall PD, Melzack R, eds. *Textbook of pain.* Edinburgh: Churchill Livingstone, 1984;110–118.

Hari R, Hämäläinen M, Ilmoniemi R, Kaukoranta E, Reinikainen K. Magnetoencephalographic localisation of cortical activity evoked by somatosensory and noxious stimulation. In: Bromm, B, ed. *Pain measurement in man. Neurophysiological correlates of pain.* Amsterdam: Elsevier, 1984;317–326.

Hari R, Hämäläinen H, Hämäläinen M, Kekoni J, Sams M, Thonen J. Separate finger representations at the human second somatosensory cortex. *Neuroscience* 1990;37:245–249.

Helmholtz H. Über einige Gesetze der Verteilung elektrischer Stroeme in koerperlichen Leitern, mit Anwendung auf die thierisch-elektrischen Versuche. *Ann Phys Chem* 1853;89:211–233.

Henderson CJ, Butler SR, Glass A. The localization of equivalent dipoles of EEG sources by the application of electrical field theory. *Electroencephalogr Clin Neurophysiol* 1975;39:117–130.

Huttunen J, Kobal G, Kaukoranta E, Hari R. Cortical responses to painful CO_2 stimulation of nasal mucosa: a neuromagnetoencephalographic study in man. *Electroencephalogr Clin Neurophysiol* 1986;64:347–349.

Jones AK, Brown WD, Friston KJ, Qi LY, Frackowiak BS. Cortical and subcortical localization of response to pain in man using positron emission tomography. *Proc R Soc Lond [B]* 1991;244: 39–44.

Joseph J, Howland EW, Wakai R, Backonja M, Baffa O, Poteni RM, Cleeland CS. Late pain related magnetic fields and electric potentials evoked by intracutaneous electric finger stimulation. *Electroencephalogr Clin Neurophysiol* 1991;80:46–52.

Kazarians H, Scharein E, Bromm B. Repeated measurements of laser-evoked potentials in human pain *Intern J Neurosci* 1995;81:111–122.

Kenshalo DR, Willis WD. The role of cerebral cortex in pain perception. In: Peters, A, and Jones, E.G. (eds.) *The cerebral cortex,* vol. 9. New York: Plenum Press, 1991;153–212.

Laudahn R, Bromm B. Topography of pain related magnetic field evoked by short pulses of infrared laser-radiation. *Advances in biomagnetism.* 9th International Conference on Biomagnetism, Vienna, 1993;19:32.

Lehmann D. From mapping to analysis and interpretation. In: Maurer K, ed. *Topographic brain mapping of EEG and evoked potentials.* Heidelberg: Springer, 1989;53–75.

Levin HS, Eisenberg HM, Benton AL. *Frontal lobe function and dysfunction.* New York: Oxford University Press, 1991.

Miltner W, Braun C, Johnson R, Simpson GV, Ruchkin DS. A test of brain electrical source analysis (BESA): a simulation study. *Electroenceph Clin Neurophysiol* 1994;91:295–310.

Mosher JC, Spencer ME, Leahy RM, Lewis PS. Error bounds for EEG and MEG dipole source localization. *Electroencephalogr Clin Neurophysiol* 1993;86:303–321.

Pfurtscheller G, Lopes da Silva FH, eds. *Functional brain imaging.* Stuttgart: Hans Huber, 1988.

Plendl H, Paulus W, Roberts IG, Botzel K, Towell A, Pitman JR, Scherg M, Halliday AM. The time course and location of cerebral evoked activity associated with the processing of colour stimuli in man. *Neurosci. Lett.* 1993;150:9–12.

Ponton CW, Don M, Waring MD, Eggermont JJ, Masuda A. Spatio-temporal source modeling of evoked potentials to acoustic and cochlear implant stimulation. *Electroencephalogr Clin Neurophysiol* 1993;88:478–493.

Sato S, Balish M, Muratore R. Principles of magnetoencephalography. *J Clin Neurophysiol* 1991;8:144–156.

Scherg M. Spatio-temporal modelling of early auditory evoked potentials. *Rev Laryngol* 1984;105:163–170.

Scherg M. Fundamentals of dipole source potential analysis. *Adv Audiol* 1990;6:40–69.

Scherg M. Functional imaging and localization of electromagnetic brain activity, *Brain Topogr* 1993;5:103–111.

Scherg M, Picton TW. Separation and identification of event-related potential components by brain electrical source analysis. In: Brunia CHM, Mulder G, Verbaten MN, eds. *Event-related potentials of the brain. Electroencephalogr Clin Neurophysiol* 1991;(Suppl 42):24–37.

Scherg M, Berg P. Brain Electrical Source Analysis, version 1.9. Munich: Medizinelektronik Press, 1992.

Scherg M, Vajar J, Picton TW: A source analysis of the human auditory evoked potentials. *J Cognitive Neurosci* 1989;1:336–354.

Simpson GV, Scherg M, Ritter W, Vaughan HG. Localization and temporal activity functions of brain sources generating the human visual ERP. In: Brunia CHN, Gaillard AWK, Kok A, eds. *Psychophysical brain research.* Tilburg University Press, 1990;99–105.

Stroink G. Cardiomagnetism: a historical perspective. In: Hoke M, Erné SN, Okada YC, Romani GL, eds. *Biomagnetism: clinical aspects.* Amsterdam: Elsevier, 1992;399–403.

Sutherling WW, Grandall PH, Engel J, Darcey TM, Cahan LD, Barth DS. The magnetic and electric fields agree with intracranial localization of somatosensory cortex. *Neurology* 1988;38:1705–1714.

Sweet WH. Cerebral localization of pain. In: Thompson RA, Green JR, eds. *New perspectives in cerebral localization.* New York: Raven Press, 1982;205–242.

Talairach J, Tournoux P. Co-*planar stereotaxic atlas of the human brain.* New York, Stuttgart, 1988.

Talbot JD, Marrett S, Evans EC, Meyer E, Bushnell MC, Duncan GH. Multiple representation of pain in human cerebral cortex. *Science* 1991;251:1355–1358.

Towle VL, Bolanos J, Suarez D, Tan K, Grzeszczuk R, Lein DM, Cakmur R, Frank SA, Spire JP. The spatial location of EEG electrodes: locating the best-fitting sphere relative to cortical anatomy. *Electroencephalogr Clin Neurophysiol* 1993;86:1–6.

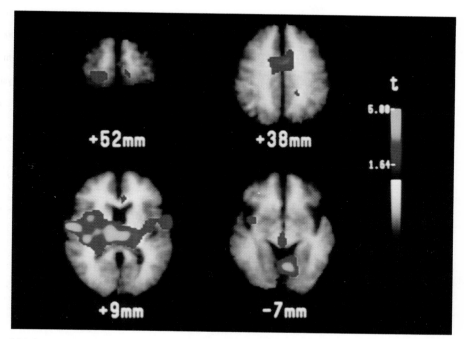

COLORPLATE 1, FIG. 13.1. Color-coded images of the sites of focal increases in rCBF associated with the perception of repetitive noxious, compared with innocuous, heat stimulation of the left forearm. The right hemisphere of the magnetic resonance brain image template is to the left of the figure. Below each image is its location with respect to a plane connecting the anterior and posterior commissures (+: superior, −: inferior). The numbers by the color bar show the *t* values corresponding to the statistical deviation of each region from the mean global rCBF increase. The colored regions in this figure include all structures showing rCBF increases above the mean at a p=0.05 level of significance, uncorrected for multiple comparisons. Those structures meeting the statistical criteria described in the text are shown in the different image planes. Upper left: Contralateral S1 cortex (captured only in a partial field of view). Upper right: Anterior cingulate gyrus. Lower left: Contralateral and ipsilateral S2 cortex and insula, and contralateral and ipsilateral thalamus (possibly including a contribution from medial and intralaminar nuclei). Lower right: dorsomedial midbrain and cerebellar vermis.

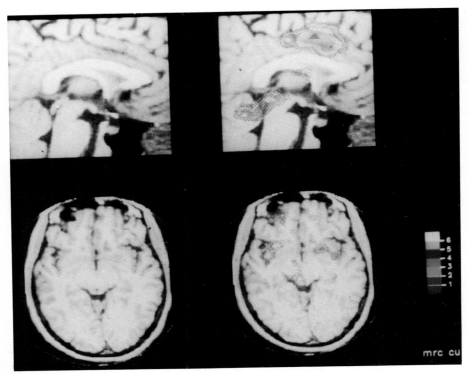

COLORPLATE 2, FIG. 14.1. Pain activation data acquired in three-dimensional mode from a single subject for whom the MR images and SPM{*t*} have been coregistered and superimposed. A transverse slice at the level of the PAG is depicted with the corresponding sagittal section above. The SPM{*t*} images are shown as coregistrations on the right and share a common color scale for their pixels' Z values, indicated on the right. The PAG, thalamus, frontal, and anterior cingulate cortex (area 24) are clearly activated.

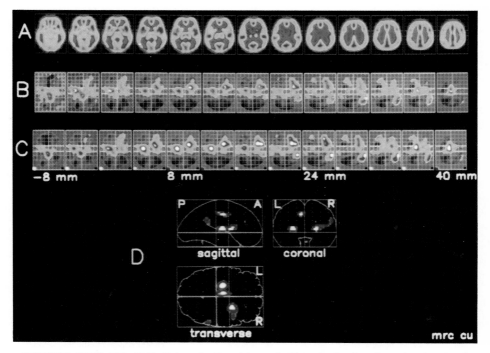

COLORPLATE 3, FIG. 14.2. Pain activation data pooled from twelve female and male normal volunteers. **A:** Averaged blood flow scans from the 12 subjects. Anatomic landmarks are clearly identified, owing to the differences between grey and white matter. **B:** The arithmetic differences between adjusted mean blood flow for painfully hot and nonpainfully hot phasic stimuli in the 12 subjects. **C:** The SPM{*t*} values derived from pixel-by-pixel comparison of the adjusted mean blood flows and variances for each condition. The color scale is arbitrary; threshold significance is indicated by the lower left pixel for each plane. **D:** The orthogonal projections of the statistical comparison at *p*<0.001 (z threshold 3.09). The areas showing significant response to the "suffering" components of pain are periaqueductal grey, thalamus/insula, thalamus/putamen, frontal (area 10) and anterior cingulate (area 24), and inferior parietal cortex (areas 39 and 40).

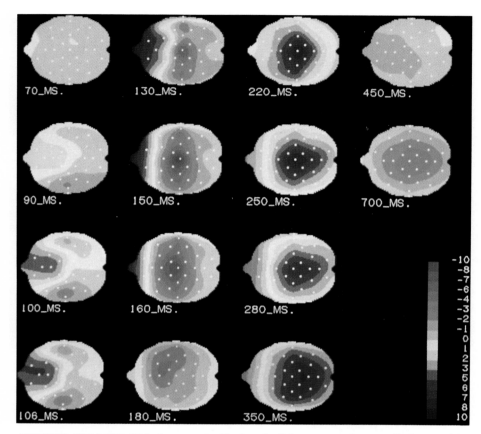

COLORPLATE 4, FIG. 16.2. Laser-evoked brain potential maps, grand means. Brain potentials in response to brief laser heat pulses applied to the right temple are recorded simultaneously at 29 scalp sites and averaged over blocks of 40 stimuli (laser-evoked potentials, LEPs). Grand mean LEPs are the averages over the four stimulus blocks per session, three repeated sessions, and 10 subjects in the study (altogether, 120 LEPs). Scalp positivity (red) emerges 90 msec after stimulation over the midline frontal cortex, disappearing at 150 msec. At 220 msec a large vertex positivity arises with a central distribution. Negativity (*blue*) appears around 90 and 130 msec over the contralateral and ipsilateral somatosensory cortex, and later at 130 to 180 msec under the vertex, with a bilateral symmetrical distribution. The late negativity starting at 450 msec may indicate the contingent negative variation.

Pain and the Brain: From
Nociception to Cognition,
edited by Burkhart Bromm and
John E. Desmedt, Advances in Pain
Research and Therapy Vol. 22.
Raven Press, Ltd., New York © 1995.

17

Magnetoencephalography in the Investigation of Cortical Pain Processing

Robert Laudahn, Holger Kohlhoff, and Burkhart Bromm

Institute of Physiology, University Hospital Eppendorf, D-20246 Hamburg, Germany

SUMMARY

Magnetoencephalography (MEG) is a new, noninvasive tool in functional research and diagnostic medicine involving the human brain. The basic idea of the technique is to identify neuronal currents by measuring their induced magnetic fields outside the skull, and to thereby localize areas of neuronal activity in their temporal development. In this context it seems to be sufficient for modeling the human head as a homogenously conducting sphere with equivalent current dipoles used for source description. By this means new possibilities of analyzing evoked responses of the brain are added to the more or less descriptive methods so far used for doing this. The challenge in MEG is to build spatiotemporal models of cerebral signal processing that explain the measured data. In the study described here we investigated late components of cerebral responses to short, painful heat pulses elicited by infrared laser radiation in seven healthy male subjects. With one equivalent current dipole used as a source descriptor, the main deflection of the magnetic signal at a group mean latency of 134 msec was localized in an area compatible with the secondary somatosensory cortex (SII). This result is in good agreement with those of other studies using painful electrical tooth-pulp stimulation, painful stimulation of the nasal mucosa by CO_2 application, and painful electrical intracutaneous stimuli.

In 1968, the American neurologist David Cohen was the first to succeed in measuring the magnetic fields arising from the human cortical alpha rhythm (Cohen 1968). Although his experiments were purely methodologic because of the poor signal-to-noise ratio (SNR) of the earliest MEG equipment, they showed the general possibility of such measurements. In view of the fact that even with some thousand simultaneously active neurons, the arising magnetic field measured over the scalp is only of about 10^{-13} Tesla (Williamson and Kaufmann 1981), which is seven to nine orders of magnitude smaller than the geomagnetic field of the Earth, the challenge of detection at the frontier of technical possibilities is obvious. With the invention of superconducting quantum interference device (SQUID) sensor technology in the 1970s, MEG has undergone rapid development. Today a number of laboratories are equipped and experienced in doing high-precision measurements of such weak magnetic fields as those induced by the electrical currents of a working brain.

For the proper detection of biomagnetic signals, it is necessary that electrical discharges appear simultaneously in a sufficiently large area of excitable tissue. If they do not, the SNR will not allow reasonable measurements (Hämäläinen et al. 1993). In the case of the myocard, where most of the tissue is active at the same time, this situation does exist and a magnetocardiogram (MCG) can be detected (Stroink 1992; Maekijaervi et al. 1993; Weismüller et al. 1993). For the cortex, simultaneous activation of a sufficiently large number of neurons is found during normal alpha rhythm and in pathologic epileptic activity. Several groups are focusing on the latter situation (Barth et al. 1984; Rose et al. 1987; Vieth 1987; Sutherling et al. 1988; Stefan et al. 1990). The idea is to localize epileptic foci by functional mapping, whereas even sophisticated imaging techniques like magnetic resonance imaging (MRI) are sensitive only to morphologic changes and fail in cases of pure functional abnormalities. Because localization of the abnormal activity is necessary for the patient to derive any benefit from the possibilities of neurosurgery, invasive methods like electrocorticography (ECoG) have so far been used for this purpose (Sutherling et al. 1988). However, with respect to the aim of avoiding invasive methods in disease diagnostics, the advantages of MEG become obvious.

The investigation of evoked cortical responses to external stimuli is another important application of MEG. In this case, the SNR is improved by averaging several tens to hundreds of poststimulus MEG segments. The functional analysis of the tonotopy of the human auditory cortex by Romani et al. (1982) and Pantev et al. (1988) is a well-known example of this. They used sine-wave tones of different frequencies as stimuli. Romani analyzed the steady-state responses, whereas Pantev investigated the 100 msec component of the responses to tone-bursts of 500-msec duration. The corresponding source localization for the evoked magnetic fields showed the presumed tonotopic organization: for lower frequencies the equivalent current dipoles were found more superficially than for higher frequencies.

Investigations of the somatosensory system were first done with the standard stimulus of neurologic diagnostics, electrical stimulation of the median nerve at the wrist. As expected, the equivalent current dipoles were located in the representation area of the hand in the primary somatosensory cortex (SI) (Wood et al. 1985; Laudahn et al. 1992). The high-resolution capabilities of this functional measurement technique were lately shown by Suk et al. (1991), who were able to separate statistically significant locations of equivalent current dipoles calculated from responses evoked by electrical stimulation of the thumb, the middle finger, and the little finger.

In pain research, the late components of cortical evoked responses to experimental phasic pain stimuli are a topic of current investigation. These bilaterally symmetrical components appear with a maximum at the vertex. They consist of a large negativity at latencies around 150 msec and a positive component, P220, depending on the body site that is stimulated and the conduction velocity of the fiber spectrum activated (see, e.g., Chapters 3 and 16). The long-latency components are supposed to reflect the cognitive processing of pain signals. The most reliable magnetic-field component corresponds to the first large negativity, N150, in the EEG. In an interindividual comparison this component can be easily identified. Hari and coworkers used electrical tooth-pulp stimulation (Hari et al. 1983), a well-established model for eliciting phasic pain (Chatrian et al. 1975). The equivalent current dipoles calculated for the main deflection at about 100 msec poststimulus were localized in SII. The same group in Helsinki investigated evoked responses to noxious CO_2 stimulation of the nasal mucosa (Kobal et al. 1985), activating nerve fibers of the middle branch of the trigeminal nerve. Locations of the equivalent current dipoles derived from the response at 350 msec turned out to be very close to those of painful tooth-pulp stimulation (Huttunen et al. 1986). Comparable dipole locations were reported by Joseph et al. (1991) using intracutaneous electrical stimuli on the fingertip (Bromm and Meier 1984).

In the study presented here, short heat pulses were used to elicit phasic pain. The latest development in the field of painful somatosensory stimuli is a portable laser unit producing short pulses of infrared radiation (see Chapter 16). The application site of this stimulus can be anywhere on the skin. The flexibility of this system, which transmits the laser beam through a glass fiberoptic element, enabled us to use it in MEG measurements.

METHODOLOGIC ASPECTS

The electrical nature of brain activity is based on the transmembrane ion currents of nerve fibers resulting from local concentration gradients created by synaptic activation. The propagation of these currents along the dendrites and axon of the nerve is described by the flow of electrical charges. As is well known, moving charges produce a magnetic field whose orientation is given by the right-hand-rule (letting the thumb of the right hand point in the direction of flow for positive charges permits the fingers to show the orientation of the magnetic field from north to south pole, denoted " + " and " − "). To obtain a measurable field it is necessary to have some thousand parallel fibers being activated simultaneously. A sensor appropriate for making biomagnetic measurements must have a high sensitivity together with a maximum rejection of environmental noise (cf. Romani and Narici 1986).

In the past quarter of this century, the development of supraconducting quantum interference device (SQUID) technology provided the possibility of precise measurements of weak magnetic fields. As a key point, this technique uses the loss by many substances of their electrical resistance at very low temperatures (e.g., niobium at −269°C, the temperature of liquid helium). Under these conditions, following Ohm's law, even very small potential differences produce high currents. Together with the quantum-mechanical tunnel effect, as applied in Josephson junctions, this fact is used to facilitate the measurement of magnetic fields arising from brain activity (for details see Williamson and Kaufmann 1981). To effect noise reduction, the sensoring coils are usually built as spatial first-order gradiometers consisting of two matched pickup loops wound in opposition to each other and connected in series. A uniform magnetic field would therefore induce currents of the same size traveling in opposite direction, leading to cancellation, whereas gradient fields (as produced by dipoles) yield net fluxes that result in measurable currents that can be amplified (Clarke and Koch 1988). Magnetically shielded chambers are commonly used to improve the SNR ratio. Additionally, higher-order gradiometers could be used to filter background noise, but at the cost of decreasing sensitivity and worsening localization properties (Hari 1990).

Today most biomagnetometers used to measure brain magnetic fields are multichannel systems consisting of 30 or more sensors covering a head area of at least 16×16 cm^2. The measurements result in a two-dimensional map of the recorded field over the scalp, as shown in Fig. 1. To evaluate these isocontour plots one has to make assumptions about the underlying physiologic system, or, in effect, to build a model. With regard to this, two main aspects need to be specified: the *source description* and the *volume conductor* in which the sources are located (for details see, e.g., van Oosterom 1991).

The cortical neuron populations activated by external stimuli (e.g., short heat or electrical pulses) are commonly identified as the large pyramidal cells, acting simultaneously in the form of the so-called cortical columns (Mountcastle and Powell 1959). These compounds of cells are understood to be the generating sources for the

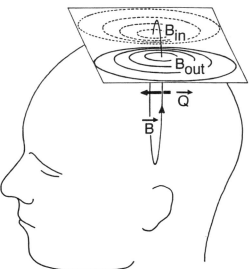

FIG. 1. Schematic drawing of a single current dipole generating a magnetic field. Q denotes the dipole moment and B the produced magnetic field. B_{in} (dashed lines, "$-$") and B_{out} (solid lines, "$+$") indicate magnetic flux into and out of the skull, respectively. In the ideal case, the current dipole is located exactly under the midline between the extremes of B_{in} and B_{out}.

magnetic field of the brain (Okada 1983), and are described as *current dipoles* (Hari and Kaukoranta 1985; Hämäläinen et al. 1993). Because of the physical nature of the situation, dipole components tangential to the volume surface contribute most greatly to the extracranial magnetic field (Melcher and Cohen 1988; Sato et al. 1991). In other words, generators in the fissures and sulci are the main sources of the magnetic field whose component normal to the surface is detected.

As a volume surrounding the brain, the head is usually simplified as a homogeneous sphere (Lütkenhöner et al. 1990) with its geometry justified for nearly every location of dipoles, although in the case of frontal or frontotemporal sources a more realistic, brain-shaped model should be applied (Hämäläinen and Sarvas 1989; Roth et al. 1993). In contrast to the evaluation of EEG data, source localization from MEG measures is largely independent of the electrical properties and homogeneity of the source environment (Kaufmann et al. 1991). As long as cortical sources are considered, even differences in the boundary conductivity differences of brain tissue do not affect the emitted magnetic field (Huang et al. 1990), allowing the use of simpler head models than are necessary in comparable EEG calculations (Kaufmann et al. 1991).

Once the physiologic sources (dipoles) of potentials and the surrounding medium have been specified, the distribution of the extracranial magnetic field can be calculated with Maxwell's equations, with the results largely following the law of Biot-Savart (Grynszpan and Geselowitz 1973). Contrary to this so-called *forward problem* is the opposite and practical question: What are the generators of the measured magnetic field? This includes the locations as well as the orientations and strengths of the responsible dipoles. It is known that, except for special, highly symmetric cases, this so-called *inverse problem* has no unique solution, as Helmholtz (1853) pointed out (for more details see Sarvas 1987). Different approaches to finding, the best solution (in the sense of a minimum norm criterion with respect to the recorded field pattern) are on the market, all of which solve the forward problem in an iterative algorithm to fix the dipole parameters. Depending on the parameters chosen to vary in time, one distinguishes between fixed and moving-dipole solutions, with the dipole locations being permanent or variable over the time period concerned (see, e.g., Fuchs et al. 1993). Ultimately, source-localization procedures result in a distribution of one or more equivalent current dipoles representing areas of activity that are investigated in terms of their time course (for a review see Hämäläinen et al. 1993).

DEWAR COORDINATES AND INDIVIDUAL HEAD COORDINATES

In our study, evoked magnetic fields were recorded with the Philips Biomagnetometer shown in Fig. 2, featuring 31 first-order gradiometers of 70 mm baseline (Dössel et al. 1991). In order to cool the SQUID sensors to their working temperature of $-269°C$, they are installed in a so-called *dewar*, which is a highly isolating cylinder filled with liquid helium. With this equipment, we measured and displayed inhomogeneous magnetic fields in the *dewar coordinate system*, which is defined by the spatial arrangement of the gradiometer coils. The subjects were lying on a bench with their heads on a vacuum cast. To keep the spatial relationship of head and dewar fixed during registration, the subjects were not allowed to move.

Dipole parameters resulting from source analyses subsequent to the measurements are calculated in the dewar-dependent coordinate system. To allow for comparisons between measurements with different dewar positions relative to the subject's head, one needs to define *individual head coordinates*. In our case, these are given in the PAN system determined by the *pre*auricular points and the *na*sion. Therewith the *x*-axis is defined as the connecting line between the left and right preauricular points emerging at the right, with the origin being calculated in such a way that the orthogonal *y*-axis emerges at the nasion and the *z*-axis is oriented perpendicular to both the *x*- and the *y*-axis, pointing upward and penetrating the scalp approximately 1 cm rostral from Cz (see Fig. 3).

To facilitate the transformation of the dipole parameters into the individual PAN system, the position of the subject's head relative to the dewar must be determined. We therefore made a position measurement with four markers, each consisting of

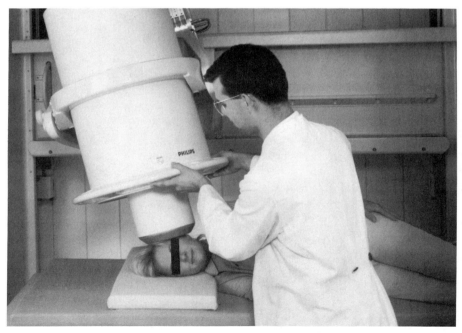

FIG. 2. Philips MEG system with subject. The large vessel contains the 31 gradiometers surrounded by liquid helium. To bring the dewar into the right position for the measurement, it can be moved up and down as well as turned around the second and third axis. The subject is lying on a bench with the head on a vacuum cast.

three orthogonally arranged coils wound around a plastic cube of 5 mm side length, which were fixed at the left and the right preauricular points, the nasion, and Cz. These markers broadcast an electromagnetic field of 25 Hz which is detected by the magnetometer. Because they behave like dipoles, the markers can be localized by referring to the dewar-dependent coordinate system (Fuchs et al. 1992). With their parameters, the individual PAN system is determined in the manner described, and the transformation matrix can be calculated. Obviously any head-dependent coordinate system based on measurements of individually located markers inherits their localization errors. In our case, by dint of its construction, the origin of the PAN-system varies with the localization accuracy of the markers. Therefore coordinate transformation gives rise to uncertainties in the dipole parameters that are typically a few millimeters in dimension (see, e.g., Fuchs et al. 1994). Because the PAN system accounts only coarsely for individual head shape and size, interindividual comparisons are expected to yield greater site deviations when compared to the intraindividual case (see, e.g., Chapter 16 by Bromm and Chen).

For an estimate of the locational reliability of the system we calculated the spatial distances of the markers, which served as a measure of the obtained precision that was independent of the coordinate system. Table 1 shows the means and standard deviations (SDs) of four repeated measurements with changing dewar position but

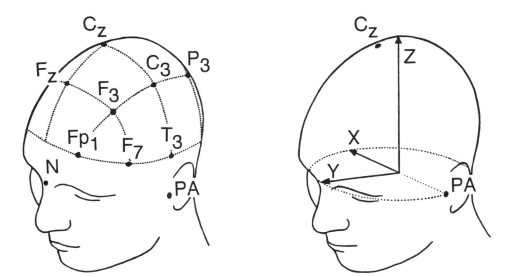

FIG. 3. Relationship between the electrode positions of the international 10/20-system and the head-dependent PAN coordinate system. On the left, the midline EEG electrode positions Fz and Cz are seen together with the left lateral Fp1 to P3, frontotemporal F7, and temporal T3. The left preauricular point and the nasion are denoted PA and N, respectively. On the right, the orthogonal PAN coordinate system is depicted with the x-axis emerging at the right preauricular point, the y-axis pointing to the nasion, and the z-axis orthogonal to both of them. Note that electrode position Cz is not used in the definition of the PAN coordinate system.

TABLE 1. *Calculated distances (mm) between position markers (nasion, preauricular points right [par] and left [pal]. Means and standard deviations (SDs) of four repeated measurements (different dewar positions, fixed markers) are shown for each subject and experimental day. Last row shows average standard deviation of position determination.*

Subject	Day	Nasion-par	Nasion-pal	Par-pal
CN	1	124.2 ± 4.4	129.9 ± 1.3	155.7 ± 2.6
	2	128.2 ± 2.2	129.5 ± 1.3	158.0 ± 0.9
HA	1	131.9 ± 3.5	129.8 ± 3.4	163.7 ± 2.4
	2	135.8 ± 0.7	126.4 ± 3.3	164.5 ± 2.3
JT	1	135.4 ± 0.8	134.1 ± 1.9	164.2 ± 1.5
	2	133.9 ± 3.8	134.4 ± 1.7	160.2 ± 1.6
MB	1	132.4 ± 0.9	123.2 ± 1.2	156.1 ± 2.0
	2	130.5 ± 1.0	127.6 ± 4.0	153.9 ± 3.2
MI	1	136.4 ± 2.3	137.1 ± 1.4	169.5 ± 3.0
	2	135.0 ± 1.9	137.9 ± 0.7	169.3 ± 1.3
RO	1	132.1 ± 2.3	131.9 ± 0.3	159.7 ± 0.9
	2	134.4 ± 1.5	133.4 ± 0.9	161.7 ± 1.4
UD	1	134.9 ± 2.3	132.6 ± 2.4	157.0 ± 1.5
	2	129.6 ± 1.0	126.7 ± 1.4	150.1 ± 1.0
Average SD		±2.0	±1.8	±1.8

fixed markers for each subject and experimental day. If the average SD of less than 2 mm is attributed to each of the markers, the resulting precision is of the same order as reported for the accuracy of stylus placement for a three-dimensional-digitizer (Towle et al. 1993); this is in perfect agreement with the values found by Fuchs et al. (1992) for the Philips Biomagnetometer. Taking the means as best estimates for the real distances, their intraindividual comparison for the first and second day mainly reflects errors in finding the individual landmarks for the coil-sets. The average difference of less than 3 mm is in good accordance with the between-session error of 2.5 mm reported by Towle et al. (1993) for repeated 10/20-electrode placement measurements. Nevertheless, neccessary coordinate transformations and marker placements remain topics under permanent study (see, e.g., Lagerlund et al. 1993; Gallen et al. 1994).

The coordinates of the four markers were further used to adjust the spherical volume conductor to the individual head. Therefore the parameters for the center and the radius were taken from the best-fitting sphere with respect to their positions. The obtained average distance of the markers from the spherical surface was less than 0.1 mm. Taking into account the results for all seven subjects and five repetitions, the center of the average sphere was located 2.2 cm anterior and 4.2 cm superior to the origin of the PAN system (see Table 2). The obtained spheres can be regarded as the corresponding sphere used in BESA calculations (see Chapter 16), with an adjusted radius.

TABLE 2. *Parameters of the best-fitting sphere for each subject and session in evaluation. The center is given in cartesian PAN coordinates. The last row shows means and standard deviations (SDs) over all subjects and sessions.[a]*

Subject	Day/block	Center			Radius
		x	y	z	
CN	1/1	−1.9	20.6	45.8	92.3
	2/4	−3.4	20.8	38.2	89.8
HA	1/1	−2.3	18.3	48.4	95.1
	2/3	5.2	20.6	43.1	94.0
JT	2/1	0.9	25.4	39.6	94.1
MB	1/1	6.0	22.5	46.2	92.1
MI	1/3	−0.7	20.0	40.1	95.1
	2/3	−3.7	19.6	35.8	93.9
RO	1/3	2.0	22.3	38.5	91.9
	2/2	3.5	23.6	34.4	91.0
UD	1/1	1.5	23.5	47.8	94.1
	2/2	2.2	26.9	44.7	91.1
Mean		0.8	22.0	41.9	92.9
SD		3.1	2.4	4.5	1.7

[a]All values in millimeters.

PAIN RELATED MAGNETIC FIELDS

Measurements were done on seven healthy male volunteers (medical students 20 to 30 years of age), each participating in two MEG sessions one week apart. In a prior EEG session the subjects were introduced to the stimulus and the experimental conditions. The subjects were selected on the basis of their ability to avoid eye movements and blink artifacts. Experimental phasic pain was induced by short infrared laser pulses of 2-msec duration. The laser pulses were transmitted through a 5 m glass fiberoptic element into the magnetically shielded room and applied to the right forehead of the subjects. Because of the long wavelength used (2μm), the applied heat pulses were completely absorbed in the most superficial skin layer (≤200 μm depth), thus activating only the Aδ- and C-afferents that terminate in this layer (Bromm and Treede 1991), producing a sharp, hot, pinprick-like pain. These stimuli were not associated with any acoustic or visual sensation. At the beginning of each experimental day the individual pain threshold was determined. The following stimulation set consisted of 40 stimuli of two different intensities around the 1.5-fold individual pain threshold, delivered in random order and with random interstimulus intervals (8 to 13 sec). With a beam diameter of 5 mm and a stimulus duration of 2 msec, the mean pain threshold strength was 316 ± 61 mJ. To avoid the possibility of tissue damage the application site was slightly changed after each stimulus. For this purpose the skin site was visualized with a constant helium laser beam parallel to the infrared beam. In each session four stimulation sets (15 min apart) were administered. The amplification unit was set to a bandpass of 0.16 to 70 Hz and the sampling rate of the A/D converter was 500 Hz. After artifact rejection,

36 to 39 stimulus responses were available for averaging. The averaged magnetic field served as the input for the source-localization procedure, which was based on a single equivalent current dipole model. To allow for inter- and intraindividual comparison, the calculated dipole coordinates were transformed into the head-dependent PAN system.

In Fig. 4 the time course of the magnetic field averaged over one stimulus block in one subject is shown for the four channels with maximum amplitudes. In agreement with EEG data (see, for example, the preceding chapter), a typical biphasic waveform appears with peak latencies of 136 msec and 192 msec, as indicated by the dashed lines. Furthermore, a phase reversal between the upper and lower two channels is found for both components. The group mean latency of the earlier component was 134 ± 7 msec, whereas the second component of 195 ± 5 msec was not identified in all cases. On the left-hand side of Fig. 4 is shown a schematic drawing of the head with the channel positions used for the measurement. For better orientation, electrode positions of the 10/20 system and marker positions are indicated.

Earlier EEG registrations, which reveal a very stable component of evoked potentials at 145 msec (group mean latency), show that this component is easy to identify in interindividual comparisons (Bromm and Chen 1995; see also Chapter 16).

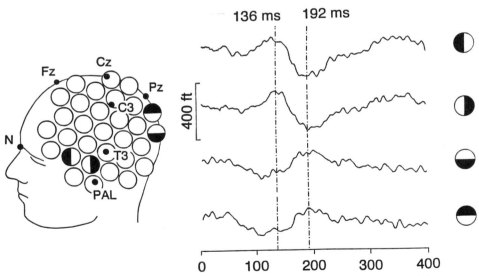

FIG. 4. Laser-evoked magnetic fields (LEFs) at selected sites, single case. On the left, an example of the spatial relationship between the head, electrode positions of the 10/20-system, and the 31 MEG channels is shown for a single case. The signals of the four MEG channels, depicted as half-filled circles, are given on the right, showing LEFs. For simplicity the four channels showing the best phase reversal for both main deflections are selected from among the 31 recording sites. The dashed lines indicate the latencies of 136 msec and 192 msec for which the best single dipole fits have been obtained.

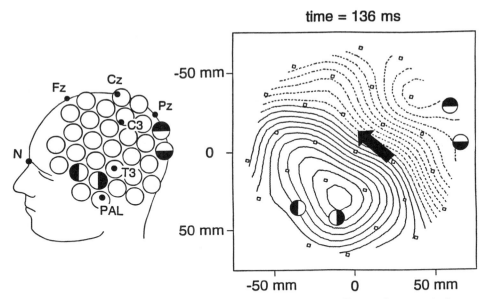

FIG. 5. Isocontour map for the m130-msec component, single case. The small squares indicate the 31 MEG channels, with the half-filled symbols corresponding to the channels shown in Fig. 4. As in Fig. 1, solid lines indicate magnetic flux out of the skull and dashed lines flux into the skull, respectively. The generating single current dipole is shown as arrow, with its center being the projection of the dipole location into the displayed plane of the registration coils in the dewar-dependent coordinate system.

Therefore, the corresponding MEG component was subjected to source analysis. From the four available averages per day, the one allowing the best dipole identification in the time range from 124 to 146 msec was chosen. In Fig. 5 the resulting dipole for the example given above (for 136-msec latency) is shown together with the measured magnetic field. As is clearly seen, the dipole is located directly below the midline, between the two field extrema, with its orientation being given by the right-hand-rule.

IDENTIFICATION OF THE m130 GENERATOR

For five of the seven subjects the field patterns registered on both experimental days allowed us to calculate a dipole for the m130 component with a goodness-of-fit of better than 78%. In two cases a reasonable dipole fit could be obtained only for the data of one session (see Table 3). For retest accuracy the spatial distances of the dipoles were evaluated. The mean and SD of the five intraindividually calculated distances between the dipoles located for the first and the second session was 11.4 ± 7.9 mm, while the comparable value for the interindividual dipole distances

TABLE 3. *Locations and orientations of calculated equivalent current dipoles for the m130 component of the LEF in seven subjects on two experimental days. Dipole orientations are given in spherical polar coordinates referring to the PAN coordinate system.*

Subject	Day/block	Latency [msec]	Dipole Pan Coordinates [mm]		Orientation [°]			Strength [µAmm]
			x	y	z	φ	θ	m
CA	1/1	140	−44.6	20.8	63.8	88.8	86.5	20.5
	2/4	144	−55.4	−2.8	65.6	103.9	61.9	22.5
HA	1/1	134	−38.7	5.5	58.5	92.2	41.9	173.2
	2/3	136	−40.4	8.6	62.0	71.6	36.6	66.5
JT	2/1	134	−61.8	−1.5	70.2	96.9	64.8	7.5
MB	1/1	128	−18.1	28.5	66.2	114.4	118.6	150.3
MI	1/3	124	−45.3	4.1	39.8	111.7	15.6	56.7
	2/3	136	−43.5	3.1	36.3	108.6	19.1	76.5
RO	1/3	146	−29.9	5.4	66.6	91.9	59.3	52.8
	2/2	136	−42.2	3.9	67.7	91.2	60.4	17.7
UD	1/1	124	−36.4	15.8	45.6	96.0	10.3	43.9
	2/2	128	−39.7	13.2	53.9	77.0	40.9	36.1
Mean		134.2	−41.3	8.7	58.0	95.4	51.3	60.4
SD		6.9	10.6	8.8	11.0	12.4	29.7	49.7

averaged over the same subjects and both sessions was found to be 20.6 ± 3.6 mm. This shows that the generator for the m130 component of the laser-evoked magnetic field (LEF) is intraindividually stable within 1.1 cm, whereas the interindividual variability is significantly larger. In reviewing these numbers one has to keep in mind that the comparison was performed in the generalized PAN system, which does not correct for the interindividual variability in anatomy. Nevertheless, the numbers are in good agreement with the results of the EEG evaluation described by Bromm and Chen in Chapter 16.

As is shown in Fig. 6, the calculated position for the generator of the pain-related magnetic field was in all cases clearly located more frontally than C3', the electrode position closest to the primary somatosensory projection area of the forehead and hand where, accordingly, the earliest somatosensory evoked responses to median-nerve stimulation were found (Wood et al. 1985; Sutherling et al. 1988; Laudahn et al. 1992). Obviously the source of the long-latency evoked responses to painful stimuli is not SI.

The central processing of pain is a complex phenomenon. To partly understand the underlying mechanisms it is necessary to find out whether or not pain perception and processing depend on the stimulus modality. The hypothesis of independence is supported by the fact that severe pain generally leads to similar vegetative reactions, no matter what the reason was for the pain perception. The investigation of evoked responses to painful stimuli may add valuable knowledge supporting this hypothesis. The results of our study indicate that the main deflection of long-latency evoked magnetic fields shows field patterns that can be well described by a single

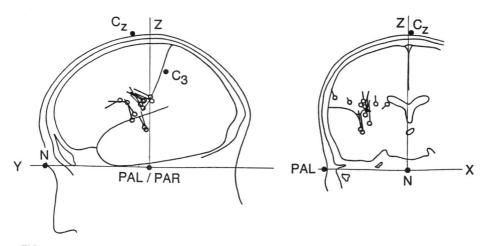

FIG. 6. Locations and orientations of equivalent current dipoles for the m130 component in seven subjects. The dipoles for all seven subjects and five experiment repetitions have been calculated in the latency range of 124 to 146 msec. They are shown in their projection onto the sagittal and coronal views of the PAN coordinate system, which serves as a generalized head model. Most of the dipoles were found along the lateral sulcus, where on the upper bank SII is located (N = nasion; PAL/PAR = preauricular point left/right; Cz, C3'-electrode positions according to the international 10/20 system).

equivalent current dipole located at the rostral end of the sylvian fissure, in SII. This is in agreement with investigations of responses to painful tooth-pulp stimulation (Hari et al. 1983) and to painful stimulation of the nasal mucosa (Huttunen et al. 1986), both of which activate the middle branch of the trigeminal nerve, as well as with the findings for median-nerve activation by intracutaneous stimulation of the fingertip (Joseph et al. 1991). Similarly, PET studies using painful heat stimuli applied to the hand have identified comparable sites of cortical activity involved in experimental pain processing (Talbot et al. 1991). In contrast, nonpainful electrical stimulation of median- and ulnar-nerve fibers leads to magnetic-field patterns of short- and long-latency responses, which give evidence for an equivalent current dipole located only in SI (Huttunen et al. 1986).

On the other hand, these results should be examined as a first step in modeling the somatosensory response. The independence of SII activation from stimulus site and modality does not necessarily mean that it is the painfulness of the stimulus that is reflected in SII. A painful stimulus should lead to an increasing state of arousal, and in an undefined inattentive condition a painful stimulus will be less ignored than a nonpainful one. Effects of changes in attention have already been shown to alter SII activation (Hari et al 1990). Further investigation of the effect of shifts in attention, arousal, and painfulness are needed to clarify their influence on evoked responses. Another step in building a more valid model of somatosensory processing is the combination of EEG and MEG measurements. Initial results of source analysis of evoked electrical potentials elicited by short heat pulses show that in the electrical case it is not possible to model the 145-msec component with only two bilateral dipoles located in SII (see Chapter 16). To arrive at a sufficient explanation of the potential distribution, it was necessary to introduce a deep-lying source that will be hardly detectable with MEG. This deep location is likely to correspond to the area of the cingulate gyrus, where activation in response to heat stimuli was shown in the PET study of Talbot et al. (1991; see also Chapters 13 and 14).

There is still a need for methodologic development in the use of MEG. The most realistic evaluation of MEG and/or EEG measures would be based on MRI data to localize the various generators within the head of the individual subject. In this context, initial results showing equivalent current dipoles located in an individual cortex have recently been published (Dössel et al. 1993; Wagner et al. 1993). Such data will provide the connection between external measurements and individual anatomy, which is clearly the direction to be followed in the near future.

ACKNOWLEDGMENT

This study was supported by grants of the Deutsche Forschungsgemeinschaft (Br310/20-1).

REFERENCES

Barth DS, Sutherling WW, Engel J, Beatty J. Neuromagnetic localization of epileptiform spike activity in the human brain. *Science* 1982;218:891–894.

Barth DS, Sutherling WW, Engel J, Beatty J. Neuromagnetic evidence of spatially distributed sources underlying epileptiform spike activity in the human brain. *Science* 1984;223:293–296.

Barth DS, Di S. The electrophysiological basis of epileptiform magnetic fields in neocortex. *Brain Res* 1990;530:35–39.

Bromm B, Chen ACN. Brain electrical source analysis of laser-evoked potentials in response to painful trigeminal-nerve stimulation. *Electroenceph Clin Neurophysiol* 1995;95:(in press).

Bromm B, Meier W. The intracutaneous stimulus. A new pain model for algesimetric studies. *Methods Findings Exp Clin Pharmacol* 1984;6:405–410.

Bromm B, Treede RD. Laser-evoked cerebral potentials in the assessment of cutaneous pain sensitivity in normal subjects and patients. *Rev Neurol (Paris)* 1991;147:10:625–643.

Chatrian GE, Canfield RC, Krauss TA, Eegt EL. Cerebral responses to electrical tooth pulp stimulation in man. *Neurology* 1992;25:745–757.

Clarke J, Koch RH. The impact of high-temperature superconductivity on SQUID magnetometers. *Science* 1988;242:217–223.

Cohen D. Magnetoencephalography: Evidence of magnetic fields produced by alpha-rhythm currents. *Science* 1968;161:784–786.

Dössel O, David B, Fuchs M, Krüger J, Kullmann WH, Lüdecke KM. A modular approach to multichannel magnetometry. *Clin Phys Physiol Meas* 1991;12(Suppl B):75–79.

Dössel O, David B, Fuchs M, Krüger J, Lüdecke KM, Wischmann HA. A modular 31-channel SQUID system for biomagnetic measurements. *IEEE Trans Mag* 1993;(in press).

Fuchs M, Dössel O. On-line head position determination for MEG measurements. In Hoke M, Erné SN, Okada YC, Romani GL, eds. *Biomagnetism: clinical aspects*. Amsterdam: Elsevier, 1992;869–873.

Fuchs M, Wagner M, Wischmann HA, Dössel O. Cortical current imaging by morphologically constrained reconstructions. Proceedings of the 9th International Conference on Biomagnetism, Vienna, August 14–20, 1993.

Fuchs M, Wischmann HA, Wagner M, Krüger J. Coordinate system matching for neuromagnetic and morphological reconstruction overlay. *IEEE Trans Biomed Eng* 1995 (in press).

Gallen CC, Schartz B, Rieke K, Pantev C, Sobel D, Hirschkoff E, Bloom FE. Intrasubject reliability and validity of somatosensory source localization using a large array biomagnetometer. *Electroencephalogr Clin Neurophysiol* 1994;90:145–156.

Grynszpan F, Geselowitz DB. Model studies of the magnetocardiogram. *Biophys J* 1973;13:911–925.

Hämäläinen MS, Sarvas J. Realistic conductivity geometry model of the human head for interpretation of neuromagnetic data. *IEEE Trans Biomed Eng* 1989;36:165–171.

Hämäläinen MS, Hari R, Ilmoniemi RJ, Knuutila J, Lounasmaa OV. Magnetoencephalography—theory, instrumentation and applications to noninvasive studies of the working human brain. *Rev Mod Phys* 1993;65:413–497.

Hari R. Neuromagnetic method in the study of the human auditory cortex. *Adv Audiol* 1990;6:222–282.

Hari R, Kaukoranta E. Neuromagnetic studies of somatosensory system: principles and examples. *Prog Neurobiol* 1985;24:233–256.

Hari R, Hämäläinen H, Hämäläinen M, Kekoni J, Sams M, Tiihonen J. Separate finger representations at the human secondary somatosensory cortex. *Neuroscience* 1990;37:245–249.

Hari R, Kaukoranta E, Reinikainen K, Huopaniemie T, Mauno J. Neuromagnetic localization of cortical activity evoked by painful dental stimulation in man. *Neurosci Lett* 1983;42:77–82.

Hari R, Kaukoranta E, Reinikainen K, Mauno J. Neuromagnetic responses to noxious stimuli. In: Weinberg H, Stroink G, Katila T, eds. *Biomagnetism: applications and theory*. New York: Pergamon Press, 1984;359–363.

Helmholtz H. Über einige Gesetze der Verteilung elektrischer Ströme in körperlichen Leibern mit Anwendung auf die tierisch-elektrischen Versuche. *Pogg Ann Phys Chem* 1853;89:211–233, 353–377.

Huang JC, Nicholson C, Okada YC. Distortion of magnetic evoked fields and surface potentials by conductivity differences at boundaries in brain tissue. *Biophys J* 1990;57:1155–1166.

Huttunen J, Hari R, Leinonen L. Cerebral magnetic responses to stimulation of ulnar and median nerves. *Electroencephalogr Clin Neurophysiol* 1987;66:391–400.

Huttunen J, Kobal G, Kaukoranta E, Hari R. Cortical responses to painful CO_2 stimulation of nasal mucosa: a neuromagnetoencephalographic study in man. *Electroencephalogr Clin Neurophysiol* 1986;64:347–349.

Joseph J, Howland EW, Wakai R, Backonja M, Baffa O, Potenti FM, Cleelands CS. Late pain-related magnetic fields and electric potentials evoked by intracutaneous electric finger stimulation. *Electroencephalogr Clin Neurophysiol* 1991;80:46–52.

Kaufmann L, Kaufmann JH, Wang J-Z. Cortical folds and neuromagnetic fields. *Electroencephalogr Clin Neurophysiol* 1991;79:211–226.

Kobal G. Pain-related electrical potentials of the human nasal mucosa elicited by chemical stimulation. *Pain* 1985;22:151–163.

Lagerlund TD, Sharbrough FW, Jack CR, Jr, Erickson BJ, Strelow DC, Cicora KM, Busacker NE. Determination of 10-20 system electrode locations using magnetic resonance image scanning with markers. *Electroencephalogr Clin Neurophysiol* 1993;86:7–14.

Laudahn R, Bromm B. Topography of pain related magnetic fields evoked by short pulses of infrared laser radiation. *Advances in biomagnetism*. Proceedings of the 9th International Conference on Biomagnetism, Vienna, August 14–20, 1993, Nr.19, 32.

Laudahn R, Tarkka IM, Kullmann WH, Fuchs M, Dössel O, Bromm B. Early somatosensory evoked magnetic fields studied with a multichannel first-order gradiometer system. In: Hoke M, Erné SN, Okada YC, Romani, GL, eds. *Biomagnetism: clinical aspects*, Amsterdam: Elsevier, 1992;259–262.

Lütkenhöner B, Pantev C, Hoke M. Comparison between different methods to approximate an area of the human head by a sphere. *Adv Audiol* 1990;6:103–118.

Maekijaervi M, Montonen J, Toivonen L, Siltanen P, Nieminen MS, Leinioe M, Katila T. Identification of patients with ventricular tachycardia after myocardial infarction by high-resolution magnetocardiography and electrocardiography. *J Electrocardiol* 1993;26(Y):117–24.

Melcher JR, Cohen D. Dependence of the MEG on dipole orientation in the rabbit head. *Electroencephalogr Clin Neurophysiol* 1988;70:460–472.

Mountcastle VB, Powell PS. Neural mechanisms subserving cutaneous sensibility, with special reference to the role of afferent inhibition in sensory perception and discrimination. *Bull Johns Hopkins Hosp* 1959;105:201–232.

Okada YC. Neurogenesis of evoked magnetic fields. NATO ASI Series: *Biomagn* 1983;66:399–408.

Pantev C, Hoke M, Lehnertz K, Lütkenhöner B, Anogianakis G, Wiesttkowski W. Tonotopic organization of the human auditory cortex revealed by transient auditory evoked magnetic fields. *Electroencephalogr Clin Neurophysiol* 1988;69:160–170.

Romani GL, Narici L. Principles and clinical validity of the biomagnetic method. *Med Prog Technol* 1986;11:123–159.

Romani GL, Williamson SJ, Kaufmann L, Brenner D. Characterization of human auditory cortex by the neuromagnetic method. *Exp Brain Res* 1982;47:381–393.

Rose DF, Smith PD, Sato S. Magnetoencephalography and epilepsy research. *Science* 1987;238: 329–335.

Roth BJ, Balisch M, Gorbach A, Sato S. How well does a three-sphere model predict positions of dipols in a realistically shaped head? *Electroencephalogr Clin Neurophysiol* 1993;87:175–184.

Sarvas J. Basic mathematical and electromagnetic concepts of the biomagnetic inverse problem. *Phys. Med. Biol.* 1987;32(1):11–22.

Sato S, Balisch M, Muratore R. Principles of magnetoencephalography. *J Clin Neurophysiol* 1991;8(2): 144–156.

Stefan H, Schneider S, Abraham-Fuchs K, Bauer J, Feistel H, Pawlik G, Neubauer U, Roehrlein G, Huk WJ. Magnetic source localization in focal epilepsy. *Brain* 1990;113:1347–1359.

Stefan H, Schneider S, Abraham-Fuchs K, Pawlik G, Feistel H, Bauer J, Neubauer U, Huk WJ, Holthoff V. The neocortico to mesio-basal limbic propagation of focal epileptic activity during the spike-wave complex. *Electroencephalogr Clin Neurophysiol* 1991;79:1–10.

Stefan H, Schueler P, Abraham-Fuchs K, Schneider S. Ictal and interictal multichannel magnetic field recordings of epileptiform activity: Quantitative description of centers of focal epileptic activity. In: Hoke M, Erné SN, Okada YC, Romani GL, eds. *Biomagnetism: Clinical aspects.* Amsterdam: Elsevier, 1992;87–91.

Stroink G. Cardiomagnetism: A historical perspective. In: Hoke M, Erné SN, Okada YC, Romani GL, eds. *Biomagnetism: Clinical aspects.* Amsterdam: Elsevier, 1992;399–403.

Suk J, Ribary U, Cappel J, Yamamoto T, Llinás R. Anatomical localization revealed by MEG recordings of the human somatosensory system. *Electroencephalogr Clin Neurophysiol* 1991;78:185–196.

Sutherling WW, Crandall PH, Cahan LD, Barth DS. The magnetic field of epileptic spikes agrees with intracranial locations in complex partial epilepsy. *Neurology* 1988;38:778–786.

Sutherling WW, Crandall PH, Darcey TM, Becker DP, Levesque MF, Barth DS. The magnetic and electric fields agree with intracranial localizations of somatosensory cortex. *Neurology* 1988;38:1705–1714.

Talbot JD, Marrett S, Evans AC, Meyer E, Bushnell MC, Duncan GH. Multiple representations of pain in human cerebral cortex. *Science* 1991;251:1355–1358.

Towle VL, Bolaños J, Suarez D, Tan K, Grzeszczuk R, Levin DN, Cakmur R, Frank A, Spire JP. The spatial location of EEG electrodes: locating the best-fitting sphere relative to cortical anatomy. *Electroencephalogr Clin Neurophysiol* 1993;86:1–6.

Van Oosterom A. Mathematical aspects of source modeling. *Acta Otolaryngol* (Suppl 491):70–79.

Vieth J. Magnetoencephalography and epilepsy. In: Wieser HG, Elger CE. 1987; *Presurgical evaluation of epileptics.* Heidelberg: Springer, 1987;117–127.

Wagner M, Fuchs M, Wischmann H-A, Ottenberg K, Dössel O. Cortex segmentation from 3D MR images for MEG reconstruction. *Proceedings of the 9th International Conference on Biomagnetism.* Vienna, August 14–20, 1993.

Weismüller P, Richter P, Abraham-Fuchs K, Haerer W, Schneider S, Hoeher M, Kochs M, Edrich J, Hombach V. Spatial differences of the duration of ventricular late fields in the signal-averaged magnetocardiogram in patients with ventricular late potentials. *Pac Clin Electrophysiol* 1993;16(1 Pt 1):70–79.

Williamson SJ, Kaufmann L. Biomagnetism. *J Magnetism Magnet Mater* 1981;22:129–201.

Wood CC, Cohen D, Cuffin BN, Yarita M, Allison T. Electrical sources in human somatosensory cortex: identification by combined magnetic and potential recordings. *Science* 1985;227:1051–1053.

Pain and the Brain: From
Nociception to Cognition,
edited by Burkhart Bromm and
John E. Desmedt, Advances in Pain
Research and Therapy Vol. 22.
Raven Press, Ltd., New York © 1995.

18

The Affective Dimension of Pain: A Model

C. Richard Chapman

Department of Anesthesiology, University of Washington, Seattle, Washington 98195

SUMMARY

Emotion is a fundamental part of the pain experience and not a reaction to the sensory appreciation of pain. Emotions evolved to foster survival, and both emotional responses to injury and emotional expression assist biologic adaptation. The affective dimension of pain imputes immediate biologic significance to the injurious event for the injured individual. From the perspective of emotion, pain is a state of the individual that has as its primary defining feature awareness of and homeostatic adjustment to tissue trauma. Rich literatures on the neurophysiology of emotion and the neuroendocrinology of stress demonstrate methods for studying emotion that may apply to the affective component of pain. Nociceptive centripetal transmission engages spinoreticular as well as spinothalamic pathways. Evidence exists that tisMMsue trauma: (a) excites both spinoreticular and spinothalamic pathways; (b) generates concomitant affective and sensory processes that subserve complementary adaptive functions; and (c) activates predominantly noradrenergic limbic structures to produce negative affective arousal; and that (d) the hypothalamically mediated stress response is an important feature of clinically significant pain and a mechanism of its emotional dimension. Moreover, psychological research and theory in these areas also provides a valuable resource for new investigation. Integrating knowledge from these fields with that gleaned from the study of nociceptive transduction and transmission should yield a comprehensive and truly multidisciplinary understanding of pain.

INTRODUCTION

Many, perhaps most, health-care professionals think of pain as an unpleasant, distressing sensation that originates in traumatized tissues and courses its way along neural pathways to the brain and consciousness. This simplistic and anachronistic view persists in part because some neurophysiologists implicitly equate nociception with pain. But the days are gone when one could speak of pain as a coded noxious sensory message in an electronic circuit: It is unequivocally a complex perceptual process that originates in the brain; typically, but not uniquely, in response to a specific type of sensory message. In the formation of the perception that we recognize as pain, the brain inextricably intertwines sensory information with emotion and cognition.

In recognition of this complexity, the International Association for the Study of pain (IASP) acknowledged the central role of affect in its keystone definition that: "Pain [is] an unpleasant sensory and *emotional* experience associated with actual or potential tissue damage, or described in terms of such damage" (Merskey 1979, p. 250, italics added).

The definition clearly emphasizes the role of affect as an intrinsic component of pain. Emotion is not simply a consequence of pain sensation that occurs after a noxious sensory message arrives at higher brain centers, but is a fundamental part of the pain experience. Curiously, however, this conspicuous and oft-quoted definition has merited only lip service. To date, researchers concerned with basic mechanisms of pain have addressed sensory processing almost exclusively, and we know little about why pain disturbs us and compels us to seek relief.

I argue here that we must turn our attention to the affective characteristics of pain in order to bridge knowledge gained in laboratory research to clinical pain phenomena. Literature on the neurophysiology of emotion and the neuroendocrinology of stress, both rich sources of literature, suggests approaches for studying the affective component of pain. Moreover, psychological research and theory in these areas also provides a rich resource and a fresh perspective. By bringing knowledge from these fields together with what we know about the sensory features of pain, we may be able to build a comprehensive, and truly multidisciplinary, understanding of pain.

In this chapter I offer a model to account for the affective dimension of pain. Models are, by definition, intentional oversimplifications, and I put this one forth as a point of departure for future thinking rather than as a strong declarative statement. In brief, I propose that tissue trauma: (a) excites both spinoreticular and spinothalamic pathways; (b) generates concomitant affective and sensory processes that subserve complementary adaptive functions; and (c) activates predominantly noradrenergic limbic structures to produce the affective dimension of pain; and that (d) the hypothalamically-mediated stress response is an important feature of pain and a mechanism of its emotional dimension. Admittedly, one finds it difficult to integrate these possibilities with our current sensory perspective on pain. I contend that we should shift our emphasis away from pain as a sensory message to pain as the dominant perceptual state of an organism during and after tissue trauma.

Below, I briefly review current concepts of emotion, certain pertinent aspects of emotional behavior, and the relevant central neuroanatomy and endocrinology of negative emotion. From this I construct a model to account for the presence of emotional arousal in the experience of pain.

EMOTION, ITS FUNCTIONS, AND ITS EXPRESSIONS

Definitions of Emotion

In order to entertain the concept of emotion as a component of pain, we need a clear notion of what emotion is. Each of us knows emotions as sensation-like feeling states that compel us to act in certain ways, but few of us profess to understand such states. Despite a large literature on the psychophysiology of emotion, poor consensus exists on a formal definition for emotion; multiple theorists have created myriad meanings for the term, perhaps because the concept of emotion encompasses a wide range of animal and human phenomena. For example, Rolls (1986, p. 126) stated that "Emotions can be usefully defined as states elicited by reinforcing stimuli." Fonberg (1986, p. 302) contended that "Emotion is the nervous process that determines what kind of stimuli coming from the inner and outer environments are desirable for the organism and what are not." Averill (1980, p. 312) asserted that "An emotion is a transitory social role (a socially constituted syndrome) that includes an individual's appraisal of a situation and that is interpreted as a passion rather than as an action." Such seemingly unrelated definitions of the term reflect the divergent theoretical frameworks within which emotion researchers work, and they investigate markedly different subjective, behavioral, and social phenomena.

The problem of defining emotion has provided a bone of contention since ancient times; the Greeks debated issues relating to it that persist today. One such issue is whether there exist a few fundamental emotions from which all others derive. Several contemporary theorists argue for this assumption. For example, Plutchik (1980) listed eight basic emotions. The subjective feeling, associated behaviors, and sociobiologic functions associated with these emotions are as follows:

Feeling	Behavior	Function
Fear	Escape	Protection
Anger	Attack	Destruction
Joy	Mate	Reproduction
Sadness	Cry	Reintegration
Acceptance	Groom	Incorporation
Disgust	Vomit	Rejection
Expectation	Map	Exploration
Surprise	Stop	Orientation

None of these affects relates to pain directly, but given that Plutchik views emotions as cognitively mediated and future focused, the basic emotion clearly associated with pain must be fear.

Lazarus (1993), who sees emotions as feelings linked to thoughts (and pain as a sensation), holds that people appraise events and persons that they encounter, and that the emotions these produce represent personal significance. He postulates 15 basic emotions. Of these, four are positive feelings: happiness, love, pride, and relief. The other nine are negative: anger, anxiety, disgust, envy, fright, guilt, jealousy, sadness, and shame. Three others that represent mixed hedonic qualities may qualify for the list of basic feeling states: hope, compassion, and gratitude. Each emotion characterizes a relationship between the person and the environment, and signifies the individual's way of adapting to the environment.

In contrast, MacLean (1990) postulated three classes of affects: basic, general, and specific. Basic affects derive from basic needs such as hunger, the urge to urinate, or sexual expression. General affects are complex feelings aroused by situations, other people, or things. Specific affects correspond to specific sensory experiences such as smells or sounds. Pain falls into this class of experience, since we experience it as a bodily sensation. Ictal aura phenomena often provide striking examples of emotions in this class, and MacLean noted many instances of ictal emotions involving bizarre pain states.

These striking differences in theory typify the lack of professional consensus about basic emotions. One could belabor this point by drawing many other lists of fundamental feelings from the literature, but this will yield little additional insight. The basic point is clear: many theorists contend that basic emotions exist, but they cannot agree on what these are, and this undermines their contention. Some theorists contest the assumption that basic emotions exist (Ortony and Turner, 1990).

Despite the poor consensus about basic concepts of emotion, I believe that sufficient agreement exists among mainstream emotion researchers on the following points:

1. Emotional responses to stimuli and emotional expression subserve biologic adaptation and emotional phenomena evolved to foster survival of the individual and the species.
2. Emotions impute positive or negative hedonic qualities to a stimulus in accordance with the biologic importance and meaning of that stimulus.
3. The central neuroanatomy for emotion corresponds to the limbic brain.
4. Emotions activate—they produce impulses to act or to express one's self.
5. Emotions communicate, and the negative emotional expression of one individual will tend to produce negative emotion in another.
6. Human cognitions and emotions function interdependently.

These points of agreement help to clarify what science currently means by emotion, but a conclusive, consensual definition for emotion still eludes us. Without this, our definition of pain remains incomplete.

In approaching the emotional dimension of pain, I favor a sociobiologic (evolutionary) framework that interprets feeling states, related physiology, and behavior in terms of adaptation and survival. Nature has equipped us with the capability for negative emotion for a purpose; bad feelings are not simply accidents of human consciousness. By understanding the emotional dimension of pain from this perspective, we may gain some insight into how to prevent or control emotions that foster suffering. Implementation of this approach as a world view of pain requires that we dispense with conventional language habits that involve describing pain as a transient sensory event. Instead, I argue that we construe pain as a state of the organism that has as its primary defining feature awareness of and homeostatic adjustment to tissue trauma.

Adaptive Functions of Emotion

Emotions and the emotional dimension of pain characterize mammals exclusively, and appear to foster mammalian adaptation. MacLean (1990, p. 425) contended that emotions "impart subjective information that is instrumental in guiding behavior required for self-preservation and preservation of the species. The subjective awareness that is an affect consists of a sense of bodily pervasiveness or feelings localized to certain parts of the body." As emotion evolved to facilitate adaptation and survival, negative emotion plays an important defensive role. The ability to impute threat to certain types of environmental events protects against life-threatening injury.

Within consciousness, threat manifests as a feeling state, and in humans, threatening events that are not immediately present can exist as emotionally colored sensory images. We can react emotionally to the mental image of a painful event before it happens (e.g., venipuncture), or for that matter we can respond to the sight of another person's tissue trauma. The emotional intensity of such a feeling marks the adaptive significance of the event that produced the experience. The threat of a minor injury provokes less feeling that the threat of one that incurs a high risk of death. The emotional magnitude of a pain is therefore the internal representation of the threat associated with the event that produced the pain. The key point is that emotional arousal indicates and expresses a perceived threat to the biologic integrity of the individual.

Emotions and Behavior

Emotions compel action and also expression through vocalization, posture, variations in patterns of facial musculature, and alterations of activity. This enhances communication and social support, thus contributing to survival. Darwin (1872), observing animals, noted that emotions enable communication through vocalization, startle, posture, facial expression, and specific behaviors. Contemporary investigators who study emotions and human or animal social behavior emphasize that communication is a fundamental adaptive function of emotion (Ploog 1986). Social mammals, including humans, use one another or their social group as resources for adaptation and survival. The emotional expression of pain in the presence of supportive persons is socially powerful; it draws upon a fundamental sociobiologic imperative: communicating threat and summoning assistance.

Central Neuroanatomy of Emotion

The limbic brain represents an anatomic common denominator across mammalian species (MacLean 1990, p. 257), and this suggests that emotion represents a common feature in consciousness across mammals. Early investigators focused on the role of olfaction in limbic function. Papez (1937) linked the limbic brain to emotion, stating that: "It is proposed that the hypothalamus, the anterior thalamic nuclei, the gyrus cinguli, the hippocampus and their interconnections constitute a harmonious mechanism which may elaborate the functions of central emotion, as well as participate in emotional expression." Emotion may have evolutionary roots in olfactory perception.

MacLean (1952) introduced the term "limbic system" four decades ago, and characterized its functions. Currently, he identifies three main subdivisions of the limbic brain: the amygdalar, septal, and thalamocingulate (MacLean 1990). Fig. 1 illus-

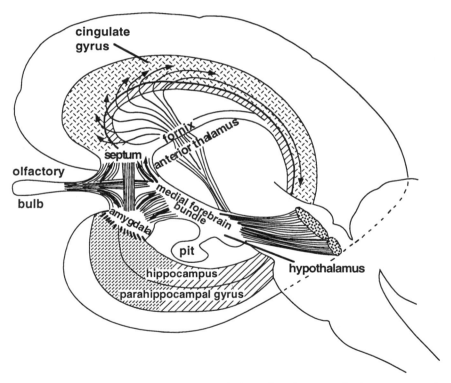

FIG. 1. Three subdivisions of the limbic brain. MacLean (1990) proposed a three-part grouping of limbic structures and functions: amygdalar, septal, and thalamocingulate subdivisions. These groupings appear as shadings. The figure, derived from MacLean's illustration (1990, p. 315), portrays the hippocampus as an upright arch joining the septum at one end and the amygdala at the other. ⎯⎯ Amygdalar ⎯ Septal ▓ Thalamocingulate

trates these three main subdivisions of the limbic brain. These represent sources of afferents to parts of the limbic cortex (MacLean 1990, p. 311). MacLean also postulated that the limbic brain responds to two basic types of input: interoceptive and exteroceptive. In the tradition of Sherrington, these terms refer to sensory information from internal and external environments, respectively.

Traditionally, pain research has ignored potential links between nociception and limbic processing. However, one can find anecdotal evidence that implicates limbic structures in the distress of pain. Radical frontal lobotomies, once done on patients for psychosurgical purposes, typically interrupted pathways projecting from the hypothalamus to the cingulate cortex and putatively relieved the suffering of intractable pain without destroying sensory awareness (Fulton 1951). Such neurosurgical records help clarify recent positron-emission tomographic (PET) and magnetic resonance imaging (MRI) observations of human subjects undergoing painful cutaneous heat stimulation: noxious stimulation activates the contralateral anterior cingulate gyrus as the well as primary (S1) and secondary somatosensory (S2) cortices (Talbot et al. 1991).

Emotion in Learning and Memory

Organisms that can learn readily from experience have adaptive advantages over those that cannot. The affective component of pain fosters adaptation through operant (instrumental) learning as well as classical conditioning (learning by association). Operant learning requires reinforcers, and reinforcers are events accompanied by emotions. Classical conditioning represents the formation of an association between a normally neutral event and the negative emotion associated with the onset of pain. Memory of past events, like learning, depends heavily upon emotion, and memories of past experience tend to shape expectations for the present and future.

Operant learning can occur in any setting in which patients are active and reinforcing events take place. A reinforcer is an event that alters the future likelihood of a behavior recurring when it follows an instance of that behavior (Fordyce 1990). Positive reinforcing events that create pleasure function as rewards; negative ones that produce pain are punishments (i.e., they suppress behaviors). The positive or negative nature of reinforcers, and their personal significance, occur in conscious awareness as feelings (Rolls 1986). Put another way, reinforcing events are those that are emotionally prominent. Emotion-free events have no reinforcing properties and therefore cannot contribute to adaptive learning.

Fear accompanying pain can become associated with non-noxious stimuli through classical conditioning. In fear conditioning, the repeated pairing of a neutral stimulus with a noxious one can condition the perceiver so that the neutral stimulus, occurring alone, acts as a trigger to elicit fear. Biologically, fear conditioning supports survival by fostering avoidance of potentially dangerous situations. Through conditioning, ordinarily neutral stimuli become warning cues for danger (Staddon 1983). Fear also helps the individual martial a flight-or-fight response to a challenge after prior exposure to it. Osborne et al. (1975) found that 3-methoxy-4-hydroxyphenylglycol (MHPG), an indicator of norepinephrine turnover in the brain, provided a marker of fear conditioning; exposure to a painful event increased MHPG in a manner that tracked the conditioning process.

Conditioned emotional responses are essentially sensory–affective associations. The amygdala appears to be the key structure in the linking of sensory experience to emotional arousal and in the conditioning of negative emotional associations (Gray 1982; Fonberg 1986; LeDoux et al. 1990). It probably contributes to the emotional evaluation of cognitive events (via corticofugal pathways) as well as sensory events that reach it via the dorsal noradrenergic bundle (DNB) or sensory thalamus. Aggleton and Mishkin (1986) described the amygdala as a gateway to the emotions for stimuli (simple or complex) in all sensory modalities, both conditioned and unconditioned.

LeDoux and colleagues (1988; 1990), working with auditory stimuli, determined that projections from the acoustic thalamus to the amygdala allow the classical conditioning of emotional responses to normally neutral auditory stimuli in experimental animals. To condition subjects, they paired tones with footshock, evaluating autonomic responses and emotional behaviors. Lesion work implicated separate efferent projections from the amygdala in the conditioning of autonomic and behavioral responses. These and other observations suggest that emotion is a complex process sustained by several mechanisms; under controlled circumstances, individual mechanisms can be independently conditioned.

Fear conditioning almost certainly occurs in cancer patients who undergo repeated painful procedures. Fear conditioning can exacerbate the affective dimension of pain in cases in which minor pain and intense affective arousal have been paired. Moreover, it can form associations between the environment of a painful event and affective processing of that event so that the environment alone can elicit elements of the affective dimension of pain. Fear conditioning may contribute to phobic behavior patterns in pediatric patients.

Emotion associated with pain also influences memory. Memory researchers surmise that both limbic and nonlimbic mechanisms contribute to memory processes (Gabriel et al. 1986). Emotional significance controls at least some and perhaps much memory formation: evidence exists that the brain preferentially stores information that has strong emotional loading (Bower 1981; Tucker et al. 1990). Heath (1986, p. 6) proposed that learning and memory are "rooted in feeling and emotion," and identified the hippocampus, cortical medial amygdala, and cingulate gyrus as key areas involved in negative emotions.

In sum, the emotional component of pain seems to support adaptation and survival by facilitating learning, memory, and related cognitive processes. It provides a bridge by which pain can affect the psychological status of the individual and the individual's behavioral tendencies.

Emotion and Cognition

Negative emotions appear to be much more than reactions to undesirable events; in nature they help an individual to determine which things benefit and which things threaten its survival, and they compel behavior consistent with such evaluations. Moreover, emotional expression allows the individual to communicate this judgment to others, and to thus set up group approach or avoidance behaviors. As noted above, MacLean (1990) described emotion as a process that imparts subjective information. In these respects, emotion approximates a crude intelligence. If emotion is a proto-intelligence, then evolutionarily newer structures, namely those derived from the later stages of cortical development, should have demonstrable links with limbic structures and functions.

Such interconnections exist. Parts of the frontal lobe (the dorsal trend) appear to have developed from the rudimentary hippocampal formation, while other parts (the paleocortical trend) originated in the olfactory cortex. While these two areas are anatomically interconnected, the former analyzes sensory information while the latter contributes emotional tone to that sensory information (Pandya et al. 1987, pp. 66–67). Pribram (1980), noting that limbic function involves the frontal and temporal cortices, offered a bottom-up concept for how cognition relates to feelings, maintaining that emotion determines cognition. However, the multimodal neocortical association areas project corticofugally to limbic structures (Turner et al. 1980), and this suggests that cognitions may drive emotions. Plutchik (1980) argued that cognitions (evaluations) always precede emotions and may be based on information provided by internal or external stimuli. These points of view may not be as diametrically opposed as they appear. Plutchik has postulated that emotions precede cognitions in evolution, and that cognitions evolved in the service of emotions. The sociobiologic purpose of cognition, for Plutchik, is to predict the future. Good agreement exists among theorists that human thinking involves intimate interplay with emotions.

A BASIS FOR THE EMOTIONAL DIMENSION OF PAIN

Nociception and Central Noradrenergic Processing

Central sensory and affective pain processes share common sensory mechanisms in the periphery: Aδ- and C-fibers serve as tissue-trauma transducers (nociceptors) for both types of pain process: the chemical products of inflammation sensitize these nociceptors, and peripheral neuropathic mechanisms such as ectopic firing excite both processes. Differentiation of sensory and affective processing begins at the dorsal horn of the spinal cord, with sensory transmission following spinothalamic pathways and transmission destined for affective processing taking place in spinoreticular pathways. Since others have already described the sensory processing of nociception well, it need not be reviewed here (see Willis 1985; Fields 1987; Peschanski and Weil-Fugacza 1987; Bonica 1990).

Nociceptive centripetal transmission engages spinoreticular as well as spino-thalamic pathways (Villanueva et al. 1989). The spinoreticular tract contains so-matosensory and viscerosensory afferent pathways that arrive at different levels of the brain stem. Spinoreticular axons have receptive fields that resemble those of spinothalamic-tract neurons projecting to the medial thalamus, and, like their spino-thalamic counterparts, transmit tissue-injury information (Fields 1987; Bonica 1990; Villanueva et al. 1990). Most spinoreticular neurons carry nociceptive signals and many of them respond preferentially to noxious input (Bowsher 1976; Willis 1985; Abou-Samra 1987; Bing et al. 1990).

Processing of nociceptive signals to produce affect begins in reticulocortical path-ways. Four extrathalamic afferent pathways project to the neocortex: the DNB, originating in the locus coeruleus (LC); the serotonergic fibers that arise in the dorsal and median raphe nuclei; the dopaminergic pathways of the ventral tegmental tract that arise from the substantia nigra; and the acetylcholinergic neurons that arise principally from the nucleus basalis of the substantia innominata (Foote and Mor-rison, 1987). Of these, the noradrenergic pathway links most closely to negative emotional states (Gray 1982, 1987). The set of structures receiving projections from this complex and extensive network corresponds to the classic defintion of the lim-bic brain (Papez 1937; Isaacson 1982; Gray 1987; MacLean 1990).

Although other processes governed predominantly by other neurotransmitters probably play important roles in the complex experience of emotion during pain, I focus here on the role of central noradrenergic processing. This processing involves two central noradrenergic pathways: the dorsal and ventral noradrenergic bundles.

The Locus Coeruleus and the Dorsal Noradrenergic Bundle

The pontine nucleus known as the locus coeruleus (LC) resides bilaterally near the wall of the fourth ventricle. The locus has three major projections: ascending, descending, and cerebellar. The DNB, which is the ascending projection, is the most extensive and important (Fillenz 1990), as Fig. 2 illustrates. The DNB projects from the LC throughout the limbic brain and to all of the neocortex, accounting for about 70% of all brain norepinephrine (Watson et al. 1986; Svensson 1987). The LC gives rise to the majority of central noradrenergic fibers in the spinal cord, hypothal-amus, thalamus, and hippocampus (Levitt and Moore 1979; Aston-Jones et al. 1985), in addition to its projections to the limbic cortex and neocortex. Conse-quently, this seemingly inauspicious nucleus may exert an almost global influence on brain activity.

The LC reacts to signaling from sensory stimuli that potentially threaten the bio-logic integrity of the individual or signal damage to that integrity. Nociception inevitably and reliably increases activity in neurons of the LC, and LC excitation appears to be an inevitable response to nociception (Korf et al. 1974; Stone 1975; Morilak et al. 1987; Svensson 1987). Notably, this does not require cognitively mediated attentional control, since it occurs in anesthetized animals. Foote et al.

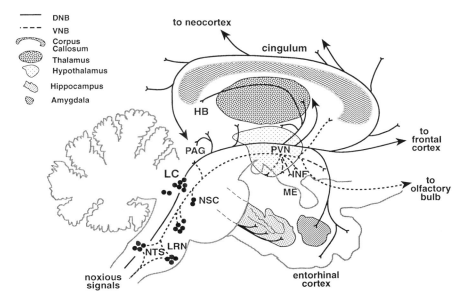

FIG. 2. Central corticopetal noradrenergic transmission in a primate brain (parasagittal view). The cell bodies of neurons that produce norepinephrine appear as black circles. The major projections of these cell bodies are the dorsal noradrenergic bundle (DNB) and the ventral noradrenergic bundle (VNB). Tissue-trauma signals from spinoreticular pathways excite the primarily noradrenergic locus coeruleus (LC), activating the DNB, which extends throughout the limbic brain and to the neocortex. ME = median eminence; PAG = periaqueductal grey; HB = habenula; NSC = nucleus subcoeruleus; LRN = lateral reticular nucleus; NTS = nucleus tractus solitarius; INF = infundibulum; PVN = paraventricular nucleus.

(1983) reported that slow, tonic spontaneous activity at the LC in rats changed under anesthesia in response to noxious stimulation. Experimentally induced phasic LC activation produces alarm and apparent fear in primates (Redmond and Huang 1979; Charney et al. 1990), and lesions of the LC eliminate normal heart rate increases to threatening stimuli (Redmond 1977).

Although the LC responds consistently, it does not react exclusively to noxious sensory input. LC activity increases following nonpainful threatening occurrences, such as strong cardiovascular stimulation (Elam et al. 1985; Morilak et al. 1987), and certain visceral events, such as distention of the bladder, stomach, colon, or rectum (Elam et al. 1986b; Svensson 1987). Thus, while it reacts to nociception consistently, the LC is not a nociceptive-specific nucleus. Rather, it responds to biologically threatening events, of which tissue injury is a significant subset. One can describe the LC as a central analog of the sympathetic ganglia (Amaral and Sinnamon 1977).

Invasive studies confirm the linkage between LC activity and threat. Direct activation of the DNB and associated limbic structures in laboratory animals produces a sympathetic nervous response and elicits emotional behaviors such as defensive threat, fright, enhanced startle, freezing, and vocalization (McNaughton and Mason 1980). This indicates that enhanced activity in these pathways corresponds to negative emotional arousal and behaviors appropriate to perceived threat.

Under normal circumstances, activity in the locus increases alertness; tonically enhanced LC and DNB discharge corresponds to hypervigilance and emotionality (Foote et al. 1983; Butler et al. 1990). Vigilance and orientation to affectively relevant and novel stimuli can occur because of the DNB; it also regulates attentional processes and facilitates motor responses (Elam et al. 1986a; Foote and Morrison 1987; Gray 1987; Svensson 1987; Calogero et al. 1988). In this sense the LC influences the stream of consciousness on an ongoing basis, and readies the individual to respond quickly and effectively to threat when it occurs.

Biologically the LC and DNB foster survival by allowing the individual to exercise global vigilance for threatening and harmful stimuli. Siegel and Rogawski (1988) hypothesized a link between the LC noradrenergic system and vigilance, focusing on rapid-eye-movement (REM) sleep. They noted that LC noradrenergic neurons maintain continuous activity in both the normal waking state and non-REM sleep, but that during REM sleep these neurons virtually cease their discharge activity. Moreover, an increase in REM sleep ensues after either lesioning of the DNB or the administration of clonidine, an alpha-2 adrenoceptor agonist. Because LC inactivation during REM sleep permits rebuilding of noradrenergic stores, REM sleep may be necessary preparation for sustained periods of high alertness during subsequent waking. Siegel and Rogawski (1988, p. 226) contended that "a principal function of NE (norephinephrine) in the CNS is to facilitate the excitability of target neurons to specific high-priority signals." Conversely, reduced periods of LC activity (REM sleep) allow time for a suppression of sympathetic tone.

Collectively, these findings suggest that the affective dimension of pain shares central mechanisms with vigilance, a biologically important process. Vigilance, intensified by injury signals from within the organism, distressing environmental events from outside the organism, or a combination of these, can generate a state that progresses to hypervigilance and panic. As a subjective experience, the emotional quality of pain therefore seems to be most accurately described as awareness of immediate biologic threat.

The Ventral Noradrenergic Bundle and the Hypothalamo-Pituitary-Adrenocortical (HPA) Axis

The ventral noradrenergic bundle (VNB), like the DNB, is an ascending noradrenergic system; it enters the medial forebrain bundle (see Fig. 2). Neurons in the medullary reticular formation project to the hypothalamus via the VNB (Sumal et al. 1983; Bonica 1990). Sawchenko and Swanson (1982) identified two VNB-linked noradrenergic and adrenergic pathways to the paraventricular hypothalamus in the rat, and described them with the Dahlström and Fuxe (1964) designations: the

A1 region of the ventral medulla (lateral reticular nucleus, LRN), and the A2 region of the dorsal vagal complex (the nucleus tractus solitarius, NTS), which receives visceral afferents. These medullary neuronal complexes supply 90% of catecholaminergic innervation to the paraventricular hypothalamus via the VNB (Assenmacher et al. 1987). Regions A5 and A7 make comparatively minor contributions to the VNB.

The VNB is important for emotion research as well as the study of pain, because it innervates the hypothalamus. The noradrenergic axons in the VNB respond to noxious stimulation (Kanosue et al. 1984), as does the hypothalamus (Svensson 1987). Moreover, nociception-transmitting neurons at all segmental levels of the spinal cord project to the medial and lateral hypothalamus and several telencephalic regions (Burstein et al. 1988). These projections provide the neurophysiologic link between tissue injury and the hypothalamic response; hormonal messengers may also play a part in some circumstances.

The coordinating center for the HPA axis is the hypothalamic paraventricular nucleus (PVN). Neurons of the PVN receive afferent information from several reticular areas, including the ventrolateral medulla, dorsal raphe nucleus, nucleus raphe magnus, LC, dorsomedial nucleus, and the nucleus tractus solitarius (Sawchenko and Swanson 1982; Peschanski and Weil-Fugacza 1987; Lopez et al. 1991). Still other afferents project to the PVN from the hippocampus and amygdala. Nearly all hypothalamic and preoptic nuclei send projections to the PVN.

The PVN responds to potentially or frankly injurious stimuli by initiating a complex series of events regulated by feedback mechanisms (see Fig. 3). These processes ready the organism for extraordinary behaviors that will maximize its chances to cope with an immediate threat (Selye 1978). Cannon (1929) described this "flight or fight" capability as an emergency reaction. Contemporary writers such as Henry (1986) and LeDoux et al. (1988) hold that neuroendocrine arousal mechanisms are not limited to emergency situations, even though most research emphasizes that such situations elicit them. In complex social contexts, submission, dominance, and other transactions can elicit neuroendocrine and autonomic responses, modified perhaps by learning and memory. This suggests that neuroendocrine processes accompany all sorts of emotion-eliciting situations.

Strong links exist between the hypothalamus and autonomic nervous reactivity (Panskepp 1986). Psychophysiologists hold that diffuse sympathetic arousal reflects, albeit imperfectly, negative emotional arousal (Lacey and Lacey 1970). The PVN invokes autonomic arousal through neural as well as hormonal pathways. It sends direct projections to the sympathetic intermediolateral cell column in the thoracolumbar spinal cord, and to the parasympathetic vagal complex, sources of preganglionic autonomic outflow (Krukoff 1990). In addition, it signals release of epinephrine and norepinephrine from the adrenal medulla. Adrenocorticotrophic hormone (ACTH) release by the adrenal medulla, while not instantaneous, is relatively rapid, occurring within about 15 sec (Sapolsky 1992). These considerations implicate the HPA axis in the neuroendocrinologic and autonomic manifestations of emotion during pain states.

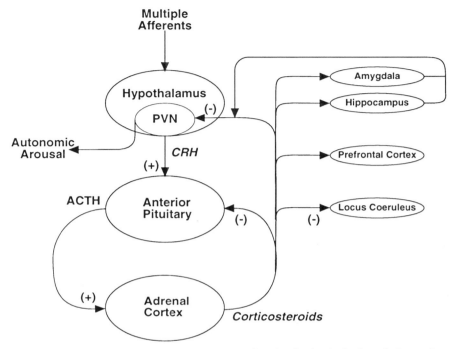

FIG. 3. Schematic representation of feedback-mediated activation in the hypothalamo-pituitary-adrenocortical (HPA) axis. In response to afferent input, including noxious stimulation, the hypothalamic paraventricular nucleus (PVN) synthesizes corticotropin-releasing hormone (CRH), and secretes CRH into the portal circulation, thus stimulating the anterior pituitary. This leads to neurohypophyseal secretion of several pro-opiomelanocortin-derived neuropeptides, including adrenocorticotrophic hormone (ACTH), into the systemic circulation. ACTH stimulates the adrenal cortex to release corticosteroids such as hydrocortisone and corticosterone. Corticosteroids provide feedback to regulatory processes by inhibiting the anterior pituitary, and this represses pro-opiomelanocortin gene expression, thereby attenuating further ACTH secretion. Corticosteroid receptors exist on parvocellular PVN neurons, and in addition corticosteroids bind to the amygdala, hippocampus, and prefrontal cortical areas. In binding to the hippocampus and amygdala, corticosteroids initiate further inhibitory feedback to the hypothalamic PVN, and also restrain the activity of the locus coeruleus (LC). (−) = inhibition; (+) = excitation

In addition to controlling neuroendocrine and autonomic nervous reactivity, the HPA axis coordinates emotional arousal with behavior (Panskepp 1986). Direct stimulation of the hypothalamus can elicit well-organized patterns of behavior, including defensive threat behaviors, accompanies by autonomic manifestations (Hess 1954; Mancia and Zanchetti 1981; Janig 1985a,b). The existence of demonstrable behavioral subroutines in animals suggests that the hypothalamus plays a key role in matching behavioral reactions and bodily adjustments to challenging circumstances or biologically relevant stimuli. Moreover, at high levels, stress hormones, especially glucocorticoids, may affect central emotional arousal, reducing startle thresholds and influencing cognition (Sapolsky 1992). Saphier (1987) observed that cortisol altered the firing rate of neurons in the limbic forebrain. In short, the HPA axis appears to take an executive responsibility for coordinating behavioral readiness with physiological capability, awareness, and cognitive function.

PAIN AND STRESS

Tissue trauma, through its impact on the HPA axis, produces a complex adaptive stress response involving neural and endocrinologic changes. This process lends itself to the physiologic investigation of stress. Concomitantly, the perception of tissue trauma (pain) produces parallel changes in consciousness and behavior. These changes constitute psychological stress and invite study from a psychological perspective. In contrast to the field of emotion, in which little consensus exists, physiologists and psychologists agree substantially on the nature of stress, and their theories complement one another. Indeed, these areas overlap. They meet on the common, albeit controversial, scientific ground of emotion research.

Physiologists investigating stress focus on the primarily endocrinologic, feedback-dependent, HPA axis. Sapolsky (1992, p. 3), primarily concerned with the effects of the acute and chronic stress response on the process of aging, defined the primary concepts of stress research in these terms: "A *stressor* can be defined in a narrow, physiological sense as any perturbation in the outside world that disrupts homeostasis, and the *stress-response* is the set of neural and endocrine adaptations that help reestablish homeostasis." Psychologists by and large accept this perspective, but emphasize psychological rather than physiologic reactions to personal threats and injuries that originate in the individual's environment. Both physiologic and behavioral perspectives are essential for a comprehensive description of stress.

Lazarus (1993, p. 4) distinguished between physiologic and psychological focus: "What generates physiologic stress—that is, what is noxious to tissues—is not the same as what is stressful psychologically." This suggests that the complex psychological dimension of pain requires a different level of inquiry than its underlying physiologic processes. In the Lazarus framework, the focus of psychological inquiry must be on personal meaning. Stress depends on cognitive appraisal of personal harms and threats. Behavior associated with stress is an adaptive effort based on appraisal, and Lazarus calls this "coping behavior." If appraisal indicates that the individual can do something to help himself, he engages in *problem-focused coping*. But if there are no apparent ways to engage the problem, *emotion-focused coping* ensues. As I have already noted, the expression of emotion is an active process with potentially significant effects on the social environment.

Taken together, these considerations lead us to a picture of stress as a state of the individual that has both physiologic and psychological manifestations. A stressor is any event or circumstance that threatens the biologic or psychological integrity of the individual. In nature, tissue trauma threatens the biologic viability of the individual by definition, and it constitutes a stressor. Physiologic stress responses therefore accompany tissue trauma like a shadow, and apart from the first few seconds after injury, when the body is mobilizing such responses, they coexist with pain. Psychological responses occur as well; these are complex and involve both cognition and emotion. Most psychological stress is cognitively mediated, and psychological coping often determines the behavior of a person in pain.

In complex ways, physiologic stress responses interact with the sensory qualities of pain and with psychological coping. For example, glucocorticoids released by the HPA axis during the stress response diminish inflammation and block the sensitization of nociceptors in injured tissue. At the same time, HPA arousal releases ACTH and other pro-opiomelanocortin-derived peptides, including β-endorphin, into the bloodstream (see Fig. 3). Conclusive information eludes us, but sufficient evidence exists to entertain the hypothesis that the stress response may concomitantly increase β-endorphinergic activity at the hypothalamic infundibular nucleus and thus modulate the sensory aspect of pain. These changes facilitate fight or flight and energize psychological coping.

SUMMARY AND IMPLICATIONS OF THE MODEL

The model of the affective dimension of pain construes pain as a complex perceptual state and not a transient sensory phenomenon. Noxious stimulation excites central noradrenergic pathways associated with hypervigilance and fear (the LC and the DNB), as well as spinothalamocortical pathways. Consequently, the experience of pain includes negative emotional arousal. As emotional expression exists primarily for social communication, pain expression is an emotional phenomenon and a social stimulus.

The HPA axis adds to arousal by exciting neuroendocrine and autonomic mechanisms concomitantly. This axis mobilizes and coordinates a global physiologic stress response and prepares the individual for flight-or-fight behavior. Both physiologic and psychological stress contribute to pain states. Psychological stress, largely cognitively mediated, interacts with physiologic stress. Collectively, central noradrenergic and hypothalamic mechanisms determine the distress that an injured or sick person in pain experiences to a much greater degree than the does the sensory intensity of the pain.

The model holds that pain is a state of discomfort and distress, and not a transient event. It accounts for the complex nature of clinical pain, emphasizing the negative affect of pain above, but not to the exclusion of, its sensory qualities. It identifies the complaint of pain as an emotional expression in contradistinction to a psychophysical report, and suggests that interventions for patients in pain should target emotional as well as sensory processes.

REFERENCES

Abou-Samra AB. Mechanisms of action of CRF and other regulators of ACTH release in pituitary corticotrophs. In: Ganong WF, Dallman MF, Roberts JL, eds. *The hypothalamic-pituitary-adrenal axis revisited.* New York: Annals of the New York Academy of Sciences, 1987;512:67–84.

Aggleton JP, Mishkin M. The amygdala: sensory gateway to the emotions. In: Plutchik R, Kellerman H, eds. *Emotion: theory, research and experience*, vol. 3. Orlando, FL, Academic Press; 1986;281–299.

Amaral DB, Sinnamon HM. The locus coeruleus: neurobiology of a central noradrenergic nucleus. *Prog Neurobiol* 1977;9:147–196.

Assenmacher I, Szafarczyk A, Alonso G, Ixart G, Barbanel G. Physiology of neuropathways affecting CRH secretion. In: Ganong WF, Dallman MF, Roberts JL, eds. *The hypothalamic-pituitary-adrenal axis revisted*. *Ann NY Acad Sci* 1987;512:149–161.

Aston-Jones G, Foote SL, Segal M. Impulse conduction properties of noradrenergic locus coeruleus axons projecting to monkey cerebrocortex. *Neuroscience* 1985;15:765–777.

Averill JR. A constructivist view of emotion. In: Plutchik R, Kellerman H, eds. *Emotion: theory, research, and experience*, vol. 1. New York: Academic Press, 1980;305–339.

Bing Z, Villanueva L, Le Bars D. Ascending pathways in the spinal cord involved in the activation of subnucleus reticularis dorsalis neurons in the medulla of the rat. *J Neurophysiol* 1990;63:424–438.

Bonica JJ, ed. *The management of pain*. 2nd ed. Philadelphia: Lea & Febiger, 1990.

Bower GH. Mood and memory. *Am Psychol* 1981;36:129–148.

Bowsher D. Role of the reticular formation in responses to noxious stimulation. *Pain* 1976;2:361–378.

Burstein R, Cliffer KD, Giesler GJ. The spinohypothalamic and spinotelencephalic tracts: direct nociceptive projections from the spinal cord to the hypothalamus and telencephalon. In: Dubner R, Gebhart GF, Bond MR, eds. *Proceedings of the 5th World Congress on Pain*. New York: Elsevier, 1988;548–554.

Butler PD, Weiss JM, Stout JC, Nemeroff CB. Corticotropin-releasing factor produces fear-enhancing and behavioral activating effects following infusion into the locus coeruleus. *J Neurosci* 1990;10:176–183.

Calogero AE, Bernardini R, Gold PW, Chrousos GP. Regulation of rat hypothalamic corticotropin-releasing hormone secretion in vitro: potential clinical implications. *Adv Exp Med Biol* 1988;245: 167–181.

Cannon WB. *Bodily changes in pain, hunger, fear, and rage*, 2nd ed. New York: Appleton, 1929.

Charney DS, Woods SW, Nagy LM, Southwick SM, Krystal JH, Heniger GR. Noradrenergic function in panic disorder. *J Clin Psychiatry* 1990;51(Suppl A):5–11.

Dahlström A, Fuxe K. Evidence for the existence of monoamine-containing neurons in the central nervous system. *Acta Physiol Scand* 1964;62:1–55.

Darwin C. *The expression of the emotions in man and animals*. London: John Murray, 1872.

Elam M, Svensson TH, Thoren P. Differentiated cardiovascular afferent regulation of locus coeruleus neurons and sympathetic nerves. *Brain Res* 1985;358:77–84.

Elam M, Svensson TH, Thoren P. Locus coeruleus neurons and sympathetic nerves: activation by cutaneous sensory afferents. *Brain Res* 1986a;366:254–261.

Elam M, Svensson TH, Thoren P. Locus coeruleus neurons and sympathetic nerves: activation by visceral afferents. *Brain Res* 1986b;375:117–125.

Fields HL. *Pain*. New York: McGraw-Hill, 1987.

Fillenz M. *Noradrenergic neurons*. Cambridge: Cambridge University Press, 1990.

Fonberg E. Amygdala, emotions, motivation, and depressive states. In: Plutchik R, Kellerman H, eds. *Emotion: theory, research and experience*, vol. 3. Orlando, FL: Academic Press, 1986;301–331.

Foote SL, Bloom FE, Aston-Jones G. Nucleus locus ceruleus: new evidence of anatomical and physiological specificity. *Physiol Rev* 1983;63:844–914.

Foote SL, Morrison JH. Extrathalamic modulation of corticofunction. *Annu Rev Neurosci* 1987;10:67–95.

Fordyce WE. Contingency management. In: Bonica JJ, ed. *The management of pain*, 2nd ed. Philadelphia: Lea & Febiger, 1990;1702–1710.

Fulton JE, ed. *Frontal lobotomy and affective behavior*. New York: WW Norton and Company, 1951.

Gabriel M, Sparenborg SP, Stolar N. The neurobiology of memory. In: LeDoux JE, Hirst W, eds. *Mind and brain: dialogues in cognitive neuroscience*. Cambridge: Cambridge University Press, 1986;215–254.

Gray JA. *The neuropsychology of anxiety: an enquiry into the functions of the septo-hippocampal system*. New York: Oxford University Press, 1982.

Gray JA. *The psychology of fear and stress*, 2nd ed. Cambridge: Cambridge University Press, 1987.

Heath RG. The neural substrate for emotion. In: Plutchik R, Kellerman H, eds. *Emotion: theory, research, and experience*, vol. 3. New York: Academic Press, 1986;3–35.

Henry JP. Neuroendocrine patterns of emotional response. In: Plutchik R, Kellerman H, eds. *Emotion: theory, research, and practice*, vol. 3. Orlando, FL: Academic Press, 1986;37–60.

Hess WR. *Diencephalon: autonomic and extrapyramidal functions*. New York: Grune & Stratton, 1954.

Isaacson RL, ed. *The limbic system*, 2nd ed. New York: Plenum Press, 1982.

Jänig W. The autonomic nervous system. In: Schmidt RF, ed. *Fundamentals of neurophysiology*. New York: Springer-Verlag, 1985a;216–269.

Jänig W. Systemic and specific autonomic reactions in pain: efferent, afferent and endocrine components. *Eur J Anaesth* 1985b;2:319–346.

Kanosue K, Nakayama T, Ishikawa Y, Imai-Matsumura K. Responses of hypothalamic and thalamic neurons to noxious and scrotal thermal stimulation in rats. *J Thermobiol* 1984;9:11–13.

Korf J, Bunney BS, Aghajanian GK. Noradrenergic neurons: morphine inhibition of spontaneous activity. *Eur J Pharmacol* 1974;25:165–169.

Krukoff TL. Neuropeptide regulation of autonomic outflow at the sympathetic preganglionic neuron: anatomical and neurochemical specificity. *Ann NY Acad Sci* 1990;579:162–167.

Lacey JI, Lacey BC. Some autonomic-central nervous system interrelationships. In: Black P, ed. *Physiological correlates of emotion*. New York: Academic Press, 1970;205–227.

Lazarus RS. From psychological stress to the emotions: a history of changing outlooks. *Annu Rev Psychol* 1993;44:1–21.

LeDoux JE, Iwata J, Cicchetti P, Reis DJ. Different projections of the central amygdaloid nucleus mediate autonomic and behavioral correlates of conditioned fear. *J Neurosci* 1988;8:2517–2529.

LeDoux JE, Farb C, Ruggiero DA. Topographic organization of neurons in the acoustic thalamus that project to the amygdala. *J Neurosci* 1990;10:1043–1054.

Levitt P, Moore RY. Origin and organization of the brainstem catecholamine innervation in the rat. *J Comp Neurol* 1979;186:505–528.

Lopez JF, Young EA, Herman JP, Akil H, Watson SJ. Regulatory biology of the HPA axis: an integrative approach. In: Risch SC, ed. *Central nervous system peptide mechanisms in stress and depression*. Washington, DC: American Psychiatric Press, 1991;1–52.

MacLean PD. Some psychiatric implications of physiological studies on frontotemoral portion of limbic system (visceral brain). *Electroencephalogr Clin Neurophysiol* 1952;4:407–418.

MacLean PD. *The triune brain in evolution: role in paleocerebral functions*. New York: Plenum Press, 1990.

Mancia G, Zanchetti A. Hypothalamic control of autonomic functions. In: Morgane JP, Panksepp J, eds. *Handbook of the hypothalamus: behavioral functions of the hypothalamus*, vol. 3. New York: Dekker, 1981;147–202.

McNaughton N, Mason ST. The neuropsychology and neuropharmacology of the dorsal ascending noradrenergic bundle—a review. *Prog Neurobiol* 1980;14:157–219.

Merskey H. Pain terms: a list with definitions and a note on usage. Recommended by the International Association for the Study of Pain (IASP) Subcommittee on Taxonomy. *Pain* 1979;6:249–252.

Morilak DA, Fornal CA, Jacobs BL. Effects of physiological manipulations on locus coeruleus neuronal activity in freely moving cats. II. Cardiovascular challenge. *Brain Res* 1987;422:24–31.

Ortony A, Turner TJ. What's basic about basic emotions? *Psychol Rev* 1990;97:315–331.

Osborne FH, Mattingley BA, Redmon WK, Osborne JS. Factors affecting the measurement of classically conditioned fear in rats following exposure to escapable versus inescapable signaled shock. *J Exp Psychol* 1975;1:364–373.

Pandya DN, Barnes CL, Panksepp J. Architecture and connections of the frontal lobe. In: Perecman, E, ed. *The frontal lobes revisited*. Hillsdale, NJ: Lawrence Erlbaum Associates, 1987;41–72.

Panksepp J. The anatomy of emotions. In: Plutchik R, Kellerman H, eds. *Emotion: theory, research, and experience*, vol. 3. Orlando, FL: Academic Press, 1986;91–124.

Papez JW. A proposed mechanism of emotion. *Arch Neurol Psychol* 1937;38:725–743.

Peschanski M, Weil-Fugacza J. Aminergic and cholinergic afferents to the thalamus: experimental data with reference to pain pathways. In: Besson JM, Guilbaud G, Peschanski M, eds. *Thalamus and pain*. Amsterdam: Excerpta Medica, 1987;127–154.

Ploog D. Biological foundations of the vocal expressions of emotions. In: Plutchik R, Kellerman H, eds. *Emotion: theory, research, and experience [biological foundations of emotion]*, vol. 3. New York: Academic Press, 1986;173–198.

Plutchik R. A general psychoevolutionary theory of emotion. In: Plutchik R, Kellerman H, eds. *Emotion: theory, research, and experience*, vol. 1. New York: Academic Press, 1980;3–33.

Pribram KH. The biology of emotions and other feelings. In: Plutchik R, Kellerman H, eds. *Emotion: theory, research, and experience [theories of emotion]*, vol. 1. New York: Academic Press, 1980; 245–269.

Redmond DE Jr, Huang YG. Current concepts. II. New evidence for a locus coeruleus-norepinephrine connection with anxiety. *Life Sci* 1979;25:2149–2162.

Redmond DE Jr. Alteration in the functions of the nucleus locus coeruleus: a possible model for studies of anxiety. In: Hannin I, Usdin E, eds. *Animal models in psychiatry and neurology*. New York: Pergamon Press, 1977;293–306.

Rolls ET. Neural systems involved in emotion in primates. In: Plutchik R, Kellerman H, eds. *Emotion: theory, research, and experience*, vol. 3. New York: Academic Press, 1986;125–144.

Saphier D. Cortisol alters firing rate and synaptic responses of limbic forebrain units. *Brain Res Bull* 1987;19:519–524.

Sapolsky RM. *Stress, the aging brain, and the mechanisms of neuron death*. Cambridge, MA: The MIT Press, 1992.

Sawchenko PE, Swanson LW. The organization of noradrenergic pathways from the brain stem to the paraventricular and supraoptic nuclei in the rat. *Brain Res Rev* 1982;4:275.

Selye H. *The stress of life*. New York: McGraw-Hill, 1978.

Siegel JM, Rogawski MA. A function for REM sleep: regulation of noradrenergic receptor sensitivity. *Brain Res Rev* 1988;13:213–233.

Staddon JER. *Adaptive behavior and learning*. London: Cambridge University Press, 1983.

Stone EA. Stress and catecholamines. In: Friedhoff AJ, ed. *Catecholamines and behavior*, vol. 2. New York: Plenum Press, 1975;31–72.

Sumal KK, Blessing WW, Joh TH, Reis DJ, Pickel VM. Synaptic interaction of vagal afference and catecholaminergic neurons in the rat nucleus tractus solitarius. *J Brain Res* 1983;277:31–40.

Svensson TH. Peripheral, autonomic regulation of locus coeruleus noradrenergic neurons in brain: putative implications for psychiatry and psychopharmacology. *Psychopharmacology* 1987;92:1–7.

Talbott JD, Marrett S, Evans AC, Meyer E, Bushnell MC, Duncan JH. Multiple representations of pain in human cerebral cortex. *Science* 1991;251:1355–1358.

Tucker DM, Vannatta K, Rothlind J. Arousal and activation systems and primitive adaptive controls on cognitive priming. In: Stein NL, Leventhal D, Trabasso T, eds. *Psychological and biological approaches to emotion*. Hillsdale, NJ: Lawrence Erlbaum Associates, 1990;145–166.

Turner BH, Mishkin M, Knapp M. Organization of the amygdalopedal projections from modality-specific cortical association areas in the monkey. *J Comp Neurol* 1980;19:515–543.

Watson SJ, Khachaturian H, Lewis ME, Akil H. Chemical neuroanatomy as a basis for biological psychiatry. In: Berger PA, Brodie HKH, eds. *Biological psychiatry*, vol. 8. (Arieti S, ed. *American handbook of psychiatry*, 2nd ed.). New York: Basic Books, 1986;4–33.

Willis WD Jr, ed. *The pain system: the neurobasis of nociceptive transmission in the mammalian nervous system*. New York: Karger, 1985.

Villanueva L, Bing Z, Bouhassira D, Le Bars D. Encoding of electrical, thermal, and mechanical noxious stimuli by subnucleus reticularis dorsalis neurons in the rat medulla. *J Neurophysiol* 1989;61:391–402.

Villanueva L, Cliffer KD, Sorkin LS, Le Bars D, Willis WD Jr. Convergence of heterotopic nociceptive information onto neurons of caudal medullary reticular formation in monkey (Macaca fascicularis). *J Neurophysiol* 1990;63:1118–1127.

Pain and the Brain: From
Nociception to Cognition,
edited by Burkhart Bromm and
John E. Desmedt, Advances in Pain
Research and Therapy Vol. 22.
Raven Press, Ltd., New York © 1995.

19

From Nociception to Pain: The Role of Emotion

Kenneth D. Craig

Department of Psychology, University of British Columbia, Vancouver, V6T 1Z4, British Columbia Canada

SUMMARY

Understanding the complex interactions among pain, emotion, and consciousness is a profoundly complex challenge, but an examination of their interrelationships informs our understanding of each. While each is known through personal experience, their definition and measurement are difficult, given their status as subjective states. Pain has a powerful capacity to command conscious attention, even to the extent of disrupting other activities, with emotional qualities empirically discriminable and representing the salient, "hot" side of thoughts and images during pain. The biologic primacy of painful experience and the threat to well-being it represents motivate defensive and recuperative action. This formulation of the role of emotion during pain is consistent with current concepts that emphasize emotions as action dispositions which organize and direct appetitive/aversive experience and behavior. While pain is ordinarily construed as disruptive and disorganizing, it can be seen as focusing attention and mobilizing resources. Unfortunately, only in recent decades has serious attention been devoted to emotional qualities of pain, relative to the sensory qualities largely emphasized in the early 20th century. This chapter reviews a number of controversies in the study of emotions that parallel issues in the current understanding of pain: Should we emphasize the biologic, inherent, and universal features of pain or emotions, or attend to their qualities as social constructions and events that vary with personal histories and the situational context? Should emotional and painful behavior be construed as indicative of internal states or as forms of communication that have an impact on observers? Evidence for a substantial impact of the social context on pain and illness behavior argues for greater attention to the communicative domain. Finally, are anxiety and depression discriminable conditions that are relatively specific to acute and chronic states? Our recent studies indicate greater difficulty than expected in discriminating between patients in acute and chronic states, with patterns of emotional distress, preoccupation with harm, and medically incongruent pain persisting in certain patients in chronic states. These findings suggest new approaches to the prevention of, and intervention into debilitating pain.

INTRODUCTION

Pain, emotion, and consciousness each are profoundly complex topics. All have long represented core preoccupations of scholars of the human condition, yet all continue to defy total comprehension, and the task of attempting to understand their relationships is daunting. In part, this reflects the status of each of these complex states as subjective experiences. While these states are well known through personal experience, they can only be known to others through inference. Subjective experiences cannot be observed directly by others, but require indirect measurement that is often subject to ambiguous interpretation.

Our current understanding of pain emphasizes the key role we assign to conscious experience. Consciousness itself is easier to illustrate in personal experience than it is to define. Whatever the individual is experiencing at the moment effectively represents consciousness, but the defining characteristics of the experience, and the processes regulating it, resist easy understanding (Baars 1988). A working definition of consciousness would characterize it as a state of experience in which events are attended to at a level of focal awareness and are addressed in the thoughts of the individual. The structures and events needed in a theory of consciousness must address both the cognitive processes involved in the acquisition and use of knowledge (the rational, logical, "cool" side) and the motives and emotions that organize, disrupt, and give meaning to our lives (the irrational, less predictable, and "heated" side). The experience of consciousness is very complex, and comprises a dynamic flow of turbulent, intimate feelings, images, and thoughts that are not readily reduced to descriptive language. Events capture our attention because they are interesting, with this quality in turn reflecting whether a particular event is anomalous (unexpected) or affectively arousing (Bower 1992).

Consideration must also be given to the opposite of consciousness, the role of the unconscious as a determinant of behavior. There is evidence that people are influenced by internal and external events that they have not noticed, or whose impact on their thoughts, feelings, and behavior they do not seem to comprehend (Bowers 1987). For example, Lazarus (1987) observed that personal well-being can be appraised in a primitive, unconscious, subcortical manner, perhaps through some form of precognition, in contrast to the meaningful, analytic appreciation of events. Concepts of the unconscious are not without criticism, but the role of unconscious mechanisms and events as determinants of conscious experience and behavior arising from noxious events must be considered.

Pain certainly falls within the class of events that has the capacity to capture conscious attention and to direct behavior. In the course of evolution, humans became endowed with a capacity to detect and evaluate noxious internal states, with conscious experience emerging later rather than sooner. The pain system has biologic primacy and importance, since it has the capacity to interrupt and even disrupt ongoing activity, and demands and maintains attention, with affective distress its most salient feature. The captured attention should allow the organism to solve the urgent crisis through defensive behavior, escape, and efforts to recuperate. From this perspective, the sensory changes instigated by tissue-damaging events operate to capture the attention of the organism, and the emotional responses would reflect dispositions to defensive action.

Current thinking accepts the proposition that it is inappropriate to characterize peripheral physiologic events as pain, with this term instead referring to the conscious experience of pain. We distinguish between nociception, or the processes regulating the transduction, transmission, and modulation of noxious stimuli in the nervous system, and pain (Fields 1987), which by convention is reserved for the perceptual experience. Only when the nociceptive assault is processed at the level of conscious experience do we characterize the event as pain.

Our understanding of pain would be dramatically enhanced if we knew how nociception gave rise to the subjective experience of pain, but the puzzle of consciousness remains a serious problem for neurobiology (e.g., Crick and Koch 1992). In the absence of such knowledge, an understanding of the experience of pain in its own right will allow us to better know what the biologic substrates of pain should be able to explain. Reducing the conscious experience of pain to biologic events will have to include a broad range of phenomena. It is also important to recognize that biologic and psychological interpretations of pain should not entail dualistic thinking. The two are different perspectives on the same process. The physiologic explanations are not restricted to an account of the events that give rise to the sensation of pain, while the psychological explanations address the way in which some immaterial mind inspects the sensory information of pain and perceives the sensation with affect, memories, and interpretations (Wall 1989). Only after we understand how the brain constructs the experience of pain by integrating nociceptive afferents with past experience will the major issues on the neurobiologic basis of pain be settled. If we are to seek biologic substrates, then, in terms of contemporary tripartite models of pain, the biologic substrates of the sensory, affective, cognitive appraisal, and behavioral components of pain will also have to be understood (e.g., Derryberry and Tucker 1992).

EMOTION IN DEFINITIONS OF PAIN

The fundamental role of affective distress in pain is clearly identified in the International Association for the Study of Pain (IASP) definition of pain as "an unpleasant sensory and emotional experience associated with actual or potential tissue damage, or described in terms of such damage" (IASP 1979, p. 250). It is evident that the sensory experience would not be pain if there were no perception of emotional distress. As the IASP Committee on Taxonomy (IASP 1979) put it, "(Pain) is unquestionably a sensation in a part or parts of the body but it is also always unpleasant and therefore also an emotional experience" (p. 250).

These distinctions are important. Fernandez and Turk (1992) recently examined a basic premise arising from these efforts to establish the experience of pain as comprising different and distinct qualities. They ask whether it is empirically valid to distinguish sensory from affective experiential properties. To what extent is sensation actually distinct from affect in the conscious experience of pain? The review advances our understanding beyond theoretical debate based on introspection to encompass diverse empirical research methodologies that have been brought to bear on the issue. These have included multivariate statistical analyses, applications of signal-detection theory, and unidimensional scaling studies. Fernandez and Turk conclude that it is possible to tease apart separate sensory and affective-distress aspects of pain, but that they remain highly intercorrelated and not distinct, and state that there is a "less-than-tidy separation of sensory and affective components of pain." The sensory experience may give rise to the emotional distress of pain, but the emotional distress can also amplify the sensory experience. It remains uncertain what operations differentially influence the various qualities, and what their separate and interactive contributions are to the overall conscious experience of pain. Answers to these questions should greatly enhance the development of interventions that selectively modify certain features of the overall pain experience. There is substantial evidence that patients describe different forms of pain in very different ways (for a review, see Craig 1993). The capacity to discriminate different qualities of the pain experience is also consistent with observations that these qualities have at least partially separate neuroanatomic substrates (Fields 1987).

This distinction has a key bearing on research we are planning in collaboration with emergency-room physicians (Grunfeld et al. 1992). Patients presenting with acute abdominal pain are often required to wait without analgesics for protracted periods until surgeons can examine them. Surgeons object to the use of analgesics because they may mask pain and the courts may deem the patient's capacity to provide consent for surgery, should it be needed, as being impaired. Emergency-care physicians, on the other hand, argue that analgesics do not necessarily mask the salient qualities of pain, pain itself may impair both the capacity to report symptoms and provide consent, and that it is humane to control pain. These are interesting propositions amenable to empirical study.

EMOTION IN MODELS OF PAIN

Most clinicians and pain researchers would generally agree with the centrality of emotional distress to the experience of pain, but the degree of importance attached to understanding and treating the emotional qualities of the experience has varied widely over time. The characterization of pain as having distinctively unpleasant qualities is a time-honored point of view that dates back at least to Aristotle and his antecedents. He described pain as a feeling state rather than a sensation (Dallenbach

1939; Keele 1957). To the ancient Greeks, pain was an essential emotional component of the human spirit—the negative counterpart to pleasure. Enduring concepts
recognized pain as an affective experience, like sadness or bitterness, signaling
something to be avoided or terminated, but not as a sense, because it was not
referable to any specific quality of external objects. Wall (1979) similarly noted the
limited information available about the nature of the stimulus in the experience of
pain. Rey (1993) concluded that in antiquity one of the consequences of the emerging use of medical language to understand and master pain was to separate it from
its powerful emotional effect.

At the end of the last and the beginning of this century there was a vigorous
debate about whether pain should be characterized as an emotion or a sensation. For
example, Marshall (1894) asserted that "pleasures and pains can in no proper sense
be classed with sensations." The debate was largely won by those who focused on
pain as a sensation arising from tissue damage.

This century has seen many major advances in the understanding of peripheral
and central biologic mechanisms in pain, and successes in efforts to control pain
that have focused on the sensory mechanisms. In terms of current conceptualiza-
tions of pain, this focus on the sensory mechanisms in pain has helped us to understand pain in terms of its temporal, spatial, pressure, thermal, and related properties
(Melzack, 1975), while leaving the roles of affective tension, fear, and stress uncertain. Thus, understanding of the sensory processes in pain was achieved at the cost
of relegating other complexities of the subjective experience to a subordinate role.

With progress through the 20th century, renewed attention was devoted to affective qualities of pain (Rey 1993). A variety of factors led to this change in approach.
We have often failed to provide adequate, comprehensive care for patients when an
exclusively biophysical model of pain has been used. It also became clear that the
substantial individual differences and varying needs for treatment in response to
apparently similar nociceptive events can be best understood by addressing cognitive and emotional features of the individual's experience of pain and disability.

Midway through the 20th century, a tentative role had been assigned to the complexities of subjective experience as theories of pain came to distinguish between
sensory components that were deemed primary, causal, and antecedent to secondary
qualities, and these secondary or reactive qualities that reflected distress and subjective feelings (Beecher 1959; Hardy et al. 1952). The reactive component was construed as subject to influence by more than the sensory component. Thus, Beecher
effectively attracted attention to placebos and the key roles of anxiety and personal
control in the experience of pain.

More recently, evidence for descending inhibitory and facilitative processes in
the central nervous system (CNS) has indicated that affective and cognitive mechanisms play an early role in the nociceptive afferent barrage. Our model of pain has
now become a complex, systems-oriented formulation that can account for many
phenomena. Emphasis has been on concurrent rather than sequential processes,
with sensory, affective, and cognitive qualities all characterized as potentially arising in parallel and interacting with each other. Thus, Melzack and Casey (1968)

proposed a model of pain that includes a sensory–discriminative dimension focusing on spatial and temporal properties, a motivational–affective dimension involving tension, fear, and autonomic events, and an evaluative dimension incorporating the individual's appraisal of the situation. Leventhal and Everhart (1979) proposed that sensory and affective qualities of pain are processed almost simultaneously (Fernandez and Turk 1992).

These formulations are abstract and seem remote from the experiences of the patients with whom we work, but they are of direct relevance to understanding and managing pain. For example, most physicians find it awkward to fully address emotional distress in patients' lives. Moving outside the domain of diagnosing and treating physical pathology often creates unfamiliar demands, and physicians may not have the time, energy, or competence to address patients' emotional concerns in the detail they require. It is easier to listen to complaints of pain if they are interpreted as keys to physical pathology than it is to open the door to a patient's psychosocial woes. This willingness to listen to complaints of pain and to be less interested in emotional distress may promote somatization of emotional distress. Generally, if the thoughts and feelings of patients are important determinants of painful distress and associated disability, they need to be addressed.

EMOTION

Given its complexity, emotion may be even more difficult to define than pain. The term "emotion" is generic, and includes many different subjective states. One can observe vast individual differences in the emotional behavior of patients. With regard to this, the emphasis in this chapter has been on the affective distress that is integral to the experience of pain, but there are also emotional components of the experience that are provoked by concurrent events or which can be brought to the situation. Fear, anxiety, and depression are most often observed, but anger, guilt, subservience, and even sexual arousal have been implicated. To understand the complex role of emotion in pain, one must also consider emotional distress as a cause of pain, a consequence of pain, and a state concurrent with pain (Craig 1993).

There are many different theories of emotion (e.g., Frijda 1986; Izard 1979). For example, Izard and Blumberg (1985) observed that "the emotion system is viewed as the principal motivational system for human beings. The emotions are seen as adaptive and motivating organizers of experience and behavior." From this perspective, pain-instigated emotion represents disruption and a redirection of activity. This would reflect the position of Frijda (1988, p. 351), who noted that emotions "can be defined in terms of some form of action tendency or some form of activation or lack thereof." Lang et al. (1990, p. 377) similarly defined emotions as "action dispositions, founded on brain states that organize behavior along a basic appetitive-aversive dimension," and concluded that "The efferent system as a whole (including exteroceptive reflexes) is presumably tuned according to the current status of this central affect-motivational organization" (p. 377). While the affective distress associated with pain is usually seen as disruptive and disorganizing, these perspectives permit a focus on the motivational properties of emotions and their capacity to mobilize the resources of the individual.

The intensity of the emotional distress provoked by pain most often appears to lead to relatively automatic, less well-considered activity, and leaves the individual less capable of well-considered action plans (Kanfer in press).

With painful injury, this is evident in fast, preemptive, preprogrammed reflexes, most of which are difficult to inhibit, that may include startle, flinching, facial grimaces, screaming, autonomic changes, or withdrawal from the noxious stimulus (Craig et al. 1991; 1992). It is these signs of emotional distress that best allow us to recognize that someone is in pain. Moreover, even basic reflexes, such as startle (Lang et al. 1990) or the newborn's reaction to heel lancing (Grunau and Craig 1987) are well-integrated with CNS states and reflect the individual's ongoing emotional and biologic status.

It is instructive to examine ongoing controversies in the study of emotions, since they provoke a different perspective on the nature of pain.

CULTURAL INFLUENCES ON EMOTIONAL EXPERIENCE

There is ongoing research on whether the various emotions are universal (i.e., inherent and immutable) or predominantly cultural (Mesquita and Frijda 1992). The contrasting perspectives resemble a similar diversity of opinion in research on pain. The current and dominant perspective on pain would appear to emphasize its sensory, biologic, and universal qualities, ignoring its plasticity. Since emotional distress is fundamental to the experience of pain, a conclusion that emotions are at least in part social constructions would be consistent with the proposition that the experience of pain also has elements of social construction (e.g., Craig 1986). Mesquita and Frijda (1992) reviewed evidence for cultural determinants of emotion, and support the position that they are important. Parallel arguments can be generated for pain, as discussed in the following sections.

Is Tissue Damage the Invariant Antecedent Event for Pain?

Complaints of pain invariably lead to efforts to identify the tissue damage or stress responsible for the experience. This usually works. Pain most often is not mysterious or esoteric. People suffer injuries or identifiable disease, experience pain in consequence, and are treated for both the disease and pain. Fortunately, they get better and the pain goes away. However, "occult" pain is also a significant problem. Frequently, a source of pain cannot be identified. Similarly, there are patients for whom the accompanying emotional distress and disability are excessive or minimal relative to the severity of an injury, and those whose pain persists beyond the time at which healing should have taken place. But this is occult or beyond human understanding only to those who fail to appreciate that psychosocial events are potent determinants of the experience and expression of pain.

Injuries, disease, and somatic experiences affect individuals in different ways in a manner that is consistent with their personal backgrounds, family experiences, and cultural assimilation. These learning experiences affect the manner in which we appraise painful events, with the end product often vastly different among individuals. At the level of the individual, this is well illustrated by the clinical problem of panic attacks, in which chest pains are appraised as affecting the individual's well-being in strikingly different ways, with efforts to cope with the threat also varying dramatically. Patients with panic disorder are organically healthy, but they experience attacks of severe somatic symptoms, such as palpitations, dyspnea, or faintness, that are accompanied by severe fear or discomfort (Clark 1986; Ehlers and Breuer 1992).

Cultural Influences on Overt Behavior During Emotion and Pain

Both emotional states and pain include variations in activation and readiness for action. For example, fear involves being alerted to protect oneself from danger, and the individual may be predisposed biologically or through experience to be self-protecting, avoidant, aggressive, or help-seeking. Similarly, the observation that pain resembles a need state rather than a sensory experience (Bolles and Fanselow 1980; Wall 1979) is parallel to the observation that emotion has a capacity to provoke readiness for action. Wall (1979) characterized pain as a drive state, stating that "pain signals the existence of a body state (in which) recovery and recuperation should be initiated."

Emphasis on readiness for action implies that overt behavior should permit inference of the subject's motivational state. Indeed, motivational and emotional states are commonly inferred from spontaneous expressive behavior and activity designed to control events provocative of an emotion. The sensitivity of the behavior to the immediate context of a situation implies subtle variations in the individual's emotional reaction. The operant perspective (Fordyce 1976; Keefe and Dunsmore 1992) effectively illustrates the subtle but powerful shaping impact of social influence and reinforcement mechanisms on illness behavior, but has had relatively little to say about emotional processes.

In contrast, research on relationships between facial activity and emotional processes has a long and productive history (e.g., Ekman et al. 1972). Current controversy about the way in which facial activity during emotion-provoking events should be interpreted illustrates interest in cultural influences. Beginning with Darwin (1872/1965), facial actions have been conceptualized as expressive of internal states. Several patterns of facial activity have been shown to be reliably associated with specific emotions across a wide variety of literate and preliterate societies. These apparently universal facial expressions include happiness, sadness, surprise, fear, anger, disgust (Ekman et al. 1969), and contempt (Ekman and Friesen 1986).

But these well-established findings have been questioned with suggestions that emphasis should be redirected toward the role of facial activity as a form of influence on other people, or as a form of communication (Fridlund 1991; Gilbert et al. 1987). Stressing the communicative importance of facial activity again puts the emphasis on situational specificity and social contexts of pain.

The role of the face as a communicator of emotional distress during pain has become conspicuous in studies of pain in newborns. We have consistently observed in the neonate a relatively stereotypic reaction to tissue-damaging events (e.g., heel sticks for blood sampling, or needle injections) that resembles activity in the older child and adult (Grunau and Craig 1987; Craig et al. 1993). This reaction therefore appears to be reasonably interpreted as pain, but pain differing in quality from the pain experienced by older children and adults. The newborn has neither the necessary capabilities nor the requisite prior experience to cognize the meaning of the experience. Hence, the reaction is perhaps better interpreted as signifying some combination of somatosensory experience and emotional distress. If, as in adults, the inability to predict termination of the painful event adds distress, then one would infer that the newborn's experience could approach raw terror (Craig and Grunau 1993).

The complex interactions between painful distress and related emotional experiences in adults have been effectively illustrated by LeResche and Dworkin (1988). They identified concurrent expressions of fear, anger, disgust, contempt, and sadness overlapping the facial display of pain in patients with provoked pain from temporomandibular joint disorder (TMJD). Facial displays and reports of pain were more severe for persons showing a greater number of different negative affects.

We have examined in detail elsewhere evidence that pain experience and behavior (Craig 1986; Craig et al. 1993), and the capacity to cope with pain (Bennett-Branson and Craig 1993), are subject to influences of socialization in the course of development. The end products are specific ways of thinking and behaving during pain that reflect the individual's cultural and familial background. A recent investigation (Walker et al. 1993) of probable psychosocial origins of recurrent abdominal pain (RAP) in children effectively illustrates the case. Walker and associates found that relative to healthy children, those with RAP and those suffering from gastrointestinal illness had more severe emotional and somatic symptoms and families characterized by a high incidence of illness and greater encouragement of child-illness behavior. The presence of more first-degree relatives with current or past abdominal disorders and more relatives with other serious health conditions living in the home might reflect physical vulnerability as a result of genetic or environmental factors, but is also consistent with social psychological explanations, including influences of social modeling and the vicarious learning of illness behavior in these families. It is also noteworthy that particular psychosocial factors were associated with pediatric pain that both had and did not have an organic etiology, underscoring the need to address these factors even when physical pathology is present.

From a broader anthropologic perspective, it should be noted that somatic events can have different socially shared meanings across cultures and give rise to different emotional states. A paper by Sargent (1984) effectively illustrates this. She provided an ethnographic description of reactions to such apparently painful events as childbirth, wounds, and initiation ordeals in the Bariba peoples, a major ethnic group in West Africa. The Bariba folklore is replete with examples of stoicism in the face of pain, and Sargent (1984) provides several dramatic illustrations of these. For example, writes Sargent, "the woman in childbirth is expected to endure labor and delivery without any expression of discomfort. Ideally, she will not display to friends or relatives that she is in labor, will deliver alone and call for help with cutting the umbilical cord" (p. 1300). The context of ritual circumcision for 9- to 11-year-old boys is described as follows. "They are told in detail the nature of the procedure to which they will be subjected, the feelings they will experience, the response which they are expected to manifest. Although not all children have observed initiations prior to their own, they have had ample opportunity to observe adults and other children reacting to other types of pain-provoking experiences. Moreover, they have been exposed to mockeries of those who complain and praises of those who perform with courage, and have received corresponding admonitions or praises when hurt or sick themselves" (p. 1302). Concepts of pain in the Bariba peoples are intimately linked to those of honor and shame. The ideal expression of courage dictates indifference, minimal response, and efforts to continue with routines despite debility and pain. Socialization practices involving praise and chastisement and the use of parables and heroic tales, together with social modeling, encourage a particularly stoical response to painful experiences such as circumcision and clitoridectomy.

There is other ample evidence for cross-cultural variation in emotional reactions to pain and illness. For example, pain was less likely to represent an antecedent to sadness among the Japanese than among European and American groups (Scherer et al. 1988). In this survey of the antecedents to emotions, bodily pains or illnesses were reported to represent antecedents to sadness among 10% of American and European respondents to a survey, but among no more than 5% of the Japanese.

The Anxiety-Depression Relationship

Anxiety and depression are often described as discrete psychological entities, with anxiety presumably reflecting preoccupation with injury and harm and depression concerning loss or failure to achieve goals. The research literature makes it increasingly clear that these are not discrete states (Dobson 1985). This is particularly true for the diagnostic categories treated as anxiety or depressive disorders, in which there is a striking overlap in symptoms (Kendall and Clarkin 1992), and the term "negative affectivity" is increasingly used (Watson et al. 1988). Symptoms of anxiety are often characteristic of people described as depressed (Kendall et al. 1992).

Parallel distinctions need to be made about the role of anxiety and depression in pain disorders. Certain time-honored, clinically based propositions about relationships between pain and emotions are beginning to be questioned. For example, it has been proposed that anxiety states are primarily associated with acute pain, reflecting the subject's apprehension that pain may continue to intensify or could be interminable, or that the tissue-damaging source of pain may be life-threatening. In contrast, persistent or chronic pain has been seen as more commonly associated with sadness and depression (Sternbach 1974). Similarly, there have been pervasive assumptions that pain that persists and becomes chronic involves a greater psychological cost to the individual, with emergent depression, disability, and invalidism (Melzack 1988; Sternbach 1974, 1984; Turk, in press). Despite the importance of these assumptions, few studies have contrasted patients with acute and chronic pain, although those that are available indicate greater variability within each group and more overlap between the two groups than was expected (Ackerman and Stevens 1989; Philips and Grant 1991).

We recently explored similarities and differences among patients with acute and chronic low back pain (Hadjistavropoulos and Craig 1994). The latter group was categorized as either "medically congruent," or having signs and symptoms of pain consistent with known pathophysiologic mechanisms, or "medically incongruent" (Reesor and Craig 1988), on the basis of inappropriate symptom complaints (e.g., vague and poorly localized symptoms, lacking in patterns of symptom progression) (Waddell and Main 1984), nonorganic physical signs (e.g., overreaction, unusual tenderness, unexpected patterns of straight leg raising, regional disturbances) (Waddell et al. 1980), and unusual drawings of parts of the body in which pain is experienced (e.g., exaggerated or nonanatomic) (Ransford et al. 1976). Note that the distinction here is not based on earlier problematic distinctions between psychogenic and organic pain (Dworkin 1992), nor is it the unfortunate practice of "diagnosis by exclusion," in which psychological dysfunction is presumed because there is no adequate pathophysiologic basis for a complaint. The distinction between medically congruent and incongruent pain is based on verbal reports of symptoms and on the presence of behavior, during a physical examination of behavior, that could not have a basis in pathophysiologic mechanisms given current understanding of the anatomy and physiology of pain (Waddell et al. 1989).

A review of the literature indicates that patients who can be characterized as medically incongruent utilize more health-care resources; have poorer outcomes and response to surgery, rehabilitation, and acupuncture; and are more likely to display ineffective coping, dysfunctional cognition, high levels of anxiety, reports of stronger pain sensations, dysfunctional personality traits identified by the Minnesota Multiphasic Personality Inventory (MMPI), depression, and stronger tendencies toward disease affirmation and somatic preoccupation than patients with congruent signs and symptoms (Hadjistavropoulos and Craig 1994).

Our findings indicated greater similarity between the incongruent patients with acute and chronic pain than the literature would lead one to expect. These groups expressed their pain emotionally, were more likely to use passive coping strategies, and more frequently reported dysfunctional catastrophizing cognitions, among other distinctions, than did the congruent patients with chronic pain. Discriminant function analyses indicated that congruent and incongruent patients with chronic pain could be distinguished primarily by the latter group's tendency to negatively interpret their pain (i.e., to respond emotionally, catastrophize, and describe the pain as unpleasant), collect compensation, and use analgesics regularly.

These findings make clear the emotional, evaluative, and behavioral complexity of both acute and chronic pain. Excessive emotional distress, inadequate coping in the form of passivity and catastrophizing, and excessive or inappropriate behavioral reactions during pain may be identified and treated during early stages. Preventive interventions (e.g., Linton et al. 1989) could forestall persistence or development of the medically incongruent pain pattern and related dysfunctional behavior as described above.

INTERACTIONS BETWEEN PAIN AND EMOTION

It is reasonable to conceptualize pain and emotions as independent states having a substantial impact on each other. For example, in examining the complex relationships between pain and depression, Romano and Turner (1985) noted that depression can provoke pain by increasing pain sensitivity and by reducing pain tolerance, and that pain can serve as a stressor that evokes subsequent depression.

Recently, the deleterious impact of pain on the immune system has been documented (Liebeskind 1991). There are also other routes by which pain can influence immune functioning. Herbert and Cohen (1993) applied meta-analytic procedures to the research literature in examining the relationship between depression and immune-system function. They examined both 35 available studies and did an analysis of a smaller subset of 14 research studies, using a particularly rigorous methodology. Clinical depression was clearly associated with robust and moderate to major decreases in all measures of lymphocyte function (an important and broad-spectrum measure of immune-system competence). The effect suggested a linear relationship between the intensity of depressive affect and immune-system function.

THERAPY

An objective of this symposium was to shed light on new approaches to pain relief. The traditional focus in medicine has been heavily on sensory processes in pain, with emotional processes seen as requiring control by means other than those designed to control the more fundamental problem of pain itself. Recognition of the integral role of affect in the experience of pain could support innovative practices. Specific treatment modalities can have an impact on sensory, affective, or both features of the experience of pain. Both pharmacologic and cognitive/behavioral therapies can be conceptualized in this manner. Targeting emotional properties of the experience of pain may prove to be a cost-effective intervention strategy. It also is possible that instigating emotional states inconsistent with pain, such as a pleasant state of affairs, will inhibit or attenuate defensive reflexes during pain (Lang et al.

1990); the observation that providing newborns with a sugar solution prior to heel lancing and circumcision inhibits pain is consistent with this proposition (Blass and Hoffmeyer 1991). It has also been suggested that therapeutically induced arousal of affect may facilitate the resolution of conflicting emotions and also reactivate biologic systems that ward off pain and depression (Beutler et al. 1986).

ACKNOWLEDGMENTS

The author's research reported in this chapter was supported by grants from the Social Sciences and Humanities Research Council of Canada and the Natural Sciences and Engineering Research Council of Canada.

REFERENCES

Ackerman MD, Stevens M. Acute and chronic pain: pain dimensions and psychological status. *J Clin Psychol* 1989;45:223–228.

Baars BJ. *A cognitive theory of consciousness.* Cambridge: Cambridge University Press, 1988.

Beecher HK. *Measurement of subjective responses: Quantitative effects of drugs.* Oxford: Oxford University Press, 1959.

Bennett-Branson SM, Craig KD. Postoperative pain in children: developmental and family influences on spontaneous coping strategies. *Can J Behav Sci* 1993;25:355–383.

Beutler LE, Engle D, Oro'-Beutler ME, Daldrup R, Meredith K. Inability to express intense affect: a common link between depression and pain. *J Consult Clin Psychol* 1986;54:752–759.

Blass EM, Hoffmeyer LB. Sucrose as an analgesic for newborn infants. *Pediatrics* 1991;87:215–218.

Bolles RC, Fanselow MS. A perceptual-defensive-recuperative model of fear and pain. *Behav Brain Sci* 1980;3:291–323.

Bower GH. How might emotions affect learning? In: Christianson SA, ed. *The handbook of emotion and memory research and theory.* Hillsdale, NJ: Lawrence Erlbaum, 1992;3–31.

Bowers KS. Revisioning the unconscious. *Can Psychol* 1987;28:93–104.

Clark DM. A cognitive approach to panic. *Behav Res Ther* 1986;24:461–470.

Craig KD. Social modeling influences: pain in context. In: Sternbach R, ed. *The psychology of pain*, 2nd ed. New York: Raven Press, 1986:67–96.

Craig KD. Emotional aspects of pain. In: Wall PD, Melzack R, eds. *Textbook of pain*, 3rd ed. Edinburgh: Churchill Livingstone, 1993.

Craig KD, Bennett-Branson SM. Developmental factors, psychological coping processes and parental influence. In: Merskey H, Prkachin KM, eds. *The prevention of postoperative pain.* London, Ontario: The Canadian Pain Society, 1993:44–76.

Craig KD, Grunau RVE. Neonatal pain perception and behavioral measurement. In: Anand KJS, McGrath PJ, eds. *Neonatal pain and distress.* Amsterdam: Elsevier, 1993.

Craig KD, Hyde SA, Patrick CJ. Genuine, suppressed, and faked facial behavior during exacerbation of chronic low back pain. *Pain* 1991;46:295–305.

Craig KD, Prkachin KM, Grunau RVE. The facial expression of pain. In: Turk DC, Melzack R, eds. *Handbook of pain assessment.* New York: Guilford Press, 1992:255–274.

Craig KD, Whitfield, MF, Grunau RVE, Linton J, Hadjistavropoulos HD. Pain in the pre-term neonate: behavioral and physiological indices. *Pain* 1993;52:201–208.

Crick F, Koch C. The problem of consciousness. *Sci Am* 1992;267:153–159.

Dallenbach KM. Pain: history and present status. *Am J Psychol* 1939;52:331–347.

Darwin C. *The expression of the emotions in man and animals.* Chicago: University of Chicago Press, 1872–1965.

Derryberry D, Tucker DM. Neural mechanisms of emotion. *J Consult Clin Psychol* 1992;60:329–338.

Dobson KS. The relation between anxiety and depression. *Clin Psychol Rev* 1985;5:307–324.

Dworkin SF. Perspectives on psychogenic versus biogenic factors in orofacial and other pain states. *Am Pain Soc J* 1992;1:172–180.

Ehlers A, Breuer P. Increased cardiac awareness in panic disorder. *J Abnorm Psychol* 1992;101:371–382.

Ekman P, Friesen WV. A new pan-cultural facial expression of emotion. *Motiv Emot* 1986;10:159–168.

Ekman P, Friesen WV, Ellsworth P. *Emotion in the human face*. Elmsford, NY: Pergamon Press, 1972.

Ekman P, Sorenson RE, Friesen WV. Pan-cultural elements in facial displays of emotion. *Science* 1969;164:86–88.

Fernandez E, Turk DC. Sensory and affective components of pain: separation and synthesis. *Psychol Bull* 1992;112:205–217.

Fields HL. *Pain*. New York: McGraw-Hill, 1987.

Fordyce WE. *Behavioral methods for chronic pain and illness*. St. Louis: CV Mosby, 1976.

Fridlund AJ. Evolution and facial action in reflex, social motive, and paralanguage. *Biol Psychol* 1991;32:3–100.

Frijda NH. *Emotions*. New York: Cambridge University Press, 1986.

Frijda NH. The laws of emotion. *Am Psychol* 1988;43:349–358.

Gilbert AN, Fridlund AJ, Sabini J. Hedonic and social determinants of facial displays to odors. *Chem Senses* 1987;12:355–363.

Grunau RVE, Craig KD. Pain expression in neonates: facial action and cry. *Pain* 1987;28:395–410.

Grunfeld A, Simpson K, Craig KD, Davies N. *Analgesia for acute abdominal pain: effects on diagnostic assessments and cognition*. Research grant application unpublished. University of Vancouver, Canada, 1992.

Hadjistavropoulos HD, Craig KD. Acute and chronic low back pain: Cognitive, affective and behavioral dimensions. *J Consult Clin Psychol*.

Hardy J, Wolff H, Goodell H. *Pain sensations and reactions*. Baltimore: Williams & Wilkins, 1952.

Herbert TB, Cohen S. Depression and immunity: a meta-analytic review. *Psychol Bull* 1993;113:472–486.

International Association for the Study of Pain. Pain terms: a list with definitions and notes on usage. *Pain* 1979;6:249–252.

Izard CE, ed. *Emotion in personality and psychopathology*. New York: Plenum Press, 1979.

Izard CE, Blumberg SH. Emotion theory and the role of emotions in anxiety in children and adults. In: Tuma AH, Maser JD, eds. *Anxiety and the anxiety disorders*. Hillsdale, NJ: Lawrence Erlbaum, 1985:109–129.

Kanfer FH. Motivation and emotion in behavior therapy. In: Dobson KS, Craig KD, eds. *State of the art in cognitive/behavioral therapy*. New York: Sage. (In press).

Keefe FJ, Dunsmore J. Pain behavior: Concepts and controversies. *Am Pain Soc J* 1992;1:92–100.

Keele KD. *Anatomies of pain*. Springfield, IL: Charles C Thomas, 1957.

Kendall PC, Kortlander E, Chansky TE, Brady EU. Comorbidity of anxiety and depression in youth: treatment implications. *J Consult Clin Psychol* 1992;60:869–880.

Kendall PC, Clarkin JF. Introduction to special section: comorbidity and treatment implications. *J Consult Clin Psychol* 1992;60:833–834.

Lang PJ, Bradley MM, Cuthbert BN. Emotion, attention, and the startle reflex. *Psychol Rev* 1990;97:377–395.

Lazarus RS. Revisioning the unconscious. *Can Psychol* 1987;28:105–106.

LeResche L, Dworkin SF. Facial expressions of pain and emotions in chronic TMJD patients. *Pain* 1988;35:71–78.

Leventhal H, Everhart D. Emotions, pain and physical illness. In: Izard CE, ed. *Emotions in personality and psychopathology*. New York: Plenum Press, 1979:261–299.

Liebeskind JC. Pain can kill. *Pain* 1991;44:3–4.

Linton SJ, Bradley LA, Jensen E, Spangfort E, Sundell L. The secondary prevention of low back pain: a controlled study with follow-up. *Pain* 1989;36:197–207.

Marshall HR. Are there special nerves for pain? *J Nerv Ment Dis* 1894;21:71–94.

Melzack R. The McGill Pain Questionnaire: major properties and scoring methods. *Pain* 1975;1:277–299.

Melzack R. The tragedy of needless pain: a call for social action. In: Dubner R, Gebhart GF, Bond MR, eds. *Proceedings of the Vth World Congress on Pain*. Amsterdam: Elsevier, 1988:1–11.

Melzack R, Casey KL. Sensory, motivational and central control of determinants of pain: a new conceptual model. In: Kenshalo DL Jr, ed. *The skin senses*. Springfield, IL: Charles C Thomas, 1968:423–436.

Mesquita B, Frijda NH. Cultural variations in emotions: a review. *Psychol Bull* 1992;112:179–204.

Philips HC. Changing chronic pain experience. *Pain* 1988;32:165–172.

Philips HC, Grant L. The evolution of chronic back pain problems: a longitudinal study. *Behav Res Ther* 1991;29:435–441.

Ransford AO, Cairns D, Mooney V. The pain drawing as an aid to the psychologic evaluation of patients with low back pain. *Spine* 1976;1:127–134.

Reesor KA, Craig KD. Medically incongruent chronic back pain: physical limitations, suffering, and ineffective coping. *Pain* 1988;32:35–45.

Rey R. *History of pain.* Paris: La Decouverte, 1993.

Romano JM, Turner JA. Chronic pain and depression: does the evidence support a relationship? *Psychol Bull* 1985;97:18–24.

Sargent C. Between depth and shame: dimensions of pain in Bariba culture. *Soc Sci Med* 1984;19:1299–1304.

Scherer KR, Walbott HG, Matsumoto D, Kudoh T. Emotional experience in cultural context: a comparison between Europe, Japan, and the United States. In: Scherer KR, eds. *Facets of emotions.* Hillsdale, NJ: Lawrence Erlbaum, 1988:5–30.

Sternbach RA. *Pain patients, traits, and treatments.* New York: Academic Press, 1974.

Sternbach RA. Acute versus chronic pain. In: Wall PD, Melzack R, eds. *Textbook of pain.* Edinburgh: Churchill Livingstone, 1984:173–177.

Turk DC. Cognitive factors in chronic pain and disability. In: Dobson KS, Craig KD, eds. *State of the art in cognitive/behavioral therapy.* New York: Sage. (*In press*).

Waddell G, Main CJ. Assessment of severity in low back pain disorders. *Spine* 1984;9:204–208.

Waddell G, McCulloch JA, Kummel E, Venner RM. Nonorganic physical signs in low back pain. *Spine* 1980;5:209–213.

Waddell G, Pilowsky I, Bond MR. Clinical assessment and interpretation of abnormal illness behavior in low back pain. *Pain* 1989;39:41–53.

Walker LS, Garber J, Greene JW. Psychosocial correlates of recurrent childhood pain: a comparison of pediatric patients with recurrent abdominal pain, organic illness, and psychiatric disorder. *J Abnorm Psychol* 1993;102:248–258.

Wall PD. On the relation of injury to pain. *Pain* 1979;6:253–264.

Wall PD. Introduction. In: Wall PD, Melzack R, eds. *Textbook of pain.* Edinburgh: Churchill Livingstone, 1989:1–18.

Watson D, Clark LA, Carey G. Positive and negative affectivity and their relation to anxiety and depressive disorders. *J Abnorm Psychol* 1988;97:346–353.

Pain and the Brain: From Nociception to Cognition, edited by Burkhart Bromm and John E. Desmedt, Advances in Pain Research and Therapy Vol. 22. Raven Press, Ltd., New York © 1995.

20

Hierarchical Clustering of Pain and Emotion Descriptors: Toward a Revision of the McGill Pain Questionnaire

*W. Crawford Clark, †J. David Fletcher, †Malvin N. Janal, and ‡J. Douglas Carroll

Department of Psychiatry, College of Physicians and Surgeons, Columbia University, New York, New York 10032, †Department of Biopsychology, New York State Psychiatric Institute, New York, New York 10032, and ‡Department of Biopsychology, Rutgers University, Newark, New Jersey 07102

SUMMARY

Improvement in the measurement and understanding of pain and related emotions requires the replacement of "armchair" taxonomies with one based on objective multidimensional scaling (MDS) techniques. We studied 270 Pain/Suffering and Health/Happiness words taken from the McGill Pain Questionnaire (MPQ) and other sources. The additional words were selected because: (a) the MPQ does not contain enough words describing the emotional and motivational component of the pain/emotion experience; and (b) positive as well as negative descriptors must be included to ensure broad, well-defined clusters and dimensions of pain/emotion. A hierarchical clustering model, Average Linkage Between Groups, which assumes a discrete rather than a continuous spatial structure, was used to analyze similarity judgments (pile-sort technique) made by seven experienced pain researchers. Analysis produced a dendrogram with 50 subclusters subsumed within the following 18 primary clusters: Penetrating Wounds, Pains Without Wounds, Fatigue, Mechanical, Temporal, Cold, Depression, Passivity, Fear/Anxiety, Hostility, Pure Sensory Pain, Suffering, Somatic/Emotional Distress, Heat, Pleasant Sensations, Affiliative Behavior, Positive Feelings, and Healthy Behaviors. Clearly, there are many more clusters or dimensions of pain and emotion than the three major groups containing 22 subgroups of the MPQ. No evidence was found to support the validity of the MPQ Evaluative group, since each MPQ word was found to belong to a different MDS cluster. Furthermore, since many of the MPQ subclasses contain words that belong to different MDS clusters, one must conclude that the words within a subclass are heterogeneous, and hence cannot be ordered with respect to intensity along a single continuum. Thus, the MPQ test requirement that the patient check but one word (the most intense) per subclass of the MPQ is misguided. The MPQ Present Pain Intensity (PPI) scale is heterogeneous since it mixes items from the MDS Pure Sensory Pain and Somatic/Emotional Distress clusters. Consequently, the scale is completely confusing to any patient trying to locate him- or herself at a single point on it. Some of the MDS subclusters in the present study contained an excess of words, while other had too few. Thus, the next step will be to prune old and graft new words into the MPQ until a set of 100 to 150 more evenly distributed descriptors are available for further MDS analysis.

INTRODUCTION

The goal of the MDS approach is to replace the essentially "armchair" taxonomies of pain and emotion with an objectively determined taxonomy. This will permit the reduction of the hundreds of words used by patients and practitioners to describe states of pain, mood, arousal, stress, and other states to the minimum number required to define the pain and emotion space. A detailed map of the structure of this space in place of conventional questionnaire responses will help diagnosis and treatment in the same way that a map is a better aid to navigation than is a list of cities. Present pain questionnaires and verbal magnitude-estimation scales resemble a list of cities, not a map.

The first step toward quantification of the pain/emotion experience is to obtain a better understanding of its dimensions (in a continuous space) or its clusters (in a discrete space). Our previous work (Clark 1984; Clark et al. 1989a; Clark et al. 1989b; Janal et al. 1993) assumed a continuous space, and the individual differences scaling (INDSCAL) spatial distance model was used to analyze the similarity judgments. The present study assumed a discrete space and used a hierarchical clustering model, Average Linkage Between Groups, to analyze similarity estimates made by the subjects (graphically represented by a dendrogram).

Once the underlying structure of the pain and emotion space is determined, it becomes possible to relate an individual patient's description of pain and emotion to a particular location within a common multidimensional universe. To discover these dimensions and clusters, the investigator must put aside preconceptions and allow the patient to provide the information. MDS accomplishes this because the subjects, not the investigator, determine the pain and emotion space. In contrast, unidimensional scales devised by the investigator impose an arbitrary structure. Thus, procedures used in traditional psychophysics, such as sensory decision theory and magnitude estimation, are of little help because they cannot reveal in an unbiased manner the number or types of dimensions that underlie pain and emotion. The MDS procedure avoids this problem of experimenter bias by allowing the subject to determine the attributes underlying a set of stimuli by making similarity judgments. Since no request is made to rate the stimuli according to pain, affect, fear, or other possible attributes, the subject generates the types and number of dimensions in his or her experiential world; the dimensions are discovered, not imposed. Experimenter influence remains, however, in the selection of the descriptors in the present study, this was minimized by selecting a large number of words from a wide variety of sources.

Clark et al. (1989) reviewed studies utilizing MDS methods to explore a variety of pain and emotion dimensions. Wack and Turk (1984) examined a large number of pain-coping strategies and found three dimensions: (a) sensation acknowledging/avoidance; (b) coping relevance; and (c) behavioral/cognitive. Turk et al. (1985) used a hierarchical clustering model and a different set of stimuli and found four primary clusters: (a) distorted posture or ambulation; (b) negative affect; (c) facial expression; and (d) avoidance of activity. Vlaeyen et al. (1987) used a broad definition of pain behavior based on observations of patients in pain interacting with their environment. Their list of 78 behaviors described patient actions that were hampering wellness behavior. Cluster analysis yielded nine groups: anxiety, attention seeking, verbal pain complaints, medication use, general verbal complaints, distorted posture and mobility, fatigue, insomnia, and depressed mood. Keefe et al. (1990) used clustering techniques to analyze data related to the behavior of patients with low back pain. They found that this group of patients could be separated into four subgroups based on their pain behavior: (a) patients who displayed low levels of all pain behaviors; (b) patients who displayed a high level of guarding, a moderate level of rubbing, but low levels of other pain behaviors; (c) patients who displayed high levels of guarding and bracing and moderate levels of rubbing; and (d) patients who displayed high levels of rubbing and guarding and moderate levels of bracing. They argued that the variability in pain behaviors among a relatively homogeneous group of pain patients could be described through the use of MDS techniques. Two studies (Kwilosz et al. 1983; Verkes et al. 1989), like the present study, contained descriptors related to the MPQ and are discussed later.

METHOD

Subjects were seven experienced pain researchers (two female). The descriptors were 270 Pain/Suffering and Health/Happiness words taken from the MPQ, the Zuckerman Multiple Affect Adjective Check List, and other sources. The additional words were selected because: (a) the MPQ does not contain enough words describing the emotional and motivational components of the pain and experience; and (b) pleasant as well as unpleasant descriptors must be included to ensure broad, well-defined clusters and dimensions of pain and emotion. The task of the subjects was to sort the 270 descriptors into as many piles of similar items as they chose; the number of piles varied from 28 to 46. The data were analyzed by various hierarchical cluster algorithms, but, as predicted, the most interpretable and robust solution was obtained using Euclidean distances and the Average Linkage Between Groups algorithm (Sokal and Michener 1958).

RESULTS

Primary clusters were all defined at the uppermost level of aggregation in the dendrogram and subclusters at lower levels of aggregation. The 18 primary clusters, which contained a total of 50 subclusters, appear in Table 1.

Primary Cluster 1, Penetrating Wounds, contains three subclusters involving very painful penetrating wounds; it contains many words from the sensory group of the MPQ. **Primary Cluster 2**, Pains Without Wounds, contains words describing moderate pain, and describes sensations of internal origin that do not involve (external) injury; it also contains many sensory words from the MPQ. **Primary Cluster 3**, Fatigue, is clearly related to the MPQ "Affect-Tension" subclass. **Primary Cluster 4**, Mechanical Stimulation, refers to mechanical receptors that mediate pressure and stretch. It contains a number of words from a variety of MPQ sensory subclasses. **Primary Cluster 5**, Temporal, contains a number of subclusters: The Periodic Intense subcluster describes distinctly painful sensations, generally referring to headaches, that vary in intensity and time, and is closely related to MPQ subclass 1; Movement includes radiating-type pains; and the Intermittent and Continuous subclusters refer to general temporal sensory qualities rather than to specifically painful qualities, including many of the nine words in the Temporal subclass (21) of the MPQ. **Primary Cluster 6**, Cold, groups words from MPQ miscellaneous subclasses 18 and 19. **Primary Cluster 7**, Depression, contains 22 words related to negative emotional states. It contains only two words from the MPQ. **Primary Cluster 8**, Passivity, with its subclusters Lassitude, Isolation, and Passive Behavior, provides an example of an important component of the pain/emotion experience that is missed entirely by the MPQ. **Primary Cluster 9**, Fear/Anxiety, is another important component of pain/emotion in which only two "fear" words from the MPQ appear. **Primary Cluster 10**, Hostility, contains the subclusters Anger, Antisocial Behavior, and Distress. In view of the recent findings about chronic pain patients' hostility and anger toward health-care providers, the absence of these elements from the MPQ constitutes a serious omission. **Primary Cluster 11**, Pure Sensory Pain, with its two subclusters Severe Pain and Mild Pain, includes the poles of a Pure Sensory Pain dimension. These descriptors form a homogeneous continuous scale and should replace the heterogeneous items contained in the Present Pain Intensity (PPI) scale of the MPQ. **Primary Cluster 12**, Suffering, contains descriptors similar to the Frightening and Excruciating subclusters of Primary Cluster 13, which are represented in the MPQ Affective group. **Primary Cluster 13**, Somatic/Emotional Distress, contains two subclusters describing intense autonomic/visceral responses (e.g., Choking, Nauseating). The four other Somatic/Emotional subclusters are of two types: those that describe moderate stimuli (e.g., Discomforting, Nagging), and those that describe intense stimuli which induce very strong somatic/emotional responses (e.g., Excruciating, Grueling, Torturing). Some of these words appear in the MPQ, but are scattered into quite different subclasses. **Primary Cluster 14**, Heat, contains two subclusters: Intense Heat, which is also found in the MPQ, and Mild Heat, which serves to define the other pole of this dimension.

1 PENETRATING WOUNDS
[1] *Punctate:*
Penetrating(17)
Drilling(3)
Piercing(17)
Stabbing(3)
Lancinating(3)
Digging[b]
Splitting(10)
[2] *Cutting:*
Nipping
Biting[b]
Lacerating(4)
Tearing(18)
Cutting(4)
Sharp(4)
[3] *Friction:*
Grinding[b]
Gnawing(5)
Rasping(10)
2 PAINS WITHOUT WOUNDS
[4] *Cutaneous Weak:*
Brush
Itchy(8)
Tickling
Tingling(8)
[5] *Cutaneous Strong:*
Rough
Smarting(8)
Pricking(3)
Stinging(8)
[6] *Irritating:*
Irritating
[7] *Contraction/Twisting:*
Wrenching(6)
Cramping(5)
Spasm
[8] *Aching:*
Sore Sensation(9)
Tender Sensation(10)
Hurting(9)
Aching(9)
3 FATIGUE
[9] *Fatigue:*
Tiring(11)
Fatiguing[b]
Exhausting(11)
Wilted
Dragging[b]
4 MECHANICAL STIMULATION
[10] *Pressure Sensation:*
Heavy(9)
Pressing(5)
Crushing(5)
[11] *Traction:*

Pulling(6)
Tugging(6)
Drawing(18)
Taut(10)
Drawing(18)
[12] *Constrictive:*
Gripping[b]
Binding[b]
Gripping[b]
Pinching(5)
5 TEMPORAL
[13] *Periodic Intense:*
Pulsing(1)
Throbbing(1)
Pounding(1)
Thumping[b]
Beating(1)
Rhythmic(21)
[14] *Blurred:*
Blurred
[15] *Movement:*
Darting
Jumping(2)
Radiating(17)
Spreading(17)
Shooting(2)
[16] *Intermittent:*
Quivering(1)
Flickering(1)
Flashing(2)
Intermittent(22)
Periodic(22)
Rhythmic(22)
[17] *Continuous:*
Transient(22)
Momentary(22)
Brief(22)
Constant(22)
Continuous(22)
6 COLD
[18] *Cold:*
Cold(19)
Freezing(19)
Cool(19)
[19] *Numbing:*
Numb(18)
7 DEPRESSION
[20] *Depression:*
Displeased
Discontented
Helpless
Defeated
Discouraged
Sunk
Forlorn
Lost
Hopeless
Melancholy

Gloomy
Blue
Sad
Unhappy
Miserable(16)
Low
Depressing
Wretched(15)
Sullen
Destroyed
Grim
Worrying
8 PASSIVITY
[21] *Lassitude:*
Quiet
Tame
Sleepy
Bored(3)
Dull(9)
Apathetic
[22] *Isolation:*
Alone
Lonely
Rejected
[23] *Passive Behavior:*
Shy
Timid
Meek
Bashful
Cautious
Passive
9 FEAR/ANXIETY
[24] *Fear:*
Frightened(13)
Afraid
Fearful(13)
Terrified
Panicky
Horrified
[25] *Anxiety:*
Anxious
Nervous
Tense
Shaky
Agitated
10 HOSTILITY
[26] *Anger:*
Stormy
Violent
Wild
Stubborn
Impatient
Aggressive
Willful
Offended
Annoyed(16)
Indignant
Outraged

TABLE 1. *Continued*

Incensed	(36) *Excruciating:*	
Cross	Excruciating(21)	17 POSITIVE FEELINGS
Furious	Agonizing(20)	[43] *Elation:*
Enraged	Punishing(14)	Delighted
Angry	Killing(14)	Amused
Mad	Grueling(14)	Cheerful
Vexed	Torturing(20)	Merry
Hostile	Blinding(15)	Happy
Upset	Racking[b]	Joyful
[27] *Antisocial Behavior:*	14 HEAT	Gay
Mean	[37] *Intense Heat:*	Glad
Cruel(14)	Searing(7)	Pleased
Vicious(14)	Burning(7)	Lucky
Wicked[b]	Scalding(7)	[44] *Positive Mood:*
Critical	Hot(7)	Peaceful
Savage[b]	[38] *Mild Heat:*	Unfrightened
Contrary	Warm Sensation	Satisfied
Jealous	15 PLEASANT	Fulfilled
Unsociable	SENSATIONS	Contented
Disagreeable	[39] *Pleasant Sensations:*	[45] *Confident Mood:*
Bitter	Ameliorate	Secure
[28] *Distress:*	Mollify	Safe
Distressing(21)	Soft Sensation	Relaxed Mood
Ugly	Soothing	Calm
Complaining	Stroking	Soothed[b]
11 PURE SENSORY PAIN	Caress	[46] *Trustworthy:*
[29] *Severe Pain:*	Relaxed Muscle	Frank
Intolerable Pain[b]	Pleasant	Steady(22)
Unbearable Pain(16)	16 AFFILIATIVE	18 HEALTH BEHAVIORS
Bearable Pain	BEHAVIOR	[47] *Healthy:*
[30] *Mild Pain:*	[40] *Affiliative Behavior:*	Strong
Mild Pain(21)	Wanted	Intense(16)
Moderate Pain	Loved	Powerful
No Pain(21)	Needed	Fit
12 SUFFERING	Affectionate	Healthy
[31] *Torment:*	Devoted	Clean
Tormented	Tender	Fine
Suffering	Gentle	[48] *Arousal:*
Desperate	Warm	Arousing
13 SOMATIC/EMOTIONAL	[41] *Compassionate*	Startling
DISTRESS	*Behavior:*	Alarming
[32] *Respiratory Distress:*	Touching	[49] *Optimism:*
Choking[b]	Merciful	Hopeful
Suffocating(12)	Amiable	Inspired
[33] *Nauseous:*	Agreeable	Heartened
Sickening(12)	Friendly	Interested
Nauseating(20)	Kindly	[50] *Active Behavior:*
Disgusting	Patient	Whole
[34] *Bothersome:*	Polite	Free
Troublesome(16)	[42] *Friendly:*	Daring
Discomforting(21)	Cooperative	Reckless
Distracting[b]	Understanding	Adventurous
Nagging(20)	Sympathetic	Young
(35) *Frightening:*	Obliging	Alive
Terrible	Thoughtful	Enthusiastic
Dreadful(20)	Good-natured	Active
Terrifying(13)	Good	Energetic
Horrible(21)	Mild	

[a]The numbers in parentheses refer to the subclass of the MPQ.
[b]Words added to the MPQ by Kwilosz et al. (1983).

Primary Clusters 15, Pleasant Sensations; 16, Affiliative Behavior; 17, Positive Feelings; and 18, Healthy Behaviors represent opposite poles to the Pain/Suffering clusters, and will prove important in defining the various poles of the Pain/Suffering and Health/Happiness dimensions. These contrasting poles are needed if bipolar scales are to be developed for estimating the exact location of a patient along these dimensions.

The relationship of the MDS clusters to the MPQ groupings appears in Table 2. A few MPQ subclasses were in complete agreement with the MDS clusters: Thermal, (MPQ subclass 7); Brightness (MPQ Subclass 8); Tension (MPQ Subclass 11); Fear (MPQ subclass 13); and Cold (MPQ Subclass 19). A second set of MPQ subclasses were in relative agreement. For example, the MPQ Temporal subclass (subclass 1) includes words from both the Intermittent and the Periodic Intense subclusters.

DISCUSSION

Cluster analysis of 270 descriptors of pain, suffering, health, and happiness yielded three important findings. First, there are a number of categories, including Depression, Passivity, Hostility, Fear/Anxiety, Antisocial Behavior, and Somatic/ Emotional Distress, which are missing or poorly represented by conventional pain scales (e.g., visual analogue and magnitude-estimation scales) as well as pain questionnaires (e.g., the MPQ). Second, the inclusion of positive affect items in the present study resulted, not surprisingly, in the appearance of additional major clusters not found in the MPQ. The use of such items in future tests will make it possible to identify a number of dimensions, extending from Health to Illness, along which individual patients can be located. Present questionnaires fail to include items that describe the positive pole (representing health and happiness) in addition to the negative pole (representing pain and suffering) of various dimensions. The present study, because it included opposites, revealed a number of clusters that formed the poles of various dimensions. These included: No Pain–Intolerable Pain, Warm–Burning, Active–Apathetic, Affiliative–Antisocial Behavior, Friendly–Hostile, Positive Feelings–Depression. Typically (e.g., for the MPQ) the patient answers "Yes" or "No"; this dichotomous decision fails to yield the quantified information available from a response to a continuous bipolar scale. With respect to data analysis, the difference is between a crude nominal scale and far more quantifiable ordinal and interval scales.

The third finding concerns the structure of the MPQ. The 270 descriptors studied included all of the items from the MPQ (see Table 2). Although one might expect a somewhat different semantic structure to emerge from such an expanded set of stimuli, it is striking how much the locations of these items in the various clusters, which were derived objectively from the dendrogram of the Average Linkage Between Groups analysis, differ from that of the more subjectively derived groups and subclasses of the MPQ. The descriptors in the MPQ are held to fall into three major groups: Sensory, containing subclasses 1 to 10; Affective, containing sub-

TABLE 2. *Location of McGill Pain Questionnaire items in the 50-cluster space[a] determined by hierarchical cluster analysis*

1 SENSORY-TEMPORAL		**9 SENSORY-DULLNESS**	
Flickering	(intermittent 16)	Dull	(lassitude 21)
Quivering	(intermittent 16)	Sore	(aching 8)
Pulsing	(periodic intense 13)	Hurting	(aching 8)
Throbbing	(periodic intense 13)	Aching	(aching 8)
Beating	(periodic intense 13)	Heavy	(pressure 10)
Pounding	(periodic intense 13)		
		10 SENSORY-MISCELLANEOUS	
2 SENSORY-SPATIAL		Tender	(aching 8)
Jumping	(temporal/spatial 15)	Taut	(traction 11)
Flashing	(intermittent 16)	Rasping	(friction 3)
Shooting	(temporal/spatial 15)	Splitting	(punctate 1)
3 SENSORY-PUNCTATE		**11 AFFECTIVE-TENSION**	
Pricking	(cutaneous sharp 5)	Tiring	(fatigue 9)
Boring (Bored)	(lassitude 21)	Exhausting	(fatigue 9)
Drilling	(punctate 1)		
Stabbing	(punctate 1)	**12 AFFECTIVE-AUTONOMIC**	
Lancinating	(punctate 1)	Sickening	(nauseous 33)
		Suffocating	(respiratory distress 32)
4 SENSORY-INCISIVE			
Sharp	(cutting 2)	**13 AFFECTIVE-FEAR**	
Cutting	(cutting 2)	Fearful	(fearful 24)
Lacerating	(cutting 2)	Frightful (Frightened)	(fearful 24)
		Terrifying	(frightening 35)
5 SENSORY-CONSTRICTIVE			
Pinching	(constrictive 12)	**14 AFFECTIVE-PUNISHMENT**	
Pressing	(pressure 10)	Punishing	(excruciating 36)
Gnawing	(friction 3)	Gruelling	(excruciating 36)
Cramping	(contraction/twisting 7)	Cruel	(antisocial behaviors 27)
Crushing	(pressure 10)	Vicious	(antisocial behaviors 27)
		Killing	(excruciating 36)
6 SENSORY-TRACTION			
Tugging	(traction 11)	**15 AFFECTIVE-MISCELLANEOUS**	
Pulling	(traction 11)	Wretched	(depression 20)
Wrenching	(contraction/twisting 7)	Blinding	(excruciating 36)
7 SENSORY-THERMAL		**16 EVALUATIVE**	
Hot	(heat 37)	Annoying (Annoyed)	(anger 26)
Burning	(heat 37)	Troublesome	(bothersome 34)
Scalding	(heat 37)	Miserable	(depression 20)
Searing	(heat 37)	Intense	(healthy 47)
		Unbearable	(severe pain 29)
8 SENSORY-BRIGHTNESS			
Tingling	(cutaneous diffuse 4)	**17 MISCELLANEOUS**	
Itchy	(cutaneous diffuse 4)	Spreading	(temporal/spatial 15)
Smarting	(cutaneous sharp 5)	Radiating	(temporal/spatial 15)
Stinging	(cutaneous sharp 5)	Penetrating	(punctuate 1)
		Piercing	(punctuate 1)

TABLE 2. *Continued*

18 MISCELLANEOUS		21 PRESENT PAIN INTENSITY	
Tight	(traction 11)	0 No pain	(mild pain 30)
Numb	(numbing 19)	1 Mild pain	(mild pain 30)
Drawing	(traction 11)	2 Discomforting	(bothersome 34)
Squeezing	(constrictive 12)	3 Distressing	(distress 28)
Tearing	(cutting 2)	4 Horrible	(frightening 35)
		5 Excruciating	(excruciating 36)
19 MISCELLANEOUS			
Cool	(cold 18)	22 TEMPORAL SENSATIONS	
Cold	(cold 18)	Brief	(continuous 17)
Freezing	(cold 18)	Momentary	(continuous 17)
		Transient	(continuous 17)
20 MISCELLANEOUS		Rhythmic	(intermittent 16)
Nagging	(bothersome 34)	Periodic	(intermittent 16)
Nauseating	(nauseous 33)	Intermittent	(intermittent 16)
Agonizing	(excruciating 36)	Continuous	(continuous 17)
Dreadful	(frightening 35)	Steady	(trustworthy 46)
Torturing	(excruciating 36)	Constant	(continuous 17)

[a]Name and number of the cluster from Table 1 follow the MPQ word. Numbers in the subclass headings are those of the MPQ. Left column: MPQ items; right column: subcluster location.

classes 11 to 15; and Evaluative, containing subclass 16. In addition, there are Miscellaneous subclasses, 17 to 20, as well as the PPI scale, and a set of Temporal words (Melzack 1983). The present cluster analysis strongly challenges the homogeneity claimed for the MPQ Evaluative group, because each MPQ word was found to belong to a different MDS cluster, a finding that agrees closely with that of Kwilosz et al. (1983). Although Holroyd et al. (1992), in a factor-analytic study of a very large number of back-pain patients, found "some support" for an Evaluative factor, Leavitt et al. (1978), Reading (1979, 1989), and Prieto et al. (1980) failed to find a factor that represented the MPQ Evaluative group.

Another serious problem revealed by cluster analysis was that the PPI scale was heterogeneous, mixing items from Primary Cluster 11, Pure Sensory Pain, and Primary Cluster 13, Somatic/Emotional Distress. This heterogeneity means that the PPI is not a monotonic intensity scale, but is rather a scale that mixes sensory and emotional dimensions, to the utter confusion of any patient forced to locate him- or herself at a single point on the scale. Cluster analysis further revealed that most of the Sensory, Affect, and Evaluative groups of the MPQ contained words from different MDS clusters. Heterogeneity of words within a group means that they cannot be ordered with respect to intensity along a single continuum. Thus, the MPQ test instruction that the patient check only one word (the most intense) in each subgroup is mistaken.

In the present study, different parts of speech were used for three of the MPQ words in order to fit them in with the other 200 or so descriptors. Boring, Frightful, and Annoying were replaced by Bored, Frightened, and Annoyed. This change probably caused Boring to be located in the Lassitude subcluster of Primary Cluster

8, Passivity. Relabeling the concepts Frightful and Annoying does not appear to have affected their category location. The inclusion of a large number of psychological terms evidently caused the subjects to reinterpret the meaning of some MPQ words; for example, Steady (MPQ Temporal subclass 22) was interpreted as a psychological quality and appeared in the Trustworthy subcluster of Primary Cluster 17, Positive Feelings. Similarly, Dull (MPQ Sensory subclass 9) appeared in the Lassitude subcluster of Primary Cluster 8, Passivity. Cruel and Vicious (MPQ subclass 14) were not interpreted as sensory or affective qualities of pain, but were included in the subcluster Antisocial Behaviors of Primary Cluster 10, Hostility. Intense (MPQ Evaluative subclass 16) was not interpreted as referring to pain but was located in the subcluster Healthy of Primary Cluster 18, Health Behaviors. It may be concluded that a number of words in the MPQ and other questionnaires are extremely ambiguous, and that there is no way the investigator can know how a patient interprets them. This confusion can be alleviated by improved instructions and, when necessary, by placing the word in a sentence (e.g., "My skin feels warm" or "I have warm feelings toward people").

Two MDS studies, in addition to the present one, have included items from the MPQ. Kwilosz et al. (1983) had 51 college students sort 104 pain descriptors, from the MPQ as well as from other sources, on the basis of similarity. A cluster analysis found two major clusters, Sensory and Affective, as well as 22 minor clusters. The Evaluative group of the MPQ was not found. In general, however, the clusters derived by Kwilosz et al. were not nearly as compelling as those obtained in the present study. A likely cause for this was the clustering algorithm that they used (Johnson 1967). This method is overly sensitive to ordering effects of the stimuli in the algorithm, and the cluster solutions are not stable. Verkes et al. (1989) did a cluster analysis of pile-sort data of 176 Dutch pain descriptors. They found 32 clusters of words among which the subclasses of the MPQ "could be easily identified." Their solution contained three Evaluative, eleven Affective, seven Sensory, seven Temporal, and four Locational clusters. This contrasts with our 18 primary cluster and 50 subcluster solution. Since their study contained words that we did not use, and vice versa, some differences would be expected. However, their conclusions, especially with respect to their Evaluative clusters, fail to agree with the results of the present study. Furthermore, although some of our clusters were congruent with those of the MPQ, we do not agree that most of the subclasses of the MPQ "could be easily identified."

CONCLUSION

The pain-suffering-pleasure space contains many more components of the pain experience than are represented by the MPQ. When Melzack and Torgerson (1971) introduced the MPQ, they commented with great prescience that once appropriate mathematical scaling models were developed, the subjectively determined grouping of descriptors in the MPQ would be replaced with an objectively based questionnaire.

The multidimensional scaling models employed here have proven successful in this regard, and work continues on selecting the precise set of words that will best reveal the patient's experience. We expect that some descriptors will serve as poles of dimensions in a continuous space; these will be used to construct bipolar ordinal or interval visual analog scales. Other descriptors will appear in clusters in a discrete space and provide qualitative, nominal scale information. The location of descriptors in this mixed continuous-discrete space will require application of the MDS hybrid model now being developed.

ACKNOWLEDGMENTS

The work described in this chapter was supported by grants NINDS20248 and NIMH30906, and by the Nathaniel Wharton Fund for Research and Education in Brain, Body and Behavior.

REFERENCES

Clark WC. Application of multidimensional scaling to problems in experimental and clinical pain. In: Bromm B, ed. *Pain measurement in man: neurophysical correlates of pain.* Amsterdam: Elsevier, 1984;349–369.

Clark WC, Ferrer-Brechner T, Janal MN, Carroll JD, Yang JC. The dimensions of pain: a multidimensional scaling comparison of cancer patients and healthy volunteers. *Pain* 1989a;37:23–32.

Clark WC, Janal MN, Carroll JD. Multidimensional pain requires multidimensional scaling. In: Loeser JD, Chapman CR, eds. *The measurement of pain.* New York: Raven Press, 1989b;285–325.

Holroyd KA, Holm JE, Keefe FJ, Turner JA, Bradley LA, Murphy WD, Johnson P, Anderson K, Hinkle AL, O'Malley WB. A multi-center evaluation of the McGill Pain Questionnaire: results from more than 1700 chronic pain patients. *Pain* 1992;48:301–311.

Janal MN, Clark WC, Carroll JD. Multidimensional scaling of painful electrocutaneous stimulation: INDSCAL dimensions, signal detection theory indices, and the McGill Pain Questionnaire. *Somatosens Motor Res* 1993;10:31–39.

Johnson SC. Hierarchical clustering schemes. *Psychometrika* 1967;32:241–254.

Keefe FJ, Bradley LA, Crisson JE. Behavioral assessment of low back pain: identification of pain behavior subclass. *Pain* 1990;40:153–160.

Kwilosz DM, Green BP, Torgerson WS. *Qualities of hurting: The language of pain.* Chicago, IL: American Pain Society, 1983.

Leavitt F, Garron DC, Whisler WW, Sheinkop MB. Affective and sensory dimensions of back pain. *Pain* 1978;4:273–281.

Melzack R. The McGill Pain Questionnaire. In: Melzack R, ed. *The McGill Pain Questionnaire.* New York: Raven Press, 1983;41–47.

Melzack R, Torgerson WS. On the language of pain. *Anesthesiology* 1971;34:50–59.

Prieto EJ, Hobson L, Bradley LA, Byrne M, Geisinger KF, Midax D, Marchisello PJ. The language of low back pain: factor structure of the McGill Pain Questionnaire. *Pain* 1980;8:11–19.

Reading AH. A comparison of the McGill Pain Questionnaire in chronic and acute pain. *Pain* 1989; 13:185–192.

Reading AE. The internal structure of the McGill Pain Questionnaire in dysmenorrhoea patients. *Pain* 1979;7:353–358.

Sokal R, Michener CD. A statistical method for evaluating systematic relationships. *Univ Kansas Sci Bull* 1958;38:1409–1438.

Turk DC, Wack JT, Kerns RD. An empirical examination of the "pain behavior" construct. *J Behav Med* 1985;8:119–130.

Verkes RJ, Van der Kloot WA, Van der Meij J. The perceived structure of 176 pain descriptive words. *Pain* 1989;38:219–229.

Vlaeyen JWS, Van Eek H, Groenman NH, Schuerman JA. Dimensions and components of observed chronic pain behavior. *Pain* 1987;31:65–75.

Wack JT, Turk DC. Latent structure of strategies used to cope with nociceptive stimulation. *Health Psychol* 1984;3:27–43.

Pain and the Brain: From Nociception to Cognition, edited by Burkhart Bromm and John E. Desmedt, Advances in Pain Research and Therapy Vol. 22. Raven Press, Ltd., New York © 1995.

21

The Corticalization of Chronic Pain

*Niels Birbaumer, †Hertha Flor, *Werner Lutzenberger, and ‡Thomas Elbert

Institute of Medical Psychology and Behavioral Neurobiology, University of Tübingen, D-72074 Tübingen, Germany, †Department of Psychology, Humboldt University, D-10117 Berlin, Germany, ‡Institute of Experimental Audiology, University of Münster, D-48129 Münster, Germany,

SUMMARY

Extensive experimental evidence in healthy subjects and patients with chronic pain indicates widespread and probably permanent changes in cortical responsivity to pain-related processing, as revealed by electroencephalographic (EEG) and magneto-encephalographic (MEG) recordings. Increased pain-evoked potentials and pain-induced magnetic fields were found in chronic-pain patients, demonstrating facilitation of the processing of noxious information at an early stage (70 to 125 msec). In amputees with phantom sensations, signs of massive reorganization of central brain areas could explain the long-lasting memories of pain. The process of the "corticalization" of specific peripheral-muscular pathologies in chronic pain consists of a classical conditioning of pain responses that is accompanied by a characteristic sequence of slow cortical potentials during the acquisition and extinction of pain-related responses. These electrocortical patterns may be predictive of the future chronicity and stability of pain memories.

CHRONIC PAIN IS A LEARNED PERIPHERAL-CENTRAL RESPONSE PATTERN

Pain is a response pattern involving three interacting response systems: the psychologic–cognitive, the motor–behavioral, and the physiologic–organic (Birbaumer and Flor, in press a). Any separation of these three response systems, whether experimentally or clinically, and any single cause-effect model such as an exlusively peripheral–physiologic or purely central-cognitive model of chronic pain, must lead to artificial results. At any time, in any individual, and for any given pain syndrome, a specific pattern of the interaction of the three response systems plays a decisive role in the instigation, maintenance, and extinction of chronic pain syndromes including sensations of pain, pain behaviors, and sustained nociceptive input.

Plastic changes in the central nervous system (CNS) and learning play substantial roles in the development of chronic pain, independent of any coexisting pathophysiology of the nociceptive system, such as lesions, inflammation, or trauma (Flor and Turk, 1984). Most chronic pain syndromes do not show a specific pathology of the nociceptive system that could explain the continued presence of the pain response. Low-back pain, tension headaches, and facial pain are the most frequent examples of such syndromes. Other pain syndromes, such as cancer pain and arthritis, have a clear pathophysiology, but learning plays an important role in the exacerbation or reduction of pain responses in these syndromes (Leventhal and Everhart, 1979). Thus, the title of this section constitutes a truism, but one that is largely ignored by the scientific community, which is still primarily concerned with the peripheral pathophysiology of the nociceptive system. In addition, the exact role and extent of the influence of learning mechanisms is largely unknown for the various pain syndromes. In this chapter we provide experimental evidence for peripheral–physiologic, behavioral, and CNS processes involved in the learned chronicity of pain.

A RESPONSE STEREOTYPY OF SELECTIVE MUSCLE GROUPS IS LEARNED THROUGH CLASSICAL AND INSTRUMENTAL CONDITIONING IN CHRONIC PAIN PATIENTS

In a diathesis-stress model of chronic pain (Flor et al., 1990), we proposed that at the peripheral–physiologic level, pain patients develop excessive muscular tension when exposed to personally relevant stressful situations and episodes of pain. The excessive contraction was hypothesized to be localized to those muscle-fiber groups in which the patients subjectively perceive the pain response. The activation of nociceptors in this situation is a consequence of tension- and inflammation-related local sensitization of nociceptors or of the direct activation of nociceptors in contracted muscle.

A series of experiments using electromyographic (EMG) recordings of several muscle groups in patients with chronic low back pain and others with temporomandibular joint disorder (TMJD) exposed to real and imagined general and personally stressful situations clearly confirmed our predictions (Flor et al. 1992; Flor et al. 1991; Flor et al. 1985). An increased muscular responsivity in comparison to matched controls is localized to the site of pain, it occurs only in personally relevant stressful situations and episodes of pain, and is maintained for a prolonged period by patients as compared to healthy controls. Furthermore, pain patients exhibit a reduced capacity to consciously perceive and voluntarily regulate their levels of muscular tension (Flor et al. 1992).

In our model this stereotypy of muscular response is contingently preceded by psychological, motor, or physical stimuli that were originally neutral with regard to their pain-eliciting properties (classical conditioning of pain responses to pain cues). The pain response is followed by body-positions of relief and the avoidance of aversive activities, as well as by direct positive reinforcement, mainly through attention from significant others. This constitutes the *instrumental* learning element in the maintenance process of the classically conditioned pain response (cf. Fordyce, 1976). Indeed, we found indirect experimental evidence for both learning mechanisms (Flor and Birbaumer, 1994a; Flor and Birbaumer, 1994b; Flor and Birbaumer 1994c). (Direct evidence for this is difficult to obtain in humans; only longitudinal lifespan measurement before and after development of the pain behavior would provide a final answer).

First, classical conditioning of muscular and subjective pain responses to previously neutral tones and slides was demonstrated in the laboratory with healthy subjects. Second, comparison of the acquisition and extinction of a conditioned, painful EMG response in a group of young healthy subjects at high risk for the development of chronic pain as compared to matched controls revealed faster and more stable acquisition of the conditioned response and more resistance to extinction in the high-risk subjects (Fig. 1).

The role of operant, instrumental factors was illustrated by comparing verbal expressions of pain in patients during the presence and absence of reinforcing or nonreinforcing spouses, resulting in significantly more pain behaviors in the presence of a reinforcing (attending) spouse (Flor et al. in press).

THE "CENTRALIZATION" OF PAIN IS CHARACTERIZED BY AN INCREASED PLASTICITY OF THE BRAIN FOR UNCONDITIONED AND CONDITIONED PAIN STIMULI

The amplitude of the pain-evoked electrical brain potential and of the pain-evoked magnetic field of the somatosensory cortex was used as an indicator of CNS responsivity and plasticity to pain stimuli in patients with chronic low-back pain and in controls (Flor et al., 1994a; Flor et al. 1994b). Previously, Bromm and collaborators (Bromm 1984) had established the negative-positive deflection of the event-related brain potential (ERP) at about 150 to 260 msec (N150–P260) as a cortical reflection of experienced pain intensity. The greater the N150–P260 amplitude the greater the subjective pain of electrical or laser stimuli briefly applied to the skin of the fingers.

In our laboratory, we compared the pain-evoked brain potential in response to intracutaneous electrical stimuli (below and above tolerance) in 16 patients and 16 controls. The late pain-evoked response had the same amplitude to below tolerance stimuli in the patients as to above tolerance intensities in the controls. Furthermore, the controls showed a clear dependence of amplitude size on stimulus intensity, as shown by Bromm and others, whereas the patients showed the same increased amplitude to below and above tolerance, thus stimulation was lacking the usual psy-

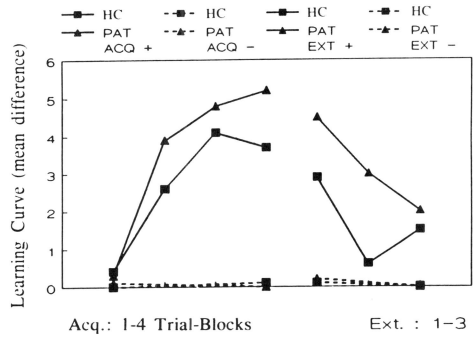

FIG. 1. Acquisition (Acq) and extinction (Ext) of classically conditioned muscular tension in a group of 12 healthy controls (HC) and a group of 12 matched subjects with a high risk for the development of chronic pain (PAT). Electromyographic (EMG) responses to a neutral tone (conditioned stimulus, CS = 800 Hz) averaged across five trials each for four acquisition blocks and three extinction blocks. The conditioned EMG responses (CR) of the left forearm are depicted as difference-values from 10 habituation trials in microvolts (μV). Responses to CS that were followed after 5 sec by an aversive electrical shock during acquisition (*solid line*, CS$^+$) are contrasted with CRs to (counterbalanced) tones, which were never followed by a shock (*dotted line*, CS$^-$). ACQ$^+$ = acquisition to CS$^+$; = ACQ$^-$ = acquisition to CS$^-$; EXT$^+$ = extinction to CS$^+$; EXT$^-$ = extinction to CS$^-$.

chophysical relationship between brain response and the conscious experience of pain (Flor et al. 1994a).

The specificity of the increased sensitivity of the CNS of patients with chronic pain was further elucidated with MEG recordings, which allow a more precise localization of cortical generators than does EEG mapping (Flor et al. 1994b). A group of 10 patients with low-back pain received painful and nonpainful electrical stimuli at the site of pain (left low back) and a control site (finger). The strength of their cephalic magnetic fields was measured above the right centroparietal region using a 37-channel MEG. The late (250 msec) magnetic field showed significantly higher field strengths in chronic-pain patients independent of the site of stimulation,

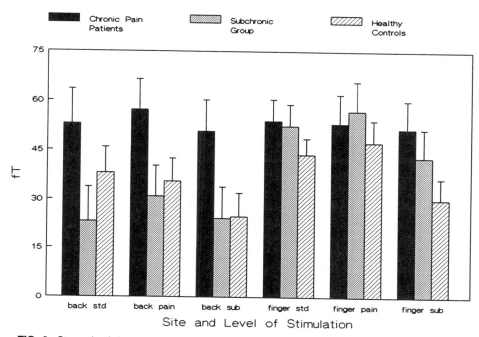

FIG. 2. Strength of the magnetically evoked field (root mean square, RMS, in femtotesla) to electrical stimuli in the 80- to 125-msec range at the postcentral region for the chronic ($n=5$) and subchronic ($n=5$) back-pain patients and the healthy controls ($n=9$). Painful (pain), nonpainful (sub), and standard (std) electrical stimuli were applied at the site of pain (left, low back) and control site (right, finger). See text for explanation. (From Flor et al. 1994c, with permission.)

pointing to a nonspecific increase in responsivity for later (evaluative–cognitive) processing in these patients. The earlier fields, at 100 msec after stimulation, revealed a site-specific increase in the field strength for stimuli applied to the low back as compared to finger stimulation only in patients with chronic pain (Fig. 2).

These data provide the first neurophysiologic evidence that the peripheral physiologic specificity we found for the muscular response in chronic pain may have an unexpected early cortical correlate: since conscious evaluation of pain stimuli at 100 msec after presentation can be excluded, we regard this site-specific increase in the early pain response in chronic pain patients as an increased (learned) facilitation for pain-related information by the primary cortical projection areas outside conscious control. Localization of the source of this early component by dipole analysis also points to an origin of this activity in the primary somatosensory cortex (S1).

Together with the ERP results, these data suggest that pain patients have both an early site-specific and a late nonspecific overexcitation of cortical areas involved in the processing of painful stimuli.

REMAPPING OF CORTICAL PROJECTION AREAS FOR SOMATOSENSORY STIMULATION AFTER AMPUTATION DEMONSTRATES EXTENSIVE REORGANIZATION OF THE ADULT HUMAN NERVOUS SYSTEM

Ramachandran et al. (1992) have reported that they could elicit painful and non-painful sensations in phantom limbs by stimulating the ipsilateral face or the proximal stump in upper-limb amputees. The authors suggested that this phenomenon, which they called "remapping," might be a perceptual correlate of changes in the cortical representation of the amputated limb. They hypothesized that the face and the stump representation "invaded" the region of the somatosensory cortex that had been formerly occupied by the amputated limb. Thus, neuronal pools that were responsive before amputation to afferents from the fingers may have become additionally excited by stimulation from the face and stump. The development of phantom pain and phantom sensations could at least partly be related to these mechanisms. Increased responsivity of somatosensory neurons representing the hand area, produced by additional input from other body areas such as the face, may be the basis for an altered "neuromatrix" in phantom-limb patients, as proposed by Melzack (1991). Such plastic ("learned") modification of cortical somatosensory representation should accordingly change the localization of electrical and magnetic field maxima. Stimulation of the stump and face should lead to a displacement of the respective fields toward the adjacent cortical areas contralateral to the amputated limb. We tested this hypothesis with a 37-channel BTI® magnetometer in addition to conventional EEG recordings in order to obtain better localization of cortical dipoles. Ten healthy male subjects with accident-related unilateral hand or arm amputations done 5 to 30 years earlier were investigated. All five patients had recurrent phantom sensations and pain. The presence of "remapping" in all five patients was documented by touching the skin of all body regions with small swabs (Q-tips) and asking the patient to report any sensation within or outside the touched region. Subsequent light tactile stimuli were applied to the first and fifth digits of the intact arm, and bilaterally to the regions of the upper arm and face. Normally, the field localizations of both hemispheres are comparable. Examination of the evoked magnetic fields contralateral to the intact and to the phantom side showed that the response from the "remapped" stump was much more similar to the response from the finger than that from the corresponding contralateral upper arm.

For the mouth this became even more evident: the locations of the representational areas of the finger and mouth on the intact site and of the mouth on the amputated side of one patient were superimposed on an MRI scan. The mouth region obviously "moved" closer to the region in which the amputated finger used to be represented (Fig. 3).

A statistical analysis for the Euclidean distances between the representational areas of the mouth and the fifth digit and the mouth and the first digit yielded a highly significant result, indicating a 1- to 2-cm shorter distance of the representations of the fifth digit and the mouth in the somatosensory cortex contralateral to the

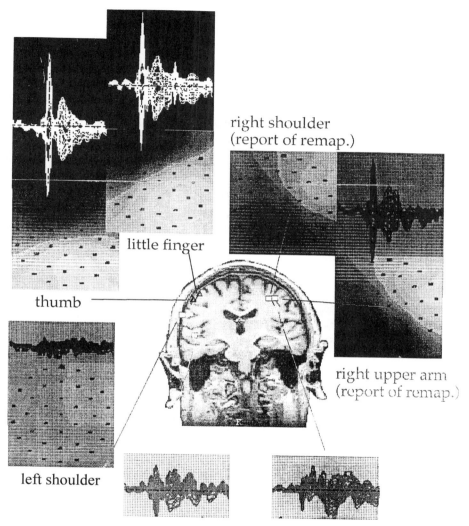

FIG. 3. MRI and MEG overlay of the presumed localization of various stimulation sites in a patient with phantom limb pain and remapping in the shoulder region. Thirty-seven channels of MEG responses to tactile stimuli and their respective contour plots over the left and right postcentral region (S1, S2) are depicted in femtotesla. Each channel constitutes an average across 100 stimuli. Note the marked difference in magnetic-field waveforms for the right (remapped) and left shoulder, and the great similarity of the right shoulder and the digit representation.

amputated side than on the intact side (cf. Elbert et al. 1994a). The amount of remapping correlated n = 0.9 with the intensity of phantom pain. These results support the hypothesis that plastic changes in cortical responsivity may play an important role in the processing of tactile and painful stimulation. Still unresolved are whether these modifications are caused by synaptic or axonal growth ("invasion") leading to the formation of Hebb synapses at pain-responsive neurons, or whether they are signs of a disinhibition of normally inhibited neuronal responsivity. In any case, the data clearly demonstrate that central cortical processes are involved in the development of pain, and that exclusively peripheral models of the chronicity of pain are incomplete.

SLOW POTENTIALS CONSTITUTE THE CORTICAL REPRESENTATION OF THE CONTINGENCY BETWEEN PAIN CUES AND LEARNED PAIN RESPONSES

The data on cortical overexcitability and changes in cortical representation reported so far provide evidence for plastic changes in the adult CNS. Plasticity in the nervous system can be caused by growth and developmental changes that do not depend on learning processes such as classical or instrumental learning or explicit declarative memory (Squire and Zola-Morgan 1991). The experiments reported above on stereotypies in muscular response to personally stressful memories, and the demonstration of classical conditioning of physiologic and psychological pain responses, point toward the involvement of learning in the maintenance of pain. Despite the fact that some "automatic" classically conditioned responses such as the blink reflex do not necessarily have a cortical representation (cf. Daum et al. 1993), the classical conditioning of a personally stressful event must have a cortical origin.

In a series of studies with healthy subjects and subjects at risk for developing pain, we have shown that the organization, maintenance, and extinction of conditioned muscular and subjective pain responses are characterized by a highly reproducible pattern of electrocortical changes (cf. Flor et al. 1994c; Larbig et al. 1982; Rockstroh et al. 1989; Rockstroh et al. 1979).

The formation of associations between conditioned stimuli (CS) and unconditioned stimuli (US) and conditioned responses (CR) is reflected in negative slow brain potentials with a specific topographic distribution. Each of the components represents a different stage of sensory processing in the preparation and execution of the motor or cognitive response (for a detailed review see Birbaumer et al. 1990). The amplitude of the negativity preceding the conditioned pain response is proportional to the cortical (attentional) responses necessary to form a particular association between two stimuli or a stimulus–response contingency (Fig. 4). In the classical terminology of Hullian learning theory, the amplitude of the negativity preceding the CR reflects the "reaction potential" (Hull 1951) or "cortical potentiality" (Birbaumer et al. 1990), $P_R = D \times H$, which corresponds to the product of drive (D) and habit strength (H). The latter increases with the repetition of re-

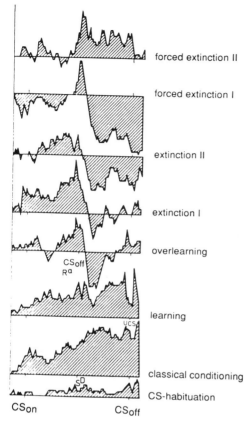

FIG. 4. Slow cortical potentials (SCP) of the vertex electrode (C$_z$) averaged across nine subjects over the course of learning of an instrumental avoidance response to painful shocks. Each curve represents the average of 10 trials from habituation (below) to forced extinction (top). At CS (conditioned stimulus), a light was turned on for 14 sec. During conditioning, learning, and overlearning trials, the light was followed by a shock at the CS off point (right). Subjects learned to avoid the painful shock by pressing a button (R^a) after 7 sec when they heard a tone (S^D). One hundred percent avoidance was achieved during overlearning trials. During extinction no shock was presented; during forced extinction subjects were instructed to withhold the avoidance response. Only two-thirds of the subjects complied with this instruction; the remaining subjects continued to respond. (From Birbaumer N. *Psychophysiologie der Angst*, 2nd ed. München: Urban 1977, with permission.)

sponses, while D is a function of the period of deprivation of a positively reinforcing event such as food, or the "aversiveness" of the unconditioned stimulus (measured by psychophysic scaling in humans).

Figure 4 shows the typical changes in cortical negativities and positivities in the course of the habituation, acquisition, and extinction of a pain-related conditioned avoidance response. The greatest cortical activity occurs in the first acquisition trials; with stabilization and automatization of the conditioned response the negativity is slightly reduced. However, since habit strength increases with repetition, the cortical response never entirely disappears, even after thousands of repetitions (see also Pauli et al. 1994). During extinction (presentation of CS alone), the negative potential disappears only in those subjects who cease to show the conditioned avoidance response. Those continuing to avoid the (no longer existing) anticipated pain exhibit the typical cortical pattern of the acquisition trials even during extinction: an anticipatory negative slow potential before the conditioned avoidance response, followed by a larger (reinforcing) inhibitory positive slow potential after the response. The stability of this cortical pattern is predictive of the stability of the behavioral or peripheral physiologic pain-avoidance response. The same cortical pattern in aversive conditioning has been demonstrated in rats (Nakamura et al. 1993).

Thus, the corticalization of pain memories may be reflected in a characteristic sequence of depolarization (negativity) and repolarization (positivity) of widespread cell assemblies responsible for the storage and retrieval of pain memories.

THE DYNAMICS OF CORTICAL OSCILLATORS ARE CHANGED IN CHRONIC-PAIN PATIENTS

The data reported up to this point clearly demonstrate plastic changes in the response to pain stimuli and pain conditioning in the CNS of patients with chronic pain. They do not reveal any information about constant or tonic modifications of the dynamics of CNS activity. At a peripheral level (i.e., in the muscular and cardiovascular system), pain patients generally do not differ from healthy controls except for their responses to specific situational cues such as those described above. The possibility remains, however, that the widespread plastic modifications described here permanently change the responsivity and dynamics of the cortical networks. In order to test this possibility we analyzed spontaneous EEG activity with classical power spectra and more recent nonlinear mathematical procedures that describe the inherent dynamics of a biologic process such as the EEG or MEG (for a detailed description of the methods, see Elbert et al. 1994b; Lutzenberger et al. 1992).

The relationship of the dimensional complexity and power spectra of the EEG to the actual experience of pain as well as to memory for pain was assessed in nine patients with chronic pain and nine matched, healthy controls (Lutzenberger et al. 1994). During a resting phase and various heat and heat-pain induction phases as well as pain recall and imagery conditions, the EEG was recorded from 15 scalp sites. Nonlinear analysis, based on the theory of deterministic chaos, revealed no differences in the complexity of the EEG for the painful as compared to the nonpainful stimulation, but confirmed previous findings of increased complexity for pain-related imagery as compared to other types of imagery. The personal pain situation induced more complex and widespread EEG activity in the patients than in the healthy controls. The self-controlled pain exposure led to a marked hemispheric difference in complexity.

Subjects with high pain thresholds showed more EEG activity in the delta and theta ranges and lower dimensional complexity when exposed to painful stimulation than subjects with low pain thresholds (Fig. 5). The power-spectra measures generally revealed few consistent effects except for the previously reported increase in beta activity during painful stimulation and an increase in the theta band frontally, related to differences in pain sensitivity.

In earlier work (Lutzenberger et al. 1992; Birbaumer et al. in press b), we demonstrated that dimensional complexity ("unpredictability") of the EEG is a highly stable characteristic of the electrocortical dynamics of an individual. In various cognitive and emotional tasks we found that dimensional complexity decreases with the

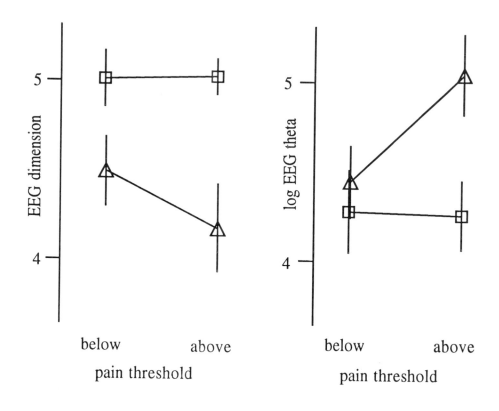

△ high threshold

☐ low threshold

FIG. 5. Dimensional complexity of the EEGs of subjects with high (△) and low pain thresholds (☐) during thermal stimulation exceeding and below the pain threshold (left), and log power spectra of EEG theta rhythms (3.5–7.5 Hz). For explanation see text.

involvement of cortical assemblies engaged in the focused processing of particular external events, but increases with the frequency and amount of interaction among assemblies during periods of external environmental quiescence. With regard to the results in pain patients, it can be hypothesized that particularly during pain-related imagery, the number and/or the interaction of cortical cell assemblies involved in the processing of pain-related memories increases. We found an impoverished picture of cortical dynamics during states of intensive emotions, lower intelligence, and increased focusing of attention to external events, among other circumstances. Chronic pain seems to fundamentally change the way in which the cortex processes painful stimulation. What specific aspect of the cell-assembly dynamics is modified remains to be elucidated.

CONCLUSION

The reported research on muscular activity and brain responses in chronic pain clearly establishes that classical and instrumental learning of a stereotypy in muscular response plays a major role in the maintenance and acquisition of chronic pain. The "corticalization" of these learning processes into a stable pain memory independent of the tissue lesions constitutes the central step in the enduring behavioral and subjective suffering of the patient. Event-related brain potentials and cortical magnetic fields recorded during painful stimuli in pain patients revealed an increased plasticity of brain structures involved in the processing of pain signals that was specific to stimulation at the site of pain. In addition, the brain electrical activity of persons in pain shows a habitual change in cortical dynamics that suggests a fundamental pathology after the formation of cortical memories of pain.

ACKNOWLEDGEMENT

The work described in this chapter was supported by grants to the participating authors from the Deutsche Forschungsgemeinschaft (DFG). This chapter is devoted to Burkhart Bromm, the pioneer in the electrophysiology of pain.

REFERENCES

Birbaumer N, Elbert T, Canavan AGM, Rockstroh B. Slow potentials of the cerebral cortex and behavior. *Physiol Rev* 1990;70:1–41.

Birbaumer N. Psychologische Analyse und Behandlung des Schmerzes [Psychological analysis and treatment of chronic pain]. In: Zimmermann M, Handwerker H, eds. *Schmerz. Konzepte und ärztliches Handeln. [Concepts and medical action]*, Berlin: Springer Verlag, 1987.

Birbaumer N, Flor H, Lutzenberger W, Elbert T. Chaos and order in the human brain. In: Karmos G, Molnar M, eds. *Event related potentials of the brain. Electroencephalograph and clinical neurophysiology*. Amsterdam: Elsevier, (*In press* b).

Bromm B. Pain-related components in the cerebral potential. Experimental and multivariate statistical approaches. In: Bromm B, ed. *Pain measurement in man. Neurophysiological correlates of pain*. Amsterdam: Elsevier, 1984;257–290.

Daum I, Schugens MM, Ackermann H, Lutzenberger W, Dichgans J, Birbaumer N. Classical conditioning after cerebellar lesions in humans. *Behav Neurosci* 1993;107:411–419.

Elbert T, Flor H, Birbaumer N, Hampson S, Taub E, Knecht U, Larbig W. Plastic changes in the adult somatosensory cortex. Extensive reorganization of the somatosensory cortex in adult humans after nervous system injury. *Neuroreport* 1994a;5:2593–2597.

Elbert T, Ray WJ, Kowalik ZJ, Skinner JE, Graf KE, Birbaumer N. Chaos and physiology. Deterministic chaos in excitable cell assemblies. *Physiol Rev* 1994b;74:1–47.

Flor H, Birbaumer N. Basic issues in the psychobiology of pain. In: Gebhart, G, et al. eds. *Proceedings of the VIIth World Congress on Pain*. Seattle: ISAP Publications, 1994a;113–125.

Flor H, Birbaumer N. Psychophysiological methods in the assessment and treatment of chronic pain. In: Carlson J, Seifert R, Birbaumer N, eds. *Clinical Applied Psychophysiology*, New York: Plenum Press, 1994b;171–184.

Flor H, Birbaumer N. Acquisition of chronic pain: psychophysiological mechanisms. *Amer Pain Soc J* 1994c;32:119–127.

Flor H, Birbaumer N, Braun C, Elbert T, Ross M, Hoke M. Chronic pain enhances the magnitude of the magnetic field evoked by painful stimulation. In: Deeke L, Baumgartner C, Stroink G, Williamson SJ, eds. *Recent advances in biomagnetism. Ninth International Conference on Biomagnetism,* Vienna (in press).

Flor H, Birbaumer N, Fürst M, Lutzenberger W, Elbert T, Braun C. Evidence of enhanced peripheral and central responses to painful stimulation in chronic pain. *Psychophysiology* 1993b;30:9.

Flor H, Birbaumer N, Schugens MM, Lutzenberger W. Symptom-specific responding in chronic pain patients and healthy controls. *Psychophysiology* 1992;29:452–460.

Flor H, Birbaumer N, Schulte W, Roos R. Stress-related EMG responses in patients with chronic temporomandibular pain. *Pain* 1991;46:145–152.

Flor H, Birbaumer N, Turk DC. The psychobiology of chronic pain. *Adv Behav Res Ther* 1990;12: 47–84.

Flor H, Breitenstein C, Birbaumer N, Fürst M. A psychophysiological analysis of operant reinforcement, spouse interaction and pain perception, 1994.

Flor H, Roberts L, Birbaumer N, Fürst M, Lutzenberger W, Herrmann C. Cortical correlates of Pavlovian conditioning. Submitted for publication. 1993c;

Flor H, Schugens MM, Birbaumer N. Discrimination of muscle tension in chronic pain patients and healthy controls. *Biofeedback Self-Regul* 1992;17:165–177.

Flor H, Turk DC. Etiological theories and treatment for chronic back pain. I. Psychological models and interventions. *Pain* 1984;19:105–121.

Flor H, Turk DC, Birbaumer N. Assessment of stress-related psychophysiological reactions in chronic back pain patients. *J Consult Clini Psychol* 1985;53:354–364.

Fordyce WE. *Behavioral concepts of chronic pain and illness.* St. Louis: CV Mosby, 1976.

Hull CL. *Essentials of behavior.* New Haven, CT: Yale University Press, 1951.

Larbig W, Elbert T, Lutzenberger W, Rockstroh B, Schnerr G, Birbaumer N. EEG and slow cortical potentials during anticipation and control of painful stimulation. *Electroencephalogr Clin Neurophysiol* 1982;53:298–309.

Leventhal H, Everhart D. Emotion, pain and physical illness. In: Izard CE, ed. *Emotion and psychopathology.* New York: Plenum Press, 1979.

Lutzenberger W, Elbert T, Birbaumer N, Ray W, Schupp H. The scalp distribution of the fractal dimension of the EEG and its variation with mental tasks. *Brain Topogr* 1992;5:27–36.

Lutzenberger W, Flor H, Birbaumer N. Dimensional and spectral analysis of the EEG during experimentally induced and recalled pain in chronic pain patients and healthy controls. Submitted for publication.

Melzack RA. The gate-control theory 25 years later: new perspectives on phantom limb pain. In: Bond MR, Charlton JE, Woolf CJ, eds. *Proceedings of the VIth World Congress on Pain.* Amsterdam: Elsevier, 1991;9–21.

Nakamura M, Ozawa N, Shinba T, Yamamoto K. CNV-like potentials on the cortical surface associated with conditioning in head-restrained rats. *Electroencephalogr Clin Neurophysiol* 1993;88:155–162.

Pauli P, Lutzenberger W, Rau H, Birbaumer N, Rickard TC, Yaroush RA, Bourne LE Jr. Brain potentials during mental arithmetic effects of extensive practice and problem difficulty. *Cognitive Brain Research* 1994;2:21–29.

Ramachandran VS, Stewart M, Rogers-Ramachandran DC. Perceptual correlates of massive cortical reorganization. *Neuroreport* 1992;3:583–586.

Rockstroh B, Elbert T, Canavan A, Lutzenberger W, Birbaumer N. *Slow brain potentials and behavior II,* 2nd ed. München: Urban & Schwarzenberg, 1989.

Rockstroh B, Elbert T, Lutzenberger W, Birbaumer N. Slow cortical potentials under conditions of uncontrollability. *Psychophysiology* 1979;16:374–380.

Squire LR, Zola-Morgan S. The medial temporal lobe memory system. *Science* 1991;253:1380–1389.

Pain and the Brain: From
Nociception to Cognition,
edited by Burkhart Bromm and
John E. Desmedt, Advances in Pain
Research and Therapy Vol. 22.
Raven Press, Ltd., New York © 1995.

22

Pain and Depression

Hans Christoph Diener, Rudolf van Schayck, and Oliver Kastrup

Department of Neurology, University of Essen, D-45122 Essen, Germany

SUMMARY

Pain and depression often occur simultaneously and may have common causal mechanisms. Exact history taking allows the classification of both according to operational criteria. The exact classification of pain and depression improves the scientific knowledge of their overlap and influence on each other. Pain can be classified as acute, chronic, nociceptive, or neuropathic. Two clinical presentations of depression are of particular interest: major depression according to the criteria of the Diagnostic and Statistical Manual of Mental Disorders, Third Edition (Revised) (DSM-III-R 1987), and depressive syndromes following chronic painful conditions. In different pain states, major depression is no more frequent than expected, whereas depressive symptoms are common in chronic pain. Modern concepts of pain therapy therefore encompass a combined analgesic and antidepressive regimen with medical and pharmacologic as well as psychological methods.

INTRODUCTION

Pain and depression are problems frequently encountered in the daily work of physicians. A recent survey in Germany indicated that the most frequent disorders that neurologists and psychiatrists see in private practice are depression (40%) and chronic pain (33%), followed by neurasthenic syndromes (25%) and sleep disturbances (22%) (Bochnik and Koch 1990). Pain and depression may occur simultaneously, but may also influence each other. Chronic pain of organic origin may result in a depressive mood. Major depression, on the other hand, may result in chronic pain (Fig. 1). This chapter aims to define "pain" and "depression," and tries to show how prior history, signs, and symptoms may help to differentiate the relative contribution of the two states in circumstances of their combined occurrence.

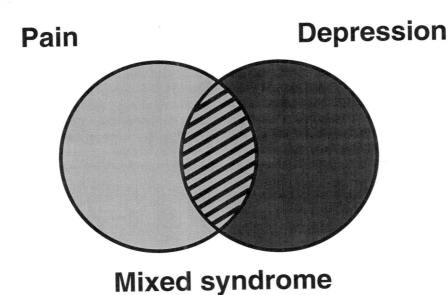

FIG. 1. Conjunction of pain and depression. Combined syndromes encompass predominantly somatic illnesses with depressive symptoms.

CLASSIFICATION OF PAIN AND DEPRESSION

Two systems are used to identify and characterize depressive symptoms or major depression. The International Classification of Diseases (ICD-10, World Health Organization 1991) and the Diagnostic and Statistical Manual of Mental Disorders, Third Edition (Revised) (DSM-III-R, 1987) give operational criteria for the diagnosis of depression. Pain can be characterized according to a classification published in 1986 by the International Association for the Study of Pain (IASP 1986), headache and facial pain according to the International Headache Society (IHS 1988), and back pain according to the Quebec Task Force on Spinal Disorders (1987). This, however, does not replace a careful and proper history and examination in a particular patient. These systems are most helpful for identifying homgeneous patient groups for scientific studies.

PAIN

The definition of pain according to the World Health Organization is: "An unpleasant sensory and emotional experience associated with actual or potential tissue damage, or described in terms of such damage" (Merskey 1986). This definition indicates that pain not only includes pathologic afferent sensory information, but also unpleasant affective sensation. Tissue damage is not a necessary prerequisite for the generation of pain. Pain resulting from the stimulation or irritation of peripheral pain receptors, the nociceptors, is called nociceptive pain. Damage to peripheral nerves, posterior roots, the spinal cord, or certain regions of the brain (e.g., the pathways involved in pain transmission) may cause so called neuropathic pain. In many pain conditions, nociceptive and neuropathic pain coexist. In contrast to acute pain, chronic pain is defined as pain persisting longer than 6 months. Epidemiologic studies show the importance of chronic pain in the general population (von Korff et al. 1988, 1990; Taylor and Curran 1985): 10% of patients in the care of practitioners, internists, or neurologists complain of chronic pain. The respective number of patients seen by orthopedic surgeons is 30%. In a survey in the United States, patients were asked whether they had suffered from any pain during the previous year: 41% complained of back pain, 26% of headache, 17% of abdominal pain, 12% of chest pain, and 12% of facial pain (von Korff et al. 1988).

DEPRESSION

The lifetime probability of experiencing a "major depression" in a western country is 20 to 30%. "Major depression" as defined by the DSM-III-R is characterized by a depressive mood, loss of interest and joy, loss or increase in weight, sleep disturbances, restlessness or tiredness, loss of energy, feeling of worthlessness, sense of guilt, and lack of concentration. Psychotic symptoms such as hallucinations or thought disturbances should be excluded. Major depression may manifest itself as so called monopolar depression, consisting of recurrent depressive phases only, or as bipolar depression, consisting of alternating depressive phases and/or manic phases. The sex ratio for major depression is 4:1 for women and men (Klerman 1988). Major depressive illness is characterized by a deep sadness with inability to experience joyful feelings. Emotions are flattened or absent. Additional symptoms include loss of initiative and interest, combined with a feeling of worthlessness and suicidal ideation. Autonomic dysfunctions include sleep disturbances, constipation, loss of appetite, impotence, and loss of libido (Klerman 1988). Sleep disturbances are common with early-morning awakening and disrupted sleep. The disturbed circadian rhythm is reflected by an accentuation of the depression in the morning, with improvement during the day. Depressive phases may occur without external triggers and may end spontaneously. Family studies show a genetic risk for depression. A transition toward psychotic depression is characterized by delusions of guilt as well as nihilistic ideation. The diagnostic category of major depression according to the newer diagnostic manuals (i.e., DSM-III-R and ICD-10) and recently developed research criteria in current use shows a considerable overlap with older European diagnoses, notably with the entity of the so called "endogenous" depression, that originates from an older German psychologic classification implying a common psychopathologic mechanism, and does not use operational criteria. However big the clinical overlap of these diagnoses, the fact that several diagnostic classifications are still in use (Lopez-Ibor 1972) and have been applied differently in the past makes it difficult to draw comparisons and parallels between existing clinical studies. So called "reactive" depression calls for a significant major life event being followed by a monophasic depression, with a tendency of improvement toward remission. "Neurotic" depression is characterized by a lesser disturbance of biorhythm and autonomic function. The history may show a life event as a biographic trigger (e.g., a conflict, a separation, or unresolved conflicts during childhood or adolescence). It is important to note that overlap between the categories may be marked.

DEPRESSION AND PAIN

Chronic pain is a frequent symptom of depression. Several studies using different diagnostic criteria showed that between 15% and 90% of patients with depression complain of chronic pain (Cassidy et al. 1957; Diamond 1964; Ierodiakonou and Iavocides 1987; Lehrl et al. 1980). The location of the pain is variable (Table 1), with the predominant site being the head. Earlier studies, however, did not apply the operational criteria proposed by the IHS to classify headache (Headache Classification Committee of the International Headache Society 1988). Pain is reported more often by patients with neurotic depression than by those with monopolar or bipolar depression (von Knorring et al. 1983). Some depressed patients may present complaints about pain only if specifically asked. The concomitant appearance of depression and pain is not surprising, considering the psychological and biochemical factors that are sometimes codependent in depression and pain and show mutual aggravation. On a psychological and emotional basis, clinically depressed patients may be more likely to develop chronic pain, whereas chronic pain should not as a rule cause a phasic monopolar depression, although clinicians have sometimes seen this. A major point is the heightened susceptibility of depressed patients over that of nondepressed patients to experience an existing, if slight, pain as more unpleasant and sometimes unbearable. This can be regarded not only as a functionally reduced central pain threshold, but also as weakened or sometimes nonexistent strategies for

TABLE 1. *Pain in depressive illness[a]*

Localization of pain	
Head	49%
Back	39%
Abdomen	38%
Chest	36%
Joints	30%
Extremities	25%

[a]Modified according to Cassidy et al. 1957.

coping with pain on a behavioral level. It is tempting to speculate that the biochemical and pharmacologic factors parallel to these psychological and behavioral factors in patients with simultaneous pain and depression may lie in the serotonergic system of the central nervous system (CNS). Pharmacologically, both pain and depression experience beneficial effects from the administration of tricyclic antidepressants, most of which are serotonin-reuptake-inhibitors. Concentrating on the serotonergic model of pain and depression alone, however, oversimplifies the complex interaction and "cross-talk" of the multiple receptor and transmitter axes. Moreover, reuptake inhibitors of other transmitters (i.e., norepinephrine) are sometimes effective. Even the anticholinergic side effects of older tricyclic drugs (experienced as side effects by patients) may actually be beneficial therapeutic activity.

OTHER PAIN SYNDROMES

In many patients with chronic pain, no organic correlate can be found. This fact, and the lack of concepts about the exact causal and pathophysiologic as well as psychopathologic factors in chronic pain, have led to the creation of a variety of diagnostic labels that have been applied to these patients. The diagnoses have been called idiopathic pain disorder, pain-prone disorder, or somatoform pain disorder, and it is not always easy to tell where the overlap with psychogenic pain (DSM-III) begins. According to Blumer and Heilbronn (1982), there are no operational criteria for the pain-prone disorder. Most of the patients with this disorder are middle-aged. The symptoms begin after a serious life event, and the intensity and duration of pain increase over time. Typical complications are multiple surgeries or dependency on analgesic drugs. If surgery was performed, it is likely that a neurogenic pain has developed. Somatoform pain disorder does have operational criteria according either to DSM-III-R or to the so-called idiopathic pain disorder (Williams and Spitzer 1982) that will be presented in detail later in this chapter (see Table 2). In general, the diagnosis of "psychogenic" pain (Valdes et al. 1989) should be made with great care. One working hypothesis stresses that the interval between a trauma or nerve injury and the beginning of chronic pain may be quite long. Recent neurophysiologic data from animal experiments clearly showed that chronic pain can induce changes in spinal and supraspinal pathways and in receptor sensitivity, resulting in an increase, beyond the anatomic limits of the original lesion, in the afferent area in which pain can be provoked (Devor et al. 1991; Jänig 1988).

DEPRESSION IN CHRONIC PAIN STATES

A review of the literature shows that between 5% and 87% of patients with chronic pain exhibit symptoms of a depression. The populations, however, are very inhomogeneous (Fishbain et al. 1986; France et al. 1987; Haley et al. 1985; Haythornthwaite et al. 1991; Hendler 1984; Kramlinger et al. 1983; Lindsay et al. 1981; Pilowsky et al. 1977; Pilowsky 1988; Reich et al. 1983). According to Williams and

TABLE 2. *Operational criteria of idiopathic pain disorder according to*
Williams and Spitzer (1982)

Constant occupation with and rumination about pain for a period longer than 6 months as the
    predominant disturbance.
Pain does not fit anatomic distribution or representation of the nervous system. No pathologic
    findings on examination and tests. If organic findings are present, the complaint of pain
    appears disproportional to the nonrelevant organic findings.
Schizophrenia or major depression are exclusion criteria.

Spitzer (1982) 80% of the patients with an idiopathic pain disorder are depressed.
The following discussion will give a more detailed description of the correlation
between pain and depression for different pain patients.

DEPRESSION AND HEADACHE

The prevalences of both depression and headache are high. The prevalence of
migraine is 14% for women and 7% for men between the ages of 18 and 65 (Pryse
Phillips et al. 1992; Rasmussen 1992; Rasmussen et al. 1991; Stang and Osterhaus
1993). The prevalence of episodic tension-type headache is 25% and 3% for chronic
tension-type headache (i.e., more than 15 headache days per month; Diener and
Edmeads 1993). Major depression occurs in the same age range in 5 to 25% of
women and 2 to 12% of men (Linet and Stewart 1984). This implies that a considerable overlap of the two conditions may exist (Diamond 1964). Despite the fact that
migraine and depression have a genetic component (Merikangas et al. 1988), no
study has yet been able to show a common causal mechanism for the two disorders.
Headaches is the most commonly reported manifestation of pain in depressed patients. The headache resembles tension-type headache and is diffuse, dull, and without autonomic disturbances (Lehrl et al. 1980).

DEPRESSION AND ATYPICAL FACIAL PAIN

Atypical facial pain is characterized by a unilateral, orofacial, chronic pain and
normal neurologic and dental examination. All other tests are invariably normal,
including X-rays of the sinuses. The prior history may reveal minor trauma, such as
small injuries, injections, or dental operations. Several studies found a higher prevalence of depression than in matched subjects without facial pain. Psychological
testing found higher values for hypochondriasis, hysteria, depression, and perfec-
tionism. Despite the high prevalence of depressive symptoms, ranging from 62 to
96%, the diagnosis of a major depression can only be made in 13% of patients with
atypical facial pain (Delaney 1976; Eversole et al. 1985; Hampf et al. 1987; Remick
et al. 1983; Remick and Blasberg 1985).

DEPRESSION AND NEUROPATHIC PAIN

Neuropathic pain is due to structural damage of peripheral or central pain-mediating systems. The pain is characterized by its burning and tearing nature. Typical examples are postherpetic neuralgia, diabetic polyneuropathy, and phantom-limb pain. A recent study showed that phantom pain is associated with depressive symptoms in 72% of cases (Sherman et al. 1987). Major depression is again not more frequent than in the general population (Lindsay 1985; Parkes 1973; Shukla et al. 1982).

DEPRESSION AND LOW-BACK PAIN

Chronic low-back pain is the most frequent manifestation of pain and one of the leading causes of early retirement. The "failed back" syndrome encompasses patients with repeated unsuccessful low-back surgery (Burton et al. 1981; Wilkinson 1983). The prevalence of depressive symptoms in this subgroup is 85% (Krishnan et al. 1985; Long 1988). In a smaller group of patients with a single lumbar-disc protrusion, only 18% had some depressive symptoms (Hasenbring and Ahrens 1987).

DEPRESSION AND CANCER PAIN

Malignant tumors lead to chronic pain in about 50% of the cases. In advanced stages, this percentage rises to 74% (Bonica 1985). With progressing tumor stages, the incidence of depressive symptoms increases (Bukberg et al. 1984; Derogatis 1983; Massi and Holland 1990). Whether this is due to the prognosis of the underlying disease or to the pain itself is not clear. The prevalence of major depression is not higher in patients with malignancies than in those without them (Derogatis 1983).

PATHOGENESIS OF PAIN AND DEPRESSION

Chronic pain can be quantified by pain diaries and pain scales, the latter consisting either of visual analogue scales or step scales. Depression can be quantified by the Beck Depression Inventory (1979). The diagnosis, however, has to be confirmed by a psychiatrist.

If two conditions overlap, such as chronic pain and depression, the search for biologic markers or common biochemical changes is of special importance. The investigation of relatives of patients with depression or idiopathic pain showed an increased prevalence of depressive symptoms and tension, increased muscle tone, and latent aggession (Chaturverdi 1989; Katon et al. 1985; Valdes et al. 1989). Both groups of patients more often show a reduced rapid-eye-movement (REM-)phase during sleep, an increase in plasma cortisol, a pathological dexamethasone-test, and low 5-hydroxy indoleacetic acid (5-HIAA) levels in the cerebrospinal fluid (CSF) (Eberhard et al. 1989). These changes may be nonspecific, and could as well be the consequence as the cause of pain, stress, and depression.

TREATMENT OF PAIN AND DEPRESSION

Older publications have already presented the concept of pain as a psychophysical phenomenon afflicting the whole person (Melzack and Wall 1965). Therefore, many authors have advocated a combination of medical and pharmacologic as well as psychological treatment for it. These measures are not seen as exclusive; their combination presents a rational and effective therapeutic approach to pain. Different nonpharmacologic therapies have been proposed. The behavioral approach stresses the importance of the development of coping strategies to reinforce so called "healthy" traits and patterns of behavior (Block et al. 1980; Fordyce 1976). The physiologic approach presents different relaxation techniques (biofeedback, Jacobson technique) that draw their efficacy not from muscle relaxation itself, but from a heightened sense of being in control (Stuckey et al. 1986). Cognitive therapy aims at readjusting the cognitive importance attributed to the experienced pain (Turk and Meichenbaum 1989). The mainstay of pharmacologic treatment for pain is antidepressive medication. Tricyclic antidepressant drugs are used to treat chronic pain. A success rate of 30 to 50% in easing pain was shown in 34 of 40 placebo-controlled trials (Magni 1991; Tura and Tura 1991; Zitman et al. 1990). The rate of patients who respond is between 40 and 65%. This corresponds to the numbers seen in the treatment of depression. Amitriptyline, amitriptylinoxide, doxepine, imipramine, and clomipramine are the drugs most widely used. All of these substances are inhibitors of serotonin (5HT) reuptake. Inhibitors of noradrenaline reuptake also seem to be effective (e.g., desipramine, maproptyline, nortryptiline). 5HT and noradrenaline are important neurotransmitters in the central modulation of pain. Both of these substances have a central analgesic effect and in higher doses an antidepressive action. The onset of the analgesic action is earlier (3 to 10 days) than that of the antidepressive effect (14 to 21 days). The greatest success rates can be obtained in patients with neuropathic pain. In cancer pain, thymoleptic drugs often have to be combined with minor or major analgesics. For practical reasons, the following recommendations should be followed:

1. If a rapid effect is required, treatment with antidepressants should be initiated parenterally, with an overlapping dose scheme in which increasing oral doses are exchanged for decreasing i.v. doses.
2. Therapy should start with low or very low doses (e.g., 10–25 mg amitriptyline). Patients must be informed that they may first experience the unpleasant anticholinergic side effects (sedation, dry mouth) and only with considerable delay the positive pain-reducing effects of the drug.
3. Patients should be informed that the analgesic action of antidepressants is not mentioned in the patient information sheet and that they are not being treated

with such a drug because the treating physician considers them as being primarily depressive.

4. In cases in which a major depression and chronic pain coexist, the treatment should include doses that are antidepressive.

5. If patients complain about sleep disturbances and restlessness, sedating antidepressants should be given in the evening.

REFERENCES

American Psychiatric Association Staff. *Diagnostic and statistical manual of mental disorders*, 3rd ed., revised. Washington, DC: American Psychiatric Association, 1987.

Beck Depression Inventory. In: Beck AT, Rush AJ, Shaw BF, Emery G, eds. *Cognitive therapy of depression*. New York: Guilford Press, 1979.

Block A, Kremer E, Gaylor M. Behavioral treatment of chronic pain: The spouse as a discriminative cue for pain behavior. *Pain* 1980;9:243–252.

Blumer D, Heilbronn M. Chronic pain as a variant of depressive disease. The pain-prone disorder. *J Nerv Ment Dis* 1982;170:361–372.

Bochnik HJ, Koch H. *Die Nervenarztstudie*. Köln: Deutscher Ärzte-Verlag, 1990.

Bonica JJ. Treatment of cancer pain: current status and future needs. In: Fields HL, Dubner R, Cervero F, eds. *Advances in pain research and therapy*, vol. 9. New York: Raven Press, 1985;589–616.

Bukberg J. Penman D, Holland J. Depression in hospitalized cancer patients. *Pychosom Med* 1984; 43:199–212.

Burton CV, Kirkaldy-Willis WH, Yong-Hing K, Hinthoff KB. Cause and failure of surgery on the lumbar spine. *Clin Orthop* 1981;157:191–201.

Cassidy WL, Flanagan NB, Spellman M, Cohen ME. Clinical observation in manic-depressive disease. *JAMA* 1957;164:1535–1547.

Chaturverdi SK. Psychalgic depressive disorder: a descriptive and comparative study. *Acta Psychiatr Scand* 1989;79:98–102.

Delaney JF. Atypical facial pain as a defense against psychosis. *Am J Psychiatry* 1976;133:1151–1154.

Derogatis LR. The prevalence of psychiatric disorders among cancer patients. *JAMA* 1983;249:751–757.

Devor M, Basbaum AJ, Bennett GJ, Blumberg H, Campbell JN, Dembowsky KP, Guilbaud, G, Jänig W, Koltzenburg M, Levine JD, Otten UH, Portenoy RK. Mechanisms of neuropathic pain following peripheral injury. In: Basbaum AJ, Besson J-M, eds. *Towards a new pharmacotherapy of pain. Dahlem Workshop Reports*. Chichester: John Wiley & Sons, 1991;417–440.

Diamond S. Depressive headaches. *Headache* 1964;4:255–261.

Diener HC, Edmeads J. Tension-type headache. General approach to treatment. In: Olesen J, Tfelt-Hansen P, Welch KMA, eds. *The headaches*. New York: Raven Press, 1993;513–514.

Eberhard G, von Knorring L, Mellerup ET, Nilson HL, Plenge P, Sundequist U. ^{3}H-imipramine binding in idiopathic pain syndromes. Basal values and changes after treatment with antidepressants. *Pain* 1989;38:261–267.

Eversole LR, Stone CE, Matheson D, Kaplan H. Psychometric profiles and facial pain. *Oral Surg Oral Med Oral Pathol* 1985;60:269–274.

Fishbain DA, Goldberg M, Meagher BR, Steele R, Rosomoff H. Male and female chronic pain patients categorized by DSM-III psychiatric diagnostic criteria. *Pain* 1986;26:181–194.

Fordyce WE. *Behavioral methods for chronic pain and illness*. St. Louis: CV Mosby, 1976.

France RD, Krishnan KRR, Trainor M, Pelton S. Chronic pain and depression IV. DST as a discriminator between chronic pain and depression. *Pain* 1987;28:39–47.

Haley WE, Turner JA, Romano JM. Depression in chronic pain patients: relation to pain, activity and sex differences. *Pain* 1985;23:337–348.

Hampf G, Vikkula J, Ylipaavalniemi P, Aalerg V. Psychiatric disorders in orofacial dysaesthesia. *Int J Oral Maxillofac Surg* 1987;16:402–407.

Hasenbring M, Ahrens S. Depressivität, Schmerz-wahrnehmung und Schmerzverarbeitung bei Patienten mit lumbalem Bandscheibenvorfall. *Psychother Psychosom Med Psychol* 1987;37:149–155.

Haythornthwaite JA, Sieber WJ, Kerns RD. Depression and the chronic pain experience. *Pain* 1991; 46:177–184.

Headache Classification Committee of the International Headache Society. Classification and diagnostic criteria for headache disorders, cranial neuralgias and facial pain. *Cephalalgia* 1988;8(Suppl 7):1–93.

Hendler N. Depression caused by chronic pain. *J Clin Psychiatry* 1984;45:30–38.

Ierodiakonou CS, Iavocides A. Somatic manifestations of depressive patients in different psychiatric settings. *Psychopathology* 1987;20:136–143.

International Association for the Study of Pain (IASP) Subcommittee of Taxonomy. Classification of chronic pain. Description of chronic pain syndromes and definitions of pain terms. *Pain* 1986;(Suppl 3):1–225.

Jänig W. Pathophysiology of nerve following mechanical injury In: Dubner R, Gebhart GF, Bond MR, eds. *Pain research and clinical management*, vol. 3. Amsterdam, New York, Oxford: Elsevier, 1988; 89–108.

Katon W, Egan K, Miller D. Chronic pain: lifetime psychiatric diagnoses and family history. *Am J Psychiatry* 1985;142:1156–1169.

Klerman G. Depression and related disorders of mood. In: *The new Harvard guide to psychiatry*. Cambridge, MA: Belknap Press, 1988;309–336.

Kramlinger GG, Swanson DW, Maruta T. Are patients with chronic pain depressed? *Am J Psychiatry* 1983;140:747–758.

Krishnan KRR, France RD, Pelton S, McCann UD, Davidson J, Urban BJ. Chronic pain and depression. I. Classification in chronic low back pain patients. *Pain* 1985;22:279–287.

Lehrl S, Zenglein R, Gallwitz A. Schmerzangaben bei Schizophrenie sowie endogener und psychischer Depression im Verleich zu Schmerzangaben bei definierten Körperkrankheiten. *Krankenhausarzt* 1980;53:55–62.

Lindsay PG, Wyckhoff M. The depression-pain syndrome and its response to antidepressants. *Psychosomatics* 1981;22:571–578.

Lindsay JE. Multiple pain complaints in amputees. *J R Soc Med* 1985;78:452–455.

Linet MS, Stewart WF. Migraine headache: epidemiologic perspectives. *Epidemiol Rev* 1984;6:107–139.

Long DM. Genesis of the failed back syndrome. In: Dubner R, Gebhart EF, Bond MR, eds. *Proceedings of the Vth World Congress on Pain*. Amsterdam, New York, Oxford: Elsevier, 1988;244–247.

Lopez-Ibor JJ. Masked depressions. *Br J Psychiatry* 1972;120:245–253.

Magni G. The use of antidepressants in the treatment of chronic pain. A review of the current evidence. *Drugs* 1991;42:730–748.

Massi MJ, Holland JC. Depression and the cancer patient. *J Clin Psychiatry* 1990;51:12–17.

Melzack R, Wall P. Pain mechanisms: a new theory. *Science* 1965;50:971–979.

Merikangas KR, Risch NJ, Merikangas JR. Migraine and depression: Association and familial transmission. *J Psychiatr Res* 1988;22:119–129.

Merskey H. Classification of chronic pain, descriptions of pain syndromes and definitions of pain terms. *Pain* 1986;(Suppl 3):217.

Parkes CM. Factors determining the persistence of phantom pain in the amputee. *J Psychosom Res* 1973; 17:97–108.

Pilowsky J, Chapman CR, Bonica JJ. Pain, depression and illness behaviour in a pain clinic population. *Pain* 1977;4:183–195.

Pilowsky J. Affective disorders and pain. In: Dubner R, Gebhart GF, Bond MR. eds. *Proceedings of the Vth World Congress on Pain*. Amsterdam, New York, Oxford: Elsevier, 1988;263–275.

Pryse Phillips W, Findlay H, Tugwell P, Edmeads J, Murray TJ, Nelson RF. A Canadian population survey on the clinical, epidemiologic and societal impact of migraine and tension-type headache. *Can J Neurol Sci* 1992;19:333–339.

Quebec Task Force on Spinal Disorders. Scientific approach to the assessment and management of activity-related spinal disorders, ch. 3. Diagnosis of the problem. *Spine* 1987;(Suppl):16–21.

Rasmussen BK. Migraine and tension-type headache in a general population: psychosocial factors. *Int J Epidemiol* 1992;21:1138–1143.

Rasmussen BK, Jensen R, Schroll M, Olesen J. Epidemiology of headache in a general population —a prevalence study. *J Clin Epidemiol* 1991;44:1147–1157.

Reich J, Tupin JP, Abramowitz SJ. Psychiatric diagnosis of chronic pain patients. *Am J Psychiatry* 1983;140:1495–1502.

Remick RA, Blasberg B, Campos PE, Miles JE. Psychiatric disorders associated with atypical facial pain. *Can J Psychiatry* 1983;28:178–181.

Remick RA, Blasberg B. Psychiatric aspects of atypical facial pain. *Can Dent Assoc J* 1985;51:913–916.

Sherman RA, Sherman CJ, Bruno GM. Psychological factors influencing chronic phantom limb pain: an analysis of the literature. *Pain* 1987;28:285–295.

Shukla GD, Sahu SC, Tripathi RP, Gupta DK. A psychiatric study of amputees. *Br J Psychiatry* 1982;141:54–58.

Stang PE, Osterhaus JT. Impact of migraine in the United States: data from the National Health Interview Survey. *Headache* 1993;33:29–35.

Stuckey SJ, Jacobs A, Goldfarb J. EMG biofeedback training, relaxation training, and placebo for the relief of chronic pain. *Percept Mot Skills* 1986;63:1023–1036.

Taylor H, Curran NM. *The Nuprin pain report*. New York: Louis Harris, 1985.

Tura B, Tura M. The analgesic effect of the tricyclic antidepressants. *Brain Res* 1991;518:19–23.

Turk DC, Meichenbaum DH. A cognitive-behavioral approach to pain management. In: Wall PD, Melzack R, eds. *Textbook of pain*. London: Churchill Livingstone, 1989;1001–1009.

Valdes M, Garcia L, Treserra J, De Pablo J, De Flores T. Psychogenic pain and depressive disorders: an empirical study. *J Affect Disord* 1989;16:21–25.

Violon A. The onset of facial pain: a psychological study. *Psychother Psychosom* 1980;34:11–16.

von Knorring L, Perris C, Eiseman M, Perris H. Pain as a symptom in depressive disorders. I. Relationship to diagnostic subgroup and depressive symptomatology. *Pain* 1983;15:19–26.

von Korff M, Dworkin SF, Le Resche L, Kruger A. An epidemiologic comparison of pain complaints. *Pain* 1988;32:173–183.

von Korff M, Dworkin SF, Le Resche L. Graded chronic pain status: an epidemiologic evaluation. *Pain* 1990;40:279–291.

Weddington WW, Blazer D. Atypical facial pain and trigeminal neuralgia. A comparison study. *Psychosomatics* 1979;20:348–356.

Wilkinson HA. *The failed back syndrome*. New York: Harper & Row, 1983.

Williams JB, Spitzer RL. Idiopathic pain disorder: a critique of pain-prone disorder and proposal for a revision of the DSM-III category psychogenic pain. *J Nerv Ment Dis* 1982;170:415–424.

World Health Organization. *Tenth Revision of the International Classification of Diseases*. World Health Organization, 1991.

Zitman FG, Linssen ACG, Edelbroek PM, Stijnen T. Low dose amitriptyline in chronic pain: the gain is modest. *Pain* 1990;42:35–42.

*Pain and the Brain: From
Nociception to Cognition,*
edited by Burkhart Bromm and
John E. Desmedt, Advances in Pain
Research and Therapy Vol. 22.
Raven Press, Ltd., New York © 1995.

23

Evidence that Secondary Hyperalgesia Involves Increased Pain To Input from Nociceptors

*Fernando Cervero, †Richard A. Meyer, and †James N. Campbell

*Department of Physiology and Pharmacology, University of Alcalá de Henares,
E-28871 Madrid, Spain, and †Department of Neurosurgery, Johns Hopkins University,
Baltimore, Maryland, 21287

SUMMARY

Substantial evidence suggests that the hyperalgesia to mechanical stimuli that occurs in an area of normal skin surrounding a site of injury (area of secondary hyperalgesia) arises from activity in low-threshold mechanoreceptors (LTMs). In this study we investigated whether activity in mechanically sensitive nociceptors also contributes to this secondary hyperalgesia. It is known that all woolen fabrics excite LTMs, but that only the prickly ones activate mechanically sensitive nociceptors. We therefore conducted a psychophysical study using a range of prickly and non-prickly woolen fabrics applied to normal and hyperalgesic skin in order to assess the roles of LTMs and nociceptors in secondary hyperalgesia. We studied the sensations of fabric-evoked prickle and pain in normal and hyperalgesic skin in 10 normal volunteers. Secondary hyperalgesia was produced by intradermal injection of capsaicin (25 µg) into the volar skin of the forearm. Five woolen fabrics (two non-prickly, two very prickly, and one intermediate) were presented, in a blind manner, to the skin before and after the capsaicin injection. The sensation of fabric-evoked prickle was not changed in hyperalgesic skin. On the other hand, little if any pain was evoked by the fabrics when applied to normal skin, but substantial pain was produced by all of the fabrics when applied to hyperalgesic skin. The pain ratings were graded with the ratings of prickle so that fabrics that evoked the greatest prickle also evoked significantly more pain. The magnitude of pain increased linearly with prickle sensation; the slope of this regression function increased substantially in hyperalgesic skin. The increased pain produced by prickly fabrics in the hyperalgesic skin exceeded that which could be predicted by the acquired capacity of LTMs to evoke pain plus the pain produced by the prickly fabrics in normal skin.

We conclude that the central alterations responsible for secondary hyperalgesia involve two components: an acquired capacity of LTMs to evoke pain and an increased responsiveness of central neurons to input from mechanically sensitive nociceptors.

INTRODUCTION

Mechanisms underlying the development of pain have been studied intensely for decades, but it is only relatively recently that some of the pathways are becoming clearly delineated. Much of this work has been done on skin because it is easily accessible for study. Injury to the skin results in hyperalgesia, with a reduced threshold for pain and enhanced pain with suprathreshold stimuli. Stated differently, hyperalgesia refers to a leftward shift in the stimulus–response function that relates the magnitude of pain to stimulus intensity. Hyperalgesia develops in normal subjects after a cutaneous injury (Meyer et al. 1985; Raja et al. 1984), and may also become evident in skin in certain neuropathic pain conditions (Campbell et al. 1988b).

Hyperalgesia produced by an injury to the skin includes two zones: a zone that incorporates the injury site (zone of primary hyperalgesia), and a much larger area extending well beyond the site of injury (zone of secondary hyperalgesia). Primary and secondary hyperalgesia differ in that the zone of primary hyperalgesia is characterized by hyperalgesia to heat and mechanical stimuli, whereas secondary hyperalgesia is characterized only by an increased painfulness of mechanical stimuli (Raja et al. 1984; Simone et al. 1989). Consequently, it is not surprising that the neural mechanisms that account for secondary hyperalgesia are different from those that account for primary hyperalgesia.

In primary hyperalgesia, pain is evoked by low-intensity heat stimuli; this is probably due to the sensitization of nociceptors to heat stimuli that develops after a cutaneous injury (Meyer and Campbell 1981; LaMotte et al. 1991). Nociceptor sensitization, however, does not occur in the zone of secondary hyperalgesia. For example, in primates, the thresholds to mechanical stimulation of nociceptors (measured with von Frey hairs) are not changed either by adjacent heat, mechanical injuries, or antidromic nerve stimulation (Campbell et al. 1988a; Meyer et al. 1988; Thalhammer and LaMotte, 1983). Thus, nociceptor sensitization in the secondary zone does not account for secondary hyperalgesia. Rather, touch-evoked pain, which partly characterizes secondary hyperalgesia, appears to be mediated by an alteration in central processing in such a way that activation of LTMs evokes pain (LaMotte et al. 1992; Torebjörk et al. 1992). In this regard, in nociceptive neurons in the spinal cord of experimental animals, the input properties and functional responses change dramatically after noxious stimulation of the skin, muscles, joints, and viscera (McMahon and Wall 1984; Schaible et al. 1987; Hylden at al. 1989; Hoheisel and Mense 1989; Laird and Cervero 1989; Cervero et al. 1993; Simone et al. 1991).

Since secondary hyperalgesia is characterized by increased pain in response to mechanical but not to heat stimuli, it does not seem likely that the central alterations discussed above include increased pain to input from polymodal nociceptors (i.e., nociceptors that respond to both heat and mechanical stimuli). If central sensitization to polymodal nociceptors did occur, secondary hyperalgesia would be expected to be characterized by heat and mechanical hyperalgesia. Nevertheless, it is conceivable that input from nociceptors sensitive only to mechanical stimuli could contribute to the altered central processing and aspects of the hyperalgesia to mechanical stimuli in the secondary zone.

It is noteworthy that two types of mechanical hyperalgesia have been demonstrated in the zone of secondary hyperalgesia (LaMotte et al. 1991; Koltzenburg et al. 1992): stroking hyperalgesia (demonstrated by gentle stimulation with a cotton swab) and punctate hyperalgesia (evoked by application of a stiff von Frey probe). This raised the question of whether there are two different neural mechanisms that underlie the two processes.

The following evidence suggests that punctate and stroking hyperalgesia are mediated by different neural mechanisms: (a) the zone of punctate hyperalgesia is consistently larger than that of stroking hyperalgesia (LaMotte at al. 1991; Koltzenburg et al. 1992; Cervero et al. 1994); (b) whereas stroking hyperalgesia induced by capsaicin injection lasts for 1 to 2 hours, punctate hyperalgesia lasts for 13 to 24 hours (LaMotte et al. 1991); and (c) after capsaicin injection, punctate but not stroking hyperalgesia developed in a patient with severe loss of large myelinated fibers (Treede and Cole 1993). It is therefore possible that stroking hyperalgesia is mediated by an altered central processing of inputs from LTMs, whereas punctate hyperalgesia is mediated by an increased sensitivity to inputs from nociceptors sensitive to mechanical but not to heat stimuli.

Evaluation of this hypothesis required a method of distinguishing the responses to stimulation of LTMs and nociceptors. For this purpose we used a psychophysical approach based on the study of the sensation of fabric-evoked prickle. It has been shown that the responses of LTMs are similar for all grades of woolen fabrics, prickly or nonprickly, whereas the responses of nociceptors to woolen fabrics are greater for fabrics that evoke a prickle sensation (Garnsworthy et al. 1988). Therefore, alterations in the kinds of sensations evoked by prickly and nonprickly woolen fabrics in areas of secondary hyperalgesia could help to determine which types of peripheral receptors are involved in initiating these sensations.

The results of this study have been reported previously (Cervero et al. 1994).

METHODS

The prickle paradigm that we developed involved testing responses to pain and prickle evoked by a variety of woolen fabrics in normal and hyperalgesic skin in 10 normal volunteers. Five samples of woolen fabric were chosen with textures that were judged to vary from nonprickly in two cases to mildly prickly in one case and very prickly in two others. The fabrics were applied to the skin in such a manner that volunteers had no visual clue about the nature of the material. Subjects were asked to rate the intensities of the fabric-evoked sensations of prickle and pain on two scales presented consecutively on a computer screen.

The following protocol was used: after mock testing to familiarize the subject with the procedure, a test of the five fabrics was administered. The fabric test consisted of presentation of the five fabrics, five times in a random order. The next day the complete fabrics tests was repeated, followed by injection of capsaicin. Following this a second fabrics test was performed in the region of secondary hyperalgesia. One or 2 days after the capsaicin study, the subject was retested without capsaicin. In this manner, three control tests on normal skin and one test on hyperalgesic skin were performed for each subject.

Although individual subjects generally gave consistent ratings of the fabrics, there was some intersubject variability in the range over which ratings were made. Data were therefore normalized in order to combine results from the group of subjects. The mean ratings for each fabric by an individual subject were calculated for a given fabric test. These means were added to obtain a measure of total reported sensation for each subject for a given test. The biggest sum for the four tests on each subject was then determined, and all data for the subject were then normalized by dividing each mean rating by this biggest sum. A separate normalization was performed for the prickle and pain data.

RESULTS

Assessment of the Fabrics Test

The fabrics test gave extremely consistent results across the control sessions. No statistically significant differences were detected between the three control tests.

Capsaicin Injections

Capsaicin has been widely used in studies of secondary hyperalgesia (Koltzenburg et al. 1992; LaMotte et al. 1992, 1991; Simone et al. 1989; Thalhammer et al. 1983; Treede and Cole 1993). In our subjects, injection of 25 μg of capsaicin intradermally into the volar surface of the left forearm produced a very intense sensation of burning pain that started immediately after the injection, reached a peak within 10 to 15 sec, and decreased slowly over 3 to 15 min.

Shortly after the injection and before the pain had subsided, an area of flare appeared around the injection site, reached its maximum size (15.2 ± 0.9 cm^2; mean $\pm$ SEM) within a few minutes, and remained visible for 1 to 2 hours. When the pain of the injection had dissipated, the skin was mapped for the occurrence of hyperalgesia to tactile stimuli. A large area of hyperalgesia (45.8 ± 4.4 cm^2) was detected in all subjects, and was then subjected to the fabrics test.

Prickle and Pain Sensations Before and After Capsaicin

We found that the ratings of prickle sensation in normal and in hyperalgesic skin were not significantly different (Fig. 1), although prickle sensation in hyperalgesic skin tended to be greater than that for normal skin for fabrics 1 and 2 and below that for normal skin for fabrics 4 and 5.

In contrast, all fabrics evoked significantly more pain in hyperalgesic skin than in normal skin ($p \leq 0.001$). Furthermore, the pain ratings in hyperalgesic skin for fabrics 4 and 5 were significantly greater than for fabrics 1 and 2 ($p \leq 0.02$).

These differences are shown in Fig. 2, in which the ratings for prickle are plotted against the pain ratings obtained for each of the fabrics in normal and hyperalgesic skin. It is clear that the changes in sensation induced by capsaicin not only include an upward shift in pain sensation, but also an increase in the slope of the regression line, representing an increase in the gain of the system.

Because it has been noted that cold hyperalgesia (Frost et al. 1988; Wahren et al. 1991) was a common feature in patients with neuropathic pain and mechanical hyperalgesia, we tested whether cold hyperalgesia might develop in areas of secondary hyperalgesia after capsaicin injection. There was no consistent finding for cold sensation in areas of capsaicin-induced secondary hyperalgesia: four subjects reported no change, whereas three reported increased sensation and the other three had decreased pain sensation.

In a patient with an injury to the left ulnar nerve who had an area of hyperalgesia to light touch, sensations of prickle and pain were similar to those evoked after capsaicin treatment of normal control subjects. The sensations of pain and prickle from normal skin were similar to those reported by normal subjects in the control experiment.

DISCUSSION

The experiments described above suggest several conclusions. Subjects were able to differentiate prickly from nonprickly fabrics quite clearly. The intensity of fabric-evoked prickle was not significantly changed in an area of secondary hyperalgesia. In contrast, all of the woolen fabrics used in the study evoked very little or no pain when applied to normal skin, but all evoked substantial pain when applied to hyperalgesic skin. Additionally, the prickly fabrics produced significantly more pain than did the less prickly ones.

PRICKLE AND PAIN IN HYPERALGESIC SKIN

Overall, our observations provide some insight into the nature of the sensation of fabric-evoked prickle. Previously, prickle was thought to be a very mild form of pain that results from low-level activation of mechanical nociceptors by punctate stimuli (Sinclair 1981). It was of considerable interest that our subjects were able to

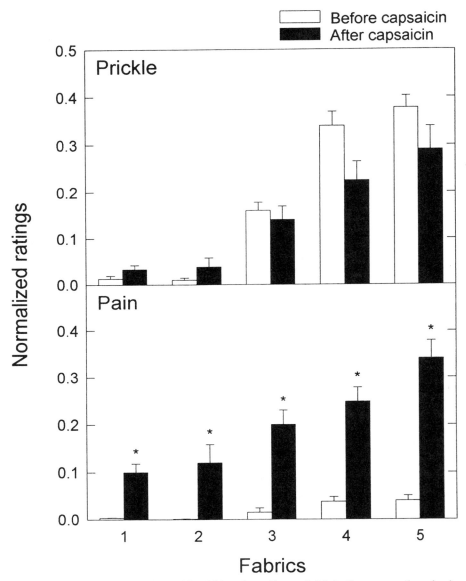

FIG. 1. Correlation of pain ratings with prickle ratings. For each fabric, the mean rating of pain sensation is plotted as a function of the mean rating of prickle sensation. The solid line corresponds to the ratings from normal skin, and the dashed line corresponds to the ratings from hyperalgesic skin. (Adapted from Cervero et al. 1994.)

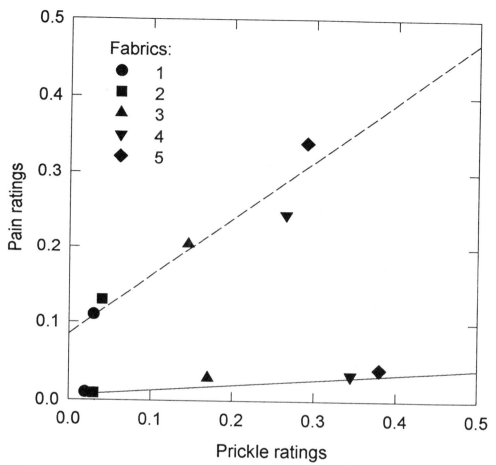

FIG. 2. Ratings of prickle (*top*) and pain (*bottom*) evoked by the five woolen fabrics before (*open bars*) and after (*filled bars*) the intradermal injection of capsaicin. The fabrics were applied in the zone of secondary hyperalgesia. The pain ratings increased significantly in the zone of secondary hyperalgesia (mean ± S.E.M., * = $p \le 0.001$. (Adapted from Cervero et al. 1994.)

discriminate the sensation of fabric-evoked prickle in hyperalgesic skin in the presence of the pain evoked by the mechanical stimulus of the fabric. Since no differences were observed between normal and hyperalgesic skin in the prickle ratings, the findings in hyperalgesic skin indicate that the sensations of prickle and pain may be associated with separate sensory channels.

The psychophysical test used in our study was based on the results of Garnsworthy et al. (1988). These authors concluded that LMTs are activated by all woolen fabrics and do not show a differential response to prickly as opposed to nonprickly fabrics, whereas the responses of Aδ- and C-fiber nociceptors are graded with respect to the prickliness of the fabric. Their results were obtained using psychophysical tests to assess prickle sensations and electrophysiologic recordings in humans and animals to study afferent-fiber discharges. From their results, we conclude that the sensation of fabric-evoked prickle implies the activation of mechanically sensitive nociceptors, whereas nonprickly fabrics mainly excite LMTs.

On the basis of these conclusions, we assume that the pain elicited by the nonprickly fabrics (fabrics 1 and 2) was due to LMT input, and that the increase in pain in response to the very prickly fabrics (fabrics 4 and 5) was due to the added input from nociceptors. However, the increase in pain for the prickly fabrics applied to hyperalgesic skin was significantly greater ($p < 0.05$) than the increase in pain for the prickly fabrics applied to normal skin (Fig. 1). Therefore, the pain produced by prickly fabrics applied to hyperalgesic skin exceeds what would be predicted by considering a linear summation of the inputs of LMTs and nociceptors.

The same conclusion was reached by a different analysis. By plotting the mean pain ratings for each fabric against the mean prickle ratings for each fabric, we found that the relationship between pain and prickle changed after the capsaicin injection (Fig. 2). If prickle sensation is an indication of nociceptor input to the central nervous system (CNS), this plot can be interpreted to represent the transfer function relating nociceptor input to pain. The slope of the transfer function for data obtained from the hyperalgesic skin is greater than the slope for data obtained from normal skin. This suggests that the gain of the central processing system (CPS) has increased. Since it is known that sensitization of nociceptors to mechanical stimuli does not occur after a capsaicin injection adjacent to the nociceptors' receptive field (RF) (LaMotte et al. 1992), this increase in slope indicates that the CNS has become more sensitive to nociceptor input.

Similar results were obtained from the patient with neuropathic pain. This suggests that the hyperalgesia to mechanical stimuli that exists in patients with neuropathic pain may also involve altered central processing of inputs from both low- and high-threshold mechanoreceptors.

We can account for these observations by assuming that with mechanical hyperalgesia, the central neurons that mediate pain sensation increase their responsiveness to input from both LMTs and nociceptors. Since a similar mechanism is thought to underlie punctate hyperalgesia (LaMotte et al. 1991), hyperalgesia to prickly fabrics may be a variant of punctate hyperalgesia. Hyperalgesia to heat is not observed in the zone of secondary hyperalgesia; hence, the altered central processing that occurs with mechanical hyperalgesia appears to involve spinal-cord cells responsive to mechanically sensitive nociceptors only (Cervero et al. 1976). An Aδ-fiber Type I nociceptor (Meyer et al. 1985) may be the receptor involved, because this type of nociceptor is sensitive to noxious mechanical stimuli but insensitive to heat stimuli.

Another possible explanation is that in the zone of secondary hyperalgesia, the pain associated with input from LTMs and nociceptors is not additive in a linear manner. Rather, coactivation of LTMs by the noxious mechanical stimulus results in a greater response to nociceptor input, perhaps due to a nonlinear transfer function relating primary afferent input to pain sensation. Such a mechanism would not require increased responsiveness of central neurons to nociceptor input. In the case of this hypothesis, the lack of response to heat in the secondary zone may be due to the lack of coactivation of LTMs by a heat stimulus. Nevertheless, this explanation does not account for the occurrence of punctate hyperalgesia following capsaicin injection observed in a patient with a neuropathic loss of large fibers (Treede and Cole 1993).

In conclusion, we suggest that secondary hyperalgesia is due to a central alteration that includes two components: (a) a switch in the type of sensation evoked by low-threshold mechanoreceptors from touch alone to both touch and pain; and (b) an increased pain sensation evoked by nociceptor activation.

ACKNOWLEDGMENTS

We appreciate the technical assistance of Timothy V. Hartke and Jennifer L. Turnquist. This research was supported by the grant NS-14447 from the U.S. National Institutes of Health. F.C. was on leave from Bristol University and was supported by the British Medical Research Council, the Wellcome Trust, and a travel grant of the British Physiological Society.

REFERENCES

Campbell JN, Khan AA, Meyer RA, Raja SN. Responses to heat of C-fiber nociceptors in monkey are altered by injury in the receptive field but not by adjacent injury. *Pain* 1988a;32:327–332.

Campbell JN, Raja SN, Meyer RA, Mackinnon SE. Myelinated afferents signal the hyperalgesia associated with nerve injury. *Pain* 1988b;32:89–94.

Cervero F, Gilbert R, Hammond RGE, Tanner J. Development of secondary hyperalgesia following nonpainful thermal stimulation of the skin: a psychophysical study in man. *Pain* 1993;54:181–189.

Cervero F, Iggo A, Ogawa H. Nociceptor driven dorsal horn neurons in the lumbar spinal cord of the cat. *Pain* 1976;2:5–24.

Cervero F, Meyer RA, Campbell JN. A psychophysical study of secondary hyperalgesia: evidence for increased pain to input from nociceptors. *Pain* 1994;58:21–28.

Frost SA, Raja SN, Campbell JN, Meyer RA, Khan AA. Does hyperalgesia to cooling stimuli characterize patients with sympathetically maintained pain (reflex sympathetic dystrophy)? In: *Proceedings of the 5th World Congress on Pain*, Dubner R, Gebhart GF, Bond MR. Amsterdam: Elsevier Science Publishers BV, 1988;151–156.

Garnsworthy RK, Gully RL, Kenins P, Mayfield RJ, Westerman RA. Identification of the physical stimulus and the neural basis of fabric-evoked prickle. *J Neurophysiol* 1988;59:1083–1097.

Hoheisel U, Mense S. Long-term changes in discharge behaviour of cat dorsal horn neurones following noxious stimulation of deep tissues. *Pain* 1989;36:239–247.

Hylden JLK, Nahin RL, Traub RJ, Dubner R. Expansion of receptive fields of spinal lamina I projection neurones in rats with unilateral adjuvant-induced inflammation: the contribution of central dorsal horn mechanisms. *Pain* 1989;37:229–243.

Koltzenburg M, Lundberg LER, Torebjörk HE. Dynamic and static components of mechanical hyperalgesia in human hairy skin. *Pain* 1992;51:207–219.

Laird JMA, Cervero F. A comparative study of the changes in receptive-field properties of multireceptive and nocireceptive rat dorsal horn neurons following noxious mechanical stimulation. *J Neurophysiol* 1989;62:854–863.

LaMotte RH, Lundberg LER, Torebjörk HE. Pain, hyperalgesia and activity in nociceptor C units in humans after intradermal injection of capsaicin. *J Physiol* (Lond) 1992;448:749–764.

LaMotte RH, Shain CN, Simone DA, Tsai E-FP. Neurogenic hyperalgesia: Psychophysical studies of underlying mechanisms. *J Neurophysiol* 1991;66:190–211.

McMahon SB, Wall PD. The receptive fields of rat lamina I projection cells move to incorporate a nearby region of injury. *Pain* 1984;19:235–247.

Meyer RA, Campbell JN. Myelinated nociceptive afferents account for the hyperalgesia that follows a burn to the hand. *Science* 1981;213:1527–1529.

Meyer RA, Campbell JN, Raja SN. Peripheral neural mechanisms of cutaneous hyperalgesia. In: Fields HL, Dubner R, Cervero F, eds. *Advances in pain research and therapy*, vol. 9. New York: Raven Press, 1985;53–71.

Meyer RA, Campbell JN, Raja SN. Antidromic nerve stimulation in monkey does not sensitize unmyelinated nociceptors to heat. *Brain Res* 1988;441:168–172.

Raja SN, Campbell JN, Meyer RA. Evidence for different mechanisms of primary and secondary hyperalgesia following heat injury to the glabrous skin. *Brain* 1984;107:1179–1188.

Schaible H-G, Schmidt RF, Willis WD Jr. Enhancement of the responses of ascending tract cells in the cat spinal cord by acute inflammation of the knee joint. *Exp Brain Res* 1987;66:489–499.

Simone DA, Baumann TK, LaMotte RH. Dose-dependent pain and mechanical hyperalgesia in humans after intradermal injection of capsaicin. *Pain* 1989;38:99–107.

Simone DA, Sorkin LS, Oh U, Chung JM, Owens C, LaMotte RH, Willis WD Jr. Neurogenic hyperalgesia: Central neural correlates in responses of spinothalamic tract neurons. *J Neurophysiol* 1991; 66:228–246.

Sinclair D. *Mechanisms of cutaneous sensation*. Oxford: Oxford University Press. 1981;1–63.

Thalhammer JG, LaMotte RH. Heat sensitization of one-half of a cutaneous nociceptor's receptive field does not alter the sensitivity of the other half. *Advances in pain research and therapy*, vol. 5. New York: Raven Press, 1983;71–75.

Torebjörk HE, Lundberg LER, LaMotte RH. Central changes in processing of mechanoreceptive input in capsaicin-induced sensory hyperalgesia in humans. *J Physiol* 1992;448:765–780.

Treede R-D, Cole JD. Dissociated secondary hyperalgesia in a subject with a large fiber sensory neuropathy. *Pain* 1993;53:169–174.

Wahren LK, Torebjörk E, Nystrom B. Quantitative sensory testing before and after regional guanethidine block in patients with neuralgia in the hand. *Pain*, 1991;46:23–30.

Pain and the Brain: From Nociception to Cognition, edited by Burkhart Bromm and John E. Desmedt, Advances in Pain Research and Therapy Vol. 22. Raven Press, Ltd., New York © 1995.

24

Pain Syndromes in Patients with CNS Lesions and a Comparison with Nociceptive Pain

Jörgen Boivie

Department of Neurology, University Hospital, S-581 85 Linköping, Sweden

SUMMARY

There are no nociceptors in the nervous tissue of the brain and spinal cord, but some of the tissues around and in the parenchyma are innervated by nociceptors, such as the meninges and arteries. Thus, there is no true nociception in the parenchyma of the central nervous system (CNS). Instead, lesions and other dysfunctions in the CNS may lead to central pain. Many kinds of CNS lesions can cause central pain. These lesions may be located at any level of the neuraxis from the spinal dorsal horn to the cerebral cortex. The most common causes of central pain are cerebrovascular lesions, multiple sclerosis, and traumatic spinal-cord injuries. On the basis of results from studies of these and other patient groups, it is hypothesized that only lesions that affect the spinothalamocortical pathways that are crucial for the sensibility to temperature and pain can cause central pain. These studies have also shown that central pain is usually constant, and that it can have many different qualities, the most common being burning, aching, and pricking. Most patients experience more than one quality of pain. From a comparison between nociceptive and central pain it is concluded that there are fundamental differences between the two pain categories. Nociception is the crucial mechanism for nociceptive pain, whereas this step is bypassed in central pain (i.e., central pain occurs without activation of the primary nociceptive pathways, although activation of these pathways may affect central pain).

CNS LESIONS AND PAIN

Lesions of the brain and spinal cord are usually not painful. A brain infarct, for instance, is not painful unless it leads to edema and increased intracranial pressure, which may cause headache. Since the parenchyma of the CNS lacks nociceptors, there is no true nociception in the CNS itself. The local pain that arises around CNS lesions is nociceptive pain caused by the activation of nociceptors in the surrounding meninges and in and around the walls of arteries in the region.

However, CNS lesions can cause severe pain through entirely different mechanisms, namely by inducing central pain, which often begins after a delay of weeks or months. In this chapter, some aspects of this kind of pain are discussed and compared with nociceptive pain.

Central pain is defined by the International Association for the Study of Pain (ISAP; Merskey et al. 1986) as pain caused by a lesion or dysfunction in the CNS. This definition requires that the lesion be a primary dysfunction in the CNS, which means that pain from a peripherally induced central dysfunction is not central pain. For instance, a neuralgia caused by a traumatic nerve lesion with a dominating central mechanism does not conform with the criterion for central pain.

CENTRAL PAIN CONDITIONS AND MECHANISMS

Many kinds of lesions of the brain and spinal cord can cause central pain. They vary enormously in location, size, and structure. The best-known such conditions are listed in Table 1. Among the many different disease processes that can lead to central pain, shown in the table, are vascular lesions, traumatic lesions, and inflammatory processes. The macrostructure of the lesion appears to be less important than its location with regard to its risk of causing central pain.

The largest groups of patients with central pain are those with cerebrovascular lesions (CVL), multiple sclerosis (MS), and spinal-cord injuries (SCI). Bonica, using data from the literature, calculated the probable prevalences of central pain in these conditions in the United States (Table 2; Bonica 1991). His results show that central pain affects more patients than is usually thought to be the case. This conclusion is supported by recent, previously unpublished results from studies on the prevalences of central pain in patients with CVL and MS. In a Danish study, 267 stroke patients were prospectively followed with regard to the development of central pain. It was found that 8% of them developed this kind of pain (Andersen et al. 1994). In our own group of 255 MS patients, 22% had central pain, including symptomatic trigeminal neuralgia (Österberg et al. 1994).

There has been a debate for many years over which features of a lesion are important for the induction of central pain. This question is still not answered un-

TABLE 1. *Causes of central pain*

Vascular lesions in the brain and spinal cord (infarct, hemorrhage, vascular malformation)
Multiple sclerosis
Traumatic spinal-cord injury
Syringomyelia and syringobulbia
Tumors
Abscesses
Inflammatory diseases other than MS (myelitis caused by viruses, syphilis)

TABLE 2. *Estimated prevalences of major disorders with central pain in the United States, 1989 (population around 250 million)*[a]

Disease	Total no. patients	Patients with central pain	% patients with central pain
Spinal-cord injury	225,000	68,000	30
Multiple sclerosis	150,000	35,000	23
Stroke	2,000,000	30,000	1.5

[a]See comments in the text indicating a much higher prevalence of central pain in stroke. (From Bonica 1991, with permission.)

equivocally, but studies from various groups of patients with central pain have yielded much important information. With modern imaging techniques [computed tomography (CT) and magnetic resonance imaging (MRI)], the location and structure of lesions can be roughly demonstrated; however, other methods are necessary to show the functional consequences of the lesions (see below).

Radiologic techniques have shown that lesions that induce central pain may be located at any level along the neuraxis (Boivie 1994). This includes the dorsal horn of the spinal cord, ascending pathways of the spinal cord and brain stem, thalamus, thalamocortical projection pathways, or cerebral cortex itself. Thus, it is now clear that the previous use of the expression "thalamic" pain for all central pain was inadequate, since only a minority of the lesions that cause central pain involve the thalamus. The expression came into use because the first known description of central pain involved six patients with thalamic lesions, reported in 1906 by Dejérine and Roussy (1906). Undoubtedly, thalamic lesions can cause central pain, but not all thalamic lesions do so. From the literature, it appears that only lesions involving the ventral posterior region, where the major somatosensory relay nuclei are located, can lead to central pain (Boivie 1994; Bougosslavsky et al. 1988). Bougosslavsky et al. (1988) found that three of 18 patients with such lesions developed central pain (i.e., 17%) whereas none of 22 patients with thalamic lesions outside this region developed central pain.

In our original material involving 27 patients with central poststroke pain (CPSP), one-third were found to have thalamic involvement by the lesion (Leijon et al. 1989). These results were based on CT examinations. In a later investigation with MRI localization of the lesions by Bowsher and colleagues, it was found that about half of the examined patients had lesions involving part of the thalamus (Lewis-Jones et al. 1990).

Brain-stem lesions have also been shown convincingly to cause central pain. Eight of the 27 CPSP patients mentioned above had unequivocal signs and symptoms of brain-stem infarcts (Leijon et al. 1989). These cases illustrate the fact that small but strategically located lesions can induce central pain. Other lesions are huge, damaging large parts of the cerebral hemisphere, as in the case of large supratentorial infarcts.

In the quest for the mechanisms underlying central pain, interesting information has been obtained from studies of the neurologic symptoms and signs that accompany central pain (Boivie 1994). First, these studies show that only abnormalities in somatic sensibility regularly accompany central pain, whereas other symptoms, such as paresis, incoordination, and speech disturbances may or may not be present. In two groups of patients with central poststroke pain, 48% and 38% had paresis (Leijon et al. 1989; Andersen et al. 1994, respectively). In the former group, 58% had ataxia, whereas other neurologic symptoms and signs were uncommon (Leijon et al. 1989). In a group of 33 MS patients with central pain, 51% had paresis and 37% had ataxia (Österberg et al. 1993, 1994). All stroke patients and all MS patients except one were found to have sensory abnormalities. This could perhaps be predicted because central pain is a somatosensory phenomenon. Thus, central pain is the result of lesions or other dysfunctions in structures involved in somatic sensibility.

Second, the results of these studies show that the sensory abnormalities that accompany central pain have particular features. The dominating feature is abnormal sensibility to temperature and pain.

Traditionally, sensory disturbances have been examined with clinical methods, such as with cotton wool for touch, a tuning fork for vibration, a pin for pain, and a hot and a cold object for temperature. These methods should be included in the examination, but the methods for quantitative examinations that are now available open possibilities for much more detailed analyses of the abnormalities. In these examinations one should not only look for decreased sensibility, but also for hyperesthesias and other abnormalities.

These methods have been employed in patients with central pain following stroke and patients with MS and spinal-cord injuries (SCI). Tables 3 and 4 summarize the results of examinations in stroke and MS patients. In the stroke group all patients had abnormal sensibility to temperature and/or pain (including heat pain and cold pain), whereas 49% and 60% had normal thresholds to touch and vibration, respectively (Boivie et al. 1989). Similar abnormalities were found in the 29 MS patients. All except two had abnormal temperature and/or pain sensibility, whereas 38% and 21%, respectively, had normal thresholds to touch and vibration (Österberg et al. 1993, 1994).

On the basis of these results, it has been proposed that central pain occurs only in patients who have a lesion affecting the spinothalamocortical pathways that under normal conditions are most important for the perception of temperature and nociceptive pain (Boivie et al. 1989; Boivie 1994). Central pain can thus be looked upon as a paradox: the lesions that decrease pain sensibility pose the risk of producing severe pain (i.e., central pain).

This hypothesis contradicts the one that central pain is the consequence of disinhibition resulting from lesions in the dorsal column–medial lemniscal pathway (DC–ML), which for many years was the dominating hypothesis in the literature. Results from several studies provide strong evidence that such lesions cannot be the crucial lesions causing central pain. For instance, studies of patients with central pain caused by syringomyelia and low brain-stem infarcts show that most of these

TABLE 3. *Sensory abnormalities in 27 patients with central poststroke pain (CPSP) as revealed with quantitative (Q) and clinical (CL) tests. Proportion of patients in percent*

	BS n = 8	TH n = 9	SE n = 6	UI n = 4	All n = 27
Vibration (Q)					
Moderate	0	22	0	0	7
Severe	12	56	50	0	33
Touch (Q)					
Moderate	0	22	33	50	23
Severe	25	67	0	0	29
Innoxious temperature (Q)					
Moderate	25	11	17	25	19
Severe	75	89	83	75	81
Temperature pain (Q)					
Moderate	12	0	33	25	15
Severe	75	100	50	75	78
Touch (CL)					
Hypesthesia	50	33	50	75	48
Hyperesthesia	38	56	33	0	37
Pinprick (CL)					
Hypesthesia	63	11	33	50	37
Hyperesthesia	38	89	50	50	59
Kinesthesia (CL)					
Hypesthesia	0	78	25	33	37

BS = cerebrovascular lesion in brain stem; TH = cerebrovascular lesion involving thalamus; SE = supratentorial, extrathalamic cerebrovascular lesion; UI = location of cerebrovascular lesion not identified.
(From Leijon et al. 1989, with permission.)

TABLE 4. *Sensory abnormalities in 29 MS patients with central pain: Results from quantitative sensory testing. Proportion of patients in percent*

Vibration	
Moderate	45
Severe	17
Touch	
Moderate	20
Severe	59
Innoxious temperature	
Moderate	3
Severe	69
Noxious temperature	
Decreased/lost	79

(From Österberg A, Boivie J, Henriksson A, Holmgren H, Johansson I, Thuomas K-A, unpublished results.)

patients have normal sensibility to touch and vibration, which would not be the case if they had lesions affecting the DC–ML pathway. Central pain following cordotomy is another example of a condition without a DC–ML lesion. It thus appears that a lesion of this pathway is not necessary for the occurrence of central pain, although such lesions do affect the sensory abnormalities.

The notion that the spinothalamic pathways are affected by a lesion in patients with central pain has also been investigated, using objective tests of spinothalamic-tract function in which cortically evoked potentials (somatosensory evoked potentials; SEPs) were observed following peripheral cutaneous stimuli delivered with a carbon dioxide laser. With this method, thermoreceptors and nociceptors are specifically activated, whereas low-threshold mechanoreceptors are not activated, contrary to the situation in which SEPs following electrical stimulation of peripheral nerves are studied (see Chapter 25). The SEPs produced with these two stimulation modes were examined in studies of patients with central poststroke pain. The SEPs were correlated with the sensory abnormalities. In brief, the results show that the electrically evoked SEPs correlated with a decreased sensibility to touch and vibration, but not with pain or a decreased sensibility to temperature and pain (Holmgren et al. 1990). The laser-evoked SEPs showed an entirely different pattern. The abnormalities in these SEPs correlated well with decreases in sensibility to temperature and pain, and thereby with the presence of central pain (Casey et al. 1990).

Even if central pain does not result from disinhibition due to a lesion in the DC–ML, it is conceivable that some form of disinhibition in the somatosensory pathways is important in the generation of central pain. This mechanism could lead to zones with hyperactive and hyperreactive neurons, and could be the mechanism underlying both the spontaneous pain and the painful hyperesthesias experienced by patients with central pain. Such neurons have in fact been shown to exist in the ventralposterior thalamus in patients with central pain following spinal-cord injuries (see chapter by Tasker).

PAIN CHARACTERISTICS

Central pain is often thought to be excruciating and of bizarre character. Although such central pain exists, it is not characteristic of central pain in general. Central pain can have trivial features such as an aching pain in one arm. However, it often has puzzling features, with a mixture of different pain qualities of an unusual nature. We have, for instance, had one patient with MS who clearly described three different central pains. He had burning pain in his legs and feet, a tight pressing pain around the waist, and a pressing perianal pain that caused the sensation of sitting on a tennis ball.

Central pain can thus have many qualities. Table 5 lists the qualities of pain reported in investigations of patients with central pain caused by stroke and MS. It has often been stated that central pain is almost always burning. The results show that this is not the case. Although burning pain is the type of pain most frequently

TABLE 5. *Quality of pain in patients with central pain caused by cerebrovascular lesions. Proportion of patients in percent*

	Central poststroke pain n = 27	Multiple sclerosis n = 40
Burning	59	58
Aching	30	55
Pricking	30	32
Lacerating	26	19

(Adapted from Leijon et al. 1989, and Österberg et al. 1994.)

experienced, it is far from being experienced by all patients with central pain. The studies show that central pain can have almost any quality. Most patients experience more than one quality of pain, as illustrated above. The various qualities can have the same location or be located in different areas of the painful region.

The location of central pain is determined by the location of the lesion. Thalamic lesions often lead to pain in most of the left or right side. Pain from infarcts of the low brain-stem (i.e., as part of a Wallenberg's syndrome) can have a crossed distribution, with the face affected ipsilaterally and the extremities on the contralateral side. In MS, central pain is most commonly located in the legs and feet, often bilaterally (Österberg et al. 1993, 1994).

Another well-known feature of central pain is that it may have a delayed onset. In stroke patients it is not unusual for central pain to start several months after the stroke event, even though it begins during the first post-stroke month in most patients (Andersen et al. 1994; Leijon et al. 1989; Mauguière and Desmedt 1988). Delays of up to 2 to 3 years have been reported.

Central pain is mostly constant, but paroxysmal central pain also occurs. The intensity of the pain varies from one patient to another. Some patients have pain of very great intensity, particularly patients with central pain following thalamic lesions (Leijon et al. 1989), whereas others may have low-intensity pain. However, even if patients rate their pain as being of low intensity on a visual analogue scale (VAS), they still consider the pain to be severe, probably because it is constant and very distressing. In addition to spontaneous pain, many patients have allodynia and hyperalgesia (i.e., painful overreactions to stimuli that are normally not painful, such as touch, cold, and warmth, and pain of increased intensity upon a noxious stimulus, respectively). Such overreactions are important characteristics in patients with central pain (Boivie 1994).

COMPARISONS BETWEEN NOCICEPTIVE AND CENTRAL PAIN

A comparison between nociceptive pain, the most important consequence of nociception, and central pain shows several fundamental differences between these two categories of pain. The most important differences are the following:

1. A noxious stimulus is not necessary for central pain to occur, whereas under normal conditions it is necessary for nociceptive pain.
2. Nociceptor activation is not necessary for central pain to occur, but is required for the experience of nociceptive pain. Nociceptor activation may, however, affect central pain.
3. Nociceptive pain is evoked through activity in nociceptive-specific (NS) or wide-dynamic-range (WDR) neurons of the dorsal horn. Central pain usually occurs without such activation, but it is conceivable that such activation may affect central pain in some conditions in which it exists. This can occur only if the ascending pathways have not been damaged to the extent that ascending signals have been blocked, which is the case in many patients.
4. Under normal conditions it can be postulated that the perception of nociceptive pain requires activation of thalamic centers. This does not appear to be the case in central pain in general, although it is probable that central pain caused by lesions in the lower brain stem and spinal cord may well depend on activity in thalamic regions. For example, central pain can occur even after huge thalamic lesions damaging the whole ventroposterior thalamic region, with an almost total loss of the ability to identify the location and nature of somatic stimuli in the affected body region. With regard to the question of whether or not activity in cortical centers is necessary for the perception of pain, be it nociceptive or central, I am convinced that true perception of pain requires cortical activity, whereas it is possible that reactions to somatic stimuli may well be evoked even in the decorticate state.
5. The quality of nociceptive pain is much more uniform than that of central pain, in which there is great variation, with more than one quality of pain often being experienced, which is rarely the case in nociceptive pain. Some of the qualities of pain experienced by patients with central pain are never present in conditions of nociceptive pain.
6. Central pain can start long after most other functional consequences of the lesion have subsided, which is not the case in nociceptive pain.
7. Central pain is accompanied by somatosensory abnormalities, which are usually absent in nociceptive pain. Severe alldoynia, hyperalgesia, and hyperpathia do not occur in nociceptive but do occur in central pain.
8. Nociceptive pain usually responds well to treatment with analgesics, whereas central pain responds poorly or not at all to such therapy.

This comparison shows that nociception, which is a crucial mechanism in nociceptive pain, is in many cases bypassed in central pain (i.e., central pain occurs without activation of the nociceptive pathways from the periphery or from the spinal dorsal horn). Central pain is thus independent of nociception, but its mechanisms may rest in the same brain are also sites of mechanisms underlying nociceptive pain.

ACKNOWLEDGMENTS

The studies from which unpublished results are presented in this chapter have been supported by grant No. 9058 from the Swedish Medical Research Council, the Bank of Sweden Tercentenary Foundation, the Swedish Association of the Neurologically Disabled, the 1987 Years Foundation for Stroke Research, and the County Council of Östergötland.

REFERENCES

Andersen G, Vestergaard K, Ingeman-Nielsen M, Jensen TS. Incidence of central poststroke pain. *Pain* 1995; (*In press*).

Boivie J. Central pain. In: Wall PD, Melzack R, eds. *Textbook of pain*, 3rd ed. New York: Churchill Livingstone, 1994;871–902.

Boivie J, Leijon G, Johansson I. Central post-stroke pain—a study of the mechanisms through analyses of the sensory abnormalities. *Pain* 1989;37:173–185.

Bonica JJ. Introduction: Semantic, Epidemiologic, and Educational Issues. In: Casey KL, ed. *Pain and central nervous disease: The central pain syndromes*. New York: Raven Press, 1991;13–29.

Bougosslavsky J, Regli F, Uske A. Thalamic infarcts: Clinical syndromes, etiology and prognosis. *Neurology* 1988;38:837–848.

Casey KL, Boivie J, Leijon G, Morrow TJ, Sjölund BIR. Laser-evoked cerebral potential and sensory function in patients with central pain. *Pain* 1990;(Suppl 5):204.

Dejerine J, Roussy G. La syndrome thalamique. *Rev Neurol (Paris)* 1906;14:521–532.

Holmgren H, Leijon G, Boivie J, Johansson I, Ilievska L. Central poststroke pain: somatosensory evoked potentials in relation to location of the lesion and sensory signs. *Pain* 1990;40:43–52.

Leijon G, Boivie J, Johansson I. Central post-stroke pain—neurological symptoms and pain characteristics. *Pain* 1989;36:13–25.

Lewis-Jones H, Smith T, Bowsher D, Leijon G. Magnetic resonance imaging in 36 cases of central poststroke pain (CPSP). *Pain* 1990;(Suppl 5):278.

Mauguière F, Desmedt JE. Thalamic pain syndrome of Dejérine-Roussy. Differentation of four subtypes assisted by somatosensory evoked potentials data. *Arch Neurol* 1988;45:1312–1320.

Merskey H, Lindblom U, Mumford JM, Nathan PW, Noordenbos W, Sunderland S. Pain terms. A current list with definitions and notes on usage. *Pain* 1986;(Suppl 3):217–221.

Österberg A, Boivie J, Henriksson A, Holmgren H, Johansson I. Central pain in multiple sclerosis. *Proceedings of the 7th World Congress on Pain*, 1993:407.

Österberg A, Boivie J, Holmgren H, Thuomas K-Å, Johansson I. The clinical characteristics and sensory abnormalities of patients with central pain caused by multiple sclerosis. In: Gebhart GF, Hammond DL, Jensen TS, eds. *Progress in pain research and management*, vol. 2. Seattle: ISAP Press, 1994;789–796.

Pain and the Brain: From
Nociception to Cognition,
edited by Burkhart Bromm and
John E. Desmedt, Advances in Pain
Research and Therapy Vol. 22.
Raven Press, Ltd., New York © 1995.

25

Assessment of Nociceptive Pathways with Laser-Evoked Potentials in Normal Subjects and Patients

*Rolf-Detlef Treede, †Jürgen Lorenz, ‡Klaus Kunze, and †Burkhart Bromm

*Institute of Physiology and Pathophysiology, University of Mainz, D-55099 Mainz, Germany, †Institute of Physiology, University Hospital Eppendorf, D-20246 Hamburg, Germany, ‡Clinic of Neurology, University Hospital Eppendorf, D-20246 Hamburg, Germany

SUMMARY

This chapter reviews recent approaches to studying nociceptive pathways and pain perception in humans through the use of laser-evoked cerebral potentials (LEPs). In this technique an infrared laser generates brief radiant heat pulses which, within a few milliseconds, selectively activate thin afferent nerve fibers (Aδ- and C-fibers) that project centrally via the spinothalamic tract of the spinal cord. Aδ-fiber activation leads to LEPs consisting of a middle-latency component (N170), possibly generated near the secondary somatosensory area, and late components (N250, P390) that are maximal near the vertex. C-fiber activation leads to an ultra-late potential (P1300) near the vertex. Late LEPs are used clinically to document impairment of nociceptive pathways at the peripheral, spinal, and brain-stem levels. Ultra-late potentials appear when late potentials are diminished by experimental nerve block or disease. Ultra-late LEPs may thus give indirect evidence for selective loss of Aδ-fiber afferents versus complete loss of all nociceptive afferents. When heat-pain sensitivity is pathologically increased, the amplitudes of late LEPs may also be increased.

INTRODUCTION

Sensory testing can yield valuable information for the localization of lesions in the nervous system, but is often considered less reliable and less objective than motor testing. This problem can be overcome when neurophysiologic techniques are used to test sensory pathways. One of these techniques is the methodology of evoked cerebral potentials, which are stimulus-induced changes in the electroencephalogram (EEG) that can be recorded noninvasively from the surface of the human scalp (for details see also Chapter 3). The appearance of an evoked potential gives evidence that a peripheral sensory impulse pattern has been transmitted to the brain via activation of the specific afferent system. This chapter reviews research in somatosensory evoked potentials (SEPs) in the assessment of nociceptive impulse transmission along the specific peripheral and central pathways, and in the ensuing conscious perception of pain.

Standard clinical neurophysiology uses electrical nerve stimulation to elicit an evoked potential (for a review see Desmedt 1988). For the study of nociceptive pathways in humans, the evoked potential is elicited by brief radiant heat pulses generated by an infrared laser (for a review see Bromm and Treede 1991). Fig. 1 shows that the evoked potential that follows conventional electrical nerve stimulation (SEP) differs from that which follows laser radiant-heat stimulation (LEP) with respect to the neuronal pathways activated. Electrical stimulation of mixed nerves activates Aβ-fiber tactile afferents as well as afferent and efferent fibers of the motor system. Neuronal impulses are then conducted within the dorsal column of the spinal cord, and the evoked potentials are correlates of mechanosensitivity and proprioception (for a review see Gandevia et al. 1984). In contrast, cutaneous heat pulses activate superficial terminals of thin afferents in the skin (Aδ- and C-fibers), which belong to the pain and temperature systems and project along the spin-

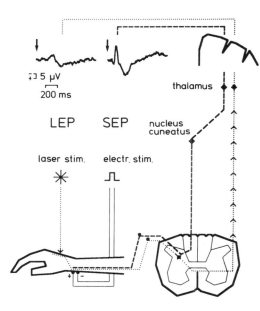

FIG. 1. Spinal pathways and late evoked potentials in response to laser radiant heat stimuli (LEP) and conventional electrical nerve stimuli (SEP). Cutaneous afferents are activated by CO_2-laser-emitted heat pulses of 200-ms duration and variable intensity. The evoked neural activity is transmitted by thin afferent nerve fibers (Aδ- and C-fibers) and is projected within the spinothalamic tract. With latencies of more than 170 msec, late cerebral potentials can be recorded (see inset). Electrical stimuli applied through surface electrodes recruit only thick afferent nerve fibers (Aβ) at the intensities used clinically. This evoked activity projects in the dorsal column/medial lemniscal system. Late potentials can be recorded with latencies beyond 80 msec. (Modified from Bromm and Treede 1991.)

othalamic tract of the anterolateral spinal cord (Bromm et al. 1984; Bromm and Treede 1987). Conventional SEP methods are sufficient for studying lesions in the nervous system if the sensory loss predominantly involves tactile and proprioceptive modalities or all somatosensory modalities to the same extent. If, however, pain and temperature sensitivity are primarily affected, conventional SEPs fail to reveal objective correlates of the sensory deficit. Such a dissociation of sensory deficits typically occurs in various diseases including polyneuropathies, syringomyelia, or Wallenberg's syndrome (for a review see Bromm and Treede 1991). Accordingly, the study of LEPs can in these cases usefully supplement standard neurophysiologic procedures as a highly sensitive test.

In addition to the "neurotopologic" approach, LEP methods can be applied in order to get a better understanding of the mechanisms of altered pain sensitivity that may underly chronic pain syndromes (see, e.g., Chapter 27). Concepts that explain abnormal pain states as a consequence of a loss of inhibition by large myelinated (Aβ-) afferents or an unbalanced interaction between Aδ- and C-fibers constitute the background against which the study of LEPs may supplement quantitative psychophysical techniques.

EVOKED-POTENTIAL CORRELATES OF PAIN PROCESSING

In pain research, late components of the SEP are evaluated (for reviews see Chudler and Dong 1983; Bromm 1989). They occur at latencies beyond 80 msec, with maximum amplitude over the vertex (Cz), and can be elicited by a variety of painful stimuli, including electrical stimulation of the tooth-pulp (Spreng and Ichioka 1964; Chatrian et al. 1975), intracutaneous electrical stimulation of the fingertip (Bromm and Meier 1984), mechanical stimulation of the skin (Bromm and Scharein 1982), thermal stimulation of the skin (Carmon et al. 1978; Bromm et al. 1983; Arendt-Nielsen and Bjerring 1988), thermal stimulation of joints (Wright and Davies 1989), and chemical stimulation of the nasal mucosa (Kobal 1984).

Many models of pain were primarily developed for algesimetry in pharmacologic studies, and are less useful for testing the integrity of nociceptive pathways because they are limited to certain body areas (i.e., tooth pulp, nasal mucosa, glabrous skin) (for a review see Chapter 3). In contrast, radiant-heat stimulation of the hairy skin that covers most of the body surface can easily be applied to almost any affected dermatome in patients with neurologic disease. We started our investigations with a CO_2 laser stimulator (Biehl et al. 1984) that generates short (e.g., 20 msec), intense pulses of long-wavelength radiation (10.6 μm) and enables the study of LEPs. Light of this wavelength is absorbed within the superficial 20- to 50-μm of the skin, and its absorption is independent of pigmentation. Because of this, CO_2 laser stimuli cause a rapid rise in skin-surface temperature (500°C/sec) and excite intraepidermal nociceptive nerve endings via temperature conduction. Several other laboratories have developed similar laser stimulators (Mor and Carmon 1975; Pertovaara et al. 1988; Kakigi et al. 1989; Gibson et al. 1991). Today we use a thulium crystal that delivers a laser beam of $2.01\,\mu$m wavelength through a flexible light conductor (see Chapter 3).

Both fine myelinated and unmyelinated nociceptors can be activated within a few milliseconds by short laser pulses (Devor et al. 1982; Bromm et al. 1984). A single laser pulse can lead to a double pain sensation, corresponding to the different velocities of these fiber types (in humans: 4–30 m/sec for Aδ-fibers and 0.4–1.8 m/sec for C-fibers; Vallbo et al. 1979): "first pain" is perceived with a latency of about 500 msec, and "second pain" after about 1,500 msec (Campbell and LaMotte 1983; Bromm and Treede 1987). As a consequence, the LEP contains late components that are related to Aδ-fiber activation (Kenton et al. 1980; Treede et al. 1994) and ultra-late components that are related to C-fiber activation (Bromm and Treede 1987).

Thresholds of laser-induced pain, measured as stimulus power in W, are inversely proportional to stimulus duration and—within limits—directly proportional to the stimulus area (Biehl et al. 1984; Pertovaara et al. 1988). Therefore, stimulus energy per unit area is the best parameter with which to characterize laser-stimulus intensity. The average pain threshold is about 10 mJ/mm^2 in healthy young adults and somewhat higher in older people (Gibson et al. 1991). The pre-pain range is very small, with a detection threshold that is about 70% of the pain threshold. Pre-pain sensations are mainly rated as tactile. Warm sensations are rare with brief CO_2-laser stimuli delivered to small areas of hairy skin (Carmon et al. 1978; Bromm et al. 1984; Pertovaara et al. 1988; Kakigi et al. 1989). Thus, the contribution of specific thermoreceptors to LEPs appears to be negligible.

LATE LEP COMPONENTS RELATED TO Aδ-FIBER ACTIVATION

The most prominent components of the LEP have peak latencies of less than 500 msec and are therefore related to activation of myelinated nociceptors. The component structure of the Aδ-fiber-related late potentials is illustrated in Fig. 2 (row A). Stimulation of the dorsal skin of the hand evokes a typical waveform consisting of a negativity at a peak latency of 250 ± 20 msec (mean $\pm$ SD) and a positivity with a peak latency of 390 ms $\pm$ 30 msec. The negative component is maximal at the vertex (Cz) and extends bilaterally into central leads. The positive component is maximal at Cz and Pz. Stimulation of the dorsal surface of the foot enlarges LEP latencies in a characteristic way (Treede et al. 1988; Kakigi and Shibasaki 1991). Primary cortical evoked potentials have not yet been identified because of considerable jitter in receptor activation times.

Since all components of LEPs are late secondary potentials, they are influenced by nonspecific mechanisms such as attention, distraction, habituation, vigilance, and expectation (for a review see Bromm 1989). Specifically, the P2 amplitude has been found to depend on the levels of attention and arousal (Beydoun et al. 1993; Siedenberg 1994). Despite its long latency, however, P2 is clearly distinct from the endogenous potential "P3," which typically occurs after rare and task-relevant stimuli (Sutton et al. 1965). In a standard "oddball" task using laser stimuli, a P3-like

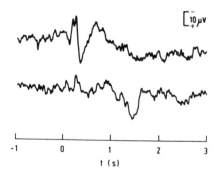

FIG. 2. Late and ultra-late LEPs in a healthy subject. Vertex versus linked earlobes (*negativity upward*). Stimulation of the back of the hand elicited a late positivity at about 400 msec (*top trace*). Preferential A-fiber block by pressure to the radial nerve at the wrist strongly attenuated the late LEP, and an ultra-late potential appeared (*bottom trace*), indicating that the latter was mediated by preserved C-fiber input.

potential has been found at peak latencies of about 600 msec (Towell and Boyd 1993; Siedenberg 1994). Nevertheless, test conditions for eliciting LEPs should minimize confusion of P2 with late cognitive components through the use of appropriate experimental paradigms. Attention should be stabilized by rating tasks and randomized interstimulus intervals. The sequence in which different skin areas are tested has to be balanced. If different stimulus properties are used within a block (e.g., different intensities or qualities), they should have equal probability and task relevance.

ULTRA-LATE LEP COMPONENTS RELATED TO C-FIBER ACTIVATION

According to the slower conduction velocity of C-fibers, LEP components related to C-fiber activation should occur about 1 sec after the late LEP. The term "ultra-late potentials" was introduced to distinguish components mediated by C-fibers from late components mediated by Aδ-fibers (Bromm et al. 1983). The ultra-late LEP consists of a vertex positivity with a peak latency of about 1,400 msec. Fig. 2 (row B) shows an example of potentials evoked in response to laser stimulation of the left hand in a healthy subject after A-fiber conduction was blocked by pressure to the radial nerve. The amplitude of the late component at about 400 msec was strongly reduced, and an ultra-late positivity at about 1,400 msec became clearly discernible. The A-fiber block was characterized by disappearance of surface electroneurogram, loss of cold sensitivity, an increase in thresholds for tactile stimulation, and loss of two-point discrimination (Bromm and Treede 1987). Preserved peripheral C-fiber function accounted for normal warm sensation and obviously for the ability to trigger an ultra-late LEP. The scalp topography of the late and ultra-late positivity in the LEP has been found to be the same (Treede and Bromm 1988). In conventional averages, the shape of ultra-late LEPs is distorted because of pronounced latency jitter, which can be corrected by appropriate digital-signal processing methods (Bromm and Treede 1987; McGillem and Aunon 1987).

Ultra-late LEPs are less reliable in recordings in which late LEPs are not suppressed by preferential A-fiber block (Bromm et al. 1983; Harkins et al. 1983). Several factors may account for this observation. Although subjects normally perceive a sequence of two pain sensations after each single laser stimulus, only the first sensation comes as a surprise, because it appears at a long and random interval after the previous stimulus. In contrast, second pain always occurs rapidly after this and is announced by the first pain. Short interstimulus intervals and certainty of stimulus timing are known to reduce the amplitudes of late cortical evoked potentials (Schafer et al. 1981; Angel et al. 1985). In the case of late LEPs, short-term habituation can explain an amplitude attenuation of about 60% when using interstimulus intervals of 900 msec (Bromm and Treede 1987). Selective attention to second pain can sometimes enhance an ultra-late LEP with the appropriate latency (Bromm and Treede 1985, see also Chapter 3). All of these factors—greater latency variability of C-fiber input, habituation, and less attention to second pain—render the ultra-late LEP smaller than with a preferential A-fiber block.

CORTICAL PROJECTION AREAS INFERRED FROM LASER-EVOKED POTENTIAL TOPOGRAPHY

Late and ultra-late LEPs have been found to have similar waveforms and scalp topography (Treede and Bromm 1988), which suggests that they have the same cerebral generators. When the scalp topography of LEPs is compared with that of evoked potentials after conventional electrical nerve stimulation, equivalent negative and positive vertex components can be identified (Treede et al. 1988). The latencies of electrically evoked vertex components are about 100 msec shorter than those of LEPs, because the latter are delayed by the time required for heat conduction to the receptor and the slower nerve-conduction velocity of Aδ-fibers than of Aβ-fibers. In general, LEPs project more posteriorly than conventional SEPs, a finding consistent with results of invasive recordings in rat somatosensory cortex, where cutaneous heat stimuli and tactile stimuli were compared (Gross-Isseroff et al. 1982).

Multilead recordings of LEPs revealed a middle-latency negative peak (N170) that could be clearly separated from the N240 and P380 components by its distinct topographic characteristics (Fig 3). Whereas the later components were symmetrical around the midline (Fig. 3, bottom left and right), the N1 was maximal over scalp regions contralateral to the stimulated hand (Fig. 3, top right). Although the N170 map covered an area close to the hand region of SI cortex (C4 for left-hand stimulation), the maximum was over temporal areas (T4). This topography may indicate a participation of SII or the insular cortex in the generation of the initial LEP negativity (Kunde and Treede 1993). Notably, some evoked potentials following direct stimulation of the spinothalamic tract have a similar topography (Taira et al. 1975). However, more studies are necessary to test whether nociceptive and non-nociceptive somatosensory pathways differ in cortical projection. Studies of patients with localized cortical lesions may yield additional information when, in the simplest

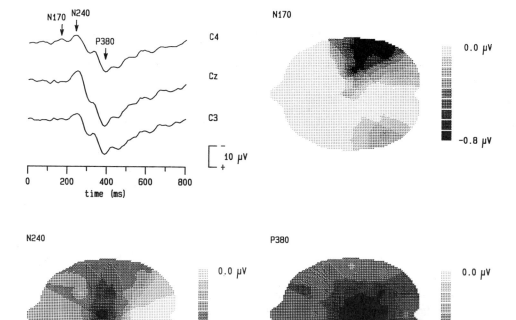

FIG. 3. Scalp distribution of cerebral potentials evoked by laser stimulation of the left-radial-nerve territory. LEP waveforms of a healthy subject display a distinct negativity at about 170 msec that appeared only at contralateral (C4) and not at vertex (Cz) or ipsilateral (C3) leads (*top left*). The spatial distribution of N170 illustrates the involvement of the somatosensory projection area, with a maximum density over temporal sites (*top right*). N240 (*bottom left*) and P380 (*bottom right*) averaged over 14 healthy subjects predominate over the vertex.

case, the lesion involves the generators of LEPs. It is likely, however, that multiple generators contribute to any LEP component, so that multilead recordings and mapping techniques are necessary for the study of such patients. Modelling techniques for source localization may then help to identify the cortical structures that are involved in the generation of pain-related LEPs (see also Chapter 14).

LEPS IN PATIENTS

Polyneuropathy

The term *polyneuropathy* (PNP) denotes a complex disease of the peripheral nervous system that is characterized by heterogeneity of etiology, histology, and clinical manifestations. It may involve the motor, sensory, and autonomic nervous systems. Differential disturbances of tactile, pain, and temperature sensitivity define the pattern of hypesthesia or dysesthesia. The type of sensory deficit that a patient displays depends upon which fiber groups are primarily affected. Comparison of LEPs with conventional SEPs provides objective information about the affected fiber groups because LEPs selectively correlate with Aδ- and conventional SEPs selectively correlate with Aβ-fiber function. Fig. 4 illustrates such selectivity of myelinated-sensory-fiber dysfunction in two patients with PNP. Patient 58 (Fig. 4, left) had a diabetic PNP. Sensory testing (Fig 4, bottom left) revealed a severe disturbance in sensitivity to mechanical, pain, and warm stimuli that had the typical distal distribution. The lower limbs were affected more than the upper limbs. Conventional SEPs were normal. In contrast, LEPs (Fig 4, top left) were absent at both 15 and 20 W intensities. These results illustrate the prevalence of dysfunction of thin myelinated rather than thick myelinated afferents. Patient 80, with PNP of unknown etiology (Fig. 4, right), displayed the opposite combination, normal LEPs and absent conventional SEPs. Accordingly, he had a reduction in mechanosensitivity with intact pain and temperature sensitivity, indicating a predominance of thick-myelinated-fiber dysfunction. Thus, in sensory PNP the extent of involvement of Aβ- and Aδ-fibers can be differentially estimated by functional neurophysiologic studies, permitting one to obtain information similar to that provided by an invasive nerve biopsy (cf. Kakigi et al. 1991b).

An unresolved issue is why some PNPs are painful and others are not. Several histologic studies of nerve biopsies have demonstrated that painfulness in PNP may be related to the rate and kind of nerve-fiber degeneration, but not to the ratio of remaining large and small fibers (Dyck et al. 1976). Patients with an acute breakdown of myelinated fibers caused either by Wallerian or axonal degeneration tended to have a higher incidence and greater intensity of pain than patients with more chronic forms of nerve-fiber degeneration. The methods used by the authors did not allow the study of degenerative changes in small unmyelinated afferents. A loss of physiologic inhibition from Aβ- or Aδ-fibers on C-fiber input has also been proposed to explain chronic pain in PNP (cf. Melzack and Wall 1965; Chung et al. 1984).

Clinical evidence for such mechanisms may be inferred from some PNP patients who show a phenomenon of abnormal summation or "wind-up" in response to repetitive pinprick stimulation at a 1-Hz rate. At such stimulation rates, healthy subjects perceive each pinprick as a single and stinging pain sensation. Some PNP patients, however, report a sensation of permanent burning pain. Fig. 5 shows the LEP pattern in the case of a 67-year-old man with PNP who displayed such marked wind-up. According to the types of sensory deficit exhibited by the patient, which were characterized by muscle weakness and impairment of position and vibration sensitivity, large myelinated nerve fibers of the lower limb were predominantly affected. This was confirmed by absent conventional tibial nerve SEPs and the results of sural nerve biopsy. A reduction in cold sensitivity and small late LEPs suggested that Aδ-fiber function was also impaired. However, Fig. 5 illustrates that

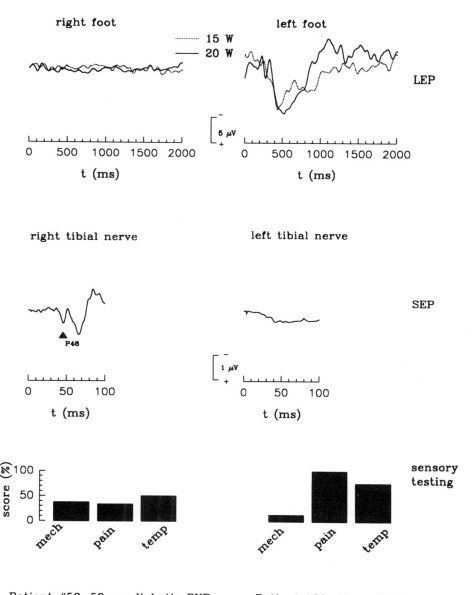

FIG. 4. LEPs in two patients with polyneuropathy (PNP). Left: In a 53-year-old man with a diabetic PNP that primarily affected small fibers, pain sensitivity was markedly reduced and the LEP was lost. Right: In a 39-year-old patient with a PNP of unknown etiology that primarily affected large fibers, mechanosensitivity and the SEP following conventional electrical nerve stimulation were impaired.

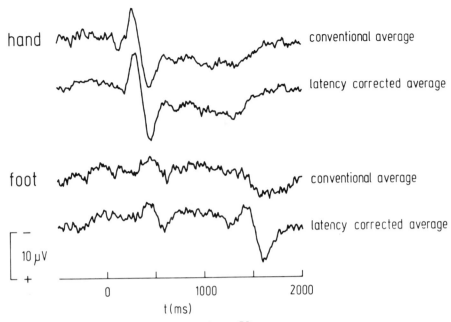

subject H.G., 67 years, polyneuropathy, laser EP

FIG. 5. Late and ultra-late LEPs in a 67-year-old man with polyneuropathy (PNP). Top traces: Following stimulation of the right hand, a normal Aδ-fiber-related late potential was recorded. Bottom traces: Following stimulation of the left foot, the late potential was markedly reduced in amplitude and a C-fiber-related ultra-late potential could be documented. The heat-pain threshold for laser stimuli was unremarkable in both areas, but a pronounced temporal summation occurred with stimulation of the foot. (From Treede, Pfeiffer, Kunze, Bromm, unpublished data.)

in this patient, C-fiber function was obviously preserved, as indicated by the large ultra-late LEP with a peak latency of about 1,600 msec, the appearance of which may be explained by unmasking. Thus, disturbed balance between A-fiber and C-fiber function in PNP may mimic effects of an experimental nerve block characterized by the attenuation or disappearance of late LEPs and unmasking of ultra-late LEPs.

The attribution of late and ultra-late LEPs to Aδ- and C-fiber input, respectively, is supported by a similar case of polyneuropathy in which late and ultra-late LEPs were found for both the upper and lower limbs (Lankers et al. 1991). Fig. 6 demonstrates that if one assumes a difference in neuronal conduction distance of 0.8 m between the hand and foot, the observed peak latencies of late and ultra-late LEPs yield conduction velocities of 16 m/sec and 1.2 m/sec, respectively. Interestingly, the patient in this second case had a reduction of pain to single pinprick, but a marked wind-up to repetitive pricks. We think that wind-up as a typical feature of spinal processing of C-fiber input (Mendell 1966) may contribute to ongoing pain in

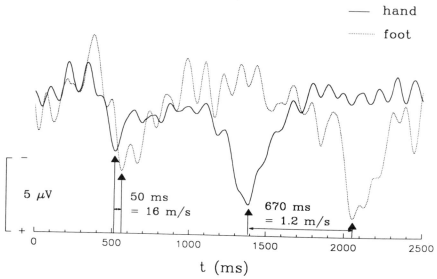

FIG. 6. Late and ultra-late LEPs in a 25-year-old man with hereditary motor and sensory neuropathy of type I. The latency differences between hand and foot stimulation indicate that late LEPs are mediated by Aδ-fibers and ultra-late LEPs by C-fibers. (Modified from Lankers et al. 1991.)

some PNP patients, and that unmasking of ultra-late LEPs in these patients may be a cortical correlate of disinhibition of C-fiber responses to noxious heat.

Spinal and Supraspinal Lesions

Interruption of nociceptive pathways anywhere between the peripheral receptor and the brain can lead to a loss of LEPs. Various lesions in the spinal cord, brain stem, and thalamus have been shown to distort or abolish LEPs (Bromm et al. 1991; Kakigi et al. 1991a; Treede et al. 1991). When LEPs were not completely absent in patients with a dissociated loss of pain sensitivity, LEP latencies were significantly delayed and LEP amplitudes significantly decreased in the affected skin areas as compared with control areas (Bromm et al. 1991).

Figure 7 shows data from a patient with a Type I Arnold-Chiari malformation and a spinal lesion due to syringomyelia ranging from C3 to Th5. Sensory testing (Fig. 7, bottom row) revealed a severe reduction in pain sensitivity and loss of temperature sensitivity in the left hand (affected site). Mechanical sensitivity was only slightly reduced. Normal sensitivity scores were found in the right hand (control site). LEPs after 15-W (dotted line) and 20-W stimuli (solid line) at the control site were highly reproducible and of normal amplitudes and latencies. The affected site,

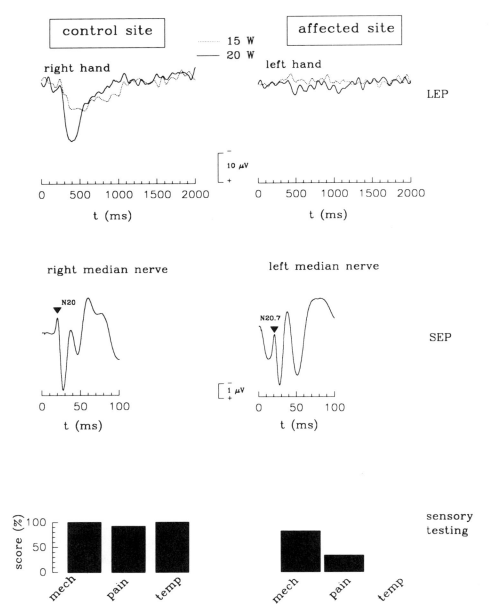

Patient #64; 52 ys; Syringomyelia C3–Th5, Arnold–Chiari I

FIG. 7. Evoked potentials in a 52-year-old woman with syringomyelia. This patient had a marked impairment of pain and temperature sensitivity of the left upper limb, whereas the right upper limb was normal (*bottom row*). This localized dissociated sensory loss was reflected in the laser-evoked potentials (*top row*), whereas the SEPs following conventional electrical nerve stimulation were unremarkable on both sides. (From Treede, Cristante, Herrmann, Bromm, unpublished data.)

however, showed a loss of LEPs at both intensities. Conventional SEPs (Fig. 7, middle row) were normal at both sites. Thus, only LEPs enabled the objective identification of the body site affected for pain and temperature sensitivity.

In a group of 10 patients with syringomyelia, we found absent LEPs in eight cases and a significantly reduced LEP amplitude in one case (Treede et al. 1991). Interestingly, in the remaining patient, who had well-configured LEPs, only temperature sensitivity was lost; pain sensitivity was intact. These results indicate that alteration of LEPs is related to disturbed pain rather than to disturbed temperature sensitivity. Inflammatory lesions in the spinal cord due to encephalitis disseminata often produced no change in LEPs, even in patients who had impaired pain sensitivity (Bromm et al. 1991). On the other hand, in one case of brain-stem encephalitis caused by herpes simplex virus, both the initial loss of pain sensitivity and later complete recovery from this impairment could be well documented by LEP analysis (Treede et al. 1992).

It has been hypothesized that LEPs might be enhanced in states of central hyperexcitability (e.g., in myoclonus epilepsy or central pain syndromes). An enhancement of LEPs in myoclonus epilepsy resembling the known enhancement of early conventional SEPs was not observed by Kakigi et al. (1990). Recently, the stimulus–response function for LEPs was found to be shifted to the left in patients with fibromyalgia (see Chapter 27). In fact, the heat-pain threshold was reduced in these patients and the area of flare in response to pinprick was increased. LEP analysis may thus also be used as a neurophysiologic test in the assessment of increased sensitivity to cutaneous pain.

CONCLUSIONS

Nociceptive pathways can be tested by the stimulation of hairy skin with brief laser radiant heat pulses and recording of the evoked cerebral potential on the scalp. The amplitude of long-latency LEPs is closely related to pain sensation. In some cases, the loss of Aδ-fiber-related late LEPs led to the appearance of C-fiber-related ultra-late LEPs. This unmasking occurred, for example, in PNPs that primarily affected myelinated fibers and thus mimicked a preferential A-fiber block. In contrast, ultra-late LEPs did not appear in any of the patients with syringomyelia or brain-stem lesions. We can thus distinguish whether the sensory deficit in a case of damage to the nervous system involves a selective loss of Aδ-fiber-related first pain or a complete loss of pain sensitivity. Selective loss of second pain cannot yet be documented because ultra-late LEPs are highly variable without nerve blocks. LEP analysis may also be used to assess increased pain sensitivity (e.g., in chronic neuropathic pain or fibromyalgia), provided that heat-pain sensitivity is involved, and not only mechanical-pain sensitivity. LEP analysis is therefore a useful neurophysiologic test in the assessment of hypalgesic and hyperalgesic dermatomes.

ACKNOWLEDGMENTS

We thank Drs. A. Frieling, T. Hölzer, S. Kief, V. Kunde, J. Lankers, and R. Siedenberg for collaboration in parts of the studies described in this chapter. This work was supported by the Deutsche Forschungsgemeinschaft (SFB 115, Br310/16).

REFERENCES

Angel RW, Quick WM, Boylls CC, Weinrich M, Rodnitzky RL. Decrement of somatosensory evoked potentials during repetitive stimulation. Electroencephalogr Clin *Neurophysiol* 1985;60:335–342.

Arendt-Nielsen L, Bjerring P. Selective averaging of argon laser induced pre-pain and pain related cortical responses. *J Neurosci Methods* 1988;24:117–123.

Beydoun A, Morrow TJ, Shen JF, Casey KL. Variability of laser-evoked potentials: attention, arousal and lateralized differences. *Electroencephalogr Clin Neurophysiol* 1993;88:173–181.

Biehl R, Treede RD, Bromm B. Pain ratings of short radiant heat pulses. In: Bromm B, ed. *Pain measurement in man.* Amsterdam: Elsevier, 1984;397–408.

Bromm B. Laboratory animal and human volunteers in the assessment of analgesic efficacy. In: Chapman CR, Loeser JD, eds. *Issues in pain measurement.* New York: Raven Press, 1989;117–143.

Bromm B, Frieling A, Lankers J. Laser evoked brain potentials in the assessment of disturbed pain and temperature sensibility. *Electroencephalogr Clin Neurophysiol* 1991;80:284–291.

Bromm B, Jahnke MT, Treede RD. Responses of human cutaneous afferents to CO2 laser stimuli causing pain. *Exp Brain Res* 1984;55:158–166.

Bromm B, Meier W. The intracutaneous stimulus: a new pain model for algesimetric studies. *Methods Find Exp Clin Pharmacol* 1984;6:405–410.

Bromm B, Neitzel H, Tecklenburg A, Treede RD. Evoked cerebral potential correlates of C-fibre activity in man. *Neurosci Lett* 1983;43:109–114.

Bromm B, Scharein E. Principal component analysis of pain related cerebral potentials to mechanical and electrical stimulation in man. *Electroencephalogr Clin Neurophysiol* 1982;53:94–103.

Bromm B, Treede RD. Evoked cerebral potential changes accompanying attention shifts between first and second pain. *Electroencephalogr Clin Neurophysiol* 1985;61:S117.

Bromm B, Treede RD. Human cerebral potentials evoked by CO_2 laser stimuli causing pain. *Exp Brain Res* 1987;67:153–162.

Bromm B, Treede RD. Laser evoked cerebral potentials in the assessment of cutaneous pain sensitivity in normal subjects and in patients. *Rév Neurol* 1991;147:625–643.

Campbell JN, LaMotte RH. Latency to detection of first pain. *Brain Res* 1983;266:203–208.

Carmon A, Dotan Y, Sarne Y. Correlation of subjective pain experience with cerebral evoked responses to noxious thermal stimulations. *Exp Brain Res* 1978;33:445–453.

Chatrian GE, Canfield RC, Knauss TA, Lettich E. Cerebral responses to electrical tooth pulp stimulation in man. *Neurology* 1975;25:745–757.

Chudler EH, Dong WK. The assessment of pain by cerebral evoked potentials. *Pain* 1983;16:221–244.

Chung JM, Lee KH, Hori Y, Endo K, Willis WD. Factors influencing peripheral nerve stimulation produced inhibition of primate spinothalamic tract cells. *Pain* 1984;19:277–293.

Desmedt JE. Somatosensory evoked potentials. In: Picton TW, ed. *Handbook of electroencephalography and clinical neurophysiology*, vol. 3. Amsterdam: Elsevier, 1988;245–360.

Devor M, Carmon A, Frostig R. Primary afferent and spinal sensory neurons that respond to brief pulses of intense infrared laser radiation: a preliminary survey in rats. *Exp Neurol* 1982;76:483–494.

Dyck PJ, Lambert EH, O'Brien PC. Pain in peripheral neuropathy related to rate and kind of fiber degeneration. *Neurology* 1976;26:466–471.

Gandevia SC, Burke D, McKeon B. The projection of muscle afferents from the hand to cerebral cortex in man. *Brain* 1984;107:1–13.

Gibson SJ, Gorman MM, Helme RD. Assessment of pain in the elderly using event-related cerebral potentials. In: Bond MR, Charlton JE, Woolf CJ, eds. *Proceedings of the VIth World Congress on Pain.* Amsterdam: Elsevier, 1991;527–533.

Gibson SJ, Littlejohn GO, Gorman MM, Helme RD, Granges G. Increased thermal pain in patients with fibromyalgia. In: Bromm B, Desmedt J, eds. *Advances in pain research and therapy.* New York: Raven Press, 1994.

Gross-Isseroff R, Sarne Y, Carmon A, Isseroff A. Cortical potentials evoked by innocuous tactile and noxious thermal stimulation in the rat: differences in localization and latency. *Behav Neural Biol* 1982; 35:294–307.

Harkins SW, Price DD, Katz MA. Are cerebral evoked potentials reliable indices of first or second pain? In: Bonica JJ, Lindblom U, Iggo A, eds. *Advances in pain research and therapy,* vol. 5. New York: Raven Press, 1983;185–191.

Kakigi R, Shibasaki H. Estimation of conduction velocity of the spinothalamic tract in man. *Electroencephalogr Clin Neurophysiol* 1991;80:39–45.

Kakigi R, Shibasaki H, Ikeda A. Pain-related somatosensory evoked potentials following CO_2-laser stimulation in man. *Electroencephalogr Clin Neurophysiol* 1989;74:139–146.

Kakigi R, Shibasaki H, Kuroda Y, Neshige R, Endo C, Tabuchi K, Kishikawa T. Pain-related somatosensory evoked potentials in syringomyelia. *Brain* 1991a;114:1871–1889.

Kakigi R, Shibasaki H, Neshige R, Ikeda A, Mamiya K, Kuroda Y. Pain-related somatosensory evoked potentials in cortical reflex myoclonus. *J Neurol Neurosurg Psychiatry* 1990;53:44–48.

Kakigi R, Shibasaki H, Tanaka K, Ikeda T, Oda KI, Endo C, Ikeda A, Neshige R, Kuroda Y, Miyata K, Yi S, Ikegawa S, Araki S. CO_2 laser -induced pain-related somatosensory evoked potentials in peripheral neuropathies: correlation between electrophysiological and histopathological findings. *Muscle Nerve* 1991b;14:441–450.

Kenton B, Coger R, Crue B, Pinsky J, Friedman Y, Carmon A. Peripheral fiber correlates to noxious thermal stimulation in humans. *Neurosci Lett* 1980;17:301–306.

Kobal G. Pain-related electrical potentials on the human respiratory nasal mucosa elicited by chemical stimuli. In: Bromm B, ed. *Pain measurement in man.* Amsterdam: Elsevier, 1984;463–468.

Kunde V, Treede RD. Topography of middle-latency somatosensory evoked potentials following painful heat stimuli and non-painful electrical stimuli. *Electroencephalogr Clin Neurophysiol* 1993;88:280–289.

Lankers J, Frieling A, Kunze K, Bromm B. Ultralate cerebral potentials in a patient with hereditary motor and sensory neuropathy I indicate preserved C-fibre function. *J Neurol Neurosurg Psychiatry* 1991;54:650–652.

McGillem CD, Aunon JI. Analysis of event-related potentials. In: Gevins AS, Rémond A, eds. *Handbook of electroencephalography and clinical neurophysiology,* vol. 1. Amsterdam: Elsevier, 1987;131–169.

Melzack R, Wall PD. Pain mechanisms: a new theory. *Science* 1965;150:971–979.

Mendell L. Physiological properties of unmyelinated fiber projections to the spinal cord. *Exp Neurol* 1966;16:316–332.

Mor J, Carmon A. Laser emitted radiant heat for pain research. *Pain* 1975;1:233–237.

Pertovaara A, Morrow TJ, Casey KL. Cutaneous pain and detection thresholds to short CO_2 laser pulses in humans: evidence on afferent mechanisms and the influence of varying stimulus conditions. *Pain* 1988;34:261–269.

Schafer EWP, Amochaev A, Russell MJ. Knowledge of stimulus timing attenuates human evoked cortical potentials. *Electroencephalogr Clin Neurophysiol* 1981;52:9–17.

Siedenberg R. Kognitive zerebrale Potentiale nach schmerzhaften Laser-Hitzereizen beim Menschen. Doctoral thesis, University of Hamburg, 1994.

Spreng M, Ichioka M. Langsame Rindenpotentiale bei Schmerzreizung am Menschen. *Pflügers Archiv* 1964;279:121–152.

Sutton S, Braren M, Zubin J, John ER. Evoked-potential correlates of stimulus uncertainty. *Science* 1965;150:1187–1188.

Taira T, Amano K, Kawamura H, Tanikawa T, Kitamura K. Cerebral evoked responses elicited by direct stimulation of the lateral spinothalamic tract in the human. *Appl Neurophysiol* 1975;48:267–270.

Towell AD, Boyd SG. Sensory and cognitive components of the CO_2 laser evoked cerebral potential. *Electroencephalogr Clin Neurophysiol* 1993;88:237–239.

Treede RD, Bromm B. Reliability and validity of ultra-late cerebral potentials in response to C-fibre activation in man. In: Dubner R, Gebhart GF, Bond MR, eds. *Pain research and clinical management* vol. 3. Amsterdam: Elsevier, 1988;567–573.

Treede RD, Hansen HC, Kunze K, Bromm B. Neurophysiologische Beurteilung der Schmerzbahnen bei Patienten mit Hirnstammläsionen. In: Schimrigk K, Haaß A, Hamann G, eds. *Verhandlungen der Deutschen Gesellschaft für Neurologie* 7, 1992;609–610.

Treede RD, Kief S, Hölzer T, Bromm B. Late somatosensory evoked cerebral potentials in response to cutaneous heat stimuli. *Electroencephalogr Clin Neurophysiol* 1988;70:429–441.

Treede RD, Lankers J, Frieling A, Zangemeister WH, Kunze K, Bromm B. Cerebral potentials evoked by painful laser stimuli in patients with syringomyelia. *Brain* 1991;114:1595–1607.

Treede RD, Meyer RA, Lesser RP. Similarity of threshold temperatures for first pain sensation, laser-evoked potentials and nociceptor activation. In: Gebhart GF, Hammond DL, Jensen TS, eds. *Proceedings of the 7th World Congress on Pain.* Seattle: IASP Publications, 1994;857–865.

Vallbo AB, Hagbarth KE, Torebjörk HE, Wallin BG. Somatosensory, proprioceptive, and sympathetic activity in human peripheral nerves. *Physiol Rev* 1979;59:919–957.

Wright A, Davies IAI. The recordings of brain evoked potentials resulting from intra-articular focused ultrasonic stimulation: a new experimental model for investigating joint pain in humans. *Neurosci Lett* 1989;97:145–150.

*Pain and the Brain: From
Nociception to Cognition,*
edited by Burkhart Bromm and
John E. Desmedt, Advances in Pain
Research and Therapy Vol. 22.
Raven Press, Ltd., New York © 1995.

26

Pain in Polyneuropathy

Allan L. Bernstein

*Department of Neurology, Kaiser Permanente Medical Center,
Hayward, California, USA 94545-4297*

SUMMARY

Painful polyneuritis is a multifactorial condition that occurs when abnormal signals are sent by the peripheral nervous system and are abnormally interpreted by the central nervous system (CNS). Many factors cause painful polyneuritis, including diabetes, alcohol abuse, toxic chemicals, and nutritional deficiency; systemic abnormalities such as peripheral myelin breakdown, axonal degeneration, and chronic nerve-sheath inflammation are thought to propagate an abnormal signal centrally or to further distort the signal that eventually reaches the neuromatrix. The central, cognitive response to pain is discussed, as is the distinction between acute and chronic pain and the healing initiated by the inflammatory reaction and increased blood flow. Metabolic abnormalities and their relation to pain levels are described. Recommend therapy for pain in polyneuropathy includes preventive measures, pharmacologic treatment, and behavioral approaches.

INTRODUCTION

The pain of polyneuritis continues to perplex both patients and their physicians. Small-fiber stimulation and large-fiber injury or dysfunction are all associated with increased perception of pain (Fields and Levine 1984; Asbury and Fields 1984). Because polyneuritis is usually chronic, the role of small-fiber stimulation in this disorder is probably minimal; study of the role of large-fiber injury is therefore more likely to reveal the cause of pain. The conditions producing polyneuritis are generally systemic, and affect the ability of the central nervous system (CNS) to interpret and modulate peripheral input.

Polyneuritis implies diffuse dysfunction of peripheral nerves. The condition has multiple causes, including toxins, metabolic disorders, ischemia, hereditary conditions, nutritional factors, infections, degeneration, and trauma (Table 1). Why some forms of neuropathy are associated with pain and others are not is poorly estab-

TABLE 1. *Forms of polyneuropathy associated with pain*

Diabetes
Postherpetic neuralgia
Posttraumatic neuralgia
Infectious/postinfectious polyneuritis
Arsenic toxicity
Thallium toxicity
Alcoholic neuropathy
Niacin deficiency
Thiamine deficiency
Pyridoxine deficiency
Medication-related
   Vincristine
   Isoniazid
   Cisplatin
   Nitrofurantoin
Ischemic neuropathy
Hereditary forms of neuropathy

lished. Myelinated fibers, usually pain-inhibitory, and unmyelinated fibers, usually pain-stimulating, are both injured in polyneuritis (Fields 1987). The ratio of stimulating to inhibitory impulses may determine whether pain is a component of neuropathy in the condition. This ratio may also determine the quality of the unpleasant sensations in polyneuritis and their response to treatment (Dyck et al. 1976).

All of the most common forms of polyneuritis (i.e., those caused by diabetes, nutritional deficiencies, toxic chemicals, infections, and vasculitis) affect the entire body and are not limited to the peripheral or central nervous systems. This systemic effect complicates the effort to isolate the "pain" component of such a condition. The emotional reaction to chronic medical conditions modulates the patient's description of pain. This phenomenon demands that treating physicians interpret such descriptions of pain as "levels of discomfort." A numb limb may be as uncomfortable to some patients as an acutely injured limb, and both may be described as painful during questioning by the investigator or treating physician.

The neuromatrix theory of pain and perception (Melzack 1990, 1991) maintains that experience is a factor in modulating pain. A thorn in a person's hand may cause the physiologic equivalent of pain but may not be described as pain by someone who has had this experience before and is aware of the benign nature of the injury. The neuromatrix thus interprets all input and modulates it on the basis of prior experience. Lack of input, which may occur in polyneuritis or even phantom-limb pain, may be interpreted as a painful or unpleasant sensation because of incomplete information. "Pain" may be the "default" setting of the neuromatrix.

Metabolic or nutritional forms of neuropathy cause symmetric injury to nerves of equal size and length. Yet painful neuropathy is not symmetric in most patients. Pathologic and electrophysiologic studies may show that the nerves tested are identical, even though one area of innervation "hurts" and the other is numb. Even more perplexing for patients and physicians is that the same nerves may alternately be described as numb or painful depending on other physical or emotional stresses. Although reversing the metabolic abnormality responsible for a neuropathy may stop the progression of injury, the chronic pain that may accompany the injury may persist if peripheral nerves have sustained significant damage.

Polyneuritis is generally considered a form of chronic pain, in that no acute injury or threat to the organism exists despite progressive, chronic nerve degeneration. The pain of polyneuritis is a learned behavior that depends on prior experience and the integration of multiple sensory inputs (Melzack 1990, 1991; Syrjala and Chapman 1984). The study of pain in polyneuritis is therefore an attempt to correlate peripheral nerve injury with the state of the central processing mechanism that defines the cognitive term "pain." Treatment of the condition ranges from attempting to modify the underlying pathologic process by pharmacologic and physical means to behavior modification.

Treatment strategies for polyneuritic pain must be of broad scope. Systemic medication directed at neurotransmitter modification has been used (Asbury and Fields 1984; Swerdlow 1984; Willner and Low 1993; Max et al. 1992); drugs that reduce hyperirritability have proved useful (Galer et al, 1993); and medication that improves the microcirculation and microenvironment at the peripheral level may also be therapeutic. Changing peripheral nerve input by such means as acupuncture, transcutaneous electric nerve stimulation (TENS), or exercise may change the way in which the neuromatrix interprets signals. Behavioral changes such as those taught in chronic-pain programs may "retrain" the neuromatrix to convert pain to "background noise."

WHAT CAUSES PAINFUL POLYNEUROPATHY AND WHY

Many factors cause painful polyneuropathy, the most clinically significant of which are diabetes, alcohol abuse, nutritional deficiency, heavy metal toxicity, and medication. Other conditions causing painful neuropathy include trigeminal neuralgia (Austin and Cubillos 1991), postherpetic neuralgia, hereditary forms of neuropathy (Dyck et al. 1983), Guillain-Barré syndrome (Ropper and Shahani 1984), and posttraumatic forms of neuropathy.

Why these conditions are associated with pain is more difficult to understand. Peripheral myelin breakdown, axonal degeneration, disordered signal transmission, chronic inflammation of nerves or perineural sheaths, impaired microvascular circulation to the peripheral nerves, and disorders of micronutrition (glucose, oxygen, amino acid, vitamin, or mineral excess or deficiency) may all lead to propagation of an abnormal signal centrally (Willner and Low 1993). The same systemic abnormalities may also affect the central nervous system (CNS) and further distort the signal that eventually reaches the neuromatrix. Thus, the abnormal peripheral nerve signal becomes progressively more disorganized as it passes through pain pathways.

THE CENTRAL COGNITIVE RESPONSE TO
PERIPHERAL NERVE INJURY

We tend to consider pain as being either acute or chronic, and to plan assessment and treatment procedures for it on this basis. Acute pain usually implies tissue injury sufficient to prompt the body to mobilize appropriate protective responses, such as the withdrawal reflex, to eliminate further threat. Healing is then initiated through an inflammatory reaction and increased blood flow. Despite knowledge of the many peripheral mechanisms of acute pain, the central, cognitive response to pain is poorly understood. This response may vary from complete inability to function after a minor injury to complete insensitivity to major injuries during stressful activities such as athletic competition or combat (Syrjala and Chapman 1984). Nociception is not always described as pain. Whether this tendency is purely biochemical, is mediated by inhibitory pathways, or is a learned behavioral response is not known. Under experimental conditions, subjects may describe sham procedures as painful and may deny experiencing pain during procedures leading to nociceptive responses, depending on instructions given before such procedures are undertaken.

Chronic pain, typified by polyneuritis, has both physiologic and emotional components. With time, the emotional aspect may overshadow the physical aspect as the pain "wears down" the patient. Input from the periphery tends to be abnormal. Chronic stimulation arises from damaged nerves and from impaired inhibitory input. Responses to this type of pain vary from mild irritation to total disability. Increased activity and stimulation of the peripheral nerves may activate inhibitory fibers, making increased activity a means of coping with chronic pain. Conversely, increased activity may stimulate the pain "loop," which may explain why some patients with chronic pain attempt to minimize all activity. Individual responses appear unpredictable. Measurable changes in neurotransmitter levels occur with chronic pain, as do changes in thresholds to stimuli experienced as "painful" by these patients (Fields and Levine 1984).

Descriptions of chronic pain vary with stimulus intensity and the communication skills of the patient. Chronic pain has a strong emotional component, and patients with such pain may use their condition to obtain secondary gains, whether emotional ("I'm a victim"), financial (posttraumatic, work-related), or social (avoidance of an unpleasant situation). Central mechanisms can "convert" a disabling chronic-pain syndrome to mild irritation at the culmination of litigation or emotionally distressing circumstances.

METABOLIC CONSIDERATIONS

Various metabolic abnormalities are associated with increased levels of pain. Increased blood glucose levels can reduce pain thresholds (Morley et al. 1984). Maintaining optimal blood glucose levels makes pain control easier. Marginal deficiency in most vitamins reduces pain thresholds (Mäder et al. 1988). Such deficiency may be more common than expected, given the tendency of patients with chronic pain to lose their appetite and appreciation of food. Toxic chemicals, including alcohol, heavy metals, and chemotherapeutic agents, may produce painful forms of neuropathy. Therapeutic agents such as metronidazole, isoniazid, phenytoin, and nitrofurantoin tend to produce painless forms of neuropathy, although some patients describe the abnormal sensation produced by these agents as painful. When the offending agent is used to treat a life-threatening disease, an alternative treatment strategy may be necessary. This strategy may include reducing doses of chemotherapeutic agents or combining them with less neurotoxic substances. Adding folic acid to phenytoin therapy or adding pyridoxine to isoniazid therapy, for example, may reduce neurotoxicity without reducing the therapeutic effect of the agents used.

PHANTOM-LIMB PAIN AND POLYNEURITIS

The high incidence of phantom-limb pain in patients with missing limbs or equivalent spinal injuries makes it likely that pain creates a homunculus-type pattern in the brain: a neuromatrix (Melzack 1990, 1991; Melzack and Loeser 1978; Loeser 1984; Conomy 1973). The activity of this pain network is modulated by constant feedback from the periphery, consisting of "normal" input such as sensations of position, pressure, movement, temperature, and vibration. Loss of input causes the neuromatrix to create the false impression of pain.

Using the analogy of the brain's predilection to seizure, the homeostatic mechanisms of both peripheral input and central modulation are designed to prevent the sensation of pain. The organism's goal is to keep peripheral nerves firing at preferred rates and in the proper balance to maintain comfort and optimal function. Loss of input from multiple stimuli may lead to a cognitive sensation of pain in a body "part" that is not physiologically attached to the body.

TREATMENT

Treatment of pain in polyneuropathy takes many forms. The most effective course has been to treat the underlying abnormality causing the neuropathy. This task may be as easy as removing a toxic chemical, changing a neurotoxic medication, or treating vitamin deficiency. On the other hand, the problem may be as complex as trying to maintain rigid glucose control in a patient with brittle diabetes or treating the ischemia of diffuse peripheral vascular disease.

On a practical basis, pain may be considered acute or chronic. Most polyneuropathic pain falls into the category of being chronic. For this group of patients, preventive treatment has proved effective and useful for prolonged periods. Surgical treatment for pain involving either spinal or peripheral nerve sectioning has not proved effective for its long-term relief (Loeser 1984; Noordenbos and Wall 1981). This limitation leaves a majority of treatments that operate pharmacologically by oral, topical, or parenteral routes (Table 2).

TABLE 2. *Treatment of painful polyneuritis*

Antidepressant medications
Antiepileptic medications
Neuroleptic medications
Antispasticity agents
Anesthetic medications
Narcotic analgesics
Nonnarcotic analgesics
Steroids
Nonsteroidal antiinflammatory drugs
Local nerve blocks
B vitamins
Topical capsaicin
Acupuncture
Biofeedback
Hypnosis
Surgical intervention at local, spinal, or brain levels

The medications most widely used for treating neuropathic pain are the tricyclic antidepressants (Max et al. 1992; Kvinesdal et al. 1984; Mendel et al. 1986). Their effectiveness seems related to their ability to increase central levels of serotonin and norepinephrine. They act by inhibiting neurotransmitter reuptake at spinal and brain-stem levels. Relatively low doses may be used, but side effects such as drowsiness, dry mouth, and bladder-neck obstruction often limit their use.

The next most used medications are the antiepileptic drugs (Swerdlow 1984; Ellenberg 1968). Phenytoin, carbamazepine, and sodium valproate have all been used to treat chronic pain with moderate success. Side effects are generally less troublesome with these agents, but again, drowsiness can be a problem. The potential of these drugs to induce hepatotoxicity and bone-marrow suppression necessitates laboratory follow-up studies during their use. Phenytoin may itself cause peripheral neuropathy.

B vitamins have been used to treat painful forms of neuropathy (Mäder et al. 1988; Bernstein and Lobitz 1988; Bernstein and Dinesen 1993; Hanck and Weiser 1985; Sharma et al. 1990; Zimmermann 1988). They appear to increase pain thresholds and serotonin levels. Their antinociceptive action appears nonspecific, and has been reported to be therapeutically effective in treating complications of diabetes, carpal-tunnel syndrome, headache, and back pain. Investigators have used varying doses of B vitamins with wide therapeutic and safety ranges. The therapeutic effect may be enhanced when B vitamins are combined with nonsteroidal antiinflammatory medications (Lettko and Bartoszyk 1990).

The effects of nonsteroidal antiinflammatory medications in treating polyneuritic pain are variable. Gastrointestinal complications limit long-term use of these drugs, but they may be appropriate for acute episodes. Their doses vary widely, depending on tolerance.

Narcotics have generally been ineffective for treating neuropathic pain because they produce tachyphylaxis. In rare instances of disabling pain, their use may be appropriate under close supervision. Narcotics have been used on a long-term basis at low levels to treat chronic headache or vertebral pain without development of drug tolerance. This approach has been less successful in treating painful polyneuropathy.

Topical lidocaine (Rowbotham and Fields 1989) and topical capsaicin (Willner and Low 1993) have been used for chronic postherpetic neuralgia. Long-term follow-up of their effects is in progress. An oral form of lidocaine, mexiletine, is being used with modest success in painful forms of diabetic neuropathy. Intravenous lidocaine has been used to treat chronic pain in peripheral polyneuritis (Galer et al. 1993), but the duration of relief from this form of treatment is unknown.

One of the most successful approaches to treating chronic pain, whether polyneuritic, posttraumatic, postsurgical, lumbar, cervical, facial, or chronic cephalic, has been a chronic pain-management program. Enrollment in this type of program provides relief through a behavioral approach to chronic pain. Progressively increasing activity, relaxation training, biofeedback, complete withdrawal from pain medication, and psychologic intervention to modify pain behavior have long-lasting effects on the ability to separate nociception from pain perception (Tulkin et al. 1992).

In summary, painful polyneuritis is a multifactorial condition that occurs when abnormal signals are sent by the peripheral nervous system and are abnormally interpreted by the CNS. The neuromatrix theory of pain and perception (Melzack 1990) suggests that a complex interaction between cognitive and physiologic components is required to distinguish the affective component, consisting of pain, from the neurochemical component, consisting of nociception. That treatment by chemical manipulation or behavioral intervention is effective and surgical ablation is ineffective in treating neuropathic pain reinforces the neuromatrix concept.

ACKNOWLEDGMENT

The Medical Editing Department, Kaiser Foundation Research Institute, provided editorial assistance with this chapter.

REFERENCES

Asbury AK, Fields HL. Pain due to peripheral nerve damage: an hypothesis. *Neurology* 1984;34:1587–1590.

Austin DG, Cubillos L. Special considerations in orofacial pain. *Dent Clin North Am* 1991;35:227–244.

Bernstein AL, Dinesen JS. Brief communication: effects of pharmacologic doses of vitamin B-6 on carpal tunnel syndrome, electroencephalographic results, and pain. *J Am Coll Nutr* 1993;12:73–76.

Bernstein AL, Lobitz CS. A clinical and electrophysiologic study of the treatment of painful diabetic neuropathies with pyridoxine. *Curr Top Nutr Dis* 1988;19:415–423.

Conomy JP. Disorders of body image after spinal cord injury. *Neurology* 1973;23:842–850.

Dyck PJ, Lambert EH, O'Brien PC. Pain in peripheral neuropathy related to rate and kind of fiber degeneration. *Neurology* 1976;26:466–471.

Dyck PJ, Low PA, Stevens JC. "Burning feet" as the only manifestation of dominantly inherited sensory neuropathy. *Mayo Clin Proc* 1983;58:426–429.

Ellenberg M. Treatment of diabetic neuropathy with diphenylhydantoin. *NY State J Med* 1968;68:2653–2655.

Fields HL. *Pain.* New York: McGraw-Hill, 1987.

Fields HL, Levine JD. Pain: mechanisms and management. *West J Med* 1984;141:347–357.

Galer BS, Miller KV, Rowbotham MC. Response to intravenous lidocaine infusion differs based on clinical diagnosis and site of nervous system injury. *Neurology* 1993;43:1233–1235.

Hanck A, Weiser H. Analgesic and anti-inflammatory properties of vitamins. *Int J Vitam Nutr Res* 1985; (Suppl 27):189–206.

Kvinesdal B, Molin J, Frøland A, Gram LF. Imipramine treatment of painful diabetic neuropathy. *JAMA* 1984;251:1727–1730.

Lettko M, Bartoszyk GD. Reduced need for diclofenac with concomitant administration of pyridoxine and other B vitamins: clinical and experimental studies. *Ann NY Acad Sci* 1990;585:510–512.

Loeser JD. Phantom limb pain. *Curr Concepts Pain* 1984;2(2):3–8.

Mäder R. Deutsch H, Siebert GK, Gerbershagen HU, Grühn E, Behl M, et al. Vitamin status of inpatients with chronic cephalgia and dysfunction pain syndrome and effects of a vitamin supplementation. *Int J Vitam Nutr Res* 1988;58:436–441.

Max MB, Lynch SA, Muir J, Shoaf SE, Smoller B, Dubner R. Effects of desipramine, amitriptyline and fluoxetine on pain in diabetic neuropathy. *N Engl J Med* 1992;326:1250–1256.

Melzack R. Phantom limbs and the concept of a neuromatrix. *Trends Neurosci* 1990;13:88–92.

Melzack R. The John J. Bonica Distinguished Lecture. The gate control theory 25 years later: new perspectives on phantom limb pain. In: Bond MR, Charlton JE, Woolf CJ, eds. *Proceedings of the VIth World Congress on Pain. Pain research and clinical management,* vol. 4. Amsterdam: Elsevier, 1991;9–21.

Melzack R, Loeser JD. Phantom body pain in paraplegics: evidence for a central "pattern generating mechanism" for pain. *Pain* 1978;4:195–210.

Mendel CM, Klein RF, Chappell DA, Dere WH, Gertz BJ, Karam JH. A trial of amitriptyline and fluphenazine in the treatment of painful diabetic neuropathy. *JAMA* 1986;256:637–639.

Morley GK, Mooradian AD, Levine AS, Morley JE. Mechanism of pain in diabetic peripheral neuropathy: effect of glucose on pain perception in humans. *Am J Med* 1984;77:79–82.

Noordenbos W, Wall PD. Implication of the failure of nerve resection and graft to cure pain produced by nerve lesions. *J Neurol Neurosurg Psychiatry* 1981;44:1068–1073.

Ropper AH, Shahani BT. Pain in Guillain-Barré syndrome. *Arch Neurol* 1984;41:511–514.

Rowbotham MC, Fields HL. Topical lidocaine reduces pain in post-herpetic neuralgia. *Pain* 1989;38:297–301.

Sharma SK, Bolster B, Dakshinamurti K. Effects of pyridoxine on nociceptive thalamic unit activity. *Ann NY Acad Sci* 1990;585:549–553.

Swerdlow M. Anticonvulsant drugs and chronic pain. *Clin Neuropharmacol* 1984;7:51–82.

Syrjala KL, Chapman CR. Measurement of clinical pain: a review and integration of research findings. *Adv Pain Res Ther* 1984;7:71–101.

Tulkin SR, Frank GW, Bernstein A, Aubel B, Lehn M. Management of chronic benign pain in a prepaid practice. In: Feldman JL, Fitzpatrick RJ, eds. *Managed mental health care: administrative and clinical issues.* Washington, DC: American Psychiatric Press, 1992;359–374.

Willner C, Low PA. Pharmacologic approaches to neuropathic pain. In: Dyck PJ, Thomas PK, Griffin JW, Low PA, Poduslo JF, eds. *Peripheral neuropathy,* 2nd ed. Philadelphia: WB Saunders, 1993; 1709–1720.

Zimmermann M. Possibilities for B-vitamins to modulate basic biological mechanisms involved in pain. In: Gerbershagen HU, Zimmermann M, eds. *B-vitamins in pain.* Symposium associated with the Vth World Congress on Pain, Hamburg, Federal Republic of Germany, August 2, 1987. Frankfurt: pmi Verlag, 1988;1–9.

Pain and the Brain: From
Nociception to Cognition,
edited by Burkhart Bromm and
John E. Desmedt, Advances in Pain
Research and Therapy Vol. 22.
Raven Press, Ltd., New York © 1995.

27

Increased Thermal Pain Sensitivity in Patients with Fibromyalgia Syndrome

*Stephen J. Gibson, †Gerald Granges, †Geoff O. Littlejohn, and *Robert D. Helme

*National Research Institute of Gerontology and Geriatric Medicine, North West Hospital, Parkville, Victoria 3052, Australia, and †Department of Medicine, Monash Medical Centre, Clayton, Victoria 3168, Australia

SUMMARY

Fibromyalgia syndrome is characterized by chronic aching and mechanical hyperalgesia, particularly over predesignated tender-point sites, yet changes in thermal pain perception in this condition have yet to be investigated. The present study examined heat-pain thresholds and cerebral event-related potentials following CO_2 laser stimulation of the dorsum of the hand in 10 pain-free controls and 10 patients with fibromyalgia. Patients with fibromyalgia exhibited a significant reduction in heat-pain threshold. In accord with previous findings, these patients also showed lower mechanical-pain thresholds and, as indexed by neurogenic flare, an increase in the efferent response of primary afferent neurons with polymodal nociceptors. These findings emphasize the multimodal nature of change in cutaneous pain sensitivity in fibromyalgia, and suggest a heightened responsivity or sensitization of polymodal nociceptors on primary afferent neurons. The fibromyalgia patients were also found to have a marked increase in the peak-to-peak amplitude of the cerebral event-related potential, indicating greater central nervous system (CNS) activation in response to a pain stimulus of threshold intensity and CO_2 laser stimulation of 1.5 times pain-threshold intensity. A significant correlation between measures of the clinical pain state and the measures of pain threshold, neurogenic flare, and cerebral event-related potential suggests that these changes in nociceptive function are strongly related to the severity of the clinical pain syndrome. However, further research is required in order to determine whether such changes are important in the etiology of fibromyalgia or are merely secondary consequences of this chronic pain disorder.

INTRODUCTION

Primary fibromyalgia syndrome (FS) is a common, chronic musculoskeletal pain condition with defined diagnostic criteria and a consistent pattern of symptoms and signs (Wolfe et al. 1990). Characteristic features include diffuse aching and soreness, a nonrestorative sleep pattern, morning stiffness, and fatigue (Yunus et al. 1989; Wolfe et al. 1990; Granges and Littlejohn 1993), and an increased neurogenic flare response following minor cutaneous injury (Littlejohn et al. 1987). Affective disturbance has also been noted among some patients with FS, particularly higher levels of anxiety, depression, hysteria, and hypochondriasis (Goldenberg 1989). Perhaps the most notable and consistent feature of this syndrome, however, is an increase in the sensitivity to mechanical stimulation (i.e., mechanical hyperalgesia). In fact, this change in sensitivity to mechanical pain, manifested clinically as tender-point sites, now constitutes one of the major defining characteristics of FS (Wolfe et al. 1990). At present, the etiology and pathophysiology of this condition is poorly understood, although both peripheral and central nervous system (CNS) factors have been implicated (Boissevain and McCain 1991).

Given the well-documented disturbance in mechanical pain perception in FS, it is perhaps surprising that changes in sensitivity to thermal pain have yet to be investigated. This is particularly relevant when one considers the recent experimental evidence of different underlying mechanisms for alterations in mechanical and thermal pain sensitivity in cases of primary and secondary hyperalgesia (Simone et al. 1991; Torebjork et al. 1992; Treede et al. 1992). Primary hyperalgesia, which occurs at a site of cutaneous injury, is characterized by an increased sensitivity to thermal and mechanical stimulation, and is thought to result from a sensitization of peripheral nociceptors on primary afferent C and Aδ fibers (Simone et al. 1991; Torebjork et al. 1992; Treede et al. 1992). In regions of secondary hyperalgesia, which surround the injury site, there is increased sensitivity to mechanical but not to thermal stimulation. Microneurographic evidence suggests that the secondary (mechanical) hyperalgesia is mediated by altered CNS processing, with a sensitization of wide-dynamic-range (WDR) neurons within the spinal cord, rather than by changes in the function of peripheral nociceptors (Simone et al. 1991; Torebjork et al. 1992; Treede et al. 1992). Thus, a finding of altered sensitivity to thermal and mechanical pain in patients with FS might well suggest different underlying mechanisms than would a finding of mechanical hyperalgesia alone. The aim of the present study was to examine heat-pain thresholds and the cerebral event-related potential (CERP) as an index of CNS processing following noxious laser stimulation in patients with FS. The clinical symptoms of fibromyalgia, mechanical pain thresholds, and the efferent response of cutaneous primary afferent fibers (as indexed by neurogenic flare) were also monitored and compared to the heat-pain threshold and CERP measures.

METHODS

Subjects

Ten female patients diagnosed by a rheumatologist as having FS and 10 pain-free, age-matched control volunteers were tested. All subjects were medication free at the time of testing.

Procedures

On the day of testing, all subjects underwent a clinical examination that included an assessment of the 18 predesignated tender-point sites used in the classification of Wolfe et al. (1990). Pain thresholds for mechanical pressure over tender-point sites and at four control sites (right and left thumb and mid-deltoid region) were assessed with a pressure algometer. A point was considered tender if the subject indicated the presence of a painful sensation at pressures of less than 4 kg/cm^2. A structured interview quantified information on pain severity, location and constancy, the presence or absence of fatigue, morning stiffness, nonrestorative sleep, paresthesia, grip strength, and skinfold tenderness. These scores were combined to provide a pseudointerval scale of symptom severity (Granges and Littlejohn 1993). A mechanically induced flare was elicited by scratching the skin with a swab stick over the upper thoracic region of the back. Neurogenic spreading flare was quantified as the width (mm) of flare 2 min after stimulation. This procedure was performed by an experimenter blinded to patient diagnosis.

The heat-pain threshold and detection threshold were determined in response to CO_2 laser stimulation of the dorsum of the right and left hand (33 msec, 5 mm beam diameter), using double random staircase procedures. The staircase procedure combines the up–down trials of the method of limits with the efficiency of the method of adjustment (see Gracely et al. 1988 for a full description). In the present study, the detection and pain thresholds were defined as the mean values of four consecutive 1-W up–down alternations in the intensity of laser stimulation. The CERP was then recorded following 36 laser stimuli presented with a random interstimulus interval (20–40 sec) and at pseudorandom intensity (pain threshold intensity or 1.5 times the pain-threshold intensity). This procedure was repeated for the right and left sides. Subjects were asked to rate each laser stimulus on a nine-item word descriptor scale (not felt, just noticeable, faint, weak, mild, moderate, strong, severe or excruciating pain) (Turskey et al. 1982). Scores (from 0, or not felt, to 8, or excruciating) were summed over the 36 trials, and a mean score was calculated for each intensity of stimulation. The EEG was recorded for 1000 msec poststimulus from Ag/AgCl electrodes attached to the vertex (Cz) versus linked ears (A1–A2), with the forehead (Fpz) as ground. Infra- and supraorbital electrodes were used to monitor gross eye movement (electrooculogram; EOG). EEG segments were amplified (100K), filtered (0.5–70 Hz), digitized (600 Hz) and stored on computer. After rejecting sweeps contaminated with EOG signals, single trial CERPs were averaged for each intensity of laser stimulation and then within each group of subjects to provide grand-mean waveforms. Measures of peak latency and peak-to-peak amplitude were calculated for each major waveform component within the averaged CERP. A computer program automatically selected the major positive and negative peaks within the 100- to 600-msec poststimulus segment of the waveform. Visual confirmation of the computer-derived values ensured correct identification of the major waveform components. Very good test-retest reliability has been demonstrated when using this method (Gibson et al. 1991).

RESULTS

On the day of testing, two patients with FS had less than 11 tender-point sites as indexed by pressure algometry with a cutoff of 4.0 kg/cm^2. This finding contrasts with the minimum number of tender-point sites required to satisfy a diagnosis of FS when using the criteria of Wolfe et al. (1990), which are based on manual palpation rather than quantitative algometry. These two subjects were not excluded from the sample because on the day of testing, both were still suffering from diffuse musculoskeletal pain and described a number of characteristic symptoms, such as a nonrestorative sleep pattern. Moreover, both patients had been attending a private rheumatology practice for over 12 months and had previously fulfilled the criteria of Wolfe et al. (1990) on a number of occasions. Finally, the determination of tender-point sites was made using pressure algometry rather than manual palpation, and in both cases there were an additional five tender-point sites with pressure-pain thresholds between 4.0 and 4.5 kg/cm^2.

Descriptive information, neurogenic flare responses, and pain-threshold data for the sample of 10 fibromyalgia patients and 10 pain-free control volunteers is shown in Table 1. An examination of Table 1 reveals that subjects were well matched for age and general mood state. FS patients reported mild to moderate levels of pain with a mean duration of over 6 years. As expected, independent-sample t-tests revealed that the number of clinical symptoms ($t_{(18)} = 7.68$, $p<0.0001$) and the number of tender-point sites ($t_{(18)} = 5.42$, $p<0.0001$) were significantly different for the fibromyalgia patients and controls.

The measures of neurogenic flare, mechanical-pain threshold, heat-pain threshold, and CERP parameters at pain-threshold intensity and 1.5 times pain-threshold intensity, taken from the right and left sides, were analyzed using multivariate analysis of variance (MANOVA). Because a significant difference was noted between the fibromyalgia patients and controls ($F_{(7,12)} = 5.33$, $p<0.01$), *post hoc* univariate ANOVA was also performed for each dependent variable. There was no significant difference between the right- and left-side measures ($F_{(7,12)} = 0.96$, $p = 0.597$), so these data were combined for the *post hoc* analyses. Univariate *post hoc* analysis of variance (ANOVA) revealed that patients with FS exhibited a significantly greater neurogenic flare response ($F_{(1,38)} = 37.64$, $p<0.0001$), as well as reduced mechani-

TABLE 1. *Descriptive information and neurogenic flare and pain-threshold data for subjects with fibromyalgia and control volunteers*[a]

	Fibromyalgia	Control
Age	28.3 (2.6)	26.6 (2.1)
VAS mood	3.6 (0.8)	3.8 (0.6)
Symptom score	10.8 (1.4)*	0.2 (0.1)
Number of TEPS	13.4 (1.5)*	3.6 (1.0)
Pain-VAS	3.8 (0.8)	—
Pain-descriptor	4.3 (0.5)	—
Pain duration	74.4 (15.4)	—
Mechanical pain threshold		
TEP sites	3.2 Kg (0.3)*	5.7 Kg (0.4)
Control sites	4.9 Kg (0.6)†	8.0 Kg (0.7)
Thermal threshold		
Detection threshold	5.3 W (0.5)	5.0 W (0.5)
Pain threshold	12.5 W (1.2)‡	18.8 W (1.4)
Neurogenic flare	16.5 mm (1.4)†	7.2 mm (0.5)

[a]Values refer to mean ± SEM
*$p < 0.001$, † $p < 0.01$, ‡ $p < 0.05$
TEPs = tender point sites
VAS = visual analogue scale
From Gibson et al. 1994, with permission.

cal pressure-pain thresholds at tender-point sites ($F_{(1,38)} = 25.25$, $p < 0.0001$) and non-tender-point sites ($F_{(1,38)} = 9.49$, $p < 0.001$) than did the controls (see Table 1). With respect to thermal stimulation, it should be noted that although the detection threshold was similar in both groups, patients with fibromyalgia exhibited a significant reduction in the laser heat-pain threshold ($F_{(1,38)} = 5.7$, $p < 0.05$; see Table 1).

Grand-mean analogue traces of the CERP for pain-threshold intensity and 1.5 times pain-threshold intensity with laser stimulation are presented in Fig. 1. The mean peak-to-peak amplitude and latency of these waveforms are shown in Table 2. Regardless of the intensity of stimulation or whether or not subjects suffered from FS, the CERP was characterized by a small negative peak at approximately 270 msec (N270) poststimulus, and a broad, high-amplitude positive peak at 370 msec (P370). *Post hoc* ANOVA revealed that the peak-to-peak amplitude of the CERP was significantly increased in patients with fibromyalgia ($F_{(1,38)} = 18.04$, $p < 0.0001$), and as expected, higher-intensity stimulation resulted in an increased peak amplitude ($F_{(1,38)} = 37.16$, $p < 0.0001$). A significant group by intensity interaction ($F_{(1,38)} = 8.12$, $p < 0.001$) suggests that while both groups displayed an increase in amplitude with high- versus low-intensity stimulation, the magnitude of this increase was greater in patients with fibromyalgia. This interaction effect is illustrated in Fig. 2. The dotted portion of the lines represents an extrapolation from the actual stimulus–response function to the point at which CERP peak-to-peak amplitude would be expected to be the same in control and FS subjects. It is of interest that this point occurs at 5 to 6 W of CO_2 laser stimulation, which corresponds almost exactly to the detection threshold for this stimulus in both groups of subjects (see Fig. 2).

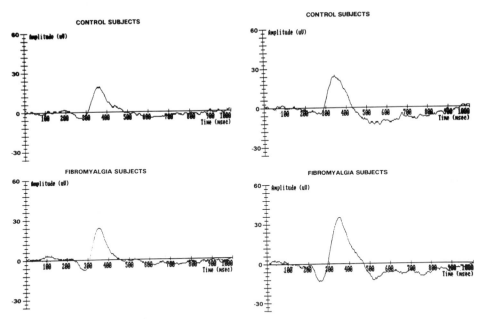

FIG. 1. Cerebral event-related potentials in response to noxious heat stimulation of pain-threshold intensity (*left panel*) and 1.5 × pain-threshold intensity (*right panel*) in subjects with fibromyalgia (*bottom panel*) and pain-free controls (*top panel*). (Modified from Gibson et al. 1994, with permission).

TABLE 2. *Latency and peak-to-peak amplitude of the cerebral potential following pain-threshold and 1.5 × pain-threshold laser stimulation*

	Fibromyalgia	Control
Pain-threshold-intensity stimulation		
Amplitude (μ volts)	34.2 (2.6)*	25.4 (1.6)
Latency N270 (msec)	269.4 (6.2)	277.5 (6.1)
Latency P370 (msec)	371.2 (6.7)	376.5 (6.5)
1.5 × pain-threshold-intensity stimulation		
Amplitude (μ volts)	50.5 (3.1)*	31.4 (1.8)
Latency N270 (msec)	267.2 (5.4)	272.5 (6.7)
Latency P370 (msec)	364.9 (6.6)	368.7 (5.8)

Values refer to mean ± SEM.
*$p < 0.0001$
Modified from Gibson et al. 1994, with permission.

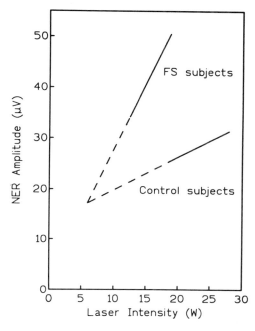

FIG. 2. Stimulus–response function of evoked-potential amplitude versus intensity of laser stimulation in subjects with fibromyalgia and pain-free controls. Dotted lines indicate an extrapolation of the stimulus–response function to the point at which evoked-potential amplitude would be expected to be equivalent in both groups.

There was no significant difference in the peak latency of the CERP for the two groups or for the two levels of stimulation.

Bivariate correlations revealed a significant positive relationship between the subjective estimate of stimulus intensity and peak-to-peak amplitude in both the fibromyalgia patients ($r = 0.72$) and controls ($r = 0.67$). Correlations between the clinical characteristics and the measures of threshold, flare, and CERP are shown in Table 3. As can be seen, multiple significant correlations were observed. To summarize these findings, it appears that the severity of clinical pain, number of

TABLE 3. *Pearson correlation coefficients for clinical characteristics and CERP, neurogenic flare, and pain-threshold measures*

	VAS pain	VAS mood	Symptom score	Pressure pain threshold	Flare
Heat-pain threshold	−0.25	−0.15	−0.33	0.46*	−0.46*
CERP amplitude	0.41†	0.29	0.64†	−0.60†	0.55†
Flare	0.53†	0.19	0.76†	−0.86†	—
VAS pain	—	−0.12	0.78†	−0.67†	0.53†
VAS mood	—	—	0.09	0.17	0.19
Symptom score	—	—	—	−0.84†	0.76†

*$p < 0.01$, †$p < 0.001$.
Modified from Gibson et al. 1994, with permission.

characteristic symptoms of FS, degree of sensitivity to mechanical-pain stimuli, size of flare, and CERP amplitude were strongly interrelated.

DISCUSSION

Previous studies have consistently documented reduced pressure-pain thresholds over predesignated tender-point sites in patients suffering from FS (Scudds et al. 1987; Yunus et al. 1989; Wolfe et al. 1990), and the presence or absence of mechanical hyperalgesia over these sites now constitutes one of the major defining characteristics of this syndrome (Wolfe et al. 1990). The present study demonstrates, for the first time, reduced heat-pain thresholds in response to CO_2 laser stimulation, thereby emphasizing a multimodal change in cutaneous pain sensitivity. The change in thermal-pain sensitivity was noted after stimulation of the dorsal surface of the hand, rather than over predesignated tender-point sites. Similarly, reduced mechanical-pressure-pain thresholds were found at both tender-point sites and non-tender-point sites. Hence, it seems likely that patients with FS exhibit a multimodal change in cutaneous pain sensitivity that is generalized rather than being restricted to predesignated anatomic sites.

In accord with previous findings (Littlejohn et al. 1987), the efferent response of primary afferent nociceptive fibers, as measured by mechanically induced flare, was also found to be significantly increased in patients with FS. Neurogenic flare follows stimulation of primary afferent $A\delta$ and C fibers with polymodal nociceptors, and is thought to be mediated by axon reflex mechanisms involving the antidromic release of substance P and calcitonin-gene-related peptide (CGRP) from primary afferent terminals (White and Helme 1985; Magi and Meli 1988). It has been suggested previously that the exaggerated neurogenic flare in FS patients might reflect an increased responsiveness or sensitization of primary afferent fibers with polymodal nociceptors (Littlejohn et al. 1987), and the present results add some support to this view. The finding of a generalized reduction in thermal- and mechanical-pain thresholds, coupled with previous findings of a reduced irritant-chemical-pain threshold (Littlejohn et al. 1987), highlights the polymodal nature of the change in cutaneous pain sensitivity. The correlational data indicate that subjects who exhibited the greatest flare response also displayed the greatest reduction in mechanical- and thermal-pain threshold and reported the greatest number of clinical symptoms as well as more severe clinical pain. The apparent strength of this association strongly suggests some common underlying mechanism for the altered efferent and afferent actions of primary afferent neurons in FS, such as an increased responsivity or sensitization of polymodal nociceptor function.

An examination of the CERP in response to noxious CO_2 laser stimulation also revealed some marked changes. Patients suffering from FS exhibited a significant increase in the peak-to-peak amplitude of this response, and this occurred with stimulation at both pain-threshold intensity and 1.5 times pain-threshold intensity. Moreover, there was a significant group by intensity interaction effect, suggesting that while FS patients exhibit higher-amplitude CERP responses with stimulation at pain-threshold intensity, there was an even greater increase relative to controls with stimulation of supra-threshold intensity. Fig. 2 illustrates this interaction and clearly demonstrates the hyperalgesic stimulus–response function for CERP amplitude in patients suffering from FS. One other interesting feature of this stimulus–response function is that if the lines are extended to the point at which one might expect the CERP amplitude to be equivalent in both groups, then they intersect at approximately 5 to 6 W of laser stimulation. This intensity is identical to the detection threshold for laser stimulation in both FS and control subjects, and it is probably more than mere coincidence that the point at which CERP responses would be expected to be of similar amplitude in the two groups is also that point at which both groups rated the intensity of laser stimulation as being the same.

The CERP is thought to provide a physiologic correlate of the CNS processing that underlies the perception of pain (Bromm and Treede 1991). In common with measures of subjective appraisal, peak amplitude is known to be influenced by factors other than supraspinal nociceptive transmission (Downman 1991), such as methodologic parameters (Chapman et al. 1981), the level of attention (Miltner et al. 1989), arousal (Bromm and Treede 1991), and anxiety (Gibson et al. 1991). These features emphasize the integrated and cognitive nature of the CERP response. Nonetheless, to the extent that this response reflects global CNS processing of nociceptive input, it is apparent that FS patients display a marked hyperalgesia in their CNS activation in response to noxious thermal input.

Considering the suggestion of a heightened responsivity of primary afferent fibers with polymodal nociceptors in FS, it is conceivable that the observed change in CNS processing may be entirely due to mechanisms of peripheral sensitization. The significant correlation between the amplitude of the CERP and the size of the concomitant neurogenic flare provides some support for this hypothesis. However, it should be noted that abnormalities in the CNS metabolism of serotonin, tryptophan, and catecholamine have been documented in FS (Boissevain and McCain 1991), and several authors have suggested that FS might represent a CNS disorder of pain modulation or pain perception (Smythe 1976; Vaeroy et al. 1989). A demonstration of decreased sound-pain threshold, hyperacusis, and vestibular hyperreactivity in FS patients has been taken to suggest a generalized disturbance in the CNS processing of sensory information (Gerster and Hadj-djilani 1984; Hadj-djilani and Gerster 1984). In the present study, care was taken to adjust stimulus intensity according to each individual's pain threshold, and the CERP was recorded with lower-intensity stimulation in patients with FS. The adjustment in stimulus intensity would be expected to control for possible differences in the strength of primary afferent input caused by peripheral sensitization, yet increased CERP responses were still noted in FS patients. On the basis of this evidence, it seems likely that while mechanisms of peripheral nociceptor sensitization may be important in explaining the increased CERP response, concomitant alterations in CNS function may also play some role.

One final implication of the present findings concerns the involvement of Aδ and C nociceptive fibers in the observed increase in pain sensitivity exhibited by FS patients. High-intensity laser stimulation is known to raise skin temperature to painful levels almost immediately, and microneurographic studies have shown a relatively selective activation of primary afferent Aδ and C nociceptive fibers with such stimulation (Devor et al. 1982; Bromm and Treede 1984). Myelinated Aβ fibers do not respond to this type of stimulus (Devor et al. 1982; Bromm and Treede 1984). Given the different conduction velocities of Aδ (approximately 8–30 msec) and C fibers (0.4–1.8 msec) (Vallbo et al. 1979), and a conduction distance of approximately 0.8 m from the dorsum of the hand to the cortex, it is apparent that the major waveform components of the CERP (i.e., N270, P370) reflect cortical processing of Aδ-fiber input (Bromm and Treede 1991; Treede and Bromm 1991). Because the latencies between stimulus onset and the major CERP components were almost identical in FS patients and pain-free controls, it seems likely that Aδ primary afferent pathways are structurally intact in patients with FS. However, the alteration in peak amplitude would suggest that patients with FS display an increase in CNS activation that is specifically associated with Aδ afferent fiber input. This finding certainly implicates Aδ-fiber function in the pathophysiology of fibromyalgic pain, particularly given the strong correlation between CERP amplitude and the severity of clinical pain and symptoms. Of course, it remains possible that CNS activation associated with C-fiber input is also altered in patients with FS, and this issue should be investigated in future studies.

Overall, the present findings demonstrate mechanical and thermal hyperalgesia in patients with FS and suggest a possible sensitization of cutaneous nociceptors with a consequent increase in pain-related CNS activity. As shown by the correlational data, these changes in nociceptive function are clearly related to the severity of the clinical pain condition. However, in the absence of demonstrable tissue injury, the precise cause(s) of cutaneous hyperalgesia is unknown, and further research is required in order to delineate whether such changes in nociceptive function are important in the etiology of FS or are merely secondary consequences of this chronic pain disorder.

ACKNOWLEDGMENT

The expert technical assistance of Mr M.M. Gorman, provided throughout the data acquisition phase of this study, is gratefully acknowledged.

REFERENCES

Boissevain MD, McCain GA. Toward an integrated understanding of fibromyalgia syndrome I: medical and pathophysiological aspects. *Pain* 1991;45:227–238.

Bromm B, Treede RD. Nerve fibre discharges, cerebral potentials and sensations induced by CO_2 laser stimulation. *Hum Neurobiol* 1984;3:33–40.

Bromm B, Treede RD. Laser-evoked cerebral potentials in the assessment of cutaneous pain sensitivity in normal subjects and patients. *Rév Neurol (Paris)* 1991;147:625–643.

Chapman CR, Colpitts YM, Mayeno JK, Gagliardi GJ. Rate of stimulus repetition changes evoked potential amplitude: dental and auditory modalities compared. *Exp Brain Res* 1981;43:246–252.

Devor M, Carmon A, Frostig R. Primary afferents and spinal sensory neurons that respond to brief pulses of intense infrared laser radiation: a preliminary study in rats. *Exp Neurol* 1982;76:483–494.

Downman R. Spinal and supraspinal correlates of nociception in man. *Pain* 1991;45:269–281.

Gerster JC, Hadj-djilani A. Hearing and vestibular abnormalities in primary fibrositis syndrome. *J Rheumatol* 1984;11:678–680.

Gibson SJ, Gorman MM, Helme RD. Assessment of pain in the elderly using event-related cerebral potentials. In: Bond MR, Charlton JE, Woolf CJ, eds. *Proceedings of the VIth World Congress on Pain.* Amsterdam: Elsevier, 1991;523–529.

Gibson SJ, Le Vasseur SA, Helme RD. Cerebral event-related responses induced by CO_2 laser stimulation in subjects suffering from cervico-brachial pain syndrome. *Pain* 1991;47:173–182.

Gibson SJ, Littlejohn GO, Gorman MM, Helme RD, Granges G. Altered heat pain thresholds and cerebral event related potentials following painful CO_2 laser stimulation in subjects with fibromyalgia syndrome. *Pain* 1994;58:185–193.

Goldenberg DL. An overview of psychologic studies in fibromyalgia. *J Rheumatol* 1989;16:12–14.

Gracely RH, Lota L, Walter DJ, Dubner R. A multiple random staircase method of psychophysical assessment. *Pain* 1988;32:55–63.

Granges G, Littlejohn GO. A comparative study of clinical signs in fibromyalgia/fibrositis syndrome, normal and exercising subjects. *J Rheumatol* 1993;20:344–351.

Hadj-djilani A, Gerster JC. Meniere's disease and fibrositis syndrome (psychogenic rheumatism). Relationship in audiometric and nystagmographic results. *Acta Octolaryngol (Stockh)* 1984;406:67–71.

Littlejohn GO, Weinstein C, Helme RD. Increased neurogenic inflammation in fibrositis syndrome. *J Rheumatol* 1987;14:1022–1025.

Magi CA, Meli A. The sensory-efferent function of capsaicin-sensitive sensory neurons. *Gen Pharmacol* 1988;19:1–43.

Miltner W, Johnson R, Braun C, Larbig W. Somatosensory event related potentials to painful and non-painful stimuli: Effects of attention. *Pain* 1989;38:303–312.

Scudds RA, Rollman GB, Harth M, McCain GA. Pain perception and personality measures as discriminators in the classification of fibrositis. *J Rheumatol* 1987;14:563–569.

Simone DA, Sorkin LS, Owens C, Chung JM, La Motte RH, Willis WD. Neurogenic hyperplasia: Central neural correlates in responses of spinothalamic tract neurons. *J Neurophysiol* 1991;66:228–246.

Smythe HA. Fibrositis as a disorder of pain modulation. *Clin Rheumat Dis* 1976;5:823–832.

Torebjork HE, Lundberg L, La Motte RH. Central changes in processing of mechanoreceptive input in capsaicin-induced secondary hyperalgesia. *J Physiol [London]* 1992;448:765–780.

Treede RD, Bromm B. Neurophysiological approaches to the study of spinothalamic tract function in humans. In: Casey KL, ed. *Pain and central nervous system disease: The central pain syndromes.* New York: Raven Press, 1991;117–126.

Treede RD, Meyer RA, Raja SN, Campbell JN. Peripheral and central mechanisms of cutaneous hyperalgesia. *Prog Neurobiol* 1992;38:397–421.

Turskey B, Jammer LO, Friedman R. The pain perception profile: a psychophysical approach to the assessment of pain report. *Behav Ther* 1982;13:376–394.

Vaeroy H, Sakurda T, Forre O, Kass E, Terenuis L. Modulation of pain in fibromyalgia: Cerebrospinal fluid (CSF) investigation of pain related neuropeptides with special reference to calcitonin gene related peptide (CGRP). *J Rheumatol* 1989;16:94–97.

Vallbo AB, Hagbarth KE, Torebjork HE, Wallin BG. Somatosensory, proprioceptive, and sympathetic activity in human peripheral nerves. *Physiol Rev* 1979;59:919–957.

White DM, Helme RD. Release of substance P from peripheral nerve terminals following stimulation of the sciatic nerve. *Brain Res* 1985;336:15–27.

Wolfe F, Smythe HA, Yunus MB, et al. The American College of Rheumatology 1990 criteria for the classification of fibromyalgia. *Arthritis Rheum* 1990;33:160–172.

Yunus M, Masi AT, Aldag JC. A controlled study of primary fibromyalgia syndrome: clinical features and association with other functional syndromes. *J Rheumatol* 1989;16:62–71.

Pain and the Brain: From
Nociception to Cognition,
edited by Burkhart Bromm and
John E. Desmedt, Advances in Pain
Research and Therapy Vol. 22.
Raven Press, Ltd., New York © 1995.

28

Brainstem Mechanisms Underlying Craniofacial Pain and its Modulation

Barry J. Sessle

Faculty of Dentistry, University of Toronto, Toronto, Ontario M5G 1G6, Canada

SUMMARY

This paper reviews recent data revealing neural mechanisms in the brain stem that contribute to conditions marked by craniofacial pain. Peripheral neural processes and crucial elements concerned with craniofacial nociceptive transmission have been identified in the brain. These elements include the convergence of deep as well as cutaneous nociceptive afferent inputs to neurons of the trigeminal (V) brain-stem complex, and neuroplastic properties of these neurons that allow these inputs to be manifested as a result of injury or inflammation. These features may contribute to the hyperalgesia and spread or referral of pain that occurs in many conditions characterized by craniofacial pain. Recent studies have also documented central neural pathways and mechanisms involved in descending modulatory influences on brain-stem nociceptive transmission. Alterations in the efficacy of these descending modulatory influences must also be considered as factors that may contribute to changes in the properties of nociceptive neurons as a result of injury to or inflammation of deep as well as superficial craniofacial tissues.

INTRODUCTION

Because other chapters in this text deal with peripheral and central mechanisms of nociception, especially in terms of vascular afferent inputs into the central nervous system (CNS) and their possible relationships to migraine, this chapter deals more broadly with mechanisms of craniofacial pain. It will focus on the properties of neurons in the trigeminal (V) brain-stem sensory complex that receive craniofacial afferent inputs from deep or cutaneous tissues, and will also review some of the intrinsic neural pathways and mechanisms controlling nociceptive transmission in the brain-stem elements of the V system.

PERIPHERAL INPUTS

Some primary afferents end in peripheral craniofacial tissues as free nerve endings, whereas others terminate as more complex corpuscular or encapsulated endings (Dubner et al. 1978; Cooper and Sessle 1992). The latter are generally associated with larger-diameter, faster-conducting primary afferents, and most provide tactile input into the V brain-stem complex. The free nerve endings, associated with small-diameter primary afferents conducting in the Aδ- (myelinated) and C-fiber (unmyelinated) range, occur in virtually all craniofacial tissues (i.e., skin, oral mucosa, temporomandibular joint [TMJ], periodontium, tooth pulp, cranial vessels, periosteum, and muscles), and many act as nociceptors. These endings can be excited by a wide range of noxious stimuli, but their sensitivity may increase following mild injury. This increased or peripheral "sensitization" is thought to be a major factor in producing hyperalgesia, and is believed to involve a number of neuropeptides and other neurochemicals found in association with these peripheral endings. It is now clear, however, that a central sensitization can also occur in V nociceptive neurons in the CNS, and probably contributes to hyperalgesia and pain spread and referral after craniofacial injury and inflammation (see below).

The small-diameter afferents conducting nociceptive information from these various craniofacial tissues may terminate centrally in laminae I, II, V, and VI of the caudal component of the V brain-stem complex, the subnucleus caudalis. The central endings of these afferents contain certain neuropeptides (e.g., substance P) and amino acids (e.g., glutamate) that may be involved in transmitting nociceptive signals from the primary afferents to second-order V nociceptive neurons (Henry et al. 1980; Wilcox 1991; Dubner and Ruda 1992). In contrast, low-threshold mechanosensitive primary afferents carrying tactile information terminate primarily in laminae III to VI of the subnucleus caudalis, as well as in more rostral components (e.g., the subnucleus oralis) of the V brain-stem complex; nociceptive cutaneous and tooth-pulp afferents also terminate in some of these rostral components, as well as in the subnucleus caudalis (e.g., Jacquin et al. 1986; Tsuru et al. 1989). Fig. 1 shows the main components of the V brain-stem complex and some of their input and output features; neurons in these components contribute to ascending nociceptive pathways involved in pain sensation, as well as to brain-stem reflex centers and regions involved in pain modulation (Dubner et al. 1978; Dubner 1985; Sessle 1986, 1987; Cooper and Sessle 1992).

BRAIN-STEM RELAY MECHANISMS

The V subnucleus caudalis has traditionally been viewed as an essential brain-stem relay site for orofacial nociceptive information to higher levels of the CNS. This laminated structure has many morphologic and functional similarities to the dorsal horn of the spinal cord, and is in fact now often designated as the medullary dorsal horn. For example, electrophysiologic investigations (see Dubner 1985; Ses-

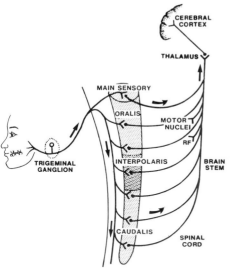

FIG. 1. Major pathways transmitting sensory information from the mouth and face to the brainstem. The first synaptic relay of information may occur on neurons at all levels of the trigeminal brain-stem sensory nuclear complex, which comprises the main sensory nucleus and the three subnuclei (oralis, interpolaris, caudalis) of the trigeminal spinal-tract nucleus. Sensory information may then be relayed directly to the thalamus and cerebral cortex, or less directly by multisynaptic pathways involving, for example, the reticular formation. The sensory information may also pass to other brain-stem structures (e.g., cranial-nerve motor nuclei involved in reflex responses to the orofacial sensory inputs). (From Sessle 1986, with permission.)

sle 1986, 1987) in anesthetized, decerebrate, or unanesthetized animals reveal neurons in the subnucleus caudalis, predominantly in laminae I and II and V and VI, that respond to cutaneous noxious stimuli. On the basis of their cutaneous (or mucosal) receptive-field (RF) properties, V nociceptive neurons have been classified into two main groups: nociceptive-specific (NS) neurons, which respond exclusively to noxious stimuli (e.g., heat, pinch) applied to a localized orofacial RF, and which receive small-diameter afferent inputs from Aδ- and usually from C-fibers; and wide-dynamic-range (WDR) or convergent neurons, which are excited by non-noxious (e.g., tactile) stimuli as well as by noxious stimuli, and which may receive both large- and small-diamter A-fiber inputs as well as C-fiber inputs (Fig. 2). The responsiveness of the WDR neurons to tactile as well as noxious stimuli results from their input from both large-diameter, rapidly conducting mechanosensitive afferents and smaller-diameter, slower-conducting nociceptive afferents, whereas the sensitivity of the NS neurons reflects a primary afferent input derived only from small-diameter afferents. The nociceptive neurons in the subnucleus caudalis have features indicating their role as critical neural elements involved in the ability to localize an acute orofacial pain to facial skin or oral mucosa, and to sense its intensity and duration (e.g., Dubner 1985). Besides these cutaneous nociceptive neurons, low-threshold mechanoreceptive (LTM) neurons also occur in the subnucleus caudalis, especially in laminae III and IV. These neurons do not respond to noxious cutaneous stimuli, but instead are activated by light tactile stimuli applied to the skin, mucosa, or teeth, and have properties comparable to those of the predominant type of neuron found in the rostral V brain-stem nuclei. These rostral and caudal LTM neurons are considered essential for the relay of orofacial touch.

Recent studies have also implicated the rostral components (subnuclei inter-

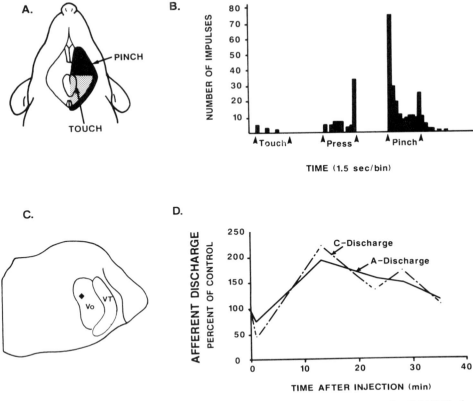

FIG. 2. Response properties of a nociceptive oralis neuron. The mechanoreceptive field (RF) of this wide-dynamic-range (WDR) neuron is shown in the face figurine **(A)**; the histogram **(B)** shows its response to touch, pressure, and pinch stimuli applied to its mechanoreceptive field. Its histologically confirmed recording locus within subnucleus oralis is shown in **C**. VT = trigeminal spinal tract. Vo = trigeminal subnucleus oralis. **D** = Facilitatory effect of the application of the inflammatory irritant mustard oil into the masseter muscle on the A- and C-fiber discharges evoked from the cutaneous RF of the same WDR neuron. Note the time course of the facilitatory effect, which affected both the A- and C-fiber cutaneous afferent inputs. (From Hu et al. 1992, with permission.)

polaris and oralis) of the V spinal tract nucleus in mechanisms of orofacial pain (for review see Sessle 1987; Cooper and Sessle 1992). Lesions of the subnucleus caudalis do not necessarily completely eliminate all reflex or behavioral responses to noxious orofacial stimuli, whereas rostral lesions may interfere with pain behavior evoked by noxious stimuli applied to intraoral or perioral tissues. Moreover, the rostral regions project to some of the same regions that are the projection sites of caudalis neurons and that are implicated in pain transmission or its control. In addition, tooth-pulp as well as cutaneous nociceptive afferents may terminate in the rostral components, and nociceptive neurons have been found in the subnuclei inter-polaris and oralis (see Fig. 2). In recent studies of the rat subnucleus oralis (Dallel et al. 1990; Hu et al. 1992), for example, 72 nociceptive neurons as well as 342 LTM neurons were documented. The 72 nociceptive neurons included 52 WDR neurons that responded to light as well as noxious mechanical stimulation, and 20 NS neurons that responded exclusively to noxious mechanical stimuli. In contrast to the LTM neurons, two-thirds of the WDR and NS neurons showed evidence of electri-cally evoked C-fiber as well as A-fiber afferent inputs from their RFs, which for 36% of the WDR and 20% of the NS neurons involved more than one V division. However, as in the case of the LTM neurons, the majority of WDR and NS neurons had RFs involving the intraoral and perioral representations of the mandibular and/or maxillary divisions; those neurons having an intraoral mandibular RF predomi-nated in the dorsomedial zone of the subnucleus oralis, whereas those with a peri-oral RF involving the maxillary division were concentrated in its ventrolateral zone. These findings add support to the gathering evidence that the rostral part of the V spinal tract nucleus represents an important element in the processing of orofacial pain, and further indicate that the subnucleus oralis may be especially involved in intraoral and perioral nociceptive mechanisms.

Another recent and important finding is that the majority of WDR and NS neu-rons, classified as above on the basis of their cutaneous RF properties, can also be excited by other types of peripheral afferent inputs. Activation of afferents supply-ing the TMJ and jaw and tongue muscles, as well as of cutaneous afferents (Amano et al. 1986; Broton et al. 1988; Hu 1990), tooth-pulp afferents, visceral afferents in cranial nerves IX and X, and even neck afferents (Sessle et al. 1986), as well as dural-vessel afferents (Dostrovsky et al. 1991), excites many WDR and NS neu-rons. For example, electrical stimulation and noxious mechanical or algesic chemi-cal (e.g., hypertonic saline, bradykinin) stimuli that activate primary afferents sup-plying jaw and tongue muscles and the TMJ may activate as many as 60% of the WDR and NS neurons in the subnucleus caudalis of the cat and rat (Amano et al. 1986; Broton et al. 1988; Hu 1990; Sessle and Hu 1991). These excitatory inputs are particularly directed at those caudalis neurons functionally identified on the basis of their cutaneous RF properties as nociceptive (WDR and NS); in contrast, LTM neurons show much less evidence of receiving these convergent inputs. More-over, in the cat, very few neurons have been found that are exclusively activated by these deep inputs. Recently, we have further analyzed the properties of these neu-rons according to their RF locations in cutaneous/mucosa or deep musculoskeletal tissues (Yu, Hu, and Sessle, unpublished observations). Of a population of over 300 neurons recorded in the rat caudalis, approximately 70% had only a cutaneous RF and were classified as LTM (86%), WDR (8%), or NS (6%). Almost 18% had both cutaneous and deep RFs, and the RFs for the great majority of these neurons were nociceptive; many also received C- and A-fiber inputs from deep as well as cu-taneous afferents. The remaining neurons (approximately 14%) were deep neurons only, and for the majority of these, the deep RF involving the TMJ or muscles was again of a nociceptive character. These and similar findings with respect to cranial-vessel afferent inputs (see, e.g., Dostrovsky et al. 1991), and analogous observations in the spinal somatosensory system of somatic-visceral-musculoskeletal afferent convergence (see Dubner and Bennett 1983; Cervero 1993), provide the basis for the view that these convergent mechanisms may explain the poor localization of deep noxious stimuli that characterizes craniofacial musculoskeletal pain and headache (Sessle et al. 1986; Dostrovsky et al. 1991; Sessle et al. 1993).

BRAIN STEM MODULATORY MECHANISMS

These convergent inputs may also contribute to the modulation of nociceptive processing, and may also explain the spread and referral of craniofacial pain. As noted above, some nociceptive neurons can be activated only by stimulation of localized parts (e.g., skin) of the craniofacial region, and thereby appear to be the critical elements in the ability to localize and discriminate pain, especially pain involving superficial tissues. Yet a particular feature of many V nociceptive neurons is their receipt of sensory inputs from nerves supplying quite widespread sites in the face, mouth, and even the neck (see above). The excitation of these neurons by several convergent afferent inputs, some of which can be demonstrated to exist only with the use of electrical stimulation, can explain how referral of pain may arise in headache, toothache, TMJ and myofascial pain, and other types of pain, and is consistent with the convergence theory of referred pain (see Cervero 1993).

It is also noteworthy that the spread of pain and hyperalgesia often seen in many peripheral injuries and inflammatory conditions may also involve these convergent afferent inputs to central nociceptive neurons. Peripherally based phenomena related to the release and spread of neurochemical substances have long been considered to underlie the spread of pain from the site of injury to adjacent tissues. Yet injury-related expansions of the cutaneous RF and heightened excitability of central nociceptive neurons can still be demonstrated even if experimental designs bypass these peripheral phenomena and sensitization. These changes have been viewed in some instances as a "central sensitization," and can be explained by a central "opening up" or "strengthening" of the convergent afferent inputs to the neurons (see, e.g., Wall 1986; Dubner and Ruda 1992). For example, the injection of algesic chemicals into muscle, or the presence of an acute localized inflammation or a chronic arthritis, can result in changes in spinal-dorsal-horn, thalamic, and somatosensory cortical neurons that reflect their enhanced responsiveness to afferent inputs not only from the site of injury or inflammation but also to other convergent inputs. The initiation and maintenance of this central sensitization process appears to involve central N-methyl-D-aspartate (NMDA) and nitric oxide (NO) receptor mechanisms as well as changes in central opioids (e.g., Dubner and Ruda 1992; Meller and Gebhart 1993). Recent studies in our laboratories (Hu et al. 1992; Sessle et al. 1993; Hu et al. 1994) have documented similar neuroplastic changes involving expanded RFs and enhanced excitability to deep as well as cutaneous inputs of V brain stem nociceptive neurons in rats (see Fig. 2). These effects are especially induced by stimulation of deep craniofacial afferent inputs (e.g., by the injection of inflammatory irritants into the TMJ or jaw or tongue muscle), and associated increases in EMG activity of the jaw muscles implicate NMDA, NO, and opioid mechanisms as contributing to or modulating this central sensitization in V nociceptive pathways. Besides their significance in revealing V central sensitization and possible neurochemical mechanisms involved in the neuroplastic changes induced by peripheral injury or inflammation, these findings are also clinically significant because they provide insights into how increased cutaneous sensitivity, spread and referral of pain, and associated neuromuscular changes may occur after craniofacial injury or inflammation. The findings also point to the need for therapeutic approaches to reduce either nociceptive inputs into the CNS (e.g., with local anesthesia) or the effects of these inputs (e.g., with opiate drugs) that can potentially prolong posttraumatic craniofacial pain by the central neuroplastic changes that they may induce.

Finally, this brief review of recent data on the central mechanisms modulating the excitability of V nociceptive pathways would not be complete without some mention of some of the intrinsic pathways and processes involved. The modulatory mechanisms noted above with respect to central changes induced by V afferent inputs associated with peripheral injury or inflammation may involve synaptic processes and interneurons intrinsic to the particular subnucleus undergoing changes in neuronal excitability. In the subnucleus caudalis, for example, inhibitory interneurons in its substantia gelatinosa have been implicated in some of these alterations (e.g., Dubner and Bennett 1983; Sessle 1987; Dubner and Ruda 1992). These interneurons, or caudalis neurons contributing to reflex or ascending pain pathways, may however receive inputs not only from peripheral afferents but also from other brainstem regions or higher brain centers implicated in the control of somatosensory transmission. These regions include the sensorimotor cerebral cortex, periaqueductal gray (PAG), nucleus raphe magnus (NRM), anterior pretectal nucleus (APT), and parabrachial area (PBA) of the pons. The effects of the inputs from these regions on V nociceptive neurons can be revealed by electrical or chemical stimulation of these regions and documentation of the stimulation-induced effects on V nociceptive neuronal responses to craniofacial afferent inputs or on associated reflex responses (e.g., jaw-opening reflex) to these afferent inputs. For example, stimulation of PAG, NRM, APT, and PBA sites, as well as of the sensorimotor cortex, can inhibit V brainstem neuronal responses as well as related jaw-muscle reflex responses to noxious cutaneous and tooth-pulp stimuli (see Sessle 1987; Chiang et al. 1992; Sessle et al. 1992). Associated studies using chemical lesions or local injections of anesthetics into the PAG, NRM, and APT have revealed that the inhibitory effects of cortical and APT stimulation are partly mediated by relays in PAG, and that APT itself is involved in mediating corticofugal modulation of V brain-stem nociceptive transmission. However, as Table 1 indicates, while these effects may be preferentially directed at nociceptive neurons, they may also act on the responses of LTM neurons to low-threshold orofacial afferent inputs; thus, nonnociceptive transmission may also be influenced by these intrinsic descending influences. Many of

TABLE 1. *Inhibitory effects of stimulation of the anterior pretectal nucleus (APT), nucleus raphe magnus (NRM), and parabrachial area of the pons (PBA) on cutaneous or deep afferent inputs of rat trigeminal brainstem neurons*

V Subnucleus	Neuron type	Afferent input	APT	NRM	PBA
Oralis/interpolaris					
	LTM	Skin	5/20	—	—
	Nociceptive	Skin	2/5	—	—
		Deep	1/1	—	—
Caudalis					
	LTM	Skin	13/24	12/16	10/16
	Nociceptive	Skin	17/20	19/22	20/22
		Deep	2/2	18/22	21/24

Each value indicates number of neurons inhibited per number of neurons tested. Neurons were recorded in the trigeminal (V) subnuclei oralis, interpolaris, or caudalis. Data obtained from Chiang et al. 1992, and Chiang, Hu, and Sessle, unpublished observations.

these modulatory influences also act on deep nociceptive transmission (e.g., electrical stimulation of the APT, NRM and PBA can suppress deep as well as cutaneously evoked responses in caudalis nociceptive neurons (see Table 1). As a consequence, alterations in the efficacy of these descending modulatory influences must also be considered as factors that may contribute to the changes in RF and response properties of V nociceptive neurons resulting from injury to or inflammation of deep as well as superficial craniofacial tissues.

ACKNOWLEDGMENTS

The cited studies done by the author were supported by Canadian Grant MT-4918 from the Medical Research Council of Canada and Grant DE04786 from the U.S. National Institutes of Health.

REFERENCES

Amano N, Hu JW, Sessle BJ. Responses of neurons in feline trigeminal subnucleus caudalis (medullary dorsal horn) to cutaneous, intraoral, and muscle afferent stimuli. *J Neurophysiol* 1986;55:227–243.

Broton JG, Hu JW, Sessle BJ. Effects of temporomandibular joint stimulation on nociceptive and non-nociceptive neurons of the cat's trigeminal subnucleus caudalis (medullary dorsal horn). *J Neurophysiol* 1988;59:1575–1589.

Cervero F. Pathophysiology of referred pain and hyperalgesia from viscera. In: Vecchiet L, Albe-Fessard D, Lindblom U, eds. *Pain research and clinical management*, vol 7. *New trends in referred pain and hyperalgesia*. Amsterdam: Elsevier, 1993;35–46.

Chiang CY, Chen IC, Dostrovsky JO, Sessle BJ. Anterior pretectal nucleus-induced modulatory effects on trigeminal brainstem somatosensory neurons. *Neurosci Lett* 1992;134:233–237.

Cooper BY, Sessle BJ. Anatomy, physiology, and pathophysiology of trigeminal system paresthesias and dysesthesias. In: LaBlanc JP, Gregg JM, eds. *Oral and maxillofacial surgery clinics of North America*. London: WB Saunders, 1992;297–322.

Dallel R, Raboisson P, Woda A, Sessle BJ. Properties of nociceptive and non-nociceptive neurons in trigeminal subnucleus oralis of the rat. *Brain Res* 1990;521:95–106.

Dostrovsky JO, Davis KD, Kawakita K. Central mechanisms of vascular headaches. *Can J Physiol Pharmacol* 1991;65:652–658.

Dubner R. Recent advances in our understanding of pain. In: Klineberg I, Sessle BJ, eds. *Oro-facial pain and neuromuscular dysfunction: mechanisms and clinical correlates*. Oxford: Pergamon Press, 1985; 3–19.

Dubner R, Bennett GJ. Spinal and trigeminal mechanisms of nociception. *Annu Rev Neurosci* 1983;6: 381–418.

Dubner R, Ruda MA. Activity-dependent neuronal plasticity following tissue injury and inflammation. *Trends Neurosci* 1992;15:96–103.

Dubner R, Sessle BJ, Storey AT, eds. *The neural basis of oral and facial function*. New York: Plenum Press, 1978;483.

Henry JL, Sessle BJ, Lucier GE, Hu JW. Effects of substance P on nociceptive and non-nociceptive trigeminal brain stem neurones. *Pain* 1980;8:33–45.

Hu JW. Response properties of nociceptive and non-nociceptive neurones in the rat's trigeminal subnucleus caudalis (medullary dorsal horn) related to cutaneous and deep craniofacial afferent stimulation and modulation by diffuse noxious inhibitory controls. *Pain* 1990;41:331–345.

Hu JW, Sessle BJ, Raboisson P, Dallel R, Woda A. Stimulation of craniofacial muscle afferents induces prolonged facilitatory effects in trigeminal nociceptive brainstem neurones. *Pain* 1992;48:53–60.

Hu JW, Yu X-M, Sunakawa M, Chiang CY, Haas DA, Kwan CL, Tsai CM, Vernon H, Sessle BJ. Electromyographic and trigeminal brainstem neuronal changes associated with inflammatory irritation of superficial and deep craniofacial tissues in rats. In: Gebhart GF, Hammond DL, Jensen TS, eds. *Proceedings of the 7th world congress on pain*. Seattle: IASP Press, 1994;325–336.

Jacquin MF, Woerner D, Szczepanik AM, Riecker V, Mooney RD. Structure-function relationships in rat brainstem subnucleus interpolaris. I. Vibrissa primary afferents. *J Comp Neurol* 1986;243: 266–279.

Meller ST, Gebhart GF. Nitric oxide (NO) and nociceptive processing in the spinal cord. *Pain* 1993;52: 127–136.

Sessle BJ. Recent developments in pain research: central mechanisms of orofacial pain and its control. *J Endodontics* 1986;12:435–444.

Sessle BJ. The neurobiology of facial and dental pain: present knowledge, future directions. *J Dent Res* 1987;66:962–981.

Sessle BJ, Chiang CY, Dostrovsky JO. Interrelationships between sensorimotor cortex, anterior pretectal nucleus and periaqueductal gray in modulation of trigeminal sensorimotor function in the rat. In: Inoki R, Shigenaga Y, Tohyama M, eds. *Processing and inhibition of nociceptive information*. Amsterdam: Excerpta Medica, 1992;77–82.

Sessle BJ, Hu JW. Mechanisms of pain arising from articular tissues. *Can J Physiol Pharmacol* 1991;69: 617–626.

Sessle BJ, Hu JW, Amano N, Zhong G. Convergence of cutaneous, tooth pulp, visceral, neck and muscle afferents onto nociceptive and non-nociceptive neurones in trigeminal subnucleus caudalis (medullary dorsal horn) and its implications for referred pain. *Pain* 1986;27:219–235.

Sessle BJ, Hu JW, Yu X-M. Brainstem mechanisms of referred pain and hyperalgesia in the orofacial and temporomandibular region. In: Vecchiet L, Albe-Fessard D, Lindblom U, eds. *Pain research and clinical management*, vol. 7. *New trends in referred pain and hyperalgesia*. Amsterdam: Elsevier, 1993;59–71.

Tsuru K, Otani K, Kajiyama K, Suemune S, Shigenaga Y. Central terminations of periodontal mechanoreceptive and tooth pulp afferents in the trigeminal principal and oral nuclei of the cat. *Brain Res* 1989;485:29–61.

Wall PD. Changes in adult spinal cord induced by changes in the periphery. In: Goldberger ME, Gorio A, Murray M, eds. *Development and plasticity of the mammalian spinal cord*. Padua: Liviana Press, 1986;101–110.

Wilcox G. Excitatory neurotransmitters and pain. In: Bond MR, Charlton JE, Woolf CJ, eds. *Proceedings of the VI World Congress on Pain. Pain research and clinical management*, vol 4. Oxford: Elsevier, 1991;97–117.

Pain and the Brain: From
Nociception to Cognition,
edited by Burkhart Bromm and
John E. Desmedt, Advances in Pain
Research and Therapy Vol. 22.
Raven Press, Ltd., New York © 1995.

29

Cerebral Mechanisms Relevant to Migraine

Peter J. Goadsby

*Institute of Neurology, The National Hospital for Neurology and Neurosurgery,
London WC1N, United Kingdom*

SUMMARY

An understanding of the basic anatomy and physiology of the cranial circulation facilitates the assessment and management of patients with headache, particularly vascular-type headache, such as migraine. At the very least, all pain is perceived and parsed in the brain. Indeed, with migraine it is likely that the fundamental problem and its clinical expression are driven by the central nervous system (CNS), and thus study of the CNS in regard to headache is warranted. As therapy evolves during the 1990s, such an understanding will be necessary as new and highly specific receptor-targeted compounds allow improvement in the treatment of headache in the many patients it affects.

INTRODUCTION

The past decade has seen major advances in the understanding of primary headache disorders. This has come both in the clinical sphere and in the basic neurosciences, and is evident in the understanding of migraine. This chapter will review these changes from the perspective of the brain, and will highlight the cerebral mechanisms that have been elucidated and explain many facets of migraine. Understanding these changes offers the clinician a sounder base on which to practice, and ultimately a better standard of clinical care. The basis for the organization of the chapter shall, therefore, be the clinical phenomenology of migraine, with the relevant mechanisms being painted onto the canvas.

DEFINITION AND CLASSIFICATION OF MIGRAINE

The conventions of the Headache Classification Committee of the International Headache Society (Olesen 1988) will be adopted throughout this chapter. In clinical practice, two varieties of migraine attacks are commonly distinguished: those associated with an aura of neurologic symptoms (previously called classical migraine), and a periodic headache without aura (common migraine). Migraine is predominantly an affliction of young people who are otherwise well, although it can be seen at virtually any age. The prevalence of a family history and early onset of the disorder suggest that there is a strong genetic component. Indeed, the first description of a genetic locus for a migraineous disease, on chromosome 19, of the gene for familial hemiplegic migraine (Joutel et al. 1993), heralds the beginning of a large effort at unraveling the functional defect(s) that lead to migraine. Taken together, these features suggest a subtle structural or functional defect that is usually not life-threatening. The female predominance of migraine and its association with menstruation do not assist in differentiating the site of the problem, since the hormonal changes described (Somerville 1972) could affect either neural or vascular structures.

PREMONITORY FEATURES

About 25% of the patients with migraine report symptoms of elation, irritability, depression, hunger, thirst, or drowsiness during the 24 hours preceding headache. Most of these manifestations can arise in the hypothalamus (Kupfermann 1985), and this suggests a central site for their evolution. In addition, the suprachiasmatic nucleus of the hypothalamus has been suggested as one of two primary oscillators in the generation of circardian rhythms (Swaab et al. 1993), and thus could easily be implicated in the periodicity that is such an important clinical feature of migraine.

PRODROME OF MIGRAINE WITH AURA

Cerebral Blood Flow and the Aura

Numerous studies over some years have confirmed that the aura phase of migraine is associated with a reduction in cerebral blood flow (CBF) (Skinhoj and Paulson 1969; O'Brien 1971; Simard and Paulson 1973; Norris et al. 1975; Mathew et al. 1976; Edmeads 1977; Hachinski et al. 1977; Sakai and Meyer 1978; Olesen et al. 1981; Staehelin-Jensen et al. 1981; Lauritzen et al. 1983; Lauritzen and Olesen et al. 1984; Skyhoj-Olsen et al. 1987). Visual disturbances (such as the scintillating scotoma, consisting of flashing lights that move across the visual field), paresthesiae, or other focal neurologic signs are associated with this reduction in CBF (Olesen et al. 1981). This change in flow moves across the cortex as a "spreading oligemia" at 2 to 3 mm/min (Lauritzen et al. 1983), corresponding to the rate that Lashley estimated from plotting the progression of his own visual aura (Lashley 1941) and to the phenomenon of cortical spreading depression (Leao 1944a, 1944b). The flow pattern that has also been seen has some common threads. First, there is a focal reduction in flow that is usually posterior, near Brodman area 7 and the superior part of area 19, although focal frontal oligemia without visual aura has been rarely reported (Friberg et al. 1987). Second, this reduction enlarges and may involve the entire hemisphere. The changes first reported by Olesen and his colleagues (1981) were seen with carotid angiography, but similar changes have been seen in spontaneous attacks with single-photon emission computed tomography (SPECT) (Lauritzen and Olesen 1984). The progression of oligemia across the cortex does not respect vascular territories and is thus unlikely to be primarily vasospastic. Vasospasm is indeed only rarely seen in patients who have an angiogram during migraine (Skinhoj 1973; Lauritzen et al. 1983; Skyhoj-Olsen et al. 1987; Symonds 1952; Connor 1962). Some vasoconstriction, however, does occur, as evidenced by retrograde flow from the carotid to the vertebrobasilar circulation in some patients (Skinhoj 1973; Norris et al. 1975; Hachinski et al. 1977). Furthermore, there are reports that the oligemia is preceded by a phase of focal hyperemia (Olesen et al. 1981; Friberg et al. 1987). Such a change is again exactly what would be expected if a phenomenon similar to cortical spreading depression was involved. Following the passage of the oligemia the cerebrovascular response to hypercapnia is blunted (Simard and Paulson 1973; Friberg et al. 1987), while autoregulation is intact (Lauritzen et al. 1983). Again, this pattern is repeated in spreading depression. Usually the flow change is accompanied by a contralateral aura, and the unilateral headache is homolateral with respect to the oligemia (Olesen et al. 1981), but patients have been reported to have unilateral headache with a homolateral aura, suggesting a mismatch of the aura with the subsequent headache (Peatfield and Rose 1991). Headache may begin while CBF is still reduced (Olesen et al. 1990), thus making untenable the concept that pain arises from a primary vascular abnormality.

Some methodologic considerations have been suggested to account for the oligemia accompanying the aura of migraine, and in particular to suggest that the observed changes in flow reach an ischemic level. Because of the errors involved, only metabolic studies will be able to satisfactorily determine whether ischemia does occur. The best estimates of flow that take into account Compton scatter (an error generated by detectors picking up a signal from a well-perfused area when positioned over a poorly perfused area, thus overestimating flow) put the flow values during the aura at 20 to 25 ml/100gm/min (Skyhoj-Olsen et al. 1987), while at this level in the awake monkey a neurologic deficit can be seen (Jones et al. 1981). Studies of oxygen utilization done with positron emission tomography (PET) in a single patient have shown that during the aura the flow reduction is balanced by an increase in oxygen extraction and that oxygen metabolism therefore is normal (Herold et al. 1985). This problem has been difficult to access because of the technologic demands of the PET studies, and for the moment it can be said that there is no hard evidence for cerebral ischemia during the aura phase of migraine.

Neural Substrates for Aura

What can be inferred from known cerebrovascular physiology concerning the aura of migraine? The cortical spreading depression of Leao was first reported to occur in the exposed rabbit cortex as a negative shift in direct-current (DC) potential, and is therefore defined electrically (Leao 1944a, 1944b). This shift corresponds ionically to a redistribution of K, Na, Cl, Ca, and H ions that has been carefully characterized by micropipette studies (Kraig and Nicholson 1978). Several features of spreading depression have been used to characterize it, including a rate of propagation of 2 to 6 mm/min, limitation to one hemisphere, and a refractory period for further spreading depression of up to 3 min. Spreading depression has been observed in a number of species, including the rat (Lauritzen et al. 1982), cat (Marshall 1959), and human (Sramka et al. 1977). The changes can involve subcortical structures, such as the caudate nucleus (Sramka et al. 1977), which seem to be quantitatively less affected (Tomida et al. 1989). Described in association with the ionic changes and shift in DC potential that are the electrophysiologic markers of spreading depression are distinct changes in CBF. Initially, flow may increase after spreading depression has been initiated; this increase has been reported to be up to 200% (Hansen et al. 1980), and is postulated to be related to the level of blood flow before spreading depression begins (Lauritzen et al. 1982). The increase is followed by a prolonged moderate reduction in CBF (Lauritzen et al. 1982; Tomida et al. 1989) that is associated with a marked blunting of cerebrovascular responses to hypercapnia (Lauritzen 1984), with normal autoregulation (Hansen et al. 1980; Lauritzen 1984). Recently it has been shown that the reduction in CBF seen after spreading depression may involve not only the cortex but also subcortical and brain-stem structures (Mraovitch et al. 1989). It has also been seen that even as hypercapnic vasodilatation is blunted or eliminated following spreading depression, stimulation of the trigeminal ganglion (Goadsby and Edvinsson 1993) or of the centromedian parafasicular thalamus (Goadsby et al. 1991) will increase blood flow. Given the suggested pathophysiologic role of spreading depression in migraine, these latter findings reinforce the view that central mechanisms can still play a role in the control of cerebrovascular tone even during the acute attack of migraine.

How can the data about aura of migraine be reconciled in the context of what is seen in humans? The neurologic changes during aura parallel those seen when the brain is directly stimulated (Penfield and Perot 1968; Brindley and Lewin 1968), and resemble what might be predicted if ocular dominance columns (Hubel and Weisel 1968) were serially activated. Taken together, the data make it likely that either spreading depression or a human homologue of it is the neurologic basis for aura in migraine. It must be said, however, that spreading depression in humans (if it exists) must be very different from what is seen in animals. Indirect measurements— indirect because spreading depression is essentially defined by electrical events— give conflicting results in humans. Welch and his colleagues, using magnetoencephalography, have shown that changes similar to those seen in rabbits undergoing spreading depression can be seen in humans, although the relative novelty of the method requires that further such observations be made (Welch et al. 1990). In two recent studies that have directly examined human cortex at surgery for epilepsy, spreading depression was not elicited as it is in animals. In a small study using laser Doppler flow probes applied directly to the cortex, the typical blood-flow changes of spreading depression (Goadsby et al. 1992; Piper et al. 1991a) were not elicited by needle-stick injury (Piper et al. 1991b), although this is never the case in animals. Recently, direct measurements of DC potential using electrocorticography (ECoG) have been made in both temporal and occipital cortex in 23 patients undergoing surgery for epilepsy. The stimuli used were KCl and mechanical and thermal injury, and again in no case was spreading depression elicited (McLachlan and Grivin 1993). Interestingly, some of the patients reported were migraineurs, although none had had aura. One possible criticism of these studies is that many of these patients had been on anticonvulsants. We have examined this question in an experimental model of spreading depression in the cat and found that pretreatment with anticonvulsants did not prevent spreading depression (Kaube and Goadsby 1994). The only other reasonable objection is that none of the patients studied were migraineurs with aura, and perhaps it is only in this group that spreading depression will be found.

Experimental evidence suggests that the trigeminovascular system promotes vasodilatation. Nerves that innervate the cerebral vessels through the trigeminovascular system contain almost exclusively vasodilatator transmitters, such as calcitonin-gene-related peptide (CGRP) and substance P (SP) (Edvinsson et al. 1986), the release of which could not provoke spreading depression. Available data suggest that lesions of the trigeminal ganglion do not affect resting CBF or glucose utilization in the cat (Edvinsson et al. 1986). They do, however, affect vasodilatator protector mechanisms such as those seen during hyperemia following ischaemia or epilepsy (Sakas et al. 1989). In addition, it has recently been shown that in subarachnoid hemorrhage with threatened cerebrovascular compromise from vasospasm, venous levels of CGRP are increased in humans (Edvinsson et al. 1990a; Juul et al. 1990; Edvinsson et al. 1990b; Edvinsson et al. 1991). Electrical stimulation of the trigeminal ganglion in both humans and the cat leads to increases in extracerebral blood flow and local release of both CGRP and substance P (Goadsby et al. 1988). In the cat trigeminal ganglion, stimulation also increases CBF by a pathway traversing the greater superficial petrosal branch of the facial nerve (Goadsby and Duckworth 1987), again releasing a powerful vasodilatator peptide, vasoactive intestinal polypeptide (VIP) (Goadsby 1989). Interestingly, the VIP-ergic innervation of the cerebral vessels is predominantly anterior rather than posterior (Matsuyama et al. 1983), and this may contribute to the vulnerability of this region to spreading depression and in part explain why the aura of migraine is so very often seen to begin posteriorly. Stimulation of the more specifically vascular-pain-sensitive superior sagittal sinus increases CBF (Lambert et al. 1988) and jugular-vein CGRP levels (Zagami et al. 1990). Human evidence that CGRP is elevated in the headache phase of migraine (Goadsby et al. 1990) and cluster headache (Goadsby and Edvinsson 1993) supports the view that the trigeminovascular system may be activated in a protective role in these conditions. Taken together, the data suggest that the trigeminovascular system is unlikely to be the source of generation of the aura, but is either activated by it or is activated in parallel by the same process that activates the aura.

Finally, it has been shown in the experimental animal that stimulation of a discrete nucleus in the brain-stem, the nucleus locus coeruleus (the main central nonadrenergic nucleus) (Amaral and Sinnamon 1977), reduces CBF in a frequency-dependent manner (Goadsby et al. 1982) through an α_2-adrenoceptor-linked mechanism (Goadsby et al. 1985). This reduction is maximal in the occipital cortex (Goadsby and Duckworth 1989). Importantly, while a 25% overall reduction in CBF is seen, extracerebral vasodilatation occurs in parallel (Goadsby et al. 1983). From the clinical standpoint, the aura of migraine can exist in isolation from the pain as "migraine equivalent"; it is thus possible that the aura originates in the CNS, with the vascular changes being a secondary feature.

THE HEADACHE

The Trigeminal Innervation of Pain-Sensitive Intracranial Structures

Surrounding the large cerebral vessels, pial vessels, large venous sinuses, and dura mater is a plexus of largely unmyelinated nerve fibers that arise from the trigeminal ganglion and in the posterior fossa from the upper cervical dorsal roots. This plexus is seen in the monkey (Ruskell and Simons 1987) and cat (Mayberg et al. 1981). Tracing studies have shown that fibers innervating cerebral vessels arise from within the trigeminal ganglion from neurons that contain substance P (Liu-Chen et al. 1983) and CGRP (Uddman et al. 1985), both of which can be released when the trigeminal ganglion is stimulated either in the human or cat (Goadsby et al. 1988). Moreover, the cell bodies in the trigeminal ganglion are of bipolar neurons that innervate the large cerebral arteries and dura mater (Liu-Chen et al. 1984) and arise largely from the first or ophthalmic division of the trigeminal nerve (Mayberg et al. 1984). Stimulation of the cranial vessels, such as the superior sagittal sinus (SSS), is certainly painful in humans (Ray and Wolff 1940). Human dural nerves that innervate the cranial vessels consist largely of small-diameter myelinated and unmyelinated fibers that almost subserve a nociceptive function (Penfield and McNaughton 1940; Feindel et al. 1960).

What then is the source of pain in migraine? Few studies answer this question directly in humans. Certainly if the carotid artery is occluded ipsilateral to the side of headache in migraineurs, two-thirds will experience relief (Drummond and Lance 1983), although this does not account for the other one-third at all. Moreover, distention of major cerebral vessels by balloon dilatation leads to pain referred to the ophthalmic division of the trigeminal nerve (Nichols et al. 1993; Martins et al. 1993). Moskowitz has provided an elegant series of experiments to suggest that the pain of migraine may be a form of sterile inflammation. Neurogenic extravasation of plasma can be seen during electrical stimulation of the trigeminal ganglion in the rat (Markowitz et al. 1987). Plasma extravasation can be blocked by ergot alkaloids (Markowitz et al. 1988), indomethacin, acetylsalicylic acid (Buzzi et al. 1989), and the serotonin (5HT)-1-like agonist sumatriptan (Buzzi and Moskowitz 1990). The pharmacology of the new migraine-abortive drugs is outside the scope of this chapter, and interested readers are referred to recent reviews (Feniuk et al. 1991; Humphrey et al. 1991). In addition, structural changes in the dura mater are seen with stimulation of the trigeminal ganglion, and include mast-cell degranulation (Dimitriadou et al. 1991) and changes in postcapillary venules, including platelet aggregation (Dimitriadou et al. 1992). While it is generally accepted that such changes, and particularly the initiation of a sterile inflammatory response, would cause pain, it is not clear whether this is sufficient of itself or requires some permissive changes in central nociceptive transmission.

The sites within the brain stem that are responsible for craniovascular pain have begun to be mapped (Table 1). Using c-fos-immunocytochemistry after meningeal irritation with blood, the expression of fos is reported in the trigeminal nucleus caudalis (Nozaki et al. 1992), while after stimulation of the superior sagittal sinus, fos-like immunoreactivity is seen in the cat in the trigeminal nucleus caudalis and in the dorsal horn at the C1 and C2 levels (Kaube et al. 1993b). These latter findings are in accord with similar data using 2-deoxyglucose measurements with superior sagittal sinus stimulation (Goadsby and Zagami 1991), and contribute to our view of the trigeminal nucleus as extending beyond the traditional nucleus caudalis to the dorsal horn of the high cervical region in a functional continuum that includes a cervical extension that could be regarded as a trigeminal nucleus *cervicalis*. The cells in the most caudal part of this relay do not merely receive a parallel input to cells in the cervicomedullary junction, since reversible cold blockade of the C1 region blocks some 50% of thalamic cells that are excited by superior sagittal sinus stimulation (Angus-Leppan et al. 1992). These data clearly demonstrate that a substantial portion of trigeminovascular nociceptive information comes by way of the most caudal cells. This concept provides an anatomic explanation for the referral of pain to the back of the head in migraine. Moreover, experimental pharmacologic evidence suggests that some migraine-abortive drugs, such as ergots (Lambert et al 1992), acetylsalicylic acid (Kaube et al. 1994), and sumatriptan (after blood–brain barrier disruption) (Kaube et al. 1993a) can have actions at these second-order neurons that reduce cell activity, suggesting a further possible site for therapeutic intervention in migraine.

Following transmission in the caudal brain stem and high cervical spinal cord, information is relayed in a group of fibers that have been termed the quintothalamic

TABLE 1. *Neuroanatomical processing of vascular head pain*

Order	Level	Structures
1st	Trigeminal ganglion	Middle cranial fossa
2nd	Trigeminal nucleus (quintothalamic tract)	Trigeminal nucleus caudalis C1/C2 dorsal horn
3rd	Thalamus	Ventrobasal complex Medial nucleus of posterior group Intralaminar complex
Final	Cortex	(?)

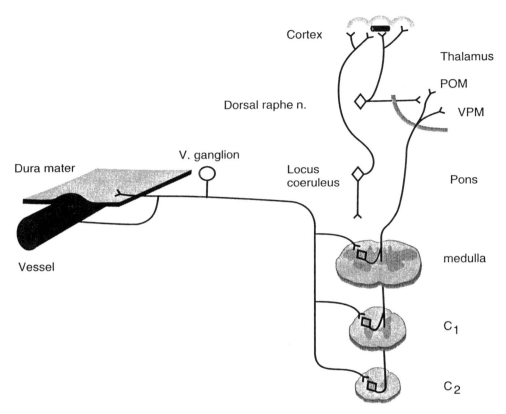

FIG. 1. Schematic summary of the neural elements required to propose a unified central neural hypothesis for migraine. The peripheral input from the trigeminovascular system that arises in the dura mater and blood vessels passes through the ophthalmic division of the trigeminal nerve and has its cell body in the trigeminal ganglion. The second-order neurons lie in the most caudal trigeminal nucleus caudalis and in the dorsal horn of the upper cervical spinal cord at the C1 and C2 levels. These cells project via the quintothalamic tract, which decussates before synapsing on third-order neurons in the ventral posteromedial thalamus (VPM) and the medial nucleus of the posterior complex of the thalamus (POM). To account for the many central-nervous-system (CNS) manifestations of migraine, the aminergic cells in the locus coeruleus (nonadrenergic) and dorsal raphe nucleus (serotonergic) are illustrated. (Reproduced from the International Association for the Study of Pain from the Headache Refresher Course of the 7th World Congress on Pain, Paris, 1993, with permission.)

tract to the thalamus (Fig. 1). Processing of vascular pain in the thalamus occurs in the ventral posteromedial thalamus, the medial nucleus of the posterior complex, and the intralaminar thalamus (Zagami and Lambert 1990; Zagami and Goadsby 1991). Zagami has shown, by applying capsaicin to the superior sagittal sinus, that transmissions from trigeminal projections with a high degree of nociceptive input are particularly processed in neurons in the ventral posteromedial thalamus and its ventral periphery (Zagami and Lambert 1991). The properties and further higher-center connections of these neurons are the subject of ongoing studies that will yield a more complete picture of the trigeminovascular pathways.

Cerebral Blood Flow Measurements During Headache

Interictal Studies

Through the use of both 133Xe inhalation and HMPAO with SPECT, regional cerebral blood flow (rCBF) has been compared in migraine patients and age- and sex-matched controls. In 92 patients (60 with aura and 32 without aura), asymmetries in interictal flow were found in about 40%, considering both modalities. The greatest asymmetries were seen in the group of patients with migraine with aura (Friberg 1993). Further studies to characterize whether these abnormalities correlate with the flow changes seen in the attack, and whether interictal physiology (such as hypercapnic vasodilatation) is normal, are awaited.

Studies During Migraine with Aura

The headache phase of migraine may be accompanied by hyperemia (Sakai and Meyer 1978), although in some studies the headache was not sufficiently characterized to determine its type (Skinhoj 1973). The pain of the headache may come during the oligemic phase, making it unlikely that dilatation of the cerebral vessels alone is responsible for the pain (Olesen et al. 1981; Lauritzen et al 1983). Differences reported in various studies in terms of the presence or absence of a flow change during the headache phase may be merely due to the study of patients at different phases of their attacks, since patients studied serially may have either oligemia, hyperemia, or no change during headache, depending upon when they are studied (Andersen et al. 1988).

Studies During Migraine without Aura

An early study suggested that in migraine without aura there is hyperemia in the headache phase (Sakai and Meyer 1978), but this has not been observed by others (Olesen et al. 1981, 1982; Lauritzen and Olesen 1984). Interestingly, hypercapnic vasodilatation may also be blunted in migraine without aura, although reports to date have demonstrated that although the change in blood flow is blunted, it is symmetrical (Sakai and Meyer 1978, 1979).

CLINICAL OBSERVATIONS OF THE TRIGEMINOVASCULAR SYSTEM

Drummond and Lance have shown that in at least one-third of patients there is a significant extracerebral vascular component to the headache of migraine (Drum-

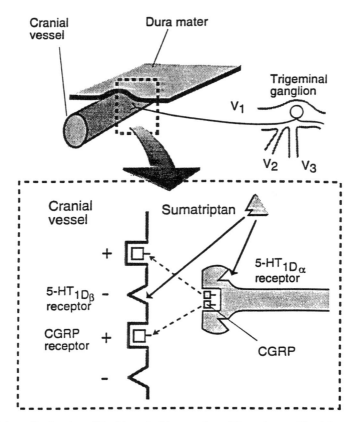

FIG. 2. Schematic drawing of the trigeminal innervation of the pain-sensitive intracranial struc-tures, the dura mater and bood vessels. They are shown innervated by axons arising from neurons in the first (ophthalmic) division of the trigeminal nerve. The presence of 5-HT receptors is illustrated both on the blood vessel (β type) (Hamel et al. 1993) and on the neuron (α type). The 5-HT receptor mediates both vasconstriction and presynaptic inhibition, thus antagonizing the vasodilator effects of calcitonin-gene-related peptide (CGRP) at both sites. (From Goadsby 1994, with permission.)

mond and Lance 1984). The level of CGRP is elevated in the external jugular venous blood of migraineurs during headache (Goadsby et al. 1990), clearly dem-onstrating some activation of trigeminovascular neurons during migraine with or without aura. Recently, these data were confirmed in adolescent migraineurs. Whether the activity is peripherally generated is again uncertain, although it is clear that such changes can be partly seen in both humans and the cat with direct stimula-tion of the trigeminal ganglion (Goadsby et al. 1988). The release of the CGRP offers the prospect of a marker for migraine that can be readily measured with a simple venous blood sample. Perhaps the most recent and challenging data in understanding the trigeminovascular system and headache come, as they should, from the clinic. In a well-conducted clinical study of patients with migraine with aura, the effect of sumatriptan was evaluated with regard to the aura (Bates 1993). The drug was administered at the onset of aura in a placebo-controlled, double-blind, parallel-group study as a 6-mg subcutaneous injection, thus assuring absorption. In this setting sumatriptan neither shortened nor prolonged the aura in comparison to the placebo.

SUMATRIPTAN AURA STUDY–FUTURE CHALLENGES

The most fascinating aspect of the sumatriptan aura study was that the incidence of headache in the placebo and in the treated group was the same, so that despite good drug delivery and a suitable drug level, with a mean length of aura of 20 min, headache still occurred. What is further and perhaps even more remarkable is that the developed headache responded to further sumatriptan injection. These data suggest that sumatriptan does not have access to a crucial receptor site during the aura of migraine, and that the drug concentration and rate of absorption, along with access to the appropriate site, are the elements required to terminate the attack. To what site in the body does sumatriptan not have ready access? The obvious suggestion is a site behind the blood–brain barrier (Kaube et al. 1993), which opens the very exciting possibility that the blood–brain barrier may not be normal in the headache phase of migraine (Fig. 2). Indeed, better access to sites within the CNS may be advantageous rather than being a drawback in drug development.

REFERENCES

Amaral, DG, Sinnamon HM. The locus coeruleus: neurobiology of a central noradrenergic nucleus. *Prog Neurobiol* 1977;9:147–196.

Andersen AR, Friberg L, Skyhoj-Olsen T, Olesen J. SPECT demonstration of delayed hyperaemia following hypoperfusion in classic migraine. *Arch Neurol* 1988;45:154–159.

Angus-Leppan H, Lambert GA, Boers P, Zangami AS, Olausson B. Craniovascular nociceptive pathways in the upper cervical spinal cord in the cat. *Neurosci Lett* 1992;137:203–206.

Bates, D. Treatment with subcutaneous sumatriptan during the migraine aura. *Cephalalgia* 1993;13 (Suppl 13):188.

Brindley GS, Lewin WS. The sensation produced by electrical stimulation of the visual cortex. *J Physiol* 1968;196:479–493.

Buzzi MG, Moskowitz MA. The antimigraine drug, sumatriptan (GR43175), selectively blocks neurogenic plasma extravasation from blood vessels in dura mater. *Br J Pharmacol* 1990;99:202–206.

Buzzi MG, Sakas DE, Moskowitz MA. Indometacin and acetylsalicylic acid block neurogenic plasma protein extravasation in rat dura mater. *Eur J Pharmacol* 1989;165:251–258.

Connor RCR. Complicated migraine. A study of permanent neurological and visual defects caused by migraine. *Lancet* 1962;2:1072–1075.

Dimitriadou V, Buzzi MG, Theoharides TC, Moskowitz MA. Ultrasonic evidence for neurogenically mediated changes in blood vessels of the rat dura mater and tongue following antidromic trigeminal stimulation. *Neuroscience* 1992;48:187–203.

Dimitriadou V, Buzzi MG, Moskowitz MA, Theoharides TC. Trigeminal sensory fiber stimulation induces morphological changes reflecting secretion in rat dura mater cells. *Neuroscience* 1991;44:97–112.

Drummond PD, Lance JW. Neurovascular disturbances in headache patients. *Clin Exp Neurol* 1984;20: 93–99.

Drummond PD, Lance JW. Extracranial vascular changes and the source of pain in migraine headache. *Ann Neurol* 1983;13:32–37.

Edmeads J. Cerebral blood flow in migraine. *Headache* 1977;17:148–152.

Edvinsson L, Ekman R, Jansen I, McCulloch J, Mortensen A, Uddman R. Reduced levels of calcitonin gene-related peptide-like immunoreactivity in human brain after subarachnoid haemorrhage. *Neurosci Lett* 1991;121:151–154.

Edvinsson L, Juul R, Uddman R. Peptidergic innervation of the cerebral circulation. Role in subarachnoid haemorrhage in man. *Neurosurg Rev* 1990a;13:265–272.

Edvinsson L, Delgado-Zygmunt T, Ekman R, Jansen I, Svendgaard NA, Uddman R. Involvement of perivascular sensory fibers in the pathophysiology of cerebral vasospasm following subarachnoid haemorrhage. *J Cereb Blood Flow Metab* 1990b;10:602–607.

Edvinsson L, McCulloch J, Kingman TA, Uddman R. On the functional role of the trigeminocerebrovascular system in the regulation of cerebral circulation. In: Owman C, Hardebo JE, eds. *Neural regulation of the cerebral circulation*. Stockholm: Elsevier 1986;407–418.

Feindel W. Penfield W, McNaughton FL. The tentorial nerves and localization of intracranial pain in man. *Neurology* 1960;10:555–563.

Feniuk W, Humphrey PPA, Perren MJ, Connor HE, Whalley ET. Rationale for the use of 5-HT1-like agonists in the treatment of migraine. *J Neurol* 1991;238:S51–S61.

Friberg L. Interictal studies of cerebral blood flow in migraine. In: Olesen J, ed. *Migraine and other headaches*: the vascular mechanisms, vol. 2. New York: Raven Press, 1993;1:245–253.

Friberg L, Skyhoj-Olsen T, Roland PE, Lassen NA. Focal ischemia caused by instability of cerebrovascular tone during attacks of hemiplegic migraine. *Brain* 1987;110:917–934.

Goadsby PJ. Diagnosis and optimum treatment of migraine. *CNS Drugs* 1994.

Goadsby PJ. Facial nerve stimulation causes local release of vasoactive intestinal polypeptide in the cat cortex. In: Seylaz J, Mackenzie ET, eds. *Neurotransmission and cerebrovascular function*, vol. 1. Amsterdam: Excerpta Medica, 1989;325–328.

Goadsby PJ, Duckworth JW. Effect of stimulation of trigeminal ganglion on regional cerebral blood flow in cats. *Am J Physiol* 1987;253:R270–R274.

Goadsby PJ, Duckworth JW. Low frequency stimulation of the locus coeruleus reduces regional cerebral blood flow in the spinalized cat. *Brain Res* 1989;476:71–77.

Goadsby PJ, Edvinsson L. The trigeminovascular system and migraine: studies characterising cerebrovascular and neuropeptide changes seen in man and cat. *Ann Neurol* 1993;33:48–56.

Goadsby PJ, Edvinsson L. Evidence of trigeminovascular activation in man during acute cluster headache. *Cephalalgia* 1993;13:30.

Goadsby PJ, Zagami AS. Stimulation of the superior sagittal sinus increases metabolic activity and blood flow in certain regions of the brainstem and upper cervical spinal cord of the cat. *Brain* 1991;114: 1001–1011.

Goadsby PJ, Kaube H, Hoskin K. Nitric oxide synthesis couples cerebral blood flow and metabolism. *Brain Res* 1992;595:167–170.

Goadsby PJ, Seylaz J. Mraovitch S. Hypercapnic but not neurogenic cortical vasodilatation is blocked by spreading depression in rat. In: Olesen J, ed. *Migraine and other headaches: the vascular mechanisms*, vol. 1. New York: Raven Press, 1991;181–186.

Goadsby PJ, Edvinsson L, Ekman R. Vasoactive peptide release in the extracerebral circulation of humans during migraine headache. *Ann Neurol* 1990;28:183–187.

Goadsby PJ, Edvinsson L, Ekman R. Release of vasoactive peptides in the extracerebral circulation of man and the cat during activation of the trigeminovascular system. *Ann Neurol* 1988;23:193–196.

Goadsby PJ, Lambert GA, Lance JW. The mechanisms of cerebrovascular vasoconstriction in response to locus coeruleus stimulation. *Brain Res* 1985;326:213–217.

Goadsby PJ, Lambert GA, Lance JW. Effects of locus coeruleus stimulation on carotid vascular resistance in the cat. *Brain Res* 1983;278:175–183.

Goadsby PJ, Lambert GA, Lance JW. Differential effects on the internal and external carotid circulation of the monkey evoked by locus coeruleus stimulation. *Brain Res* 1982;249:247–254.

Hachinski VC, Olesen J, Norris JW, Larsen B, Enevoldsen E, Lassen NA. Cerebral hemodynamics in migraine. *Can J Neurol Sci* 1977;4:245–249.

Hamel E, Lau B, Gregoire L, Ting V, Fan E, Chia LS. 5-HT1Db but not 5-HT1Da receptor MRNA is expressed in bovine and human cerebral blood vessels: pharmacological and molecular identification of the contractile 5-HT receptor. *J Cereb Blood Flow Metab* 1993;13:S265.

Hansen AJ, Quistorff B, Gjedde A. Relationship between local changes in cortical blood flow and extracellular K^+ during spreading depression. *Acta Physiol Scand* 1980;109:1–6.

Herold S, Gibs JM, Jones AKP, Brooks DJ, Frackowiak RSJ, Legg NJ. Oxygen metabolism in migraine. *J Cereb Blood Flow Metab* 1985;5,(Suppl):S445–S446.

Hubel DH, Weisel TN. Receptive fields and functional architecture of monkey striate cortex. *J Physiol* 1968;195:215–243.

Humphrey PPA, Feniuk W, Marriott AS, Tanner RJN, Jackson MR, Tucker ML. Preclinical studies on the anti-migraine drug sumatriptan. *Eur Neurol* 1991;31:282–290.

Jones TH, Morawetz RB, Crowell RM. Threshold of focal cerebral ischemia in awake monkeys. *J Neurosurg* 1981;54:773–778.

Joutel A, Tournier-Lasserve E, Biousse V. Genetic mapping of familial hemiplegic migraine. *Cephalalgia* 1993;13(Suppl 13):25.

Juul R, Edvinsson L, Gisvold SE, Ekman R, Brubakk AO, Fredriksen TA. Calcitonin gene-related peptide-LI in subarachnoidal haemorrhage in man. Signs of activation of the trigemino-cerebrovascular system? *Br J Neurosurg* 1990;4:171–180.

Kaube H, Goadsby PJ. Antimigraine compounds fail to modulate the propagation of cortical spreading depression in the cat. *Eur Neurol* 1994;34:30–35.

Kaube H, Hoskin KL, Goadsby PJ. Intravenous acetylsalicylic acid inhibits central trigeminal neurons in the dorsal horn of the upper cervical spinal cord in the cat. *Headache* 1994;(In press).

Kaube H, Hoskin KL, Goadsby PJ. Sumatriptan inhibits central trigeminal neurons only after blood-brain barrier disruption. *Br J Pharmacol* 1993a;109:788–792.

Kaube H, Keay K, Hoskin KL, Bandler R, Goadsby PJ. Expression of c-fos-like immunoreactivity in trigeminal nucleus caudalis and high cervical cord following stimulation of the sagittal sinus in the cat. *Brain Res* 1993b;33:541–544.

Kraig RP, Nicholson C. Extracellular ionic variations during spreading depression. *Neuroscience* 1978; 3:1045–1059.

Kupfermann I. Hypothalamus and limbic system II: motivation. In: Kandel ER, Schwartz JH. eds. *Principles of neural science*. Amsterdam: Elsevier, 1985;626–635.

Lambert GA, Lowy AJ, Boers P, Angus-Leppan H, Zagami AS. The spinal cord processing of input from the superior sagittal sinus: pathway and modulation by ergot alkaloids. *Brain Res* 1992;597: 321–330.

Lambert GA, Goadsby PJ, Zagami AS, Duckworth JW. Comparative effects of stimulation of the trigeminal ganglion and the superior sagittal sinus on cerebral blood flow and evoked potentials in the cat. *Brain Res* 1988;453:143–149.

Lashley KS. Patterns of cerebral integration indicated by the scotomas of migraine. *Arch Neurol Psychiatry* 1941;46:331–339.

Lauritzen M, Olesen J. Regional cerebral blood flow during migraine attacks by xenon-133 inhalation and emission tomography. *Brain* 1984;107:447–461.

Lauritzen M, Skyhoj-Olsen T, Lassen NA, Paulson OB. The changes of regional cerebral blood flow during the course of classical migraine attacks. *Ann Neurol* 1983;13:633–641.

Lauritzen M. Long-lasting reduction of cortical blood flow of the rat brain after spreading depression with preserved autoregulation and impaired CO_2 response. *J Cereb Blood Flow Metab* 1984;4:546–554.

Lauritzen M, Skyhoj-Olsen T, Lassen NA, Paulson OB. Regulation of regional cerebral blood flow during and between migraine attacks. *Ann Neurol* 1983;14:569–572.

Lauritzen M, Jorgensen MB, Diemer NH, Gjedde A, Hansen AJ. Persistent oligaemia of rat cerebral cortex in the wake of spreading depression. *Ann Neurol* 1982;12:469–474.

Leao AAP. Spreading depression of activity in cerebral cortex. *J Neurophysiol* 1944a;7:359–390.

Leao AAP. Pial circulation and spreading activity in the cerebral cortex. *J Neurophysiol* 1944b;7: 391–396.

Liu-Chen LY, Mayberg MR, Moskowitz MA. Immunohistochemical evidence for a substance P-containing trigeminovascular pathway to pial arteries in cats. *Brain Res* 1983;268:162–166.

Liu-Chen LY, Gillespie SA, Norregaard TV, Moskowitz MA. Co-localization of retrogradely transported wheat germ agglutinin and the putative neurotransmitter substance P within the trigeminal ganglion cells projecting to cat middle cerebral. *J Comp Neurol* 1984;225:187–192.

Markowitz S, Saito K, Moskowitz MA. Neurogenically mediated leakage of plasma proteins occurs from blood vessels in dura mater but not brain. *J Neurosci* 1987;7:4129–4136.

Markowitz S, Saito K, Moskowitz MA. Neurogenically mediated plasma extravasation in dura mater: effect of ergot alkaloids. A possible mechanism of action in vascular headache. *Cephalalgia* 1988;8: 83–91.

Marshall WH. Spreading cortical depression of Leao. *Physiol Rev* 1959;39:230–288.

Martins IP, Baeta E, Paiva T, Campo T, Gomes L. Headaches during intracranial endovascular procedures: a possible model of vascular headache. *Headache* 1993;33:227–233.

Mathew NT, Hrastnik F, Meyer JS. Regional cerebral blood flow in the diagnosis of vascular headache. *Headache* 1976;15:252–260.

Matsuyama T, Shiosaka S, Matsumoto M. Overall distribution of vasoactive intestinal polypeptide-containing nerves on the wall of the cerebral arteries: an immunohistochemical study using whole-mounts. *Neuroscience* 1983;10:89–96.

Mayberg MR, Zervas NT, Moskowitz MA. Trigeminal projections to supratentorial pial and dural blood vessels in cats demonstrated by horseradish peroxidase histochemistry. *J Comp Neurol* 1984;223: 46–56.

Mayberg MR, Langer RS, Zervas NT, Moskowitz MA. Perivascular meningeal projections from cat trigeminal ganglia: possible pathway for vascular headaches in man. *Science* 1981;213:228–230.

McLachlan RS, Grivin JP. Spreading depression in the human cortex. *Can J Neurol Sci* 1993;20,(Suppl 4):S54.

Mraovitch S, Calando Y, Seylaz J. Long-lasting cerebral blood flow and metabolic changes within the limbic and brainstem regions following cortical spreading depression in rat. *J Cereb Blood Flow Metab* 1989;9:S508.

Nichols FT, Mawad M, Mohr JP, Hilal S, Adams RJ. Focal headache during balloon inflation in the vertebral and basilar arteries. *Headache* 1993;33:87–89.

Norris JW, Hachinski VC, Cooper PW. Changes in cerebral blood flow during a migraine attack. *Br Med J* 1975;3:676–677.

Nozaki K, Boccalini P, Moskowitz MA. Expression of c-fos-like immunoreactivity in brainstem after meningeal irritation by blood in the subarachnoid space. *Neuroscience* 1992;49:669–680.

O'Brien MD. Cerebral blood flow changes in migraine. *Headache* 1971;10:139–143.

Olesen J, Friberg L, Skyhoj-Olsen T. Timing and topography of cerebral blood flow, aura and headache during migraine attacks. *Ann Neurol* 1990;28:791–798.

Olesen J. Classification and diagnostic criteria for headache disorders, cranial neuralgias and facial pain. *Cephalalgia* 1988;8(Suppl 7):1–96.

Olesen J, Tfelt-Hansen P, Hendriksen L, Larsen B. Spreading cerebral oligaemia in classical- and normal cerebral blood flow in common migraine. *Headache* 1982;22:242–248.

Olesen J, Larsen B, Lauritzen M. Focal hyperemia followed by spreading oligemia and impaired activation of rCBF in classic migraine. *Ann Neurol* 1981;9:344–352.

Peatfield RC, Rose FC. *New advances in headache research*, vol. 2. London: Smith-Gordon and Co., 1991;35–38.

Penfield W, Perot P. The brain's record of auditory and visual experience. *Brain* 1968;86:595–596.

Penfield W, McNaughton FL. Dural headache and the innervation of the dura mater. *Arch Neurol Psychiatry* 1940;44:43–75.

Piper RD, Lambert GA, Duckworth JW. Cortical blood flow changes during spreading depression in cats. *Am J Physiol* 1991a;261:H96–H102.

Piper RD, Matheson JM, Hellier M. Cortical spreading depression is not seen intraoperatively during temporal lobectomy in humans. *Cephalalgia* 1991b;11(Suppl 11):1.

Ray BS, Wolff HG. Experimental studies on headache. Pain sensitive structures of the head and their significance in headache. *Arch Surg* 1940;41:813–856.

Ruskell GL, Simons T. Trigeminal nerve pathways to the cerebral arteries in monkeys. *J Anat* 1987;155: 23–37.

Sakai F, Meyer JS. Abnormal cerebrovascular reactivity in patients with migraine and cluster headache. *Headache* 1979;19:257–266.

Sakai F, Meyer JS. Regional cerebral hemodynamics during migraine and cluster headaches measured by the 133-Xe inhalation method. *Headache* 1978;18:122–132.

Sakas DE, Moskowitz MA, Wei EP, Kontos HA, Kano M, Ogilvy C. Trigeminovascular fibers increase blood flow in cortical grey matter by axon-dependent mechanisms during severe hypertension or seizures. *Proc Natl Acad Sci USA* 1989;86:1401–1405.

Simard D, Paulson OB. Cerebral vasomotor paralysis during migraine attack. *Arch Neurol* 1973;29:207–209.

Skinhoj E. Hemodynamic studies within the brain during migraine. *Arch Neurol* 1973;29:95–98.

Skinhoj E, Paulson OB. Regional cerebral blood flow in the internal carotid artery distribution during migraine. *Br Med J* 1969;3:569–570.

Skyhoj-Olsen T, Friberg L, Lassen NA. Ischemia may be the primary cause of the neurological deficits in classic migraine. *Arch Neurol* 1987;44:156–161.

Somerville BW. The role of estradiol withdrawal in the etiology of menstrual migraine. *Neurology* 1972;22:355–365.

Sramka M, Brozek G, Bures J, Nadvornik P. Functional ablation by spreading depression: possible use in human stereotactic neurosurgery. *Appl Neurophysiol* 1977;40:48–61.

Staehelin-Jensen T, Vlodby B, Olivarius BF, Jensen FT. Cerebral hemodynamics in familial hemiplegic migraine. *Cephalalgia* 1981;1:121–125.

Swaab DF, Hofman MA, Lucassen PJ, Purba JS, Raadsheer FC, van de Nes JA. Functional neuroanatomy and neuropathology of the hypothalamus. *Anat Embryol* 1993;187:317–330.

Symonds C. Migrainous variants. *Trans Med Soc Lond* 1952;67:237–250.

Tomida S, Wagner HG, Klatzo I, Nowak TS. Effect of acute electrode placement on regional CBF in the gerbil: A comparison of blood flow measured by hydrogen clearance, [^{3}H]-nicotine, and [^{14}C]-iodoantipyrine techniques. *J Cereb Blood Flow Metab* 1989;9:79–86.

Trojaborg W, Boysen G. Relation between EEG, regional cerebral blood flow and internal carotid artery pressure during carotid endarterectomy. *Electroencephalogr Clin Neurophysiol* 1973;34:61–69.

Uddman R, Edvinsson L, Ekman R, Kingman T, McCulloch J. Innervation of the feline cerebral vasculature by nerve fibers containing calcitonin gene-related peptide: trigemnial origin and coexistence with substance P. *Neurosci Lett* 1985;62:131–136.

Welch KMA, D'andrea G, Tepley N, Barkeley GL, Ramadan NM. The concept of migraine as a state of central neuronal hyperexcitability. *Headache* 1990;8:817–828.

Zagami AS, Goadsby PJ. *New advances in headache research*, vol. 2. London: Smith-Gordon and Co., 1991;169–171.

Zagami AS, Lambert GA. Craniovascular application of capsaicin activates nocicpetive thalamic neurons in the cat. *Neurosci Lett* 1991;121:187–190.

Zagami AS, Lambert GA. Stimulation of cranial vessels excites nociceptive neurons in several thalamic nuclei of the cat. *Exp Brain Res* 1990;81:552–566.

Zagami AS, Goadsby PJ, Edvinsson L. Stimulation of the superior sagittal sinus in the cat causes release of vasoactive peptides. *Neuropeptides* 1990;16:69–75.

Pain and the Brain: From Nociception to Cognition, edited by Burkhart Bromm and John E. Desmedt, Advances in Pain Research and Therapy Vol. 22. Raven Press, Ltd., New York © 1995.

30

Endorphins, Pain Relief, and Euphoria

Walter Zieglgänsberger, Thomas R. Tölle, *Alexander Zimprich, *Volker Höllt, and Rainer Spanagel

*Max-Planck-Insitute of Psychiatry, D-80804 Munich, Germany, and *Institute of Physiology, University of Munich, D-808336 Munich, Germany*

SUMMARY

The three precursors for the opioid peptides, proopiomelanocortin, proenkephalin, and prodynorphin, are tissue-specifically processed. Multiple opioid receptors have been cloned. The best established opioid receptor types are μ, δ, and κ, including several subtypes. The various types of opioid receptors are differentially distributed within the central and peripheral nervous systems, and there is evidence that they show functional differences in various structures. Systemically applied opioids activate spinal and supraspinal mechanisms via μ-, δ-, and k-type opioid receptors. Their preferential effect, with few known exceptions, is a depression of spontaneous, chemically, or synaptically induced neuronal discharge. Opioids excite various groups of neurons, probably by inhibition of inhibitory GABAergic interneurons (disinhibition). A spinal opioidergic circuit exerts a tonic (inhibitory) action on spinofugally projecting neurons. Analgesic doses of systemically administered morphine, when given prior to stimulation, prevent the induction of immediate-early gene (IEG) expression in the spinal cord following noxious stimulation. Opioid analgesics, like other drugs of abuse, exert marked effects on mood and motivation. They produce euphoria in humans and are self-administered in animals. Repeated administration of opioids results in the development of tolerance and physical dependence. The activation of endogenous reward pathways determines the abuse potential of certain drugs and initiates the addictive process. The motivational effects of opioids and other drugs of abuse are affected by manipulation of dopamine (DA) neurotransmission, suggesting that dopaminergic (DAergic) systems are key components of reward pathways. The stimulus provided by these drugs is a conditioned stimulus, and the aversive effects of withdrawal, which are at least in part dependent on mesolimbic DAergic activity, contribute to drug-seeking behavior and finally to an addictive state.

INTRODUCTION

Opioidergic neurotransmission is found throughout the brain and appears to influence many central-nervous-system (CNS) functions, including nociception, cardiovascular and thermoregulation, respiration, neuroendocrine and neuroimmune activity, consummatory, sexual, aggressive, locomotor, and hedonic behavior, and learning and memory. The recent advances in pain research illustrate the analytical power of modern neurosciences in a field previously accessible only to methods of systems biology. Novel electrophysiologic, molecular, and cellular biologic techniques have changed the face of pain research by detailing the multiplicity of transducing and suppressive systems that involve neuronal and hormonal mechanisms acting in concert to help the individual to cope with pain. At present it would be unwarranted to assign an exclusive role to any neurotransmitter or neuromodulator system either in pain perception or pain modulation. The introduction of concepts of neuronal plasticity into this field of research has had important therapeutic consequences. Novel compounds and new regimens for drug treatment are emerging to prevent activity-dependent long-term changes that create or worsen pain, or to facilitate extinction in pain-related systems.

Opioid analgesics, like other drugs of abuse, exert marked effects on mood and motivation, produce euphoria in humans, and are self-administered in animals. The positive reinforcing effects of certain of these drugs, caused by the activation of endogenous reward pathways, determine their abuse potential and initiate the addictive process. Although a causal relationship between peripheral stimulation, the induction of immediate-early genes (IEGs), and long-term changes in the expression of target genes is still lacking, circumstantial evidence indicates that at least some long-term effects triggered by synaptic input may have their starting point in genetic events initiated by transactivation of IEGs. Enhancing synaptic processes mediated by excitatory amino acids (EAA) may be functionally most significant for the long-term changes induced by opioids.

RESULTS AND DISCUSSION

Opiate Receptors and Their Ligands

The opioid peptides that have been characterized in the mammalian central and peripheral nervous systems are derived from three precursors: proopiomelanocortin, proenkephalin, and prodynorphin. These precursors are tissue-specifically processed and yield numerous biologically active products (Höllt 1991). The identification of specific opioid binding in nervous tissue (Pert and Snyder 1973; Simon et al., 1973; Terenius 1973) initially indicated the existence of only one type of opioid receptor. However, soon after this landmark finding, several groups provided pharmacologic evidence for multiple opioid receptors. Today, the best established opioid receptor types are μ, δ, and κ. There is increasing pharmacologic evidence for subtypes of the major opioid receptor types, such as μ_1, μ_2 (Pasternak and Wood 1986), δ_1, δ_2 (Portoghese et al., 1992), and κ_1 and κ_2 (Devlin and Shoemaker 1990). At present the enkephalins are considered the putative ligands for the δ-receptors, β-endorphins for the μ-receptors, and dynorphins for the κ-receptors. This classification is further strengthened by binding studies employing cloned opioid receptors (see below). The various types of opioid receptors are differently distributed within the central and peripheral nervous systems. There is evidence for functional differences in these receptors in various structures (e.g., activation of μ receptors in limbic structures such as the nucleus accumbens produces reward and euphoria, whereas activation of κ receptors in this structure results in aversive symptoms and dysphoria; see Shippenberg 1993, and below. In the peripheral nervous system, opioid receptors (Stein et al., 1990; Stein 1991) are most likely localized on small-caliber nerve fibers, sympathetic endings, and immunocompetent cells, the last of which may also be a source for opioid peptides.

The Molecular Structure of Opioid Receptors

Many strategies have been employed during the past 15 years for cloning opioid receptors. However, the cloning of opioid receptors was only recently successful (Evans et al. 1992; Kieffer et al. 1992). The technique that was finally successful in identifying the structure of an opioid receptor was the expression of cloned DNA in monkey kidney cells (COS) and Chinese hamster ovary (CHO) cells. The expressed receptors were then identified by their binding of specific opioid ligands.

The δ-Receptor

The mouse δ receptor is a membrane-spanning glycoprotein with seven transmembrane sections comprising 372 amino acids. The observation that the cloned δ receptor exhibits a 500-fold higher affinity for the δ_2-selective antagonist naltriben (NTB) than for the δ_1-selective antagonist E-7-benzylidenenaltrexone (BNTX) suggests that the cloned receptor is a δ_2-subtype receptor (Kong et al. 1993) that is negatively coupled to adenylate cyclase (Evans et al. 1992).

The multiple forms of the δ receptor, with sizes ranging from 12 to 25 kb (Evans et al. 1992), may result from alternative splicing of a single gene (Evans et al. 1992; Bzdega et al. 1993). *In situ* hybridization experiments revealed high levels of the messenger ribonucleic acids (mRNAs) for the δ receptor in the olfactory bulb, hypothalamus, amygdala, and hippocampus. Moderate amounts of δ-opioid-receptor mRNA were also detected in the neocortex, caudate nucleus, and substantia gelatinosa, and unexpectedly also in the cerebellum (Keith et al. 1993). Interestingly, by far the greatest levels of δ-receptor mRNA were observed in the anterior pituitary (Bzdega et al. 1993), where affinity-purified antibodies raised against a synthetic peptide corresponding to the N-terminus of the mouse δ opioid receptor also demonstrated a high concentration of the receptor protein.

The κ-Receptor

Following the pioneering cloning of the mouse δ receptor, the structures of the rat δ receptor and of the closely related rat μ and κ receptor subtypes were soon elucidated by several groups (Meng et al. 1992; Minami et al. 1992). The rat κ receptor is a protein of 380 amino acids. Northern-blot analysis revealed a single species of mRNA of a size of 5.8 kb, which is expressed in abundance in the striatum and hypothalamus but weakly in the neocortex. *In situ* hybridization experiments showed a particularly high level of κ-receptor mRNA in the claustrum, nucleus accumbens, olfactory tubercle, hypothalamic nuclei, and substantia nigra. The cloned κ receptor displays a very high affinity for dynorphin$_{1-17}$. The relative affinities of the expressed κ receptor for various opioid ligands suggested that the cloned receptor belongs to the κ$_1$ type.

The μ-Receptor

Using strategies similar to those used for cloning the δ and κ receptors, the rat μ opioid receptor has been independently cloned by several groups (Chen et al. 1993; Fukuda et al. 1993; Thompson et al. 1993; Wang et al. 1993). The rat μ opioid receptor is a protein of 398 amino acids that displays a 63% identity to the rat δ and a 58% identity to the rat κ opioid receptor. Northern-blot analysis revealed that the size of the μ-opioid-receptor mRNA is approximately 14 to 16 kb (Fukuda et al. 1993; Thompson et al. 1993; cf. Wang et al. 1993). In ribonuclease (RNAse) protection experiments, μ-opioid-receptor mRNA levels have been measured in the thalamus, cortex, striatum, hypothalamus, midbrain, brain stem, and spinal cord, but not in the cerebellum (Wang et al. 1993). *In situ* hybridization experiments showed that μ-receptor mRNA was expressed at high levels in the striatal patches, medial septum, medial preoptic area, locus coeruleus, and interpeduncular nucleus. High levels of μ-receptor mRNA were found in the dorsal-root ganglia, but only low levels were measured in the spinal cord (Thompson et al. 1993). On the basis of the relative affinities of morphine and other selective μ agonists, the cloned receptor appears to be a μ$_2$ subtype of the μ opioid receptor (Thompson et al. 1993). A μ-opioid-receptor isoform was recently cloned (Höllt et al., unpublished data) that is identical to the described μ opioid receptor, up to amino acid 387, but contains a different and shorter C-terminus. It is very likely that this μ receptor isoform is generated by alternative splicing of the rat μ-receptor gene (Zimprich and Höllt, unpublished data). This indicates that heterogeneity of opioid receptors might not only result from the transcription of different genes, but may also result from the alternative splicing of genes.

Comparison of the amino-acid sequences of the three cloned opioid receptors reveals that the second and third intracellular loops of the opioid-receptor subtypes are highly conserved. These loops have been reported to be the G-protein-binding domain of the three receptors (Dohlman et al. 1992), suggesting that all three of the cloned receptors interact with similar G proteins.

Desensitization and Chronic Actions

The highly conserved third intracellular loop of the seven transmembrane domains of the opioid receptors contains many consensus sequences for protein kinases (sites for protein kinase C [PKC] as well as for cyclic adenosine monophosphate [cAMP]- or cyclic guanosine monophosphate [cGMP]-dependent kinases). Phosphorylation of the receptors at these sites may be involved in adaptive processes in response to prolonged treatment with opioid agonists, resembling what has been found with the β_2-adrenergic receptor (Dohlman et al., 1992). The amino acid at site 279 (threonine) in the μ receptor, which is conserved between the three cloned opioid receptors, corresponds to a similar phosphorylation site on the β_2-adrenergic receptor. This phosphorylation site is thought to be very critical in agonist-induced desensitization. Very recently, desensitization of the κ opioid receptor has been investigated in COS cells expressing the cloned receptor (Reisine and Bell 1993). The desensitization apparently involves the enzyme β-adrenoreceptor kinase (β-ARK), since it can be prevented by the coexpression of a β-ARK mutant that blocks the action of wild-type β-ARK. It remains to be established whether β-ARK is also involved in the desensitization of μ and δ receptors.

Mechanism of Opioid Action

At analgesic doses, systemically administered opioids activate spinal and supraspinal mechanisms via μ-, δ-, and k-type opioid receptors (see Duggan 1992; Morgan et al. 1992; Zieglgänsberger and Tölle 1993). Their preferential effect, with few exceptions, is a depression of spontaneous, chemically, or synaptically induced neuronal discharge. Probably by inhibition of inhibitory γ-butyratergic (GABAergic) interneurons (disinhibition), opioids excite hippocampal pyramidal neurons (Zieglgänsberger et al. 1979) and neurons in the rostral ventromedial medulla (Heinricher et al. 1992; Morgan et al. 1992). GABA and its synthesizing enzyme glutamate decarboxylase (GAD) are abundant in the superficial dorsal horn (Carlton and Hayes 1990), and GABA binding sites and GABA-containing neurons have been characterized in almost all pain-related pathways. Recent ultrastructural studies report that GABA-immunoreactive terminals are presynaptic to opioid-peptide-immunoreactive cell bodies and dendrites in the dorsal horn of the spinal cord (Carlton and Hayes 1990). It has been suggested that the blocking of these GABAergic interneurons can evoke disinhibition of opioid-containing interneurons in these pain-related circuits (see Zieglgänsberger 1986). Recently, an increase in GABA-immunoreactive neurons and GABA levels was reported in the spinal cord of rats with unilateral peripheral inflammation (Castro-Lopes et al. 1992). This effect is likely to occur in parallel with the increase in enkephalin and dynorphin in response to increased nociceptive input (Faccini et al. 1984; Millan et al. 1986; Takahashi et al. 1988). In vitro studies of neurons in the substantia gelatinosa report hyper- and depolarizing responses to morphine applied in the superfusate. It remains to be elucidated whether disinhibitory effects mediated by interneurons play a role in these responses (Magnuson and Dickenson 1991). In an *in vivo* preparation of the spinal cord it was found that the opioid agonist buprenorphine (a mixed opioid agonist-antagonist), which is widely used in treating pain, and the μ-receptor-selective agonist D-Ala^2, *N*-Me-Phe^4, Gly^5-ol enkephalin (DAMGO), facilitated C-fiber-evoked responses at low doses (Dickenson et al. 1990; Magnuson et al. 1990). Interestingly, the κ-opioid agonists dynorphin and U 50.488H increased the excitability of some nociceptive neurons in the dorsal horn, expanded their receptive fields (RFs), and reduced thresholds for mechanical and thermal stimulation (Hylden et al. 1991; cf. Skilling et al. 1992). It remains to be shown whether the κ-agonists display opioid-antagonistic properties as does dynorphin$_{1-17}$ (Vidal et al. 1984), or block (e.g., dynorphinergic) interneurons (Dubner and Ruda, 1992). In *in vitro* preparations some primary afferent neurons appear to be directly activated by opioid agonists (Crain and Shen 1992).

There is evidence that the opioid antagonist naloxone evokes hyperalgesia by reducing the efficacy of tonically active opioidergic circuits. A spinal opioidergic circuit is likely to exert most of its tonic (inhibitory) action on spinofugally projecting neurons through postsynaptically located receptors (Zieglgänsberger 1980; for a review, see Zieglgänsberger 1986; Lombard and Besson 1989; Kayser et al. 1989; Hartell and Headley 1991; Duggan 1992), although additional presynaptic actions cannot be excluded (Besse et al. 1990; Kalso et al. 1992). A reduced degradation of opioid peptides, which increases the efficacy of a tonically active opioidergic circuitry, explains why peptidase inhibitors such as Kelatorphan enhance the antinociceptive effect of opioid peptides (Dickenson et al. 1987; Kayser et al. 1989; Sullivan et al. 1989; Roques et al. 1990, 1993; Tölle et al. 1994b).

Neuroplastic Changes Induced by Noxious Stimulation are Reduced by Opioids

Activity-dependent modulation of gene expression is a characteristic feature of highly integrated neuronal systems, and greatly expands their capacity to react in a more plastic manner to environmental stimuli (Fig. 1). Increased or paroxysmal activity, such as in the spinal cord, will eventually also evoke activity-dependent adaptive changes in more rostral stuctures such as the thalamus or neocortex.

Transcriptional factors encoded by IEGs are rapidly induced by neuronal activity evoked by excitatory neurotransmitters such as L-glutamate. There is ample evidence that excitatory amino acids (EAAs) play a dominant role in the central nervous system (CNS) as excitatory neurotransmitters involved in memory acquisition and developmental plasticity. L-glutamate-receptor subtypes are present throughout the CNS, and the ligand-gated ion channels (*N*-methyl-D-aspartate[NMDA]; α-amino-3-hydroxy-5-methyl-4-isooxazole propionic acid [AMPA]; kainate) activated by EAAs are at present among the best-studied channel species (Sommer and Seeburg 1992). Molecular cloning studies suggest that ionotropic EAA receptors are heterooligomeric assemblies, and that the combination of subunits is crucial for the

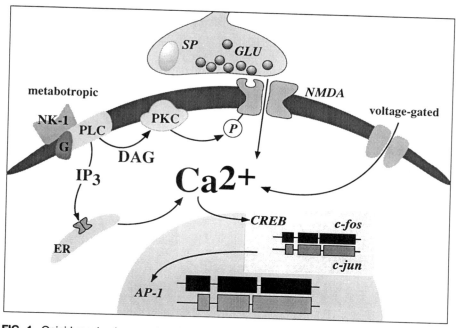

FIG. 1. Opioid mechanisms and neuroplasticity. Opioids reduce immediate-early gene (IEG) expression in central neurons through a naloxone-reversible mechanism. In cultured neocortical neurons, ionotropic and metabotropic excitatory amino acids (EAA) receptor activation induces expression of mRNAs for c-*fos*, *jun*-B, and NGF1-a, an effect that is partially blocked by a protein kinase inhibitor (Vaccarino et al. 1992). Substance P (SP) is co-localized with EAAs (such as L-glutamate) (GLU) in small-caliber primary afferent fibers and is released by high-intensity stimulation. SP activates phospholipase C (PLC) via G-protein-coupled neurokinin-1 (NK-1) receptors. Inositol 1,4,5-triphosphate (IP3) evokes the release of Ca^{2+} from intracellular stores in the endoplasmic reticulum (ER) and activates protein kinase C (PKC) through 1,2-diacylglycerol (DAG). NMDA and some AMPA receptor proteins (see text) carry consensus sequences for phosphorylation (P) by PKC or cAMP-dependent protein kinase. Phosphorylation and de-phosphorylation by kinases stimulated by second messengers such as cAMP/cGMP, Ca^{2+}, IP3/ DAG, or phosphatases alters receptor properties, ion-channel kinetics, structural proteins, or the activity of other enzymes (Swope et al. 1992). NMDA receptor activation triggers Ca^{2+} influx through ligand-gated channels. Depolarization triggered by NMDA, AMPA, and kainate receptor activation evokes Ca^{2+} influx through voltage-gated channels. Ca^{2+} influx induces the expression of *fos*/*jun* through a Ca-response element that is indistinguishable from a cAMP response element (CRE). CREB, its cognate transcription factor, is rapidly phosphorylated in response to synaptic activation, and probably integrates Ca^{2+}- and cAMP-linked signals. Opioid-receptor activation could reduce IEG expression through its hyperpolarizing action by a reduction of EAA release from terminals or by an interference with second messengers involved in the generation of transcription factors (see text). AP-1 activator protein 1.

composition and kinetics of ion fluxes through these ligand-gated channels. NMDA triggers Ca^{2+} fluxes through ligand-gated channels, whereas the AMPA/low-affinity kainate receptors preferentially activate NA^+/K^+-fluxes, provided the subunit assembly contains the GluR-B subunit. The activation of the G-protein-linked metabotropic L-glutamate receptors (mGluR) depolarizes neurons in the CNS, increases phosphoinositide hydrolysis, activates phospholipases, and alters cAMP and cGMP levels. In addition, mGluR agonists can enhance AMPA- and NMDA-receptor-mediated ionic currents (Aniksztejn et al. 1992; Ben-Ari et al. 1992; Cerne and Randic 1992; Kalso et al. 1992), and could thus also increase the intracellular Ca^{2+} concentration indirectly through activation of ligand- and voltage-gated channels.

The number of neurons that express IEGs, and the anatomic distribution as well as the time course of expression of IEGs in certain neurons, depend specifically on the parameters of the peripheral stimulus applied (Williams et al. 1990; Wisden et al. 1990; Herdegen et al. 1990, 1991a,b,c). Acute noxious stimulation triggers IEG expression (Hunt et al. 1987; Draisci and Iadorala 1989; Menétrey et al. 1989; Bullitt 1990; Presley et al. 1990; Wisden et al. 1990; Herdegen et al. 1990, 1991 a,b,c; Anton et al. 1991; Birder et al. 1991; Kehl et al. 1991; Traub et al. 1992; Tölle et al. 1990, 1991, 1994a,b,c). Analgesic doses of systemically administered morphine prevent IEG induction in the spinal cord after noxious stimulation only when given prior to stimulation (Tölle et al. 1994c). Electrophysiologic and biochemical experiments have provided strong evidence that opioid receptors: (a) increase membrane potassium conductance, (b) inhibit the voltage-dependent Ca^{2+} current, and (c) modulate second messengers and interfere with excitatory and inhibitory synaptic processes, thus affecting the expression of IEGs (for a review see Duggan and Fleetwood-Walker 1992).

In somatosensory neocortical neurons, μ-receptor-preferring opioid peptides differentially affect excitatory synaptic transmission mediated by subtypes of the L-glutamate receptor: these peptides reduce excitatory postsynaptic potentials (EPSPs) evoked by the activation of AMPA receptors and increase EPSPs mediated by the activation of NMDA receptors. The enhancement of the NMDA component is blocked by the intracellular injection of PKC inhibitors (Martin, Pawelzik, Deisz and Zieglgänsberger, unpublished results). It has been previously described that the activation of protein kinases by μ-preferring opioid agonists enhances NMDA-mediated postsynaptic currents (Chen and Huang 1991) and increases the response to L-glutamate (Greengard et al. 1991). Whole-cell patch-clamp recording from acutely dissociated dorsal horn neurons reveals that μ-opioid agonists affect NMDA responses in a complex manner. After an initial depression, the NMDA responses were potentiated for long periods (Rusin and Randic 1991). In keeping with these findings, low doses of μ-receptor-preferring agonists facilitate C-fiber-evoked firing (Magnuson et al. 1990) as well as facilitating spinal-flexor reflexes (Wiesenfeld-Hallin et al. 1991). Such an enhancing effect on NMDA-receptor-mediated synaptic processes may be functionally most significant for long-term changes induced by opioids. Several lines of evidence suggest that protein phosphorylation of

NMDA-receptor subunits by protein kinase C and cAMP-dependent protein kinase can modulate glutamate-gated ionotropic channels and thus influence synaptic plasticity (see Nairn and Shenolikar 1992; Zieglgänsberger and Tölle 1993). The link between NMDA-receptor-mediated Ca^{2+} fluxes, voltage-gated Ca^{2+} channels, and the release of Ca^{2+} ions from intracellular stores following the activation of metabotropic EAA receptors and opioid receptors remains to be elucidated.

Protein phosphorylation of ligand-gated channels appears to be a major mechanism in the regulation of neuronal plasticity (Swope et al. 1992). NMDA- and some AMPA-receptor proteins carry consensus sequences for phosphorylation by PKC (Gerber et al. 1989; Linden and Connor 1991; Chen and Huang 1991, 1992) or cAMP-dependent protein kinase (Greengard et al. 1991; Wang et al., 1991; Raymond et al. 1993). It has been shown that the inhibition of phospholipase C by neomycin, or treatment with the PKC inhibitor H-7, reduces nociceptive responses in the formalin test, whereas activation of PKC by phorbol esters enhances these responses (Coderre 1992; Mao et al. 1992). The activation of PKC increases the responsiveness of dorsal-horn neurons to glutamate (Gerber et al. 1989) and enhances NMDA-activated currents in trigeminal neurons. These findings suggest a role for PKC in synaptic plasticity related to central sensitization to noxious stimuli (Coderre 1992; Tölle et al. 1994a). The physiologic role of presynaptically located L-glutamate receptors, and the mechanism by which they modulate transmitter release, still wait to be established.

Besides EAAs, neuropeptides such as the tachykinins, calcitonin-gene-related peptide (CGRP), galanin, cholecystokinin, vasoactive intestinal polypeptide (VIP), neurotensin, and opioid peptides serve as transmitters in primary afferent fibers, including nociceptors impinging on dorsal-horn neurons. Numerous interneurons in the dorsal horn also contain neuropeptides and release them following synaptic stimulation. In recent years, various steroid hormones, cytokines, target-derived trophic factors rapidly induced by EAAs, and diffusible arachidonic-acid metabolites, as well as radicals like NO, have been considered as factors influencing neuroplasticity in pain-related structures (see Dubner and Ruda 1992).

The Positive Reinforcing Effects of Opioids and the Treatment of Chronic Pain

Opioid analgesics, like other drugs of abuse, exert marked effects on mood and motivation (Wise 1987; Herz and Shippenberg 1989). They produce euphoria in humans and are self-administered in animals. Repeated administration of opioids results in the development of tolerance and physical dependence. Although these effects of chronic drug intake may be important for the maintenance of established drug addiction, it is now generally accepted that they do not represent causal factors in the development of addiction. There is now increasing evidence that the positive reinforcing effects caused by activation of endogenous reward pathways determine the abuse potential of certain drugs and initiate the addictive process (Koob 1992).

Drug-seeking behavior is seen as the common element in all drug addictions. Three factors are thought to be critically involved in the initiation of drug-seeking behavior: (a) positive reinforcing effects of drugs; (b) discriminative effects of drugs; and (c) stimuli conditioned to effects of drugs (Stolerman 1992). These factors will be discussed in detail below in relation to the prototypically addictive opioids such as morphine and heroin.

The operant-reinforcement techniques of self-administration and intracranial self-stimulation measure the primary reinforcing processes in drug-seeking behavior and have been widely used to measure the motivational effects of drugs of abuse (Wise and Bozarth 1982; Bozarth 1987). The most interesting insights into the nature of motivational processes induced by opioids have been provided by the use of place conditioning, a technique that measures the secondary reinforcing effects of drugs. In this procedure, the association that develops between the presentation of a drug and a previously neutral stimulus (e.g., differently colored compartments of a shuttle box) is evaluated. The results obtained with this paradigm for rewarding drugs are largely identical with those obtained with the self-administration paradigm technique (Spyraki 1988; Carr et al. 1989). Besides the evaluation of rewarding properties, the place-conditioning procedure allows the detection of aversive (negatively reinforcing) properties of drugs, which is of particular importance when investigating the effects of opioids.

Mucha and Herz (1985) used the place-conditioning paradigm to demonstrate rewarding or aversive effects of opioids according to their receptor specificity. The paradigm comprised dose-dependent place preference induced by systemic administration of μ-opioid-receptor ligands such as morphine, fentanyl, or sufentanyl, and place aversion (with a tendency for reversal at higher doses) with systemic administration of the κ-receptor specific benzeneacetamide-derivatives U 50,488H and U-69593. Rewarding or aversive effects of μ- and κ-receptor ligands were obtained with intracerebroventricular (i.c.v.) injections of much lower doses of opioids, indicating the central origin of these motivational effects (Bals-Kubik et al. 1989, 1990). The motivational effects of opioids are selectively modified by several factors. In an experimental model of mild but prolonged inflammatory pain, κ-opioid receptor agonists failed to produce aversive states, whereas the positive reinforcing effects of morphine remained unaltered (Shippenberg et al. 1988; cf. Lyness et al. 1989). The clinical relevance of this finding is obvious: The chronic administration of opioids to patients with chronic pain eventually results in profound physical dependence without evidence of psychological dependence or addiction (Porter and Jick 1980; Portenoy et al. 1990). There is also evidence that the motivational properties of opioids are altered under the influence of chronic stress.

Findings showing that motivational effects of opioids and other drugs of abuse are affected by manipulation of dopamine (DA) neurotransmission and DA-receptor activation suggest that dopaminergic (DAergic) systems are key components of reward pathways (Bozarth and Wise 1981; Wise and Rompre 1989). Inactivation of these components by local injection of the neurotoxin G-hydroxydopamine (G-

OHDA) or the D_1-receptor antagonist SCH 23390 into the nucleus accumbens (NAC) abolished the rewarding as well as the aversive effects of μ- and κ-receptor ligands, respectively. These data indicate that DAergic transmission in the NAC is necessary not only for the manifestation of the rewarding but also of the aversive effects of opioids (Shippenberg et al. 1993). Interestingly, data derived on the neurochemical level by means of *in vivo* microdialysis show a dose-dependent increase in the release of mesolimbic DA after i.c.v. injections of the μ-receptor agonist DAMGO, whereas the κ-receptor ligand E-2078, a dynorphin analogue, induces a decrease in mesolimbic DA upon i.c.v. administration (Spanagel et al. 1990a,b; Longoni et al. 1991). The effective doses of the two substances in these experiments were very similar to those in the behavioral tests mentioned above. A close parallelism between the biochemical and behavioral data was particularly obvious in the case of κ-agonists, where in both experimental approaches higher doses were less effective than lower ones. These results suggest that the different effects of μ-agonists and κ-agonists on mesolimbic DA function may underlie their opposing motivational effects.

Results providing a new perspective on the modulation of the mesolimbic DA system were obtained when opioids were either microinjected into the ventral tegmental area (VTA) or infused into the NAC (through the microdialysis probe from which the samples for evaluation of DA and its metabolites were also taken) (Spanagel et al. 1992). Microinjection of the μ-receptor agonist DAMGO into the VTA increased DA release in the NAC, while the μ-receptor antagonist Cys[2], Tyr[3], Orn[5], Pen[7]amide (CTOP) decreased basal DA levels. The κ-receptor agonist U 69593 and the κ-receptor antagonist nor-binaltorphamine (nor-BNI) were ineffective at this site. Quite opposite results were obtained when these drugs were injected into the NAC: DAMGO and its antagonist CTOP did not change the basal release of DA, while U 69593 decreased and nor-BNI increased the basal release of DA. These data indicate that basal DA release is under the tonic control of both opioid systems: μ-receptor activation in the VTA (via a β-endorphin system) results in increased DA release, whereas κ-receptor activation in the NAC (via a dynorphin system) decreases basal DA release (Smith et al. 1992; Spanagel et al. 1992; Jackisch et al. 1993) (Fig. 2). Thus, after prolonged morphine exposure, there may be a compensatory increase in the activity of the functionally opposing dynorphin system located within the NAC and/or hypoactivity of the μ-system in the VTA. Either effect may play an important role in the initiation of drug-seeking behavior.

Psychoactive drugs are used to obtain their characteristic subjective effects. Drug-discrimination procedures are thought to be the closest available experimental models of the human subjective effects of psychoactive drugs in laboratory animals (Bozarth 1987). In a typical drug-discrimination procedure an animal is placed into a Skinner box (test chamber), in which its lever-pressing responses result in delivery of an operant reinforcement (e.g., food pellets). Pretreatment with a drug serves as a discriminative stimulus that indicates to the animal how a reinforcement can be obtained. An animal can, for example, be trained to press one of two levers to obtain a reinforcement after receiving an injection of drug, and to press the other

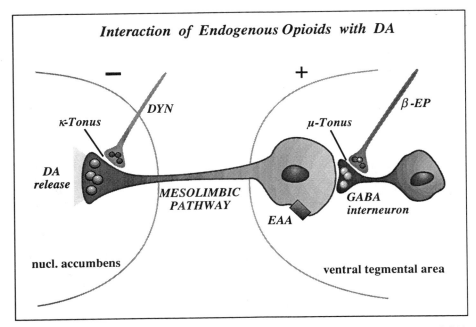

FIG. 2. Interaction of endogenous opioids with dopamine. Model for the modulation of A10 dopamine (DA) neurons by opposing, tonically active endogenous opioid systems. In the ventral tegmental area the A10 neurons are stimulated by a tonically active μ system (β-EP, β-endorphin) via disinhibition of a γ-aminobutyrate (GABA)-containing interneuron. In the nucleus accumbens the release of DA by A10 neurons is suppressed by a tonically inhibitory κ system (Dyn, dynorphin). The action of both opioid systems is necessary for the maintenance of basal DA release. EAA = excitatory amino acid.

lever to obtain a reinforcement after an injection of vehicle. After the discrimination has been learned, the animal begins pressing the appropriate lever according to whether it has received the drug or the vehicle. The discriminative effect of a drug may directly promote drug-seeking behavior because such behavior has previously been associated with the perceived reinforcing effect of the drug. With regard to opioids, for example, it has been suggested (Colpaert 1978; Overton 1987a,b) that rats may at least partly discriminate morphine by its rewarding effects. Such a linkage between the rewarding and discriminative effects of morphine would suggest that both effects are mediated by the same neuroanatomic and neurochemical substrates.

The rewarding effects of morphine are associated with the activation of μ-receptors in the VTA. Morphine administered into the VTA produced an almost complete generalization to the discriminative effects of systemic morphine (Shoaib and Spanagel 1994). Microinjection of morphine into the NAC, the major terminal region of the mesolimbic pathway, produced signs of partial generalization at a single dose, with a tendency toward vehicle-like responses at larger doses. These microinjections were behaviorally active, as evidenced by significant decreases in the rate of lever-pressing responses. In this study the striatum was examined as a control region. Doses of morphine identical to those injected into the NAC failed to generalize to the systemic morphine stimulus.

These findings suggest that the morphine stimulus may be mediated at least partially by the mesolimbic DAergic pathway, a conclusion supported by the observation that neuroleptic agents selective for the D_1 or D_2 subtypes of the DA receptor can attenuate heroin discrimination (Corrigall and Coen 1990).

It has been shown that animals can also be trained to discriminate between the presence and absence of κ-opioid agonists (Shearman and Herz 1982; Picker and Dykstra 1989). Despite their demonstration of partial generalization between κ- and μ-opioid ligands, these studies were confounded by the use of nonspecific compounds and test doses (Picker et al. 1990), and it is now accepted that the discriminative-stimulus properties of the κ-agonists relate to their action at κ-opioid receptors. Although there are few reports of study of the neurochemical substrate(s) mediating the κ-stimulus, evidence has been provided that DAergic systems are critically involved. Thus, sulpiride substitutes for U-62,066E (a highly specific κ-agonist) as a stimulus cue without reducing the response rate of the test animal (Ohno et al. 1992). A recent study also shows an involvement of serotonin in the discriminative effects of κ-agonists (Bronson et al. 1993). In summary, the κ-stimulus may not only be mediated by activation of κ-receptors and a consequent reduction in DAergic activity, but may also involve other transmitter systems.

Environmental stimuli are associated with effects of drugs by means of classical conditioning. The association of environmental stimuli with the effects of drugs can profoundly influence the acquisition of drug-seeking behavior, and is also seen as the trigger for the reinstatement (facilitation of relapse) and maintenance of drug-seeking behavior (Stewart 1983). Goldberg and Schuster (1967) were the first to show that in monkeys that self-administer morphine by pressing a lever, conditioned stimuli can maintain lever-pressing even if morphine is temporarily unavailable (context-dependent self-administration). Furthermore, a distinct environment, repeatedly paired with morphine, can elicit locomotion in the absence of morphine (Mucha et al. 1981) and can also potentiate the locomotor-stimulant and mesolimbic DA-releasing effects of morphine (Vezina et al. 1989; Kalivas and Stewart 1991). It is suggested that such context-dependent sensitization phenomena are what contribute most substantially to drug-seeking behavior.

The reinforcing and the discriminative effects of opioids are seen as the primary factors in the acquisition of drug-seeking behavior. The mesolimbic system, and particularly the DA release therein, play a critical role in the mediation of both effects. However, the modulation of the mesolimbic DAergic pathway underlies the integrity of the endogenous, tonically active, opioid systems. Thus, these systems seem to be critically involved in the initiation of the reinforcing and possibly also of the discriminative effects of morphine. After the manifestation of drug-seeking behavior, reinforcement and discrimination may play a minor role in addiction. It is the conditioned stimulus and the aversive effects of withdrawal, which depend at least in part on mesolimbic DAergic activity, that contribute to addictive behavior.

REFERENCES

Aniksztejn L, Otani S, Ben-Ari Y. Quisqualate metabotropic receptors modulate NMDA currents and facilitate induction of long-term potentiation through protein kinase C. *Eur J Neurosci* 1992;4: 500–505.

Anton F, Herdegen T, Peppel P, Leah JD. C-*fos* like immunoreactivity in rat brainstem neurones following noxious chemical stimulation of the nasal mucosa. *Neuroscience* 1991;41:629–641.

Bals-Kubik R, Herz A, Shippenberg TS. Evidence that the aversive effects of opioid antagonists and opioid agonists are centrally mediated. *Psychopharmacology* 1989;98:203–206.

Bals-Kubik R, Shippenberg TS, Herz A. Involvement of μ- and δ-receptors in mediating the reinforcing effects of β-endorphin in the rat. *Eur J Pharmacol* 1990;175:63–69.

Ben-Ari Y, Aniksztejn L, Bregestovski P. Protein kinase-C modulation of NMDA currents—an important link for LTP induction. *Trends Neurosci* 1992;15:333–339.

Besse D, Lombard ME, Zajac JM, Roques BP, Besson JM. Pre- and postsynaptic distribution of μ, δ and κ opioid receptors in the superficial layers of the cervical dorsal horn of the rat spinal cord. *Brain Res* 1990;521:15–22.

Birder LA, Roppolo JR, Iadarola MJ, de Groat WC. Electrical stimulation of visceral afferent pathways in the pelvic nerve increases *c-fos* in the rat lumbosacral spinal cord. *Neurosci Lett* 1991;129:193–196.

Bozarth MA. Intracranial self-administration procedures for the assessment of drug reinforcement. In: Bozarth MA, ed. *Methods of assessing the reinforcing properties of abused drugs*. Heidelberg: Springer, 1987;173–188.

Bozarth MA, Wise R. Heroin reward is dependent on a dopaminergic substrate. *Life Sci* 1981;29:1881–1886.

Bronson ME, Lin YP, Burchett K, Picker MJ, Dykstra LA. Serotonin involvement in the discriminative stimulus effects of κ opioids in pigeons. *Psychopharmacology* 1993;111:69–77.

Bullitt E. Expression of c-fos-like protein as a marker for neuronal activity following noxious stimulation in the rat. *J Comp Neurol* 1990;296:517–530.

Bzdega T, Chin H, Kim H, Jung HH, Kozak CA, Klee WA. Regional expression and chromosomal localization of the δ opiate receptor gene. *Proc Natl Acad Sci USA* 1993;90:9305–9309.

Carlton SM, Hayes ES. Light microscopic and ultrastructural analysis of GABA-immunoreactive profiles in the monkey spinal cord. *J Comp Neurol* 1990;300:162–182.

Carr GD, Fibinger HC, Phillips AG. Conditioned place preference as a measure of drug reward. In: Liebman JM, Cooper SJ, eds. *The neuropharmacological basis of reward*. Oxford: Clarendon Press, 1989;264–319.

Castro-Lopes JM, Tavares I, Tölle TR, Coito A, Coimbra A. Increase in GABAergic cells and GABA levels in the spinal cord in unilateral inflammation of the hindlimb in the rat. *Eur J Neurosci* 1992;4: 296–301.

Cerne R, Randic M. Modulation of AMPA and NMDA responses in rat spinal dorsal horn neurons by trans-1-aminocyclopentane-1,3-dicarboxylic acid. *Neurosci Lett* 1992;144:180–184.

Chen L, Huang LYM. Sustained potentiation of NMDA receptor-mediated glutamate responses through activation of protein kinase C by a μ-opioid. *Neuron* 1991;7:319–326.

Chen L, Huang LYM. Protein kinase C reduces Mg^2 block of NMDA-receptor channels as a mechanism of modulation. *Nature* 1992;356:521–523.

Chen Y, Mestek A, Liu J, Hurley JA, Yu L. Molecular cloning and functional expression of a μ opioid receptor from rat brain. *Mol Pharmacol* 1993;44:8–12.

Coderre TJ. Contribution of protein kinase C to central sensitization and persistent pain following tissue injury. *Neurosci Lett* 1992;140:181–184.

Colpaert FC. Theoretical review: discriminative stimulus properties of narcotic analgesic drugs. *Pharmacol Biochem Behav* 1978;9:863–887.

Corrigall WA, Coen KM. Selective D1 and D2 dopamine antagonists decrease response rates of food-maintained behavior and reduce the discriminative stimulus produced by heroin. *Pharmacol Biochem Behav* 1990;35:351–355.

Crain SM, Shen KF. After chronic opioid exposure sensory neurons become supersensitive to the excitatory effects of opioid agonists and antagonists as occurs after acute elevation of GMI ganglioside. *Brain Res* 1992;575:13–24.

Devlin T, Shoemaker WJ. Characterization of kappa opioid binding using dynorphin A1-134 and U69,593 in the rat brain. *J Pharmacol Exp Ther* 1990;253:749–759.

Dickenson AH, Sullivan AF, Fournié-Zaluski MC, Roques BP. Prevention of degradation of endogenous enkephalins produces inhibition of nociceptive neurons in rat spinal cord. *Brain Res* 1987; 408:185–191.

Dickenson AH, Sullivan AF. Differential effects of excitatory amino acid antagonists on dorsal horn nociceptive neurones in the rat. *Brain Res* 1990;506:31–39.

Dohlman HG, Thorner J, Caron MG, Lefkowitz RJ. Systems for the study of seven-transmembrane-segment receptors. *Annu Rev Biochem* 1992;60:653–688.

Draisci G, Iadarola MJ. Temporal analysis of increases in c-fos, preprodynorphin and preproenkephalin mRNAs in rat spinal cord. *Molec. Brain Res* 1989;6:31–37.

Dubner R, Ruda MA. Activity-dependent neuronal plasticity following tissue injury and inflammation. *Trends Neurosci* 1992;15:96–103.

Duggan AW. Neuropharmacology of pain. *Curr Opin Neurol Neurosurg* 1992;5:503–507.

Duggan AW, Fleetwood-Walker SM. Opioids and sensory processing in the central nervous system. In: Herz A, Akil H, Simon EJ, eds. *Handbook of experimental pharmacology.* Berlin: Springer, 1992; 731–772.

Evans CJ, Keith DE Jr, Magendzo K, Edwards RH. Cloning of a delta opioid receptor by functional expression. *Science* 1992;258:1952–1955.

Faccini E, Uzumaki M, Govoni S, Missale C, Spano PF, Covelli V, Trabucchi M. Afferent fibers mediate the increase of metenkephalin elicited in rat spinal cord by localized pain. *Pain* 1984;18: 25–31.

Fukuda K, Kato S, Mori K, Nishi M, Takeshima H. Primary structures and expression from cDNAs of rat opioid receptor δ- and μ- subtypes. *FEBS Lett* 1993;327:311–314.

Gerber G, Kangrga I, Dyu PD, Larew JSA, Randic M. Multiple effects of phorbol esters in the rat spinal dorsal horn. *J Neurosci* 1989;9:3606–3617.

Goldberg SR, Schuster CR. Conditioned suppression by a stimulus associated with nalorphine in morphine-dependent monkeys. *J Exp Anal Behav* 1967;10:235–242.

Greengard P, Jen J, Nairn AC, Stevens CF. Enhancement of the glutamate response by cAMP-dependent protein kinase in hippocampal neurons. *Science* 1991;253:1135–1138.

Hartell NA, Headley PM. The effect of naloxone on spinal reflexes to electrical and mechanical stimuli in the anaesthetized, spinalized rat. *J Physiol (Lond)* 1991;442:513–526.

Heinricher MM, Morgan MM, Fields HL. Direct and indirect actions of morphine on medullary neurons that modulate nociception. *Neuroscience* 1992;48:533–543.

Herdegen T, Leah JD, Manisali A, Bravo R, Zimmermann M. c-JUN-like immunoreactivity in the CNS of the adult rat: basal and transsynaptically induced expression of an immediate-early gene. *Neuroscience* 1991a;41:643–654.

Herdegen T, Kovary K, Leah L, Bravo R. Specific temporal and spatial distribution of JUN, FOS, and KROX-24 proteins in spinal neurons following noxious transsynaptic stimulation. *J Comp Neurol* 1991b;313:178–191.

Herdegen T, Tölle TR, Bravo R, Zieglgänsberger W, Zimmermann M. Sequential expression of JUN B, JUN D and FOS B proteins in rat spinal neurons: cascade of transcriptional operations during nociception. *Neurosci Lett* 1991c;129:221–224.

Herdegen T, Walker T, Bravo R, Leah JD, Zimmermann M. The KROX-24 protein, a new transcription regulating factor: expression in the rat nervous system following afferent somatosensory stimulation. *Neurosci Lett* 1990;120:21–24.

Herz A, Shippenberg TS. Neurochemical aspects of addiction: Opioids and other drugs of abuse. In: Goldstein A, ed. *Molecular and cellular aspects of drug addiction.* New York: Springer, 1989; 111–141.

Höllt V. Opioid peptide genes: structure and regulation. In: Almeida OFX, Shippenberg TS, eds. *Neurobiology of opoids.* Berlin: Springer, 1991;11–51.

Hunt SP, Pini A, Evan G. Induction of c-fos-like protein in spinal cord neurones following sensory stimulation. *Nature* 1987;328:632–634.

Hylden JLK, Nahin RL, Traub RJ, Dubner R. Effects of spinal kappa-opioid receptor agonists on the responsiveness of nociceptive superficial dorsal horn neurons. *Pain* 1991;44:187–193.

Jackisch R, Hotz H, Hertting G. No evidence for presynaptic opioid receptors on cholinergic, but presence of kappa-receptors on dopaminergic neurons in the rabbit caudate nucleus: involvement of endogenous opioids. *Naunyn-Schmiedebergs Arch Pharmacol* 1993;348:234–241.

Kalivas PW, Stewart J. Dopamine transmission in the initiation and expression of drug- and stress-induced sensitization of motor activity. *Brain Res Rev* 1991;16:223–244.

Kalso EA, Sullivan AF, McQuay HJ, Dickenson AH. Spinal antinociception by Tyr-D-Ser(otbu)-Gly-Phe-Leu-Thr, a selective delta-opioid receptor agonist. *Eur J Pharmacol* 1992;216:97–101.

Kayser V, Fournié-Zaluski MC, Guilbaud G, Roques BP. Potent antinociceptive effects of kelatorphan (a highly efficient inhibitor of multiple enkephalin-degrading enzymes) systemically administered in normal and arthritic rats. *Brain Res* 1989;497:94–101.

Kehl LJ, Gogas KR, Lichtblau L, Pollock CH, Mayes M, Basbaum AI, Wilcox GL. The NMDA antagonist MK-801 reduces noxious stimulus-evoked Fos expression in the spinal dorsal horn. In: Bond MR, Charlton JE, Woolf CJ, eds. *Proceedings of the VIth World Congress on Pain. Pain research and clinical management*. Amsterdam: Elsevier, 1991;307–311.

Keith DE Jr, Anton B, Evans CJ. Characterization and mapping of a delta opioid receptor clone from NG108-15 cells. *Proc West Pharmacol Soc* 1993;36:299–306.

Kieffer BL, Befort K, Gaveriaux-Ruff C, Hirth CG. The δ-opioid receptor: isolation of a cDNA by expression cloning and pharmacological characterization. *Proc Natl Acad Sci USA* 1992;89:12048–12052.

Kong H, Raynor K, Yasuda K, Moe ST, Portoghese PS, Bell GI, Reisine T. A single residue, aspartic acid 95, in the δ opioid receptor specifies selective high affinity agonist binding. *J Biol Chem* 1993;268:23055–23058.

Koob GF. Drugs of abuse: Anatomy, pharmacology and function of reward pathways. *Trends Pharmacol Sci* 1992;13:177–184.

Linden DJ, Connor JA. Participation of postsynaptic PKC in cerebella long-term depression in culture. *Science* 1991;254:1656–1659.

Lombard MC, Besson JM. Electrophysiological evidence for a tonic activity of the spinal cord intrinsic opioid systems in a chronic pain model. *Brain Res* 1989;477:48–56.

Longoni R, Spina L, Mulas A, Carboni E, Garau L, Melchiorri P, Di Chiara G. (D-Ala2) Deltorphin II:D1-dependent stereotypies and stimulation of dopamine release in the nucleus accumbens. *J Neurosci* 1991;11:1565–1576.

Lord JAH, Waterfield AA, Hughes J, Kosterlitz HW. Endogenous opioid peptides: multiple agonists and receptors. *Nature* 1977;267:495–499.

Lyness WH, Smith FL, Heavner JE, Iacono CU, Garvin RD. Morphine self-administration in the rat during adjuvant-induced arthritis. *Life Sci* 1989;45:2217–2224.

Magnuson DS, Dickenson AH. Lamina-specific effects of morphine and naloxone in dorsal horn of rat spinal cord *in vitro*. *J Neurophysiol* 1991;66:1941–1950.

Magnuson DS, Sullivan AF, Simonnet G, Roques BP, Dickenson AH. Differential interactions of cholecystokinin and FLFQPQRF-NH2 with μ and δ opioid antinociception in the rat spinal cord. *Neuropeptides* 1990;16:213–218.

Mao J, Price DD, Mayer DJ, Hayes RL. Pain-related increases in spinal cord membrane-bound protein kinase C following peripheral nerve injury. *Brain Res* 1992;588:144–149.

Martin WR, Eades CG, Thompson JA, Huppler RE, Gilbert PE. The effects of morphine- and nalorphine-like drugs in the nondependent and morphine-dependent chronic spinal dog. *J Pharmacol Exp Ther* 1976;197:517–532.

Ménétrey D, Gannon A, Levine JD, Basbaum AJ. The expression of *c-fos* protein in presumed nociceptive interneurons and projection neurons of the rat spinal cord: anatomical mapping of the central effect of noxious somatic, articular and visceral stimulation. *J Comp Neurol* 1989;285:177–195.

Meng F, Xie GX, Thompson RC, Mansour A, Goldstein A, Watson SJ, Akil H. Cloning and pharmacological characterization of a rat κ opioid receptor. *Proc Natl Acad Sci USA* 1992;90:9954–9958.

Millan MJ, Millan MH, Pilcher CWT, Czolonkowski A, Herz AA, Colpaert FC. A model of chronic pain in the rat: response of multiple opioid systems to adjuvant-induced arthritis. *J Neurosci* 1986;6:899–906.

Minami Y, Toya T, Katao Y, Maekawa K, Nakamura S, Onogi T, Kaneko S, Satoh M. Cloning and expression of a cDNA for the rat κ-opioid receptor. *FEBS Lett* 1992;329:291–295.

Morgan MM, Heinricher MM, Fields HL. Circuitry linking opioid-sensitive nociceptive modulatory systems in periaqueductal gray and spinal cord with rostral ventromedial medulla. *Neuroscience* 1992;47:863–871.

Mucha RF, Herz A. Motivational properties of μ- and κ-opioid receptor agonists studied with place and taste preference conditioning procedure. *Psychopharmacology* 1985;86:274–280.

Mucha RF, Volkovskis G, Kalant H. Conditioned increases in locomotor activity produced with morphine as an unconditioned stimulus, and the relation of conditioning to acute morphine effect and tolerance. *J Comp Physiol Psychol* 1981;95:351–362.

Nairn AC, Shenolikar S. The role of protein phosphatases in synaptic transmission, plasticity and neuronal development. *Curr Opin Neurobiol* 1992;2:296–301.

Ohno M, Yamamoto T, Ueki S. Analgesic and discriminative stimulus properties of U-62,066E, the selective kappa-opioid receptor agonist, in the rat. *Psychopharmacology* 1992;106:31–38.

Overton DA. Applications and limitations of the drug discrimination method for the study of drug abuse. In: Bozarth MA, ed. *Methods of assessing the reinforcing properties of abused drugs.* Berlin: Springer, 1987a;291–340.

Overton DA. Major theories of state dependent learning. In: *Drug discrimination and state dependent learning.* New York: Academic Press, 1987b;283–318.

Pasternak GW, Wood PL. Multiple μ opiate receptors. *Life Sci* 1986;38:1889–1898.

Pert CB, Snyder SH. Opiate receptor; demonstration in nervous tissue. *Science* 1973;179:1011–1014.

Picker MJ, Doty P, Negus SS, Mattox SR, Dykstra LA. Discriminative stimulus properties of U50, 488 and morphine: Effects of training dose on stimulus substitution patterns produced by mu and kappa opioid agonists. *J Pharmacol Exp Ther* 1990;254:13–22.

Picker MJ, Dykstra LA. Discriminative stimulus effects of mu and kappa opioids in the pigeon: analysis of the effects of full and partial mu and kappa agonists. *J Pharmacol Exp Ther* 1989;249:557–566.

Portenoy RK, Foley KM, Inturrisi CE. The nature of opioid responsiveness and its implications for neuropathic pain: new hypotheses derived from studies of opioid infusions. *Pain* 1990;43: 273–286.

Porter J, Jick H. Addiction rare in patients treated with narcotics. *N Engl J Med* 1980;302:123.

Portoghese P, Sultana M, Nagase H, Takemori A. A highly selective delta 1-opioid receptor antagonist: 7-benzylidenaltrexone. *Eur J Pharmacol* 1992;218:195–196.

Presley RW, Ménétrey D, Levine JD, Basbaum AI. Systemic morphine supresses noxious stimulus-evoked Fos protein-like immunoreactivity in the rat spinal cord. *J Neurosci* 1990;10:323–335.

Raymond LA, Blackstone CD, Huganir RL. Phosphorylation and modulation of recombinant GluR6 glutamate receptors by cAMP-dependent protein kinase. *Nature* 1993;361:637–641.

Reisine T, Bell GI. Molecular biology of opioid receptors. *Trends Neurosci* 1993;16:506–510.

Roques BP, Gacel G, Dauge V, Baamonde A, Galenco G, Turcaud S, Coric P, Fournié-Zaluski MC. Novel approaches in the development of new analgesics. *Neurophysiol Clin* 1990;20:369–387.

Roques BP, Noble F, Dauge V, Fournié-Zaluski MC, Beaumont A. Neutral endopeptidase 24.11: structure, inhibition, and experimental and clinical pharmacology. *Pharmacol Rev* 1993;45:87–146.

Rusin KI, Randic M. Modulation of NMDA-induced currents by mu-opioid receptor against DAMGO in acutely isolated rat spinal dorsal horn neurons. *Neurosci Lett* 1991;124:208–212.

Shearman GT, Herz A. Evidence that the discriminative stimulus properties of fentanyl and ethyletocyclazocine are mediated by an interaction with different opiate receptors. *J Pharmacol Exp Ther* 1982;221:735–739.

Shippenberg TS. Motivational effects of opioids. In: Herz A, ed. *Opioids I, vol. 2.* Berlin/Heidelberg: Springer-Verlag, 1993;633–650.

Shippenberg TS, Bals-Kubik R, Herz A. Examination of the neurochemical substrates mediating the motivational effects of opioids: Role of the mesolimbic dopamine system and D-1 vs. D-2 dopamine receptors. *J Pharmacol Exp Ther* 1993;265:53–59.

Shippenberg TS, Stein C, Huber A, Millan MJ, Herz A. Motivational effects of opioids in an animal model of prolonged inflammatory pain: Alteration in the effects of κ- but not μ-receptor agonists. *Pain* 1988;35:176–186.

Shoaib M, Spanagel R. Mesolimbic sites mediate the diskriminative stimulus effects of morphine. *Eur J Pharmacol* 1994;252:69–75.

Simon EJ, Hiller JM, Edelman I. Stereospecific binding of the potent narcotic analgesic ³H-etorphine to rat brain homogenate. *Proc Natl Acad Sci USA* 1973;70:1947–1949.

Skilling SR, Sun XF, Kurtz HJ, Larson AA. Selective potentiation of NMDA-induced activity and release of excitatory amino acids by dynorphin—possible roles in paralysis and neurotoxicity. *Brain Res* 1992;575:272–278.

Smith JAM, Loughlin SE, Leslie FM. kappa-Opioid inhibition of [3H]dopamine release from rat ventral mesencephalic dissociated cell cultures. *Mol Pharmacol* 1992;42:575–583.

Sommer B, Seeburg PH. Glutamate receptor channels: novel properties and new clones. *Trends Pharmacol Sci* 1992;13:291–296.

Spanagel R, Herz A, Shippenberg TS. The effects of opioid peptides on dopamine release in the nucleus accumbens: An *in vivo* microdialysis study. *J Neurochem* 1990;55:1734–1740.

Spanagel R, Herz A, Shippenberg TS. Opposing tonically active endogenous opioid systems modulate the mesolimbic dopaminergic pathway. *Proc Natl Acad Sci USA* 1992;89:2046–2050.

Spanagel R, Herz A, Shippenberg TS. Identification of the opioid receptor types mediating β-endorphin-induced alterations in dopamine release in the nucleus accumbens. *Eur J Pharmacol* 1990;190:177–184.

Spyraki C. Drug reward studied by use of place conditioning in rats. Oxford: Oxford University Press, 1988.

Stein C. Peripheral analgesic actions of opioids. *J Pain Sympt Mgmt* 1991;6:119–124.

Stein C, Gramsch C, Herz A. Intrinsic mechanisms of antinociception in inflammation: Local opioid receptors and beta-endorphin. *J Neurosci* 1990;10:1292–1298.

Stewart J. Conditioned and unconditioned drug effects in relapse to opiate and stimulant drug self-administration. *Prog Neuropsychopharmacol Biol Psychiatry* 1983;7:591–597.

Stolerman I. Drugs of abuse: Behavioural principles, methods and terms. *Trends Pharmacol Sci* 1992;13:170–176.

Sullivan AF, Dickenson AH, Roques BP. Delta-opioid mediated inhibitions of acute and prolonged noxious-evoked responses in rat dorsal horn neurones. *Br J Pharmacol* 1989;98:1039–1049.

Swope SL, Moss SJ, Blackstone CD, Huganir RL. Phosphorylation of ligand-gated ion channels: a possible mode of synaptic plasticity. *FASEB J* 1992;6:2514–2523.

Takahashi O, Traub RJ, Ruda MA. Demonstration of calcitonin gene-related peptide immunoreactive axons contacting dynorphin A(1–8) immunoreactive spinal neurons in a rat model of peripheral inflammation and hyperalgesia. *Brain Res* 1988;475:168–172.

Terenius L. Stereospecific interaction between narcotic analgesics and a synaptic plasma membrane fraction of rat brain cortex. *Acta Pharmacol Toxicol (Copenh)* 1973;32:317–320.

Thompson RC, Mansour A, Akil H, Watson SJ. Cloning and pharmacological characterization of a rat μ opioid receptor. *Neuron* 1993;11:905–913.

Tölle TR, Ableitner A, Castro-Lopes JM, Zieglgänsberger W. C-*fos* protein, prodynorphin mRNA, and protein kinase C are altered with distinct spatial and temporal patterns in the spinal cord of monoarthritic rats. In: Gebhart GF, Hammond DL, Jensen TS, eds. *Proceedings of the VIIth World Congress on Pain*, vol. 2. *Progress in pain research and management*. Seattle: IASP Press, 1994a;409–422.

Tölle TR, Castro-Lopes JM, Coimbra A, Zieglgänsberger W. Opiates modify induction of c-*fos* proto-oncogene in the spinal cord of the rat following noxious stimulation. *Neurosci Lett* 1990;111:46–51.

Tölle TR, Castro-Lopes JM, Evan G, Zieglgänsberger W. C-*fos* induction in the spinal cord following noxious stimulation: prevention by opiates but not by NMDA antagonists. In: Bond MR, Charlton JE, Woolf CJ, eds. *Proceedings of the VIth World Congress on Pain. Pain research and clinical management*. Amsterdam: Elsevier, 1991;299–305.

Tölle TR, Herdegen T, Schadrack J, Bravo R, Zimmermann M, Zieglgänsberger W. Application of morphine prior to noxious stimulation differentially modulates expression of Fos, Jun and Krox-24 proteins in rat spinal cord neurons. *Neuroscience* 1994b;58:305–321.

Tölle TR, Schadrack J, Castro-Lopes JM, Evan G, Roques BP, Zieglgänsberger W. Effects of kelatorphan and morphine before and after noxious stimulation on immediate-early gene expression in rat spinal cord neurons. *Pain* 1994c;56:103–112.

Traub RJ, Pechmann P, Iadarola MJ, Gebhart GF. Fos-like proteins in the lumbosacral spinal cord following noxious and non-noxious colorectal distention in the rat. *Pain* 1992;49:393–403.

Vaccarino FM, Hayward MD, Nestler EJ, Duman RS, Tallman JF. Differential induction of immediate early genes by excitatory amino acid receptor types in primary cultures of cortical and striatal neurons. *Mol Brain Res* 1992;12:233–241.

Vezina P, Giovino AA, Wise RA, Stewart J. Environment-specific cross-sensitization between the locomotor activating effects of morphine and amphetamine. *Pharmacol Biochem Behav* 1989;32:581–584.

Vidal C, Maier R, Zieglgänsberger W. Effects of dynorphin A_{1-17}, dynorphin A_{1-13} and D-ala^2-D-leu^5-enkephalin on the excitability of pyramidal cells in CA1 and CA2 of the rat hippocampus *in vitro*. *Neuropeptides* 1984;5:237–240.

Wang JB, Imai Y, Eppler CM, Gregor P, Spivak CE, Uhl GR. μ Opiate receptor: cDNA cloning and expression. *Proc Natl Acad Sci USA* 1993;90:10230–10234.

Wang LY, Salter MW, MacDonald JF. Regulation of kainate receptors by cAMP-dependent protein kinase and phosphatases. *Science* 1991;253:1132–1135.

Wiesenfeld-Hallin Z, Xu XJ, Hakanson R, Fend DM, Folkers K. Low-dose intrathecal morphine facilitates the spinal flexor reflex by releasing different neuropeptides in rats with intact and sectioned peripheral nerves. *Brain Res* 1991;551:157–162.

Williams S, Evan G, Hunt SP. Changing patterns of c-FOS induction in spinal neurons following thermal cutaneous stimulation in the rat. *Neuroscience* 1990;36:73–81.

Wisden W, Errington ML, Williams S, Dunnett SB, Waters C, Hitchcock D, Evan G, Bliss TV, Hunt SP. Differential expression of immediate early genes in the hippocampus and spinal cord. *Neuron* 1990;4:603–614.

Wise RA. The role of reward pathways in the development of drug dependence. *Pharmacol Ther* 1987; 35:227–263.

Wise RA, Bozarth MA. Action of drugs of abuse on brain reward systems: an update with specific attention to opiates. *Pharmacol Biochem Behav* 1982;17:239–243.

Wise RA, Rompre PP. Brain dopamine and reward. *Annu Rev Psychol* 1989;40:191–225.

Zieglgänsberger W. An enkephalinergic gating system involved in nociception? In: Costa E, Trabucchi M, eds. *Neural peptides and neuronal communication*, New York: Raven Press, 1980;425–434.

Zieglgänsberger W. Central control of nociception. In: Mountcastle VB, Bloom FE, Geiger SR, eds. *Handbook of physiology*, vol. 4. *The nervous system*. Baltimore: Williams & Wilkins, 1986;581–656.

Zieglgänsberger W, French ED, Siggins GR, Bloom FE. Opioid peptides may excite hippocampal pyramidal neurons by inhibiting adjacent inhibitory interneurons. *Science* 1979;205:415–417.

Zieglgänsberger W, Tölle TR. The pharmacology of pain signalling. *Curr Opin Neurobiol* 1993;3: 611–618.

Pain and the Brain: From Nociception to Cognition, edited by Burkhart Bromm and John E. Desmedt, Advances in Pain Research and Therapy Vol. 22. Raven Press, Ltd., New York © 1995.

31

The Pharmaco-Electroencephalogram of Analgesic and Psychotropic Drugs

Werner M. Herrmann

Laboratory of Clinical Psychophysiology, Department of Psychiatry, Free University of Berlin, D-14050 Berlin, Germany

SUMMARY

Psychotropic drugs, taken as single doses by healthy volunteers, have been successfully classified on the basis of pharmacodynamic electroencephalographic (EEG) models. Not only could a pattern of sedation and of stimulation be discriminated from the EEG pattern with placebo, but different types of EEG mechanisms causing subjective sedation have also been identified. The major mechanisms for sedation are represented by (a) a shift from a normal, reactive alpha/beta EEG pattern to more slow-wave activity (as with tricyclic antidepressants), and (b) a shift from a flexible alpha/beta EEG pattern to a more rigid beta EEG (as with minor tranquilizers), or from a flexible alpha into a more rigid sub-alpha pattern (as with neuroleptic drugs). It is well-known that analgesic drugs cause changes in the nociceptive system that can be identified by pain-evoked protentials. The question is whether changes in the background activity itself are indicators of the analgesic effect of psychotropic and analgesic drugs. Several examples suggest that in addition to specific nociceptive effects, a change in vigilance contributes to the subjective analgesic effect. The antidepressants imipramine and amitriptyline cause a transfer from alpha to polymorphic slow waves, and subjects given these drugs show a pronounced decrease in vigilance after acute medication. It is understandable that the underlying physiologic effects of tricyclic antidepressants can at least contribute to the analgesic pattern produced by these drugs. Another model is that of minor tranquilizers. If information processing is generally slowed by a forcing of the vigilance system into a rigid, spindling beta activity, it is quite understandable that at least the consciousness of pain would be changed. Some types of surgery can be done after the i.v. infusion of about 50 mg of diazepam. Subjects may show behavioral signs of pain, such as crying without later remembering pain. Obviously, changes in subjective feelings about pain also depend on memory processes. On the basis of these observations, we believe that in addition to specific nociceptive effects, various psychotropic drugs influence the perception of pain and may be valid tools in the treatment of pain.

INTRODUCTION

Analgesic research has had two traditional roots: nociceptive research and research in higher mental information processing. Since many of the known psychotropic drugs also influence the brain's processing of information, it seems a logical consequence that psychotropic drugs would be screened for their analgesic potential and tested for their utility in the treatment of pain. Among the psychotropic agents used in the treatment of pain are some with known nociceptive effects, such as tricyclic antidepressants of the imipramine type, and others without a specific nociceptive effect. However, imipramine is not an approved drug for the treatment of pain states, nor have psychotropic agents been screened systematically for their analgesic potential in human pharmacologic experiments.

The purpose of this chapter is to describe effects of psychotropic and analgesic agents on the spontaneous, waking electroencephalographic (EEG) activity of volunteers in clinical pharmacologic experiments, and to develop a hypothesis for how such effects could contribute to analgesia. It will be shown that psychotropic agents have differential effects on the spontaneous, waking EEG. Some of these effects (e.g., the vigilance effects) should influence pain perception and could explain the analgesic potential of some psychotropic drugs. It will also be shown that all analgesics so far tested, including so-called "weak" or "nonnarcotic" ones, have characteristic effects on the spontaneous waking EEG through interactions with the vigilance system. Vigilance in the neurophysiologic meaning and in context with the waking EEG is defined as the readiness of a cortical system to function and to process information. It will be hypothesized that analgesia is caused not only by nociception but also by an interaction with the vigilance system.

THE PHARMACO-EEG MODEL FOR PSYCHOTROPIC DRUGS

The basic activity of the cerebral cortex and any changes induced in it by psychotropic drugs can be measured by recording an EEG. Since Berger's suggestions for EEG evaluations, first published in 1932, and Dietsch's (1932) introduction of the Fourier analysis method, many methods of EEG analysis, both visual and computer-aided, have been developed. Automated EEG analysis, based on the power-spectrum technique, has in recent decades undergone considerable improvement and become the most commonly used method for providing a quantitative description of EEG activity. This procedure has been used for investigating most of the psychotropic drugs. Moreover, the quantitative pharmaco-EEG has been used to study the effects of cannabis (Volavka et al. 1974; Koukkou and Lehmann 1978), morphines and both their agonists and antagonists (Kubicki et al. 1977; Volavka et al. 1979), beta blockers (Wagner et al. 1981), ergot alkaloids (Itil et al. 1975), hormones (Itil et al. 1974; Itil 1968; Itil and Herrmann 1978), and the so-called nootropic drugs (Künkel and Westphal 1970; Bente 1977). The allocation of psychotropic drugs to classes, which will subsequently be referred to in terms of their classification, was first and foremost based on their therapeutic efficacy. For a long time the description of sedative-hypnotic and central nervous system (CNS)-stimulating effects received the greatest emphasis. With the discovery of the psychotropic drugs in the 1950s, new spectra of effects were defined, and increasingly specific (psychotropic) components of effects were differentiated from nonspecific sedative or stimulating effects, as occurred for the mood-elevating and the sedating antidepressants.

The current clinical classification of psychotropic drugs, which was essentially established during the 1960s and early 1970s, delineates four major classes of these drugs (Degkwitz 1967; Wandrey and Leutner 1967; Kielholz and Pöldinger 1968; Haase 1969; Arnold et al. 1970; Pöldinger 1971; Honigfeld and Howard 1973; Nahunek 1973; AMA 1977): neuroleptics, anxiolytics, antidepressants, and psychostimulants. The boundaries between the classes are drawn by means of defined effects on delimited clinical syndromes. The allocation of psychotropic drugs to particular classes has been a developmental process that has lasted for years, in which, in addition to clinical experience, structural chemical considerations, biochemical, and pharmacologic methods have participated (see: Korolkovas 1970; Fenner 1971, 1974; Creese and Snyder 1978; Guidotti 1978; Koe 1974, 1975; Fielding and Lal 1974; Randall and Kappell 1973; Niemegeers 1975; Niemegeers and Janssen 1975; Carlsson 1978; Haefely 1978; Janssen and van Bever 1978; Innes and Nickerson 1970; Jarvik 1970; Ritchie 1970; Ladinsky et al. 1973; Lidbrink et al. 1973; Stille 1976; Snyder et al. 1977; Braestrup and Squires 1978; Bunney and Aghajanian 1978; Carlsson 1978; Carlsson and Lindqvist 1978; Goodwin et al. 1978; Guidotti 1978; Iversen 1978; Longo, 1978; Murphy et al. 1978; Schildkraut 1978). With these methods, it was generally possible to differentiate the four therapeutic classes listed above. Every model for a classification is valid only within its limitations and for only those types of drugs for which it was developed. The models therefore do not necessarily describe the biochemical, pharmacologic, or electrophysiologic phenomena of the illnesses to be treated with a drug, but rather its partial effects on different systems in the CNS.

It has long been apparent that stimulants and sedatives induce different types of changes in the EEG. Moreover, clear differences have been observed in the EEG patterns produced by different classes of drugs with sedative effects, such as minor tranquilizers, 1,4-benzodiazepines, barbiturates, tricyclic antidepressants, and neuroleptic drugs. Consequently, it is possible to distinguish between the sedative compounds, since they all exhibit EEG changes that are different from one another yet typical for their particular class. In the following discussion, examples of the EEG changes in the occipital region (lead O_2–A_2) for three therapeutic drug classes (i.e., anxiolytics, neuroleptics, and antidepressants) will be given.

Chlorpromazine at a dose of 75 mg has been selected here as a representative of the sedative neuroleptics. Fig. 1A shows a well-modulated occipital alpha EEG

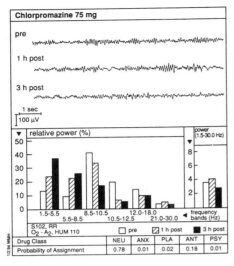

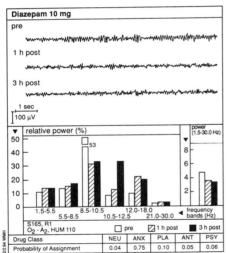
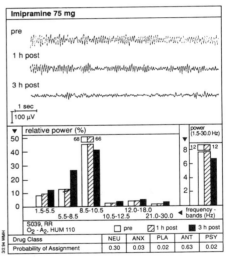

FIG. 1A–C. Pharmaco-EEG profiles of typical psychotropic substances in human pharmacologic experiments done with healthy volunteers and double-blind, placebo-controlled crossover designs. The results are from single subjects and are typical for the drug class. In the upper part of the figure are shown typical EEG segments before, at 1 hour, and at 3 hours after drug intake. The middle part of the figure contains the absolute power values as well as the relative power values in predetermined frequency classes. The lower part of the figure shows the allocation probability of this particular subject into the five-class classification system: NEU = neuroleptics; ANX = anxiolytics; PLA = placebo; ANT = antidepressants; PSY = psychostimulants.

rhythm before drug intake. One hour after dosing there are more slow waves in the delta range, together with the typical increase in the sub-alpha to fast-theta range. At the same time there is a decrease in the the occipital beta power but an increase in the frontocentral beta power. These effects are even more apparent at 3 hours after dosing. These findings show that upon treatment with neuroleptic drugs, the EEG converts to slower waves. This is apparently most typical of neuroleptic drugs and can be interpreted as a deactivation of cortical functions, with a simultaneous second apparent effect consisting of the increase in frontocentral beta power, interpreted as an activating property of these drugs (Coppola and Herrmann 1987).

Diazepam (Fig. 1B) is representative of the anxiolytic class of psychotropic drugs, which has received the greatest attention in pharmaco-EEG studies. Following the oral administration of 10 mg of diazepam, there is an apparent decrease in the alpha portion and alpha amplitude of the EEG, and an increase in the fast- and slow-beta waves. In addition to a small increase in the slow frequencies, there is a shift from slow-alpha to fast-alpha activity, generally shifting further to slow-beta spindle-like activity, as well as an increase in diffuse fast-beta activity.

Imipramine at a dose of 75 mg (Fig. 1C) is here an example of the sedative tricyclic antidepressants, which induce a destruction of the alpha rhythm, an increase in slow-wave activity of up to 8.5 Hz, and an increase in the fast-frequency range. It is characteristic of sedative tricyclic antidepressants that after their acute use they produce a marked decrease in the relative and absolute alpha power and an increase in the delta and beta power.

On the basis of these observations, the EEG should be able to discriminate not only between sedative and stimulating drugs, but also among the different psychotropic drug classes that have primarily sedative or deactivating effects.

In order to establish a classification system, we tested 16 typical psychotropic substances as well as four placebos in four basic trials (Herrmann 1982). Each trial was designed as a controlled, randomized fivefold investigation with a crossover and double-blind protocol. Accordingly, there were 15 independent young, healthy male subjects who received each substance in the indicated dose, and 60 independent subjects as representatives of the four therapeutic drug classes and placebo. The placebo served to control the interpretation of the drug effects. We anticipated having four drug classes, consisting of anxiolytics, neuroleptics, antidepressants, and psychostimulants, and the placebo class. A five-group linear discriminant analysis was applied in order to find a rule with a minimum of false reclassifications. The target variables were defined on the basis of parametrization procedures that estimate the power portions of frequency classes, and were specified as the percentage of the total power within a given frequency band. The frequency bands were defined on the basis of a structural analysis of the EEG data (Herrmann et al. 1980), which should maximize independency and minimize redundant target variables.

After the classification rule was constructed, it was applied to the 20 treatments. This procedure was called reclassification. The results of the reclassification system showed that 17 of 20 substances could be reclassified correctly.

The reclassification was conducted in order to establish the relationship between the clinical therapeutic efficacy of the drugs and their projections within the classification system. It was intended to provide information about whether psychotropic drugs, which were allocated to drug classes according to their clinical therapeutic efficacy, would project in a class-specific manner to the functional level of the EEG according to an objective rule.

In order to understand the classification rule, normalized coefficients of the discriminant function were evaluated (Fig. 2). The variables selected were factor scores (Herrmann 1982, p. 322 ff).

Although the placebo showed no preference for any variable, the psychotropic

Variables		Times of Measurement	Coefficients of the Discriminant Function				
Factor No.	Factor Name		NEUroleptics	ANXiolytics	PLAcebos	ANTidepressants	PSYchostimulants
1	delta $^F\uparrow$/alpha$_1$$^F\downarrow$	pre 1 h 3h	− 0.698 O − 0.326 o + 0.697 ●	− 0.487 O − 0.114 O + 0.652 ●	− 0.340 O − 0.182 O + 0.154 ●	− 1.050 O − 0.500 O + 1.239 ●	+ 0.177 ● − 0.428 O − 0.133 O
2	theta $^F\uparrow$/alpha$_1$$^F\downarrow$	pre 1 h 3 h	− 2.452 O − 0.264 ● + 1.795 ●	− 0.089 o − 0.089 O + 0.125 ●	− 0.779 O + 0.103 ● + 0.449 ●	− 1.286 O + 0.221 ● + 0.754 ●	− 0.764 O + 0.631 ● − 0.033 O
3	alpha$_2$$\uparrow$/alpha$_1$$^F\downarrow$	pre 1 h 3 h	− 0.410 O + 0.810 ● − 0.371 O	− 0.008 O − 0.255 O + 0.118 ●	− 0.382 O + 0.045 ● + 0.398 ●	− 0.658 O + 0.231 ● + 0.480 ●	− 0.481 O + 0.175 ● + 0.325 ●
4	beta$_1$$^F\uparrow$/alpha$_1$$^F\downarrow$	pre 1 h 3h	+ 0.468 ● + 0.320 ● − 0.962 O	− 2.034 O + 0.837 ● + 1.306 ●	− 0.292 O − 0.111 O + 0.468 ●	+ 0.085 ● − 0.183 O − 0.017 O	− 0.384 O + 0.231 ● + 0.057 ●
5	beta$_3$$^F\uparrow$/alpha$_1$$^F\downarrow$	pre 1 h 3 h	+ 0.780 ● − 0.258 O − 0.493 O	− 0.305 O − 0.132 O + 0.301 ●	+ 0.324 ● − 0.191 O − 0.132 O	+ 0.071 ● − 0.473 O + 0.569 ●	+ 0.598 ● + 0.301 ● − 0.275 O
Total Power	1.5-30.0 Hz	1h-pre	↑	Ø	, ↑	Ø	↑
		3h-pre	Ø	↓	↑	↓	↑

RR ↑ (↑) definite   ↓ (↓) (slight) — Increase or decrease — high (medium) — positive or negative loading profile — Ø no change

FIG. 2. Normalized coefficients of the discriminant-function analysis (five groups for five substance classes). The variables are factor scores of the five main bipolar factors. All of the factors also have loadings in the alpha-1-F band. The factor delta-F ↑ /alpha$_1$-F ↓ would mean that alpha rhythm is replaced by delta rhythm. The data are for 60 subjects with high resting alpha rhythms and closed eyes, on lead: O_zT_6.

agents did exhibit preferences for certain variables: Neuroleptics exhibited a preference for theta-F (shift from flexible alpha into the more rigid sub-alpha), anxiolytics for slow beta-1-F (shift from flexible alpha into synchronized beta spindle activity), antidepressants for delta-F and beta-3-F (destruction of alpha rhythm and transfer into polymorphic slow waves and diffuse fast beta activity), and psychostimulants for the same variables as the antidepressants but in the reverse direction.

If we assume that both benzodiazepine tranquilizers and tricyclic antidepressants of the imipramine type can contribute to analgesia through different neurophysiologic mechanisms, the question will be raised of whether analgesic agents exhibit pharmaco-EEG effects similar to those of psychotropic drugs.

EFFECTS OF ANALGESICS USING THE PHARMACO-EEG MODEL

As examples of analgesics, paracetamol 500 mg and 1,000 mg, flupirtine 200 mg, and pentazocine 100 mg were investigated.

Paracetamol

In a placebo-controlled human pharmacologic experiment (Herrmann et al. 1994) with 27 subjects, EEG effects of paracetamol were seen in the delta, $alpha_2$, $beta_1$ and $beta_3$ bands (Fig. 3). The increase in delta activity was seen only after 1,000 mg and in the temporal region under acoustic stimulation. The alpha-2 reduction became apparent with 500 mg and more pronounced with 1,000 mg, both in the resting EEG and with acoustic stimuli, while during videotracking there were no effects in comparison to placebo. In the $beta_1$ and $beta_3$ bands, the only tendencies exhibited were toward an increase, preferably with acoustic stimulation and in both the frontal and temporal regions.

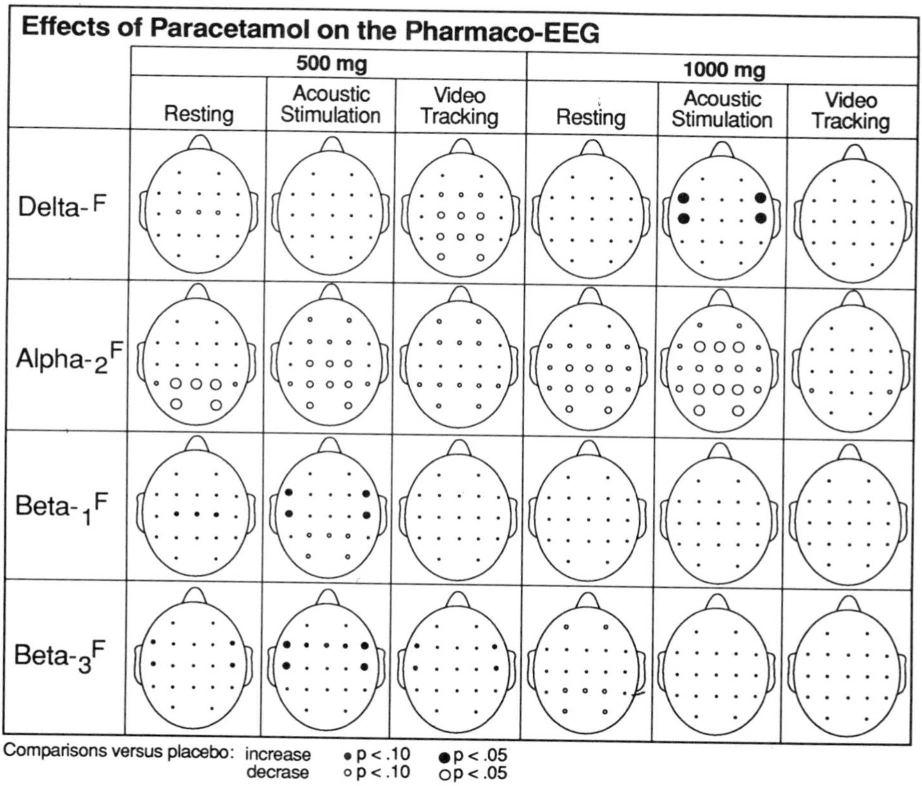

Effects of Paracetamol on the Pharmaco-EEG

Comparisons versus placebo: increase ● $p < .10$ ● $p < .05$
                          decrase   ○ $p < .10$ ○ $p < .05$

FIG. 3. Effects of 500 mg and 1,000 mg paracetamol on the pharmaco-EEG for 27 subjects. Comparisons are versus placebo; p-values are descriptive. Acoustic stimulation was done by two tones (500 and 1,000 Hz) given in randomized order. The subjects had to react and press a button. The videotracking was done by a signal moving on the screen, followed by the subject via a joystick.

Flupirtine

As described by Herrmann and Irrgang (1984) and by Bromm et al. 1987, flupirtine did not produce an increase in slow waves, but rather a massive shift from alpha to sub-alpha activity in the occipital region under acoustic stimulation (Fig. 4A), and a massive increase in the beta range in the frontocentral area in both the slow- and the fast-beta range (Fig. 4B). The slow-beta effect was an increase in synchronized activity such as that with minor tranquilizers, while the fast-beta effect was a low-voltage, desynchronized activity.

Pentazocine

The pentazocine data were obtained from the same trial as the flupirtine data (a double-blind, placebo controlled, randomized, crossover trial with 12 subjects).

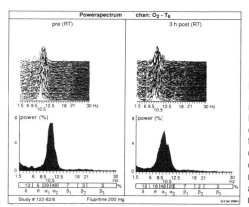

FIG. 4A–D. Effects of flupirtine 200 mg and pentazocine 100 mg on the pharmaco-EEG in 12 subjects in a double-blind, controlled trial including placebo, with a threefold crossover. RS = resting recording; RT = reaction-time recording (see legend to Fig. 5). The upper part of the figure shows the EEG power-spectrum curves for each 4-sec segment as relative power %. The middle part of the figure shows mean plot over all segments. In the lower part are given the relative power values in predetermined frequency classes.

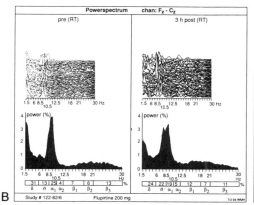

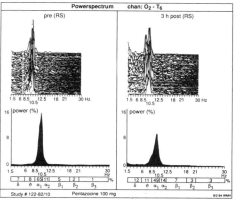

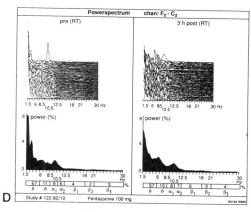

FIG. 4. *Continued.*

The results were described by Herrmann and Irrgang (1984). In this experiment pentazocine produced a massive desynchronization (the total power went from 5.5 to 2.5×10^8 $V^2 \times$ sec) of the alpha rhythm, with a relative increase in the slow- and fast-wave activity in the occipital region (Fig. 4C). A similar picture was seen in the frontocentral area. The total beta range was diffusely increased, while synchronized activity was decreased (Fig. 4D).

The conclusions derived from these pharmaco-EEG trials with substances having known nociceptive effects were that both narcotic (pentazocine) and non-narcotic (flupirtine, paracetamol) analgesics exhibit effects on the spontaneous, waking EEG after single oral doses in healthy volunteers. Earlier statements that non-narcotic (so-called "weak" or "peripherally active") analgesics have no CNS effects must be revised.

As shown in Fig. 5, there are two major pharmaco-EEG effects of the analgesics tested:

1. A decrease in alpha and an increase in polymorphic slow-wave activity, which is a typical change with a neurophysiologic decrease in vigilance. Such changes in vigilance correlate with a decrease in performance in the critical-flicker fusion test and serial addition (Pauli) test (Ott et al. 1982). It is very possible that a decrease in vigilance also has an effect on analgesic perception, and thus expresses analgesia in an indirect manner.
2. An increase in beta activity, preferentially in the frontocentral region. The effects in the beta range are twofold, comprising an increase in synchronized slow-beta activity and an increase in diffuse fast-beta activity. A shift from flexible alpha into more rigid, spindle-like beta activity is the physiologic correlate of the tranquilizing/sedative effects of benzodiazepine anxiolytics. It is understandable that this effect will change the perception of analgesia. The increase in diffuse fast-beta activity in the frontocentral area has been observed for all analgesics so

	drug and dosage	delta-F	theta-F	alpha	slow beta	fast beta	synchron-ization
	placebo	↓↑ 1)	∅	↑↓	∅	∅	∅
Analgetics	paracetamol 1000 mg	⬆	∅	↓	↑	↑	∅
Analgetics	flupirtine 200 mg	∅	∅	↓ 2)	⬆	⬆	∅
Analgetics	pentazocine 100 mg	⬆4)	∅	⬇	⬆4)	⬆4)	⬇
Psychotropics	diazepam 10 mg	↑	∅	⬇	⬆	↑	∅ 3)
Psychotropics	imipramine 75 mg	⬆	∅	⬇	∅	⬆4)	⬇

FIG. 5. Pharmaco-EEG effects of three analgesics in comparison to psychotropics with analgesic potential. The data were obtained from different pharmaco-EEG studies, all involving healthy young subjects with a high resting alpha rhythm in placebo controlled, double-blind crossover trials involving single oral doses. The test results for placebo are pre- and post-dose comparisons. The test results for psychotropic and analgesic agents are descriptive comparisons versus placebo: 1) Vigilance increase or decrease; 2) shift from alpha to subalpha; 3) transfer from synchronized alpha to synchronized slow beta, 4) relative power ∅ no significant change in comparison to placebo. ↓ ↑ tendency (p<.10); ⬇⬆increase/decrease (p<.05); ⬇ p <.01

far tested. Its importance is unknown. However, if the system were to be forced into rigid desynchronized beta activity and lose its flexibility for a rapid transition from alpha to non-alpha activity, this would correspond to the B-stages described by Bente (1977), who assumes a decrease in vigilance that corresponds with a decrease in performance. Again, it would be understandable that the cognition of pain were to be altered in this phsyiologic state.

HYPOTHESIS ABOUT PHARMACO-EEG CHANGES AND ANALGESIC POTENTIAL

On the basis of the EEG findings for the analgesics tested, and the pharmaco-EEG profile of psychotropic drugs with and without known analgesic potential, the following hypotheses are proposed:

1. Analgesics have, *a priori*, a central action as measurable by pharmaco-EEG.
2. Psychotropic drugs with analgesic potential have common pharmaco-EEG effects with analgesics.
3. In addition to nociceptive effects, a neurophysiologically defined decrease in vigilance contributes to the analgesic effects of these drugs. The mechanisms for a decrease in vigilance are: (a) an increase in polymorphic delta waves; (b) a

decrease in EEG dynamics and flexibility (transition from flexible alpha into more rigid beta spindle activity); and (c) a transition from A stages to B stages according to Bente (1977).

We therefore suggest that in future screenings of potential analgesics their effects on the waking EEG should be described in addition to testing of their nociceptive effects. It is necessary to examine the analgesic effects of such drugs both in terms of changes in the pain-evoked potential and changes in vigilance in the spontaneous waking EEG.

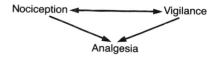

There will probably be an interaction between nociception and vigilance, and both elements will contribute to the analgesic effect. Future studies must investigate whether the concept of neurophysiologically determined vigilance is also a useful concept for the pain-relieving effects of psychotropic and analgesic drugs. This suggestion cannot, however, be a general answer to the problem of how the pharmaco-EEG can contribute to determining the analgesic potential of drugs, and how it may also change concepts relating to the development of new types of analgesics with combined nociceptive and psychotropic (cortical information process changing) properties.

REFERENCES

AMA Drug evaluations, 3rd ed. Littleton, MA: Publishing Sciences Group, 1977.

Arnold OH, Collard J, et al. Definition and classification of neuroleptics. In: Bobon DP, Janssen PAJ, et al. eds. *Modern problems of pharmacopsychiatry*, vol. 5: *The neuroleptics*. Basel: Karger, 1970;141–147.

Bente D. Vigilanz: Psychophysiologishce Aspekte. Verhandlungen der Deutschen Gesellschaft für innere Medizin. 83. Band. München: J.F. Bergmann Verlag, 1977;945–952.

Berger H. Über das Elektrenkephalogramm des Menschen. IV. Mitteilung. *Arch Psychiatr Nervenkrankh* 1932;97:6–26.

Braestrup C, Squires RF. Brain specific benzodiazepine receptors. *Br J Psychiatry* 1978;133:249–260.

Bromm B, Ganzel R, et al. The analgesic efficacy of flupirtine in comparison to pentazocine and placebo assessed by EEG parameters and subjective pain ratings. *Postgrad Med J* 1987;63:109–112.

Bunney BS, Aghajanian GK. Mesolimbic and mesocortical dopaminergic systems: Physiology and pharmacology. In: Lipton MA, di Mascio A, et al., eds. Psychopharmacology: A generation of progress. New York: Raven Press, 1978;159–169.

Carlsson A. Mechanism of action of neuroleptic drugs. In: Lipton M.A., di Mascio A, et al., eds. *Psychopharmacology: A generation of progress*. New York: Raven Press, 1978;1057–1070.

Carlsson A, Lindqvist M. Effects of antidepressant agents on monoamine synthesis. In: Garattini S, ed. *Depressive disorders*. Stuttgart-New York: Schattauer Verlag, 1978;95–106.

Coppola R, Herrmann WM. Psychotropic drug profiles: Comparison by topographic maps of absolute power. *Neuropsychobiology* 1987;18:97–104.

Creese I, Snyder SH. Behavioral and biochemical properties of the dopamine receptor. In: Lipton MA, di

Mascio A, et al. eds. *Psychopharmacology: A generation of progress.* New York: Raven Press, 1978;377–388.

Degkwitz R. *Leitfaden der Psychopharmakologie.* Stuttgart: Wissenschaftliche Verlagsgesellschaft mbH, 1967.

Dietsch G. Fourier-Analyse von Elekoenkephalogrammen des Meschen. *Pflüger's Arch* 1932;230: 106–112.

Fenner H. Strukturcharakteristika tricyclischer Psychopharmaka. *Deutsche Apotheker-Zeitung* 1971;111: 1495–1502.

Fenner H. ERP studies on the mechanism of biotransformation of tricyclic neuroleptics and antidepressant. In: Forrest IS, Carr CJ, et al. eds. *The phenothiazines and structurally related drugs.* New York: Raven Press, 1974;5–13.

Fielding S, Lal H. Pre-clinical neuropsychopharmacology of neuroleptics. 3. Screening tests using higher animals. In: Fielding S, Lal H, eds. *Industrial pharmacology*, vol. 1: *Neuroleptics.* Mount Kisco, NY: Futura Publishing, 1974;64–75.

Goodwin FK, Cowdry RW, et al. Predictors of drug response in the affective disorders: Toward an integrated approach. In: Lipton MA, di Mascio A, eds. *Psychopharmacology: A generation of progress.* New York: Raven Press, 1978;1277–1288.

Guidotti A. Synaptic mechanisms in the action of benzodiazepines. In: Lipton MA, di Mascio A, et al. eds. *Psychopharmacology: A generation of progress.* New York: Raven Press, 1978;1349–1357.

Haase HJ. *Therapie mit Psychopharmaka und anderen psychotropen Medikamenten.* Oldenburg: Gerhard Stalling AG, 1969.

Haefely WE. Behavioral and neuropharmacological aspects of drugs used in anxiety and related states. In: Lipton MA, di Mascio A, et al. eds. *Psychopharmacology: A generation of progress.* New York: Raven Press, 1978;1359–1374.

Herrmann WM. Development and critical evaluation of an objective procedure for the electroencephalographic classification of psychotropic drugs. In: Herrmann WM, ed. *Electroencephalography in drug research.* Stuttgart, New York: Gustav Fischer Verlag, 1982;249–351.

Herrmann WM, Fichte K, et al. Definition von EEG-Frequenzbändern aufgrund strukturanalytischer Betrachtungen. In: Kubicki StK, Herrmann WM, et al, eds. *Faktorenanalyse und Variablenibildung aus dem Elektroenzephalogramm. (Factor analysis and EEG variables).* Stuttgart, New York: Gustav Fischer Verlag, 1980;61–74.

Herrmann WM, Irrgang U. Characterization and classification of psychoactive drugs on a functional electrophysiological level as a basis for the interpretation of EEG effects of the two analgesics pentazocin and flupirtine. In: Bromm B, ed. *Pain measurement in man.* Amsterdam: Elsevier, 1984; 167–188.

Herrmann WM, Coper H, et al. Psychotropic and analgesic effects of paracetamol and their interaction with caffeine 1995; (submitted).

Honigfeld G, Howard A. *Psychiatric drugs. A desk reference.* New York: Academic Press, 1973.

Innes IR, Nickerson M. Drugs acting on post-ganglionic adrenergic nerve endings and structures innervated by them (sympathomimetic drugs). In: Goodman L, Gilman A, eds. *The pharmacological basis of therapeutics.* New York: Macmillan, 1970;478–423.

Itil TM. Electroencephalography and pharmacopsychiatry. In: Freyhan FA, Petrilowitsch N, et al., eds. *Modern problems of pharmacopsychiatry*, vol. 1: *Clinical psychopharmacology.* Basel: Karger, 1968; 163–194.

Itil TM, Cora R, et al. "Psychotropic" action of sex hormones: Computerized EEG in establishing the immediate CNS effects of steroid hormones. *Curr Ther Res* 1974;16:1147–1170.

Itil TM, Herrmann WM. Prediction of psychotropic properties of lisuride hydrogen maleate by quantitative pharmaco-electroencephalogram. *Int J Clin Pharmacol* 1975;12:221–233.

Itil TM, Herrmann WM. Effects of hormones on computer analyzed human electroencephalogram. In: Lipton MA, di Mascio A, et al. eds. *Psychopharmacology: A generation of progress.* New York: Raven Press, 1978;729–743.

Iversen LL. GABA and benzodiazepine receptors. *Nature* 1978;275:477.

Janssen PA, van Bever WFM. Preclinical psychopharmacology of neuroleptics. In: Clark WG, del Giudice J, eds. *Principles of psychopharmacology.* New York: Academic Press, 1978;279–295.

Jarvik ME. Drugs used in the treatment of psychiatric disorders. In: Goodman LS, Gilman A, eds. *The pharmacological basis of therapeutics.* New York: Macmillan, 1970;151–203.

Kielholz P, Pöldinger W. Antidepressive drug therapy in clinic and practice. In: Freyhan FA, Petrilowitsch N, et al., eds. *Modern problems of pharmacopsychiatry*, vol. 1: *Clinical psychopharmacology*. Basel: Karger, 1968;73–87.

Koe BK. Effects of neuroleptic drugs on brain catecholamines. In: Fielding S, Lal H, eds. *Industrial pharmacology*, vol. 1: *Neuroleptics*. Mount Kisco, NY: Futura Publishing Company, 1974;131–172.

Koe BK. Effects of antidepressant drugs on brain catecholamines and serotonin. In: Fielding S, Lal H, eds. *Industrial pharmacology*, vol. 2: *Antidepressants*. Mount Kisco, NY: Futura Publishing Company, 1975;143–180.

Korolkovas A. *Essentials of molecular pharmacology. Background for drug design*. New York: Wiley Interscience, 1970.

Koukkou M, Lehmann D. Correlations between cannabis-induced psychopathology and EEG before and after drug ingestion. *Pharmacopsychiatry* 1978;11:220–227.

Künkel H, Westphal M. Quantitative EEG analysis of pyrithioxine action. *Pharmacopsychiatry* 1970; 3:41–49.

Ladinsky H, Consolo S, et al. Increase in mouse and rat brain acetylcholine levels by diazepam. In: Garattini S, Mussini E, et al., eds. *The benzodiazepines. Monographs of the Mario Negri Institute for Pharmacological Research*. New York: Raven Press, 1973;241–242.

Lidbrink P, Corrodi H et al., The effects of benzodiazepines, meprobamate, and barbiturates on central monoamine neurons. In: Garattini S, Mussini E, et al., eds. *The benzodiazepines. Monographs of the Mario Negri Institute for Pharmacological Research*. New York: Raven Press, 1973;203–223.

Longo VG. Effects of psychotropic drugs on the EEG of animals. In: Clark WC., del Guidice J, eds. *Principles of psychopharmacology*. New York, San Francisco, London: Academic Press, 1978;247–260.

Murphy DL, Campbell I, et al. Current status of the indoleamine hypothesis of the affective disorders. In: Lipton MA, di Mascio A, et al., eds. *Psychopharmacology: A generation of progress*. New York: Raven Press, 1978;1235–1247.

Nahunek K. 1973; Antidepressants. Their classification and efficacy in endogenous depression. Universita JE Purkyne, BRNO.

Niemegeers CJE. Antagonism of reserpine-like activity. In: Fielding S, Lal H, eds. *Industrial pharmacology*, vol. 2: *Antidepressants*. Mount Kisco, NY: Futura Publishing Company, 1975;73–98.

Niemegeers CJE, Janssen PAJ. Differential antagonisms to amphetamine-induced oxygen consumption and agitation by psychoactive drugs. In: Fielding S, Lal H, eds. *Industrial pharmacology*, vol. 2: *Antidepressants*. Mount Kisco, NY: Futura Publishing Company, 1975;125–141.

Ott H, McDonald RJ, et al. Interpretation of correlations between EEG-power-spectra and psychological performance variables within the concepts of "subvigilance," "attention" and "psychomotoric impulsion." In: Herrmann WM, ed. *Electroencephalography in drug research*. Stuttgart, New York: Gustav Fischer Verlag, 1982;227–247.

Pöldinger W. *Kompendium der Psychopharmakotherapie. Wissenschaftlicher Dienst Roche*. Grenzach/Baden: Hoffmann-La Roche AG, 1971.

Randall LO, Kappell B. Pharmacological activity of some benzodiazepines and their metabolites. In: Garattini S, Mussini E, et al., eds. *The benzodiazepines. Monographs of the Mario Negri Institute for Pharamacological Research*. New York: Raven Press, 1973;27–51.

Ritchie JM. Central nervous system stimulants. II. The xanthines. In: Goodman LS, Gilman A, eds. *The pharmacological basis of therapeutics*. London, Toronto: Macmillan, 1970;358–370.

Schildkraut JJ. Current status of the catecholamine hypothesis of affective disorders. In: Lipton MA, di Mascio A, et al., eds. *Psychopharmacology: A generation of progress*. New York: Raven Press, 1978; 1223–1234.

Snyder SH, Enna SJ, et al., Brain mechanism associated with therapeutic actions of benzodiazepines: Focus on neuro-transmitters. *Am J Psychiatry*, 1977;134:662–665.

Stille G. Neurophysiological correlates to anti-psychotic drugs. In: Sedvall G, ed. *Antipsychotic drugs, Pharmacodynamics and pharmacokinetics*. Oxford: Pergamon Verlag, 1976;51–61.

Volavka J, Levine R, et al. Short-term effects of heroin in man. Is EEG related to behavior? *Arch Gen Psychiatry* 1974;30:677–801.

Volavka J, James B, et al. EEG and other effects of naltrexone and heroin in man. *Pharmakopsychiatry* 1979;12:79–85.

Wagner WW, Ott H, et al. A multidimensional concept for measuring CNS effects of beta-adrenoceptor blocking agents in human pharmacology. *Int J Clin Pharmacol* 1981;19:23–33.

Wandrey D, Leutner V. *Neuro-Psychopharmaka in Klinik und Praxis*. Stuttgart: F. K. Schattauer Verlag, 1967.

*Pain and the Brain: From
Nociception to Cognition,*
edited by Burkhart Bromm and
John E. Desmedt, Advances in Pain
Research and Therapy Vol. 22.
Raven Press, Ltd., New York © 1995.

32

Comparative Evaluation of Analgesic Efficacy of Drugs

Eckehard Scharein and Burkhart Bromm

Institute of Physiology, University Hospital Eppendorf, 20246 Hamburg, Germany

SUMMARY

This chapter describes a standardized experimental model for determining the analgesic potency of drugs that allows the comparison of results acquired in different studies. The model is based on the well-defined activation of the nociceptive system by short, intracutaneously applied currents in healthy humans. Long-latency cerebral potentials and subjective pain ratings evoked by the pain-inducing stimuli are used to assess the strength of the nociceptive activation. The degree to which this standardized activation is antagonized by a specific drug determines its analgesic potency. After presenting the physiologic basis of the *intracutaneous pain model*, the experimental and methodologic prerequisites necessary to ensure a valid interpretation of the results are discussed in detail. The chapter presents evidence that components of the cerebral response to the intracutaneous stimulus may be used: (a) as a correlate of pain sensation; (b) as an indicator of pharmacologically induced pain relief; (c) to portray the dose-dependent antagonization of opioid effects; (d) to detect central effects of "peripherally" acting analgesics; (e) to monitor the cerebral bioavailability of analgesics on a functional level; and (f) to rank the "pure" analgesic potency of drugs on an "objective" neurophysiologic scale. By simultaneously analyzing spontaneous EEG activity, cerebral potentials of other sensory modalities, subjective moods, motor reactions, and side effects, we are able to differentiate between "specific" analgesic effects and nonspecific drug-induced alterations in the vigilance system. Finally, the results of all our pharmacologic studies with the intracutaneous pain model are summarized, resulting in a ranking of analgesic potency for the most commonly used analgesics. We are convinced that the quantitative comparison of the efficacy of different analgesics is best performed under experimentally stringent, controlled conditions, in homogeneous samples of healthy, informed, and cooperative volunteers. This may be the reason why the intracutaneous pain model that we developed is now being used by several other groups (e.g., Miltner et al. 1989; Droste et al. 1991; Joseph et al. 1991; Becker et al. 1993; Wright et al. 1993).

PAIN MODELS IN ALGESIMETRY

How effective is an analgesic drug or treatment? The answer to this question is inherently connected to the problem of measuring pain. Pain is a subjective phenomenon. Moreover, pain sensation is influenced by a variety of emotional, cognitive, social, and cultural factors, as described in many chapters of this book, and pain is therefore difficult to measure.

Many attempts have been made to quantify pain sensation at both subjective and objective levels of measurement (for a review, see Melzack 1984; Gracely 1989; McGuire 1992). On the subjective level, category and analogue scales, pain dictionaries, and pain diaries have been used for the quantitative description of pain, supplemented by behavioral observations and performance tests. Such measurements have especially been applied to the assessment of pain in hospitalized patients. But the pain of a patient is always a unique event, and relief of this pain does not allow a generalization. Moreover, the clinical environment is not constant, owing to variations in the schedule of daily activities, the behavior of other patients, the medical care provided by physicians and nurses, and contact with family and visitors.

The most frequently used model of pain in clinical trials is postoperative pain (for a review, see Reading 1989; Stambaugh 1991). Here the pain strongly depends on the kind of operation performed, and is essentially different depending on whether the surgery was destructive or constructive. The best experiences in the assessment of analgesic efficacy are reported with postoperative pain after dental surgery (for a review, see Skoglund et al. 1991). But this pain model fails in attempts at the comparative evaluation of mild analgesics with justifiable sample sizes. Contradictory results have been published, perhaps because of the inhomogeneity of patients, pain states, and surgical techniques. Last but not least, there are ethical constraints that do not allow placebo-controlled double-blind studies in patients.

On the physiologic level of measurement, a great many variables have been used as indicators of patients' pain, including cardiovascular parameters, respiration, oculomotor reactions, sudomotor activity, electromyographically recorded muscle activity, trans- and intracutaneously measured neuronal activity, and changes in spontaneous electroencephalographic (EEG) activity (for a review, see Bromm 1984). But because of the aforementioned heterogeneity, an assessment of clinical pain states using physiologic variables was not feasible until now.

There is no question that nociceptive responses to experimentally induced pain are the most important measures in laboratory animal tests of the analgesic efficacy of novel drugs. Examples are the hot-plate test, in which the time interval between heat application and the animal's reaction is said to indicate pain sensitivity, the skin-twitch reaction, and the tail-flick test (for a review, see Hammond 1989). Complex behaviors of laboratory animals in response to experimentally induced pain have also been used to determine drug-induced modulations of pain sensitivity (Vierck et al. 1989).

Clearly, manipulations in algesimetry with living animals must be humane, and for ethical reasons algesimetric studies are better done directly in human volunteers, provided that the toxicologic and metabolic properties of the test drug have been documented as harmless. Simple experimental pain-inducing stimuli can easily be applied in humans, since human volunteers are able to verbalize the induced pain and disclose whether they are willing to tolerate the procedure or not. The most decisive grounds for performing analgesic tests in humans are, of course, that drugs are developed to relieve human pain (Beecher 1957; Bromm 1984). As often stated, the gap between testing analgesics in the healthy laboratory animal and their application in treating the ill human is too large. To bridge this gap, we use analgesic assessment in healthy volunteers.

THE EXPERIMENTAL PAIN MODEL

In the following sections a model of pain is described that allows documentation of the strength and time course of drug-induced analgesia in humans. Drugs are tested in a double-blind manner in a placebo-controlled, repeated-measures design. After detailed investigations of withdrawal reflexes, skin-conductance reactions, and microelectroneurographic recordings from peripheral nociceptive afferents (for details see Bromm 1984), we selected the parameters of spontaneous and stimulus-evoked EEG activity as the most powerful indicators of pain and of drug-induced pain relief. The procedure involves selectively stimulating, in a well-defined manner, nociceptive Aδ- and C-fibers by means of appropriate "pain stimuli" (see below and Fig. 1). The stimulus-induced neuronal-impulse pattern is transmitted through anterolateral-tract projections into ventrobasal thalamic nuclei and reaches primary and secondary areas of the cortex. The volunteer feels a brief prick and has to rate its intensity on analogue scales (pain estimation, E). Simultaneously, a late brain potential is evoked, consisting of a late vertex negativity (N150) and a subsequent positivity (P250). The amplitude difference between the two components is highly correlated with the subject's pain estimation (E) if decisive experimental parameters are well under control (see below). In order to differentiate specific analgesic effects on the nociceptive system from nonspecific sedative effects, parameters of the spontaneous EEG, motor-reaction times, mood scales, and brain potentials in response to other stimulus modalities are included in the evaluation of a drug. It is easy to simultaneously measure plasma concentrations of the drug in the volunteers during the analgesic test, and in this way the analgesic efficacy of the drug can be discussed in relation to the plasma value of its active metabolite. We began analgesic studies in 1980 with the model described above, and have created a data bank with the analgesic effects of the most often used mild, medium, and strong pain-relieving drugs.

The Pain-Inducing Stimulus

One of the most important factors in every model of pain is the kind of stimulus chosen to induce pain. The stimulus should activate the nociceptive system while

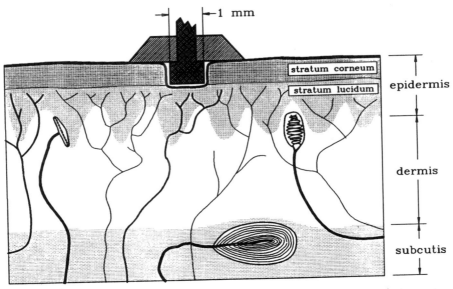

FIG. 1. The intracutaneous pain stimulus. Schematic representation of the types of receptors within hairless skin. By drilling a hole through the stratum corneum, the electrode is placed directly in the vicinity of Aδ- and C-fibers, belonging mainly to the nociceptive system. (Adapted from Bromm and Scharein 1990.)

minimizing concomitant excitation of other sensory modalities. Because of the need to average the evoked brain potentials over a series of repeated trials to build up a reliable estimate of the cerebral reaction with a satisfactory signal-to-noise (S/N) ratio, the physical properties of the stimulus should not change from one trial to another. Additionally, the stimulus should, if applied repeatedly, induce a comparable activation of nociceptive afferents without any sensitization or habituation. The stimulation should be unequivocally painful, but not "noxious," in order to avoid severe tissue damage. Long-lasting heat radiation delivered by thermodes, the cold-pressure test, the tourniquet-exercise method (ischemic pain), chemically induced pain, and repetitive application of strong mechanical pressure are stimuli that can scarcely be applied sufficiently often for response averaging (for a detailed discussion of the pros and cons of the different stimulus qualities, see Bromm 1989; Handwerker and Kobal 1993). Furthermore, for computing stimulus-locked evoked potentials, the time point of suprathreshold nociceptor activation has to be known precisely. For this purpose, stimuli with rise times in the range of milliseconds are needed.

Brief electrical skin or tooth-pulp stimulation (Benedetti et al. 1982; Buchsbaum 1984; Umino et al. 1988; Klement et al. 1992; Lekic and Cenic 1992) and short mechanical skin indentations (Bromm and Scharein 1982a; Stowell 1984) fulfil these requirements and have been successfully used. In recent years, short, radiant heat pulses elicited by infrared CO_2 or thulium YAG lasers have shown their utility, especially in repeated experiments with patients for the documentation of normal and disturbed pain sensitivity (Carmon et al. 1976; Bromm and Treede 1991; Kakigi et al. 1991). Laser stimuli in the visible range, as have been used by Arendt-Nielsen and his group (e.g., Arendt-Nielsen et al. 1990), are well known to be reflected by the skin, which should therefore be blackened, as already suggested by Hardy et al. (1952). Moreover, a stimulus duration of 100 msec or more is untenable if stimulus-locked averaging techniques are required.

For algesimetric studies in humans, we prefer the intracutaneously applied brief current pulse, particularly if the effects are to be monitored in sessions of no more than 6 hours duration. Sessions of a longer duration led to inconsistencies because of partial reepithelization (Bromm and Meier 1984), in addition to disturbances due to increased drowsiness or habituation, as described below.

In the intracutaneous pain model, the stimuli are applied to the tip of the left middle finger. A hole is drilled into the stratum corneum, usually of the tip of the left middle finger, and a specially designed electrode is inserted (Fig. 1). In this way the electrical currents are applied to the immediate vicinity of the most superficial skin afferents, the unmyelinated C-fibers and the thin myelinated Aδ-fibers, which typically display high-threshold response characteristics and belong mainly to the nociceptive system (Munger and Halata 1983). This permits stimulation of the nociceptive system while minimizing a concomitant excitation of receptors for other sensory modalities. In normal subjects the stimulus evokes a well-localized pain, characterized as a stabbing, hot, and sharp sensation that is very similar to the pain induced by tooth-pulp stimulation and in clear contrast to the unpleasant paresthesia induced by conventionally applied skin or nerve-trunk stimulation (for more detail see Bromm and Meier 1984). These responses are particularly ascribed to a selective Aδ-fiber activation. C-fiber responses are expected to appear with latencies of 1 sec and more, and are normally masked by the cerebral processing of the earlier nociceptive inputs (for details see Chapter 3). Only in patients with a selective loss of A-fiber function (see, e.g., Treede et al. 1984) can C-fiber-mediated burning-pain components be felt by the subject (see Chapters 3 and 25).

The Reactions

The standardized activation of the nociceptive system by intracutaneous stimuli is assessed on the physiological level of measurement by late somatosensory evoked cerebral potentials (SEPs), with a negativity after 150 msec (N150) and a following positivity (P250) in the case of finger stimulation. In a multivariate analysis, these SEP segments were identified as pain-related components that varied significantly with the magnitude of the subjects' pain estimation (Bromm and Scharein 1982a). A careful evaluation of analgesic effects on pain-related brain potentials should therefore be based on multivariate techniques (see below). However, in the case of well-controlled experimental surroundings (see next paragraph), measurements of the difference in amplitude of N150 and P250 may be sufficient for a quick evaluation of drug-induced effects. On the subjective level, the intensity of the pain sensation (E) induced by the intracutaneous stimulus is rated on a numerical scale ranging from 0 (no sensation) to 10 (unbearable pain), with values of 4 and more denoting increasing pain. In order to avoid contamination with motor reactions, the subjects have to scale their sensations verbally at 3 sec after stimulus application, when they are prompted by a weak tone (1,000 Hz, 30 dB SPL, 0.5 sec).

This tone was also used to assess nonspecific effects of the analgesics on auditory evoked cerebral potentials. Because of the essential importance of changes in alertness as a possible source of interference with pain sensitivity, the vigilance of the subjects was also assessed from the spontaneous EEG, mood scale, and reaction-time measurements. The ongoing EEG activity was measured continuously throughout the entire experimental session, while reaction times and mood were determined after each stimulus block, together with a description of drug effects estimated as symptoms (side effects).

Study Design

In order to achieve a high and constant level of vigilance throughout the 3- to 6-hour sessions, stimuli were given in blocks of 80, with randomized intensities and randomized interstimulus intervals. The stimulus intensities should be individually tailored, at the beginning of each session, on the basis of the subject's pain thresholds (see below). We prefer intensities of two and three times the individual pain-threshold intensity, with interstimulus intervals between 10 and 20 sec. Thus, each block lasts 20 min. Stimulus randomization is essential in algesimetric studies. Given these conditions, the vigilance level of the subject can be kept constant even during long-lasting sessions, as has been shown by the power-spectral density function of the ongoing EEG (Bromm and Scharein 1982b). If stimuli were applied in a monotonous sequence of equal intensities with equal interstimulus intervals, the vigilance level decreased, and cerebral potentials and pain ratings were attenuated (Bromm 1989). If, on the other hand, the interstimulus interval was shortened to less than 5 sec, a dissociation between cerebral potentials and pain ratings was observed: pain sensations were gradually prolonged into a "chronic" pain state, and the amplitudes of the brain potentials were markedly depressed (Jacobson et al. 1985).

Of similar importance are the requirements for homogeneity of the sample of subjects. In order to avoid discussion about effects on pain of sex, age, and socio-cultural background, our experiments were always done with healthy male medical students between 20 and 30 years of age. Before a student was included in a study, a screening examination with a thorough medical and drug history was taken. In the medical investigation, subjects had to be within standard limits for size, weight, cardiovascular parameters, and hematologic and urine values. A personality inventory based on the Freiburg Personality Inventory (FPI) (Fahrenberg and Selg 1970) was taken. This scaled the subject's emotional lability between the poles "emotionally stable" and "emotionally labile." Subjects classified as labile (depressive, anxious, sad, etc.) were excluded from the study. Furthermore, the subject's individual pain sensitivity had to be normal. For intracutaneously applied electrical pulses of 20 msec duration, the mean threshold intensity is 0.4 ± 0.2 mA. The EEG had to be a normal variant. Other exclusion criteria were regular smoking, regular use of medication, abuse of alcoholic beverages, pharmacologic treatments within the previous 3 months, and symptoms of any illness within the 4 weeks before the study.

Last but not not least, all sessions were performed at the same time of day in order to minimize influences of circadian rhythms. All subjects were familiarized with the experimental surroundings in a first complete session, the data from which were discarded from further analysis. For the same reasons, each experimental session started with an adaptation block. The adaptation periods are indispensable parts of our pain model because the subjects have to be relaxed before the analgesic test can be started.

Agents and placebos were given in a randomized treatment sequence with an intersession interval of 7 days in order to avoid crossover effects. Blood samples were taken routinely in all our experiments to determine the plasma concentration of each analgesic active metabolite. Table 1 illustrates a typical experimental session. To ensure the same resorption conditions for all subjects, a standardized breakfast was given at the beginning of each experimental session. In order to compare the analgesic efficacy of different drugs in all of our studies, a dose of double the minimal dose recommended by the manufacturer was administered.

EXEMPLARY RESULTS

In the following, some demonstrations are given on how our knowledge about the neurophysiological basis of pain sensation increases by analyzing pain-related cerebral potentials with multivariate statistical methods and new signal-processing techniques. These procedures allow us, for example, to document central analgesic effects of so-called "peripherally" acting analgesics, to relate the analgesic potency to the momentary plasma level of active metabolites, and to evaluate comparatively the pain-relieving effects of different drugs.

Pain-Related Principal Components

Principal-component analysis (PCA) is a multivariate statistical technique that is used with increasing frequency to identify components of the brain-potential waveform as covariates of cortical information-processing mechanisms (Hunt 1985; Guthrie 1990; Möcks and Verleger 1991; May et al. 1992). Mathematically, the principal components are the varimax-rotated (Kaiser 1959), orthonormalized eigenvectors of the association-matrix of similarities between all pairs of SEP ampli-

TABLE 1. *Time schedule of an experimental session from the ValoronN™ and tramadol study*

7.00	• Clinical examination	
	• Standardized breakfast	
	• Urine sample, ECG, wiring-up	
	• Placing of the butterfly	
7.40	• Introduction of the pain-inducing stimuli	
	• Determination of sensation threshold and pain threshold	
8.05–8.25	Stimulus block	Adaptation
	• Determination of reaction time	"
8.45–9.05	Stimulus block	(PRE) Baseline
	• Determination of reaction times, mood scales, and side effects	"
	• Blood sample 1	"
9.10	MEDICATION	
	• Determination of reaction times, mood scales, and side effects	
	• Blood sample 2	
9.40–10.00	Stimulus block	(POST1) 40 min[a]
	• Blood sample 3	
	• Determination of reaction times, mood scales, and side effects	
	• Blood sample 4	
10.20–10.40	Stimulus block	(POST2) 80 min
	• Blood sample 5	
	• Determination of reaction times, mood scales, and side effects	
	• Blood sample 6	
11.00–11.20	Stimulus block	(POST3) 120 min
	• Blood sample 7	
	• Determination of reaction times, mood scales and side effects	
	• Determination of sensation threshold and pain threshold	
	• Urine sample, ECG	
11.45	• Final clinical examination	

[a]Each block of stimuli lasted for 20 min. The mean time point of each stimulus block after medication is given in the last column.

tudes at different time points, multiplied by the square root of the corresponding eigenvalue. This technique replaces the coarse peak-to-peak amplitude measure, commonly used to quantify evoked cerebral potentials, with a set of independent parameters more suitable for describing the underlying brain processes. A detailed tutorial description of PCA is given in Donchin and Heffley (1978) (see also Bromm 1984).

We applied PCA to identify pain-relevant SEP components and to analyze their dependency on stimulus modality, intensity, and perception in a sample of 15 healthy male subjects by applying mechanical and electrical skin stimuli below and above the individual pain threshold (Bromm and Scharein 1982a). The main result was that six principal components (PCs) were found that were adequate to describe all variations in SEP amplitude (Table 2).

The influence of stimulus modality (mechanical, electrical) and stimulus perception (nonpainful, painful) on the PCs was evaluated by analysis of variance (ANOVA). To prove the dependence of the PCs on stimulus perception *per se* (i.e., independent of the stimulus intensity), the influence of the varying stimulus intensity was eliminated in a second step using a regression-analytical technique (see also

TABLE 2. Decomposition of somatosensory evoked potenials (SEPs) into independent components by principal-component analysis

Principal component (PC)	Loading maxima [msec]	Proportion of variance accounted for [%]
PC_1	50–80	17
PC_2	140–160	20
PC_3	180–240	19
PC_4	240–360	15
PC_5	400–500	17
PC_6	Polyphasic	3

Sen and Srivastava 1990), and the remaining variance was reanalyzed. The results are summarized as follows:

Differences between stimulus qualities (mechanical, electrical) were reflected in the early SEP components with latencies of less than 100 msec, represented by PC_1.
All six principal components (except the polyphasic PC_6) were significantly correlated with the intensity of the stimuli.
No component could be extracted that appeared only when the stimuli were rated as painful.
After eliminating the influence of stimulus intensity, two PCs were found (PC_2 and PC_4) that correlated with the intensity of the pain sensation. PC_2 describes the marked negativity in the SEP that emerges 150 msec after stimulus onset, whereas PC_4 essentially describes the positivity P250. Both PCs were elicited in the same way by mechanical as well as by electrical pain-inducing stimuli, and could be identified as modality-independent cerebral correlates of pain sensation.

In other words, all six PCs varied significantly with stimulus intensity, and also varied with the subject's verbal report of pain because of the well-known relationship between stimulus intensity and induced pain, in which an increasingly strong stimulus has a greater potency for inducing pain. But if effects of stimulus intensity were eliminated, only two PCs were correlated with the intensity of pain. Therefore, simply quantifying the peak-to-peak amplitude difference of the late components of a recorded SEP as an indicator of induced pain is only a first approach that may not be attributed directly to the subjectively perceived intensity of the pain. Only if all other relevant sources of interference are experimentally controlled can the peak-to-peak difference in N150 and P250 be used as a valid correlate of the pain.

That the two components PC_2 and PC_4 do indeed have something to do with the subjective experience of pain was additionally tested by administering analgesics. In a double-blind, placebo-controlled, randomized crossover study with 15 healthy subjects, we analyzed the effects of the opioid tilidine both alone and together with increasing amounts of its antagonist naloxone (Table 3). The effects of the treatments were evaluated at a postmedication interval of 120 min. PCA was applied to

TABLE 3. *Treatments and dosages for the tilidine/naloxone study*

T	100 mg tilidine	
TN8	100 mg tilidine	+ 8 mg naloxone
TN32	100 mg tilidine	+ 32 mg naloxone
N	32 mg naloxone	
P	placebo	

All drugs were orally administered together with 100 ml of distilled water.

decompose the cerebral potentials into independent components. Again, six principal components could be extracted (Fig. 2, left) that explained more than 90% of the total variance. They exhibited the same component structure as described in Table 2, proving the high stability of the SEP components in a different sample of subjects. The bars (Fig. 2, right) indicate the mean component scores averaged over all subjects, separately for the five treatments, describing the degree to which each PC was influenced by the specific treatment. In the lowest line on the right of Fig. 2 the mean pain ratings are given as deviations from the grand mean obtained from all subjects and sessions. Tilidine markedly decreased the pain ratings. The addition of 8 mg of naloxone did not significantly antagonize the opioid-induced analgesia, although a numerically small reduction was seen. Only after the addition of 32 mg of naloxone did the reversal of the tilidine-induced analgesia become evident. After the application of naloxone alone, the pain ratings returned to the placebo level.

As documented in the right part of Fig. 2, only the scores of the components PC_2 and PC_4 were significantly affected by the analgesic treatments. Both components exhibited the same pattern as did the pain ratings of a dose-dependent antagonization of the opioid-effect. Decomposing the SEP waveform into its components and analyzing the treatment effects separately for the single components clearly improved the sensitivity and specificity of SEP measurements in detecting pharmacologic effects.

Monitoring the Cerebral Bioavailability of Drugs

In the quantitative evaluation of centrally acting drugs, the question arises of how to continuously monitor the development of their cerebral bioavailability. In psychopharmacology, the pharmaco-EEG—the analysis of pharmacologically induced alterations in spontaneous EEG activity—is usually used to describe drug effects on a functional cerebral level (for a review, see Herrmann and Schaerer 1989). This approach seems to be suitable for psychotropic drugs, and indeed most such drugs can be classified correctly according to their effects on the ongoing EEG. The pharmaco-EEG may be considered as the most sensitive method for monitoring the functional effects of psychotropic drugs on the CNS, and is an excellent tool for detecting nonspecific effects on the arousal system. However, this approach fails in the case of analgesics. A classification of analgesics based on their effects on the

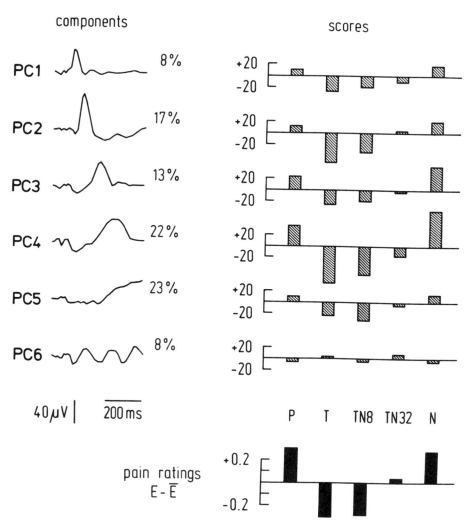

components   scores

PC1   8%   +20 / -20

PC2   17%   +20 / -20

PC3   13%   +20 / -20

PC4   22%   +20 / -20

PC5   23%   +20 / -20

PC6   8%   +20 / -20

40μV | 200 ms   P   T   TN8   TN32   N

pain ratings
E - Ē   +0.2 / -0.2

FIG. 2. Principal components reflecting the antagonism of opioid effects. The extracted PCs (*left column*), ordered with respect to their peak latencies, accounted for more than 90% of the total variance of the evoked-potential amplitudes (as indicated in the insets). In the right column are shown the mean scores of the six principal components, describing the degree to which each PC is affected by the treatments: P = placebo; T = tilidine 100 mg; TN8 = tilidine 100 mg + naloxone 8 mg; TN32 = tilidine 100 mg + naloxone 32 mg; N = naloxone 32 mg. *Below right*, the deviation of the mean pain rating E from grand mean value Ē averaged over all treatments is given for each treatment. Negative deviations denote a decrease in pain. (Adapted from Bromm 1984.)

spontaneous EEG has not been possible (see Chapter 31 for a detailed discussion), because no specific alterations in the spontaneous EEG have been seen during pain.

Repeated measurements of pain-related components of cerebral responses to pain-inducing stimuli are more suitable for monitoring the time course of the bioavailability of centrally acting analgesics. By using the stimulus-locked cerebral responses and the spontaneous EEG together, it should be possible to assess both the "specific" analgesic effects of such drugs and nonspecific CNS alterations. We tested this hypothesis in an experimental study with two different centrally acting drugs. Meperidine was chosen as a well-known narcoanalgesic and imipramine as a classical tricyclic antidepressant with an analgesic component (Bromm et al. 1986; for dosages and application see Table 4). Both drugs were given orally in a double-blind, placebo-controlled, crossover study involving 20 volunteers. Each subject participated in three sessions, with a washout interval of 7 days. After establishing the baseline values, the effects of the drugs on the spontaneous EEG and on pain-related cerebral potentials were monitored over a postmedication period of 240 min in six blocks, with pain-inducing stimuli of 20-min duration, separated by 15-min interblock intervals.

Because the spontaneous EEG is normally evaluated in the frequency domain, we evaluated the cerebral potentials evoked by pain-inducing stimuli in this same way in order to ensure a comparable quantification. EEG segments of 500-msec duration, recorded immediately before stimulation, were used to represent the spontaneous EEG, and segments of the same duration recorded directly thereafter were used to represent the evoked cerebral response. Since power-spectral density functions (PSDs) estimated by the conventional direct Fourier-transformation method have an insufficient frequency resolution of only 2 Hz if applied to EEG segments of only 500-msec duration, a new parametric spectral estimator with a higher frequency resolution had to be adapted. We chose the maximum entropy method (MEM) as a suitable spectral estimator (for details see Scharein et al. 1984).

The parametrization of cerebral potentials in the frequency domain has a distinct advantage over the usual quantification in the time domain. Since the peaks of the cerebral reactions vary considerably from one trial to another, evoked potentials are usually averaged over a set of single-trial recordings in order to improve the S/N ratio. Averaging in the frequency domain avoids the smearing of information that occurs over relatively broad ranges during quantification in the time domain.

Treatment effects on spontaneous and evoked EEG activities within the total sample of 20 subjects are summarized in Fig. 3. The grand mean PSDs of the

TABLE 4. *Treatments and dosages for the meperidine/imipramine study*

MEP	Meperidine (pethidine)	Dolantin™	Solution	150 mg
IMI	Imipramine	Tofranil™	2 capsules	100 mg
PLA	Placebo	Placebo 1 + placebo 2		

All drugs were orally administered. Since meperidine was available as solution and imipramine as capsules, a double dummy placebo was used. The dosages correspond to twice the minimal clinical doses.

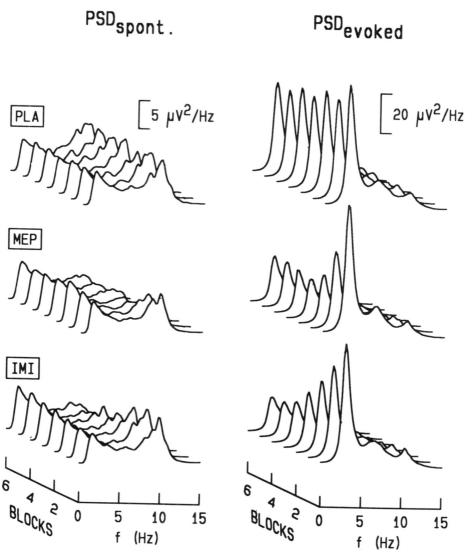

FIG. 3. Spectra of spontaneous and evoked EEG under meperidine and imipramine. Mean power-spectral density functions (PSD) of the EEG immediately before (PSD$_{spont.}$) and after (PSD$_{evoked}$) application of pain-inducing stimuli with placebo (PLA), meperidine (MEP, 150 mg p.o.), and imipramine (IMI, 100 mg p.o.). Spectra were averaged over all 20 subjects, separately for each stimulus block (0 = pre-, 1–6 = postmedication). Note the different ordinate scales of the pre- and poststimulus EEG spectra.

spontaneous EEG immediately before stimulus application are presented to the left. To the right are given the spectra of the cerebral reactions to the pain-inducing stimuli. The latter were characterized by the concentration of spectral power in the frequency band (1–4 Hz, hereinafter called delta-power, DP). The DP represents most of the stimulus-induced power in the poststimulus EEG, which amounts to more than tenfold that in the ongoing EEG immediately before stimulation (see also Chapter 3). In addition, two more peaks, between 4 and 7 Hz (theta) and between 8 and 12 Hz (alpha), were recognizable, suggesting that the classical frequency classification developed by Berger (1934) for spontaneous EEG activity may also be valid for the description of stimulus-evoked activity (for discussion see Chapter 31).

The spectra of spontaneous and evoked EEG activity were highly stable in the premedication periods. Given the constancy under placebo, differences in the effects of the two drugs were obvious. Both drugs diminished the DP in the poststimulus EEG, but the time courses of their action were different. Furthermore, in the spontaneous EEG, the power in the alpha ranges was attenuated, whereas the DP, at least with imipramine, seemed to be increased. Next, the drug effects on the power within the classical frequency bands were evaluated in detail. As documented in Table 5, meperidine decreased the power in higher frequency bands, but increased the power of the delta and theta bands in the spontaneous EEG. The effects of imipramine were similar to this but smaller. In the evoked EEG both drugs depressed the power in the delta and theta bands to below the placebo level. Although in the lower frequencies the two drugs acted in opposite direction on spontaneous and evoked EEGs, their effects in the high frequencies upon the pre- and poststimulus EEGs were parallel. Both drugs decreased the power in all EEG segments in the alpha band.

The most obvious differences between the two drugs were seen in the dynamics of their effects. The effects of meperidine began early and differed significantly from those of placebo in the first (25 min) and second (60 min) postmedication block, with maximal effects in the third block (95 min). Later, a slight recovery was seen. The effects of imipramine occurred considerably later, at about 200 min after medication. Similar differences in the time course of the pharmacologic effects of the two drugs were detected in pain ratings: meperidine rapidly decreased pain

TABLE 5. *Summary of the pharmacologic effects of meperidine and imipramine on the spontaneous and evoked EEG*

Drug	EEG	Rhythm			
		Delta	Theta	Alpha	Beta
Meperidine	Spontaneous	↑	⇑	↓	↓
	Evoked	⇓	⇓	↓	↓
Imipramine	Spontaneous	⇑	∅	↓	∅
	Evoked	⇓	↓	↓	∅

⇑, ⇓ = significant effects, denoting a pharmacologically induced change from the premedication values of more than 40%: ↑, ↓ = significant effects of less than 20%; ∅ = no significant effect.

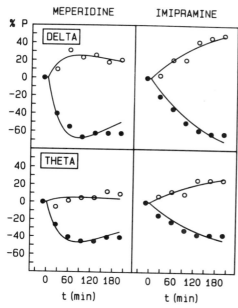

MEPERIDINE   IMIPRAMINE

FIG. 4. Expected effect kinetic and observed effect dynamics. Effects of meperidine (100 mg, p.o.) and imipramine (100 mg, p.o.) on the delta and theta power of the spontaneous (*open circles*) and evoked EEG (*filled circles*). The drug-induced percentage changes from the pre- to the postmedication blocks were compared with values estimated by a one-compartment model with fixed time constants based on plasma concentration values (*continuous lines*). Each session consisted of seven blocks (10 min before and 15, 50, 85, 120, 155, and 190 min after medication).

ratings below the pain threshold, whereas imipramine produced a slower decrease in pain ratings, beginning with values comparable to those for placebo but ending very close to the ratings with meperidine (for a detailed discussion of the analgesic properties of antidepressants, see Chapters 22 and 33).

The different pharmacodynamics of the two drugs were in agreement with their pharmacokinetic data (Fig. 4). This was shown by calculating the dynamics of expected effects (continuous lines), using values reported in the literature, and by fitting an open one-compartment model to the data (for details see Bromm et al. 1989b). As already mentioned, the spontaneous and evoked EEGs were reciprocally affected by the drugs: the delta and theta power in the prestimulus EEG was increased, whereas in the poststimulus EEG a pronounced attenuation in power was seen. The most important result documented in Fig. 4, however, was the surprisingly good agreement between expected effects and observed data for the DP of the poststimulus EEG (filled circles). Thus, the power in the 1- to 4-Hz range of the pain-related cerebral potentials seems to be a good indicator of the cerebral bioavailability of analgesically acting drugs on a functional level.

Central Effects of "Peripherally" Acting Analgesics

Another question recently discussed in the literature concerns central mechanisms of the so-called "peripherally" acting nonsteroidal antiinflammatory drugs (NSAIDs). Since the fundamental work of Vane (1971) and of Smith and Willis

(1971), most textbooks of pharmacology have ascribed the analgesic effects of the NSAIDs to their ability to prevent the synthesis of prostaglandin in the vicinity of tissue damage, thereby attenuating the nociceptive message generated by peripheral inflammation (e.g., Ferreira et al. 1978; Flower et al. 1985). However, the postulated sensitization of nociceptors by prostaglandin could not be confirmed in humans (see, e.g., Yaksh 1982; Shyu et al. 1984), and some of the NSAIDs produce pain relief irrespective of inhibition of prostaglandin synthesis (Brune et al. 1991; for a review, see Flower et al. 1985; Jurna and Yaksh 1993), for which reason additional analgesic mechanisms and sites of action are likely.

We tested three NSAIDs in two placebo-controlled, double-blind crossover studies, each with 32 subjects (Bromm et al. 1989, 1992): acetylsalicylic acid, paracetamol, and phenazone (for details see Table 6). Since the same standardized experimental design was used, and no differences were seen in the two studies in either the premedication values or placebo effects, the results were evaluated together. Acetylsalicylic acid is a salicylate, paracetamol an aniline (paraaminophenol) derivative, and phenazone a member of the group of pyrazolones. Although belonging to different pharmacologic groups, these three analgesics exhibit similar kinetics. Maximum plasma concentrations are reported to occur between 1 and 2 hours after their oral administration, and their plasma half-lives range from 1 to 3 hours (for a review, see, e.g., Flower et al. 1985). In clinical applications the drugs are known to relieve pain to about the same degree (Cooper 1981; Jackson et al. 1984). All exhibit antipyretic properties, but in contrast to acetylsalicylic acid, acetaminophen and antipyrine have practically no antiinflammatory properties. All three drugs differ in the potency of their inhibition of prostaglandin synthesis (Flower and Vane 1972) and in their spectra of side effects (for a review, see Brune 1990).

In our pain model, peripheral nociceptors are activated and brain responses are measured. In the case of an attenuation of cerebral responses to pain-inducing stimuli, the site of action has therefore to be located somewhere between the site of stimulus application and cerebral generators responsible for the evoked potentials. With respect to the nociceptor, we don't believe that the technique for delivering intracutaneous stimuli induces inflammation, since only the most superficial keratinized layers of the epidermis are affected. Furthermore, it is commonly assumed that electrical currents stimulate the cutaneous afferents without neurochemical receptor activation. Analgesic effects found in our model may thus be attributed to

TABLE 6. *Treatments and dosages for the NSAID study*

ASA	Acetylsalicylic acid	1,000 mg
PAR	Paracetamol (acetaminophen)	1,000 mg
PHE	Phenazon (antipyrine)	1,000 mg
PLA	Placebo	

All drugs were orally administered as tablets. The dosages correspond to twice the minimal clinical doses.

changes in excitability of the pain-mediating and pain-processing nervous systems between sites of stimulation and recording.

Pharmacodynamics

The effects of the three NSAIDs on pain-related potentials and pain ratings are summarized in Fig. 5. Mean values were obtained just before and 90 min after medication, 90 min being in the middle of the second postmedication stimulus block. As indicated, the premedication response values were stable in all trials. Mean pain ratings were diminished by 4% to 7% with the NSAIDs. This decrease is numerically small, but is significantly larger than the corresponding placebo effect. The peak-to-peak amplitude of the SEPs decreased by 15% to 20% after drug administration. Effects of similar magnitude were seen in the power-spectral density function of the evoked EEG. The DP declined by about 20%. Comparisons of the analgesic effects of the three NSAIDs showed a similar potency for all three drugs on both the pain ratings and the pain-related brain potentials.

These studies in healthy volunteers suggest, at least in part, a comparable mode of central action for acetylsalicylic acid, paracetamol, and phenazone: all three drugs reduced nociceptive brain activity in response to pain-inducing stimuli, as assessed by pain ratings and by late cerebral potentials. No changes in peak latencies of cerebral potentials were observed with the drugs, in agreement with findings for NSAIDs tested by painful tooth-pulp stimuli (Chapman and Jacobson 1984). Obviously the "peripherally" acting NSAIDs do not change the excitability or conductivity of peripheral nerve membranes. For these reasons we assume that our findings with the three NSAIDs might be explained by a central site of action, in the spinal cord or in the brain (for a more detailed discussion, see Bromm et al. 1993). Consequently, the term "peripherally acting analgesics" (Lim 1970) should be discarded for these NSAIDs.

Plasma Concentrations

Fig. 6 illustrates the measured plasma concentrations of the tested NSAIDs. All three drugs are rapidly absorbed. The highest plasma concentration was seen for phenazone. Paracetamol reached about half the plasma concentration of phenazone. The plasma concentration of acetylsalicylic acid was the lowest of the three drugs, amounting to about half that of paracetamol. Acetylsalicylic acid reached a steady-state concentration of about 3 μg/ml within 25 min after its oral administration. In contrast, the concentration of the metabolite salicylic acid increased steadily within the postmedication period of 105 min, to a value of 32 μg/ml. The maximum blood concentration of phenazone (15 μg/ml) occurred at 25 min after administration and remained approximately constant until the end of the session. The absorption of paracetamol was slower, and its mean maximum plasma level was only half as high (approximately 7.5 μg/ml) as that of phenazone. All of these differences were statistically significant ($p<0.01$).

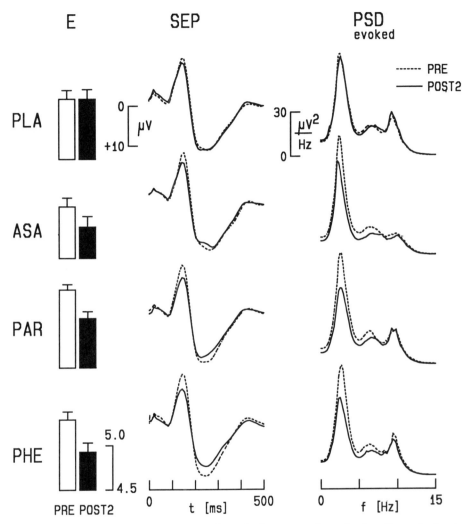

FIG. 5. Effects of NSAIDs on pain-related cerebral components and pain ratings. Analgesic effects of acetylsalicylic acid (ASA), paracetamol (PAR), and phenazone (PHE). Mean pre- and postmedication values (POST2, 90 min after oral application) are given for pain ratings (E, *left*), for pain-related somatosensory evoked potentials (SEP, *middle*), and for power-spectral densities (PSD$_{evoked}$, *right*) of EEG activity in response to pain-inducing stimuli for sessions with placebo (PLA), acetylsalicylic acid (1,000 mg), paracetamol (1,000 mg), and phenazone (1,000 mg). The data were collected in two samples of 32 subjects; placebo data were pooled from studies I and II. (From Bromm and Scharein 1993 with permission.)

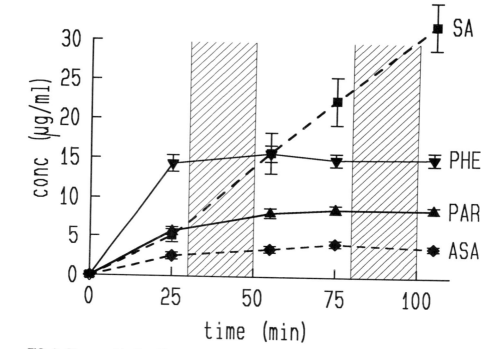

FIG. 6. Pharmacokinetics. Time course of plasma concentration of acetylsalicylic acid (ASA), salicylate (SA), paracetamol (PAR), and phenazone (PHE). The three drugs were administered orally at a dose of 1,000 mg. Mean values and their standard errors are given. *Hatched areas* indicate the time of the stimulus blocks used for testing the analgesics. (From Bromm and Scharein 1993, with permission.)

NSAIDs and the Blood–Brain Barrier

Our observations emphasize that the investigated agents, broadly classified as NSAIDs, can exert a significant effect on CNS function and should thus be able to cross the blood–brain barrier. But while cerebrospinal fluid (CSF) concentrations of some NSAIDs have been determined in various animal studies (e.g., Ochs et al. 1985; Cheney-Thamm et al. 1987), no data on this are available for humans, with the exception of one report by Bannwarth et al. (1992). We therefore measured plasma and CSF concentrations of orally administered paracetamol in 32 inpatients at the neurology clinic of the University Hospital Eppendorf who had to undergo diagnostic lumbar puncture (51.1 ± 19 years of age; 12 males, 20 females). None of the patients had disturbances of the blood–CSF barrier according to their CSF/serum ratios of albumin (Reiber and Felgenhauer 1987). Paracetamol was chosen because it does not affect blood coagulation, as does acetylsalicylic acid, and also does not increase the tendency toward bleeding after lumbar puncture.

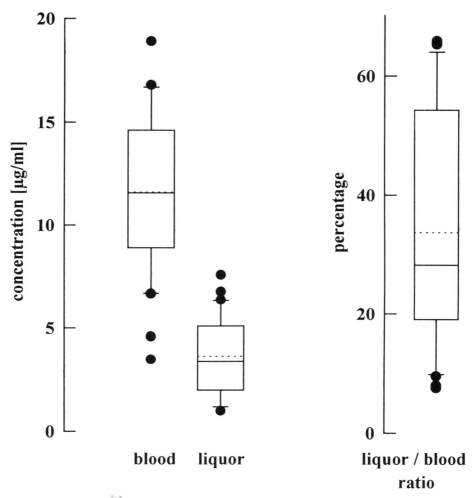

FIG. 7. Plasma and CSF concentrations of paracetamol. Distribution of plasma- and CSF concentrations in 32 inpatients at the neurologic clinic of the University Hospital Eppendorf, Hamburg, in the form of box-and-whisker plots. A dose of 1,000 mg paracetamol was given orally 90 min before the patients were subjected to a lumbar puncture for diagnostic reasons.

The distribution of the paracetamol concentration in plasma and CSF for the whole sample of patients is presented in the form of box-and-whisker-plots in Fig. 7. Mean values and medians are denoted by dotted and continuous lines within the box. The box itself encompasses the mean 50% of the data. The whiskers denote the 10th and 90th percentiles of the data distribution. At 90 min after the oral administration of 1,000 mg, the plasma concentration of paracetamol varied between 4.6 and 18.9 μg/ml, with a mean of about 12 μg/ml, while its concentration in CSF varied between 1.0 and 7.6 μg/ml, with a mean of about 3 μg/ml. In 50% of the patients a CSF/blood ratio of about 1/3 was seen (Fig. 7, right). This means that paracetamol penetrates the blood–CSF barrier to a high degree. The plasma concentration of paracetamol observed in the patients was slightly higher than in the healthy subjects (compare Fig. 4 and Fig. 6). This difference may be due to the concentrations in the healthy subjects having been measured just after a standardized breakfast, whereas the patients' blood samples were taken just before lunch.

The results of this study do not allow any direct statement about the site of action of paracetamol; however, the relatively high CSF concentrations of the drug support the hypothesis of its having a centrally mediated analgesic action.

Analyzing the Efficacy of Competitive Opioids

In a final step, the intracutaneous model of pain was used to compare the analgesic efficacy of different, competitive analgesics. We evaluated two such drugs, tramadol and ValoronN^{TM}, both used in step two of the cancer-pain-relief ladder (modestly potent opioids), as recommended by the World Health Organization (WHO) (1986). Although both agents are classified as opioids, they are available on the market by simple prescription.

Tramadol is a cyclohexanol derivative that is supposed to be a partial opiate agonist, with weak antagonistic properties, and is available on the market as Tramal^{TM}. Tramadol is well resorbed. The first effects are visible from 5 to 10 min after its oral administration, while maximal effects appear after about 60 min. The elimination half-life is about 5 hours (Lintz et al. 1986). The analgesic potency of tramadol in clinical applications is lower than that of morphine. A dose of 50 to 100 mg, given orally, corresponds to an equivalent of 10 mg morphine (Albinus and Hempel 1988). Corresponding to its low affinity for all opioid receptors, its abuse potential is relatively weak (Friderichs et al. 1978).

ValoronN^{TM} is an opioid agonist/antagonist combination (Vollmer 1988). A single dose contains the opioid agonist tilidine and the opioid antagonist naloxone in a ratio of 100:8. After oral administration, tilidine is rapidly metabolized to the analgesically active substance nortilidine. Maximal plasma concentrations of nortilidine were reached about 60 min after oral administration of ValoronN^{TM}. The elimination half-life of nortilidine varies between 3.5 and 5 hours. The analgesic efficacy of ValoronN^{TM} is about 1/5 that of 100 mg of morphine (Albinus and Hempel 1988). Naloxone was added to tilidine in order to reduce the abuse potential from non-therapeutic overdosing. After the oral administration of ValoronN^{TM} in a recommended dose, naloxone is eliminated nearly completely during passage through the liver, and has no effect. Only in the case of overdosing will naloxone reach the opioid receptors and induce withdrawal symptoms.

The same double-blind, placebo-controlled crossover design as already described was used in a sample of 32 healthy subjects (see Table 1 for the schedule of each experimental session). Both drugs were given, as is usual in our studies, in doses

TABLE 7. *Treatments and dosages for the ValoronN™/tramadol study*

VAL	100 mg tilidine + 8 mg naloxone	ValoronN™
TRA	100 mg tramadol	Tramal™
PLA	Placebo	

All drugs were orally administered. The dosages correspond to twice the minimal clinical doses.

corresponding to twice the minimum clinical dose. Details of the dosage forms and dosages are given in Table 7. The mean plasma concentrations of the two drugs, and their standard errors (SEs), are given in Fig. 8. The drugs were given orally at time point zero. The hatched areas indicate the periods in which the intracutaneous stimuli were applied. Since tilidine is transformed into the analgesically active metabolite nortilidine, the plasma concentrations for both agents are given. The nortilidine concentration reaches its maximum (about 150 ng/ml) relatively rapidly within the first 30 min after dosing, and then declines slowly, reaching a concentration of about 120 ng/ml at the end of the postmedication period. Tramadol reaches its maximum (about 280 ng/ml) significantly later, at about 50 to 70 minutes after dosing.

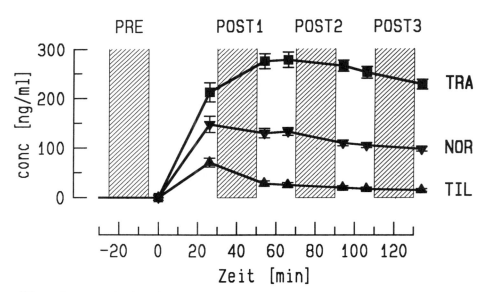

FIG. 8. Pharmacokinetics of tramadol and tilidine. The plasma concentrations of tramadol (TRA), tilidine (TIL), and nortilidine (NOR) were measured over a postmedication period of 130 min after oral administration. At time point t = 0, tramadol (100 mg) or ValoronN™ (100 mg) was given orally. The mean values and their standard errors (SEs) for a sample of 32 healthy subjects are given. The subjects received a standard breakfast 30 min before drug dosing. *Hatched areas* indicate the times of the stimulus blocks used to test the analgesics. (From Bromm et al. 1989, with permission.)

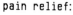

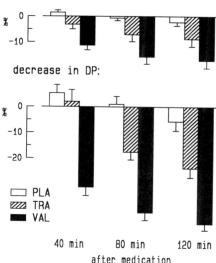

FIG. 9. Effects on pain ratings and delta power (DP) of pain-related brain potentials. The figure documents the degree of pain relief from the pre- to the postmedication periods, as a percentage of the premedication value after oral application of 100 mg ValoronN™ (VAL), 100 mg tramadol (TRA), and placebo (*PLA*). Negative values represent a decrease in pain. The mean values and their standard errors (SEs) for a sample of 32 healthy subjects are given. Upper figure: pain rating, lower figure: DP of pain-related potentials.

Although tramadol reached markedly higher concentrations than nortilidine, its analgesic effects were significantly weaker, as documented in Fig. 9. The figure shows the mean drug-induced changes from the pre- to the postmedication period, the means and SEs for the pain ratings (above), and the DP of the pain-related cerebral potentials (below). The data are given as percentages of the premedication values. With ValoronN™ the pain ratings were reduced by about 15% and with tramadol by about 5%. This difference in analgesic efficacy was highly significant during the entire postmedication period. The pharmacologically induced changes in the DP of the pain-related cerebral potentials were even higher. The different kinetics of the tested substances were also reflected in the time course of their effects. Whereas ValoronN™ exhibited a significant effect in the first postmedication period, the effects of tramadol became significant only in the second and third postmedication periods.

The evaluation of ValoronN™ and tramadol revealed that the intracutaneous model of pain can be used successfully to detect differences in analgesic efficacy, even in the case of two competitive drugs. This model may therefore provide the basis for a comparative ranking of the potency of the great variety of available analgesics in an experimentally controlled and standardized framework.

Comparative Evaluation of Analgesics by
Pain Ratings and Evoked Potentials

This chapter should not end without an attempt to present an overall view of the analgesic efficacy of all the drugs that we have so far tested. Methodologically, it is

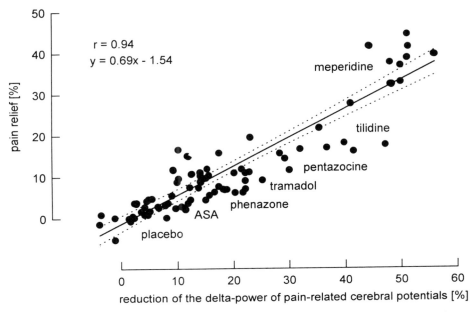

FIG. 10. Comparative evaluation of analgesic efficacy. Synoptic display of the results of 11 experimental studies with the intracutaneous pain model. The relation between the pharmacologically induced reduction of the delta power (DP) of pain-related brain potentials and the drug-induced pain relief is shown as percentages of the corresponding premedication values. Each dot represents a mean value averaged over all subjects in that study for one block of stimuli. Also plotted is the regression line of pain relief on DP reduction, and the 95% confidence interval. In the *inset*, the Pearson product-moment correlation coefficient *r* and the linear regression equation are given.

permissible to combine the results of the different pharmacologic studies described above because all were performed with the intracutaneous model of pain, using the same standardized experimental procedures, the same variables, and the same population of subjects. However, this ranking of the most commonly used analgesics should be seen in the context of the particular mode of use of each drug, its applied dosage, and the time points of measurement. Fig. 10 presents the results of 11 studies involving 16 analgesic treatments and about 250 subjects.

The ranking of analgesic potency shown in Fig. 10 has been included for two reasons. The first reason is the astonishingly high correlation between the indicators of analgesic efficacy on the physiologic and subjective levels of measurement. On the ordinate, drug-induced pain relief is plotted as a percentage of the premedication value, while on the abscissa is plotted the drug-induced decrease in the DP of pain-related cerebral potentials. Each point in the scatter diagram represents the results of one stimulus block averaged over all subjects in that study. The Pearson product-moment correlation coefficient between the two variables amounts to $r = 0.94$. This means that about 85% of the pharmacologically induced pain relief provided by each drug can be predicted from changes in the cerebral potentials, using the linear regression equation given in the inset. This high correlation suggests that pain-related components can be used in all cases in which a verbal report about analgesic effects is unavailable or may be biased.

The second reason for the ranking of analgesic potency shown in Fig. 10 is that the clinically accepted potency of the various analgesics tested is well reflected in our pain model. The results of the placebo sessions are near zero, and some new agents whose analgesic effects had been shown only in animal experiments could not be confirmed in our model. The effectiveness of the NSAIDs (e.g., acetylsali-cylic acid) is more distinct, followed by the analgesic potency of the weak opioids such as tramadol and ValoronN^{TM}, both of which are available by simple prescription. The most pronounced effects were seen for narco-analgesics licensed by the German Drug Enforcement Administration, such as the synthetic opioid meperidine (Dolantin^{TM}). This ranking of analgesic potency may be known independently of our model, but the results of our model provide some important anchor points and constitute a homogeneous framework for the classification and evaluation, in an experimentally controlled setting, of newly developed analgesic products with respect to the most familiar analgesics.

ACKNOWLEDGMENTS

The studies were supported by grants BR 310 /16 1,2,3 from the Deutsche For-schungsgemeinschaft.

REFERENCES

Albinus M, Hempel V. *Analgetika und Schmerztherapie*. Stuttgart: Wissenschaftliche Verlagsgesell-schaft, 1988.

Arendt-Nielsen L, Zachariae R, Bjerring P. Quantitative evaluation of hypnotically suggested hyper-aesthesia and analgesia by painful laser stimulation. *Pain* 1990;42:243–251.

Bannwarth B, Netter P, Lapicque F, Gillet P, Pere P, Royer RJ, Gaucher A. Plasma and cerebrospinal fluid concentrations of paracetamol after a single intravenous dose of propacetamol. *Br J Clin Pharmacol* 1992;34:79–81.

Becker DE, Yingling CD, Fein G. Identification of pain intensity and P300 components in the pain evoked potential. *Electroencephalogr Clin Neurophysiol* 1993;88:290–301.

Beecher HK. The measurement of pain: Prototype for the quantitative study of subjective responses. *Pharmacol Rev* 1957;9:59–209.

Benedetti C, Chapman CR, Colpitts YH, Chen ACN. Effects of nitrous oxide concentration on event-related potentials during painful tooth stimulation. *Anesthesiology* 1982;56:360–364.

Berger H. Über das Elektroenkephalogramm des Menschen. IX. Mitteilung. *Arch Psychiat Nervenkr* 1934;102:538–553.

Bonica JJ. The need of a taxonomy. *Pain* 1979;6:247–252.

Bromm B. Pain-related components in the cerebral potential. Experimental and multivariate statistical approaches. In: Bromm B, ed. *Pain measurement in man: Neurophysiological correlates of pain*. Amsterdam: Elsevier, 1984;233–256.

Bromm B. Laboratory animal and human volunteers in the assessment of analgesic efficacy. In: Chapman CR, Loeser JD, eds. *Issues in pain measurement*. New York: Raven Press, 1989;117–143.

Bromm B, Forth W, Richter E, Scharein E. Effects of acetaminophen and antipyrine on non-inflammatory pain and EEG activity. *Pain* 1992;50:213–221.

Bromm B, Ganzel R, Herrmann WM, Meier W, Scharein E. Pentanzocin and flupirtine effects on spontaneous and evoked EEG activity. *Neuropsychobiology* 1986;16:152–156.

Bromm B, Meier W. The intracutaneous stimulus: a new pain model for algesimetric studies. *Methods Find Exp Clin Pharmacol* 1984;6:405–410.

Bromm B, Meier W, Scharein E. Antagonism between tilidine and naloxone on cerebral potentials and pain ratings in man. *Eur J Pharmacol* 1983;87:431–440.

Bromm B, Meier W, Scharein E. Imipramine reduces experimental pain. *Pain* 1986;25:254–257.

Bromm B, Meier W, Scharein E. Pre-stimulus/post-stimulus relations in EEG spectra and their modulations by an opioid and an antidepressant. *Electroencephalogr Clin Neurophysiol* 1989;73:188–197.

Bromm B, Rundshagen I, Scharein E. Central effects of acetylsalicylic acid in healthy men. *Arzneim Forsch* 1991;41:1123–1129.

Bromm B, Scharein E. Principal component analysis of pain-related cerebral potentials to mechanical and electrical stimulation in man. *Electroencephalogr Clin Neurophysiol* 1982a;53:94–103.

Bromm B, Scharein E. Response plasticity of pain-evoked reactions in man. *Physiol Behav* 1982b;28:109–116.

Bromm B, Scharein E. Alterations in the human EEG induced by acetylsalicylic acid and related drugs. In: Jurna I, Yaksh TL, eds. Central mechanisms for analgesia by acetylsalicylic acid and [functionally] related compounds. *Progr in Pharmacol and Clin Pharmacol* 1993;10,1:23–40.

Bromm B, Treede RD. Nerve fibre discharges, cerebral potentials and sensations induced by CO2-laser stimulation. *Hum Neurobiol* 1984;3:33–40.

Bromm B, Treede RD. Laser evoked cerebral potentials in the diagnosis of cutaneous pain sensitivity. *Rév Neurol* 1991;147:625–643.

Brune K. Is there a rational basis for the different spectra of adverse affects of nonsteriodal anti-inflammatory drugs (NSAIDs)? *Drugs* 1990;40(Suppl 5):12–15.

Brune K, Beck WS, Geisslinger G, Menzel-Soglowek S, Peskar BM, Peskar BA. Aspirin-like drugs may block pain independently of prostaglandin synthesis inhibition. *Experientia* 1991;47:257–261.

Buchsbaum MF. Quantification of analgesic effects by evoked potentials. In: Bromm B, ed. *Pain measurement in man: neurophysiological correlates of pain*. Amsterdam: Elsevier, 1984;291–300.

Carmon A, Mor J, Goldberg J. Evoked cerebral responses to noxious thermal stimuli in humans. *Exp Brain Res* 1976;25:103–107.

Chapman RC, Jacobson RC. Assessment of analgesic states: can evoked potentials play a role? In: Bromm B, ed. *Pain measurement in man: neurophysiological correlates of pain*. Amsterdam: Elsevier, 1984;233–256.

Cheney-Thamm J, Alianello EA, Freed CR, Reite M. *In vivo* electrochemical recording of acetaminophen in non human primate brain. *Life Sci* 1987;40:375–379.

Cooper SA. Comparative analgesic efficacies of aspirin and acetaminophen. *Arch Intern Med* 1981;141:282–285.

Donchin E, Heffley EF. Multivariate analysis of event-related potentials data: a tutorial review. In: Otto D, ed. *Multidisciplinary perspectives in event-related brain potential research*. Washington, DC: U.S. Government Printing Office, 1978;555–572.

Droste C, Greenlee MW, Schreck M, Roskamm H. Experimental pain thresholds and plasma beta-endorphin level during exercise. *Med Sci Sports Exerc* 1991;23:334–342.

Fahrenberg J, Selg H. Freiburger Persönlichkeitsinventar (FPI). Göttingen: Hogrefe Verlag, 1970.

Ferreira SH, Lorenzetti BB, Correa FMA. Central and peripheral antialgesic action of aspirin-like drugs. *Eur J Pharmacol* 1978;53:39–48.

Flower RJ, Moncada S, Vane JR. Drug therapy of inflammation. Analgesic-antipyretics and anti-inflammatory agents; drugs employed in the treatment of gout. In: Goodman Gilman A, Goodman LS, Rall, TW, Murad F, eds. *The pharmacological basis of therapeutics*, 7th ed. New York: Macmillan, 1985;674–715.

Flower RJ, Vane JR. Inhibition of prostaglandin synthetase in brain explains the anti-pyretic activity of paracetamol (4-aceta-midophenol). *Nature* 1972;240:410–411.

Friderichs E, Felgenhauer F, Jougschaap P, Osterloh G. Pharmakologische Untersuchungen zur Analgesie, Abhängigkeits- und Toleranzentwicklung von Tramadol, einem stark wirksamen Analgetikum. *Arzneim Forsch* 1978;28:122–143.

Gracely RH. Methods of testing pain mechanisms in normal man. In: Wall PD, Melzack R, eds. *Textbook of pain*. Edinburgh: Churchill Livingstone, 1989;257–268.

Guthrie D. Intergroup and intrasubject principal component analysis of event-related potentials. *Psychophysiology* 1990;27:111–119.

Hammond D. Inference of pain and its modulation from simple behavior. In: Chapman CR, Loeser JD, eds. *Issues in pain measurement*. New York: Raven Press, 1989;69–92.

Handwerker HO, Kobal G. Psychophysiology of experimentally induced pain. *Physiol Rev* 1993;73: 639–671.

Hardy JD, Wolff HG, Goodell H. *Pain sensation and reactions*. Baltimore: Williams & Wilkins, 1952.

Herrmann WM, Schaerer E. Pharmaco-EEG: computer EEG analysis to describe the projection of drug effects on a functional level in humans. In: Lopes da Silva FH, Storm van Leeuwen W, Remond A, eds. *Handbook of electroencephalography and clinical neurophysiology, Review series*, vol. 2. 1989;385–448.

Hunt E. Mathematical models of the event-related potential. *Psychophysiology* 1985;22:395–402.

Insel PA. Analgesic-antipyretics and antiinflammatory agents; drugs employed in the treatment of rheumatoid arthritis and gout. In: Goodman LS, Gilman A, Rall TW, Nies AS, Taylor P, eds. *The pharmacological basis of therapeutics*. 8th ed. New York: Pergamon Press, 1990;638–681.

Jackson CH, MacDonald NC, Cornett JWD. Acetaminophen. *Can Med Assoc J* 1984;131:25–37.

Jacobson RC, Chapman CR, Gerlach R. Stimulus intensity and inter-stimulus interval effects on pain-related cerebral potentials. *Electroencephalogr Clin Neurophysiol* 1985;62:352–363.

Joseph J, Howland EW, Wakai R, Backonja M, Baffa O, Potenti FM, Cleeland CS. Late pain-related magnetic fields and electrical potentials evoked by intracutaneous electrical finger stimulation. *Electroencephalogr Clin Neurophysiol* 1991;80:46–52.

Jurna I, Yaksh TL eds. Central mechanisms for analgesia by acetylsalicylic acid and [functionally] related compounds. *Prog Pharmacol Clin Pharmacol* 1993;10:1.

Kaiser HF. Computer program for varimax rotation in factor analysis. *Educ Psychol Meas* 1959;3:413–420.

Kakigi R, Shibasaki H, Kuroda Y, Neshige R, Endo C, Tabuchi K, Kishikawa T. Pain-related somatosensory evoked potentials in syringomyelia. *Brain* 1991;114:1871–1889.

Klement W, Medert HA, Arndt JO. Nalbuphine does not act analgetically in electrical painful tooth pulp stimulation in man. *Pain* 1992;48:269–274.

Kobal G, Hummel C. Cerebral chemosensory evoked potentials elicited by chemical stimulation of the human olfactory and respiratory nasal mucosa. *Electroencephalogr Clin Neurophysiol* 1988;71:241–250.

Lekic D, Cenic D. Pain and tooth pulp evoked potentials. *Clin Neurophysiol* 1992;23:37–46.

Lim RKS. Pain. *Annu Rev Physiol* 1970;32:269–288.

Lintz W, Erlacin E, Frankus E, Uragg H. Metabolismus von Tramadol bei Mensch und Tier. *Arzneim Forsch* 1981;31:1932–1943.

May JG, Dunlap WP, Lovegrove WL. Factor scores derived from visual evoked potential latencies differentiate good and poor readers. *Clin Vis Sci* 1992;7:67–70.

McGuire DB. Comprehensive and multidimensional assessment and measurement of pain. *J Pain Sympt Mgmt* 1992;7:312–319.

Melzack R. Measurement of the dimension of pain experience. In: Bromm B, ed. Pain measurement in man: neurophysiological correlates of pain. Amsterdam: Elsevier, 1984;349–370.

Miltner W, Johnson R, Braun C, Larbig W. Somatosensory event-related potentials to painful and non-pain stimuli: effects of attention. *Pain* 1989;38:303–312.

Möcks J, Verleger R. Multivariate methods in biosignal analysis: application of principal component analysis to event-related potentials. In: Weikunat R, ed. *Digital biosignal processing*. Amsterdam: Elsevier, 1991;399–458.

Munger BL, Halata Z. The sensory innervation of primate facial skin. *Brain Res Rev* 1983;5:45–80.

Ochs HR, Greenblatt DJ, Abernethy DR, Arendt RM, Gerloff J, Eichelkraut W, Hahn N. Cerebrospinal fluid uptake and peripheral distribution of centrally acting drugs: relation to lipid solubility. *J Pharm Pharmacol* 1985;37:428–431.

Reading AE. Testing pain in persons in pain. In: Wall PD, Melzack R, eds. *Textbook of pain*. Edinburgh: Churchill Livingstone, 1989;269–283.

Reiber H, Felgenhauer K. Protein transfer at the blood cerebrospinal fluid barrier and the quantitation of the humoral immune response within the central nervous system. *Clin Chim Acta* 1987;163:319–328.

Scharein E, Häger F, Bromm B. Spectral estimators of short EEG segments. In: Bromm B, ed. *Pain measurement in man: neurophysiological correlates of pain*. Amsterdam: Elsevier, 1984;189–202.

Sen A, Srivastava M. *Regression analysis*. Berlin: Springer-Verlag, 1990.

Shyu KW, Lin MT, Wu TC. Possible role of central serotoninergic neurons in the development of dental pain and aspirin-induced analgesia in the monkey. *Exp Neurol* 1984;84:179–187.

Skoglund LA, Skjelbred P, Fyllingen G. Analgesic efficacy of acetaminophen 1000 mg, acetaminophen 2000 mg, and the combination of acetaminophen 1000 mg and codeine phosphate 60 mg versus placebo in acute postoperative pain. *Pharmacotherapy* 1991;11:364–369.

Smith JB, Willis AL. Aspirin selectively inhibits prostaglandin production in human platelets. *Nature (New Biol)* 1971;231:235–237.

Spreng M, Ichioka M. Langsame Rindenpotentiale bei Schmerzreizung am Menschen. *Pfluegers Arch* 1964;279:121–132.

Stambaugh JE. Multidose analgesic studies in chronic pain models. In: Max MB, Portenoy RK, Laska EM, eds. *The design of analgesic clinical trials.* New York: Raven Press, 1991;151–164.

Stowell H. Event related brain potentials and human pain: a first objective overview. *Int J Psychophysiol* 1984;1:137–151.

Treede RD, Kief S, Hölzer T, Bromm B. Late somatosensory evoked cerebral potentials in response to cutaneous heat stimuli. *Electroencephalogr Clin Neurophysiol* 1988;70:429–441.

Umino M, Sano H, Ohwatari T, Oka S, Kubota Y. Relationship between subjective pain estimation and somatosensory evoked potentials by electrical tooth stimulation. *Bull Tokyo Med Dent Univ* 1988;35: 67–74.

Vane JR. Inhibition of prostaglandin synthesis as a mechanism of action for aspirin-like drugs. *Nature (New Biol)* 1971;231:232–235.

Vierck CJ, Cooper BY, Ritz LA, Greenspan JD. Inference of pain sensitivity from complex behaviors of laboratory animals. In: Chapman CR, Loeser JD, eds. *Issues in pain measurement.* New York: Raven Press, 1989;93–116.

Vollmer KO. Pharmakologische Grundlagen des Valoron-N-Prinzips. *Fortschr Med* 1988;106:593–596.

Cancer pain relief. Geneva: World Health Organization, 1986.

Wright A, Davies I, Riddell JG. Intra-articular ultrasonic stimulation and intracutaneous electrical stimulation: evoked potential and visual analogue scale data. *Pain* 1993;52:149–155.

Yaksh TL. Central and peripheral mechanisms for the antialgesic action of acetylsalicylic acid. In: Barnett HJM, Hirsh J, Mustard JF, eds. *Acetylsalicylic acid: new aspects for an old drug.* New York: Raven Press, 1982;137–151.

Pain and the Brain: From
Nociception to Cognition,
edited by Burkhart Bromm and
John E. Desmedt, Advances in Pain
Research and Therapy Vol. 22.
Raven Press, Ltd., New York © 1995.

33

Antidepressant Drugs as Treatments for Chronic Pain: Efficacy and Mechanisms

Mitchell B. Max

*Clinical Trials Unit, Neurobiology and Anesthesiology Branch,
National Institutes of Health, Bethesda, Maryland, USA 20892*

SUMMARY

Apart from the aspirin-like drugs and opioids, tricyclic antidepressants are probably the class of drugs most commonly used to treat chronic pain. Although about 60 controlled clinical trials have been done with these drugs, evidence of their efficacy is conclusive only for diabetic neuropathy and postherpetic neuralgia, with a likely effect in fibromyalgia, tension and migraine headache, and atypical facial pain. This chapter focuses on the 16 trials of tricyclic antidepressants in neuropathic pain, from which the following conclusions may be drawn: (a) Although improvement in mood may contribute to reports of decreased pain in some patients, there is clear evidence for pain relief in patients without preexisting mood disorders. (b) Several different types of painful symptoms are relieved, including brief and steady spontaneous pains of various qualities, and light touch-evoked allodynia. (c) Drugs that block both serotonin 5-hydroxytryptamine (5HT) and norepinephrine (NE) reuptake, such as amitriptyline and imipramine, appear superior to drugs with selective actions on one of these neurotransmitters. However, the relatively selective NE reuptake blocker desipramine has consistently shown efficacy in four clinical trials. Some selective 5HT reuptake blockers (paroxetine, citalopram), but not others (fluoxetine, zimelidine), have surpassed placebo in single clinical trials. Whether other actions of the first-generation tricyclic antidepressants, such as blockade of muscarinic, adrenergic, or histaminic receptors, play a role in analgesia remains unclear, but may be elucidated by further comparisons with new and more selective agents.

Portions of this chapter are adapted, with permission, from Mitchell B. Max, Antidepressants as analgesics. In: Fields HL, Liebeskind JC, eds. *Pharmacological Approaches to the Treatment of Chronic Pain*, Seattle: IASP Publications, 1994.

INTRODUCTION

In light of the rather ambitious purpose of this book, of encouraging speculation about brain function, pain, and human experience, I must begin by saying that evidence from clinical pharmacologic studies can go only so far. The more inclusive topic of the relationship between pain and depression is fascinating (Dworkin and Gitlin 1991), and an understanding of the neural basis of that linkage would offer great benefits. Research in primary-care medicine has shown that while healthy people constantly have symptoms that go unreported to physicians, the coexistence of depression greatly increases the likelihood that the affected individual will seek a physician for treatment (Sullivan and Katon 1993); moreover, a variety of physical symptoms improve when the depression is successfully treated. Although these empirical relationships are well established, data about higher brain activity in patients with chronic pain must be correlated with the rich body of psychological literature about chronic-pain perception if we are to construct a brain-based theory of depression and pain (Price 1992), whereas suitable methods for doing this, such as brain imaging and measurement of event-related potentials, have only recently become available (see the Chapters 13 and 21).

The more modest aspiration of this chapter is to interpret the body of about 60 controlled trials that have been done with antidepressants in chronic pain, addressing recent efforts to dissect which receptor actions of these drugs are necessary for pain relief. The first-generation tricyclic antidepressants, which include amitriptyline, imipramine, desipramine, nortriptyline, clomipramine, and doxepin, have been the most frequently used and studied of this broad class of drugs. I will focus on the group of studies in patients with neuropathic pain, which provides the most coherent body of trials comparing drugs with different neurochemical mechanisms. Like most clinical pharmacology studies, these will say rather little about the site of action of tricyclic antidepressants in the nervous system. A number of animal studies have shown effects of antidepressants in models of acute pain (see references in Ardid et al. 1991), but few results have yet been published in animal models of chronic pain (Ardid and Guilbaud 1992; Fasmer et al. 1989; Ansuategui et al. 1989). Although data from clinical trials are not the firmest platform for making speculative leaps about neural mechanisms, perhaps a critical review will stimulate the thinking and research of others.

ARE ANTIDEPRESSANTS EFFECTIVE IN MOST CHRONIC PAIN SYNDROMES?

A crucial question for building an account of antidepressants' analgesic actions is whether they relieve many types of pain or just a few. Two recent reviews have examined the existing clinical data on antidepressants in chronic pain: a meta-analysis by Onghena and Van Houdenhove (1992), and a more traditional qualitative review and synthesis by Magni (1991). There have been few studies of antidepressants in acute pain conditions, most of which have focused on their interactions with opioids (Levine et al. 1986; Gordon et al. 1993; Kerrick et al. 1993; Max et al. 1992). Distilling the entire literature in this area is a difficult task, because aside from the studies in neuropathic pain, only a small number of studies have been done in each disease category. Table 1 summarizes the conclusions of the reviews by Onghena and Van Houdenhove (1992) and Magni (1991) about antidepressant efficacy in each disease category. The diagnostic categories are listed in order of decreasing magnitude of drug effect as calculated by Onghena and Van Houdenhove. The magnitude of effect is the ratio of the mean reduction in pain determined in the study (relative to placebo) divided by the standard deviation (SD) of the pain reduction; it therefore reflects the certainty that some favorable effect occurred rather than the actual magnitude of the pain reduction. Only three of the 16 published studies relating to painful neuropathy and postherpetic neuralgia were included in the meta-analysis, but those three studies are representative of the treatment effects in the other studies. The reviews concluded that antidepressant treatment appeared effective in neuropathic pain, tension and migraine headache, and atypical facial pain, but found the data to be less convincing in other disorders. The one possible exception to this were the studies of fibromyalgia, which were combined with the less responsive chronic arthritis syndromes in Onghena and Van Houdenhove's "rheumatological pain" category.

Onghena and Van Houdenhove (1992) also summarized the data regarding the importance of depressed mood as a mediator of pain relief by antidepressants (Table 2). They found the magnitudes of effect to be similar in studies that excluded depressed patients and those that included only depressed patients, in those that did and did not report a significant improvement in mood, and in those using doses below and within the dosing range considered effective for the treatment of major depression. These comparisons support the conclusions of individual studies that at least some antidepressants relieve pain independently of their effect on mood (Watson et al. 1982; Max et al. 1987; Sindrup et al. 1990b).

Although these meta-analyses suggest that a number of chronic pain conditions

TABLE 1. *Reviews of antidepressant-induced analgesia*

Diagnosis	Meta-analysis by Onghena and Van Houdenhove (1992)		Synthesis by Magni (1991)
	No. of studies	Effect size	
Diabetic neuropathy	1	1.71	Responsive
Postherpetic neuralgia	2	1.44	Responsive
Tension headache	6	1.11	Responsive
Migraine	4	0.82	Responsive
Atypical facial pain	3	0.81	Responsive
Chronic back pain	5	0.64	Minimal clinical benefit
Rheumatological pain	10	0.37	Fibrositis responsive
			Osteo- and rheumatoid arthritis, probably responsive
Not specified or mixed	7	0.23	Probable effect

From Max 1994, with permission.

TABLE 2. *Depression and antidepressant-induced analgesia*

Feature of Study	Number of studies	Effect size
Depressed patients excluded	9	0.85
Only depressed patients included	4	0.94
Mixed	26	0.52
No antidepressant effect	16	0.56
Antidepressant effect	9	0.55
Not reported	15	0.74
Doses below "antidepressant" range	22	0.75
Usual "antidepressant" doses	18	0.51

(From Max 1994, with permission, and modified from Onghena and Van Houdenhove 1992.)

may respond to antidepressants, I do not think that the data are sufficient to permit a conclusion that antidepressant drugs activate a single analgesic mechanism involved in the processing of all types of pain. Apart from the studies of neuropathic pain, the number of studies is rather small and the studies themselves lack some important design measures, such as active controls. The many side effects of tricyclic antidepressants make them clearly distinguishable from an inert placebo, and patients' belief that they are getting an active drug may produce an "active placebo" effect of the magnitude seen in some of these studies. Regarding the few conditions in which tricyclic antidepressants showed large effects, one could argue that amitriptyline and related drugs had distinct actions on several types of pathophysiologic abnormalities specific to those syndromes, such as the discharge from neuromas in nerve injury, or tight muscles in fibromyalgia, or blood-vessel or muscle abnormalities predisposing to headache.

CLINICAL TRIALS IN PAINFUL NEUROPATHY AND POSTHERPETIC NEURALGIA

The 16 controlled clinical trials of antidepressants in painful neuropathy and postherpetic neuralgia comprise the largest and most coherent body of data about the effects and mechanisms of these drugs in chronic pain. Fifteen of these trials were done by three research groups at the University of Toronto, Odense University (Denmark), and the U.S. National Institute of Dental Research (NIDR). Because these research teams used well-defined patient populations and research methods, and examined many of the same questions, their studies lend themselves to an integrated analysis.

Table 3 summarizes the 16 studies of peripheral neuropathic pain. The substantial treatment effect in these conditions is demonstrated by the fact that each of the controlled trials showed efficacy for at least one antidepressant, despite the modest sample sizes of 15 to 40 patients per group. In many of these studies, moreover, the antidepressant was superior to either an "active placebo" that mimicked antidepressant side effects (Max, 1987, 1991, 1992; Kishore-Kumar et al. 1990), to another antidepressant (Watson et al. 1985, 1992; Sindrup et al. 1992b), or to another active drug (Max et al. 1988).

TABLE 3. *Controlled antidepressant trials in painful diabetic neuropathy and postherpetic neuralgia*

Reference	Diagnosis	n	Drug	Average Dose mg/day	% Good Responders Active	% Good Responders Placebo
Watson (1982)	PHN	24	Amitriptyline	73	67%	5%
Max (1988)	PHN	34	Amitriptyline	65	47%	8%
Kishore-Kumar (1990)	PHN	19	Desipramine	167	63%	11%
Watson (1992)	PHN	32	Maprotilene	100	18%	—
			Amitriptyline	100	44%	—
Watson (1985)	PHN	15	Zimelidine	300	7%	—
			Amitriptyline	70	60%	—
Max (1987)	Diab	29	Amitriptyline	90	66%	21%
Max (1991)	Diab	20	Desipramine	201	55%	10%
Max (1992)	Diab	38	Amitriptyline	105	74%	—
		38	Desipramine	111	61%	—
		46	Fluoxetine	40	48%	41%
Kvinesdal (1984)	Diab	12	Imipramine	100	58%	0%
Sindrup (1989)	Diab	9	Imipramine	178	88%	11%
Sindrup (1990a)	Diab	15	Imipramine	25–350‡	93%	—
Sindrup (1990b)	Diab	20	Imipramine	200	89%	—*
			Paroxetine	40	60%	
Sindrup (1990c)	Diab	19	Clomipramine	75	47%	—*
			Desipramine	200	42%	
Sindrup (1992a)	Diab	15	Citalopram	40	40%	13%†
Sindrup (1992b)	Diab	18	Imipramine	150	50%	—*
			Mianserin	60	22%	
Langohr (1982)	Mixed neurop	40	Clomipramine	150	58%	15%

†Global relief scores not reported, so response defined here as >33% reduction in patient's VAS symptom score relative to baseline†, if reported, or to placebo period.

‡Prospective concentration–response study; each patient was given a series of doses, the highest of which would ensure a plasma concentration of imipramine + desipramine>120 ng/ml.

Abbreviations: Diab = painful diabetic neuropathy; PHN = postherpetic neuralgia; neurop = neuropathic pain syndromes.

Adapted from Max (1994), with pemission.

In many of these studies there was a significant pain-relieving effect even when depressed patients were excluded from the analysis (Max et al. 1987, 1992; Sindrup et al. 1990b). All three research groups have prospectively followed various qualities of pain to learn whether antidepressants selectively relieve certain pains. However, no such selective effect was observed. The antidepressants in these studies relieved brief, lancinating pains as well as constant pains (Watson et al. 1982; Max et al. 1987; Kishore-Kumar et al. 1990), and allodynia as well as spontaneous pain (Kishore-Kumar et al. 1990; Watson et al. 1992). No differences have been discerned in the relief afforded for various qualities of steady pain, such as burning, aching, sharp, or pressing pain (Max et al. 1988, 1992), or between pain, paresthesia, and dysesthesia (Sindrup et al. 1990b).

Effects of antidepressants on experimental pain are less clear. Both Max et al. (1987) and Sindrup et al. (1990b) found that chronic treatment with amitriptyline, and with imipramine and paroxetine, reduced clinical neuropathic pain but did not affect ratings of experimental thermal pain stimuli delivered to normally innervated skin. In contrast to these results following chronic antidepressant treatment, experimental pain appears to respond to acute administration of antidepressants. Bromm et al. (1986) reported that a single oral dose of 100 mg of imipramine reduced the perception of pain produced by intracutaneous electrical stimulation. In Bromm's study, the reports of reduction in pain may have been caused by the acute sedative effects of the drug, which were sufficient to produce slow waves in the electroencephalogram (EEG). Sedation was only minimal, however, in the recent report by Coquoz et al. (1993), who found that single doses of desipramine increased the pain threshold and reduced the amplitude of the R-III reflex evoked by electrical stimulation of the sural nerve. Because the R-III reflex is a spinal reflex, the authors concluded that at least part of the acute analgesic action of desipramine was mediated at that level. Poulsen et al. (1993) have presented preliminary results showing that a single dose of imipramine reduces pain evoked by heat and electrical stimuli, and the amplitude of the R-III reflex. The disparity between the results of acute and chronic treatment is perplexing. One might hypothesize that tolerance occurs to analgesic effects of tricyclic antidepressants on experimental pain, yet the clinical studies have shown no fading of relief of clinical pain after up to 6 weeks of treatment.

Selective versus Mixed Monoamine-Reuptake Blockers

The prevailing hypothesis regarding antidepressant-related analgesia is that the drugs' blockade of norepinephrine (NE) and/or serotonin (5HT) reuptake causes prolonged inhibitory effects of these neurotransmitters at central nervous system (CNS) synapses involved in the modulation of pain (Basbaum and Fields 1978; Dubner and Bennett 1983). The three laboratories investigating neuropathic pain have each pursued this reasoning by comparing drugs with selective actions on NE or 5HT to drugs with both actions.

If acute monoamine-reuptake blockade were the primary analgesic mechanism of antidepressants, one would expect the onset of pain relief to occur within minutes after dosing, just as it does in animals (Ardid and Guilbaud 1992). This would contrast with the mood effects of antidepressants, which often require several weeks to develop (Davis and Glassman 1989). Sindrup et al. (1990b) have done careful studies of the time course of antidepressant activity of tricyclic antidepressants. Preliminary studies of each patient's metabolic rate for a single dose of imipramine made it possible to use a high fixed dose during the multidose clinical trial, rather than the slow titration from a small dose that other investigators have used. Fig. 1 (upper left panel) shows that pain relief during treatment with imipramine and paroxetine approached near-maximal levels within 4 to 6 days after the beginning of treatment. This time course, which parallels the increase in plasma concentrations of these drugs, is consistent with the hypothesis that pain relief is directly linked to acute blockade of monoamine reuptake. Other studies have suggested that there may also be smaller increments in pain relief 1 or 2 weeks after amitriptyline or desipramine reach steady-state concentrations. Such an effect was described in 7 of 12 drug treatment periods in the studies by Kishore-Kumar et al. (1990) and Max et al. (1987, 1988, 1991, 1992) listed in Table 3.

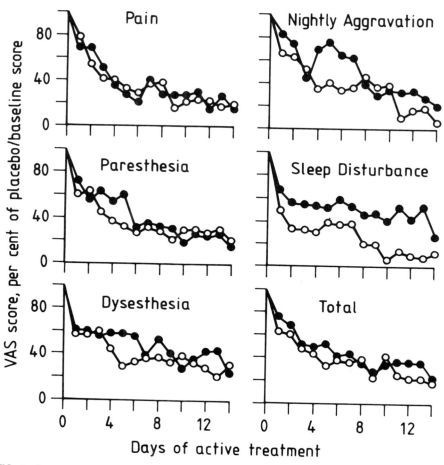

FIG. 1. Onset of action of imipramine (*open circles*) and paroxetine (*filled circles*) in a study of patients with painful diabetic neuropathy. Near-maximal reduction of pain (*upper left*) is evident as early as 4 to 6 days after beginning treatment with a fixed dose of imipramine determined by a prior dose-finding period. The time course of onset of pain relief parallels the expected time course of imipramine plasma concentrations. These results are consistent with the hypothesis that acute blockade of monoamine reuptake mediates pain relief. (From Sindrup et al. 1990b, with permission.)

I would raise several *caveats* about the assumptions underlying the clinical comparisons of selective monoamine-reuptake blockers. First, the concentrations of various antidepressants at the relevant receptors in the brain are unknown. Therefore, one cannot say with assurance whether selective blockade of central neural mechanisms is achieved. Richelson (1989) has pointed out that explanations of comparative effects of antidepressants based on affinity constants are on firm ground only for peripheral tissues, where plasma drug concentrations are relevant. In order to directly answer this question in humans, one would need to do imaging studies of the pertinent receptors, using radiolabeled noradrenergic and serotonergic ligands. A second caveat is that although particular antidepressants selectively affect reuptake of NE or 5HT, the consequences do not remain confined to each of these two particular monoamine systems, as demonstrated by Potter et al. (1985) in patients with depression. These investigators showed that a selective blocker of 5HT reuptake, zimelidine, and of NE reuptake, desipramine, produced similar alterations in the levels of cerebrospinal fluid (CSF) metabolites of both 5HT and NE.

The evidence accumulated to date about selective monoamine-reuptake blockers suggests that the potentiation of NE is the more important action of tricyclic antidepressants. Our group at NIDR has done three clinical trials of the selective NE reuptake blocker desipramine in neuropathic pain. Placebo-controlled studies of desipramine in both diabetic neuropathy (Max et al. 1991) and postherpetic neuralgia (Kishore-Kumar et al. 1990) showed analgesic effects of similar magnitude to those that we had reported with amitriptyline. In order to directly compare the effects of reuptake blockade of NE, 5HT, and both transmitters, we then performed two concomitant crossover studies (Max et al. 1992). In one study we compared amitriptyline (mean dose, 105 mg/day) to desipramine (111 mg/day) in 38 patients with diabetic neuropathy, and in the other we compared fluoxetine, 40 mg, to a benztropine active placebo in 46 diabetic patients. Most of the patients were randomly assigned to either of the studies as well as to the order of treatment, allowing a comparison among all three drugs and placebo in this subgroup.

Table 3 and Figure 2 show that amitriptyline and desipramine were each effective, resulting in "moderate" relief or better in 74% and 61% of the patients, respectively. The trend toward superiority of amitriptyline was not statistically significant. In the other crossover comparison, fluoxetine was similar to placebo, with 47% and 41% of the patients responding, respectively. The modest trend toward a fluoxetine effect apparent in Fig. 2 disappeared when the 13 depressed patients were excluded from the analysis, suggesting that this small effect was related to improvement in patients' mood. While it is possible that 40 mg was a suboptimal dose of fluoxetine, there was no greater analgesic effect in patients with relatively high or low plasma concentrations of fluoxetine or its metabolite, norfluoxetine.

We conclude from these results that desipramine approaches amitriptyline in its efficacy in relieving neuropathic pain, offering an alternative to patients unable to tolerate the sedative or anticholinergic effects of amitriptyline. Fluoxetine appears ineffective except in depressed patients. If we were to assume that drug concentrations in the brain were similar to plasma concentrations at steady state, these results would be consistent with the hypothesis that a high level of blockade of NE reuptake is required for pain relief (Table 4). Note that the plasma concentration of fluoxetine in this study, 480 nM, was well over the 280 nM required for 50% blockage of NE reuptake. In contrast, the high degree of 5HT reuptake blockade afforded by fluoxetine was insufficient to provide pain relief. This finding is consistent with Watson and Evans' (1985) report that zimelidine, another specific 5HT reuptake blocker, did not relieve pain in patients with postherpetic neuralgia who responded to amitriptyline.

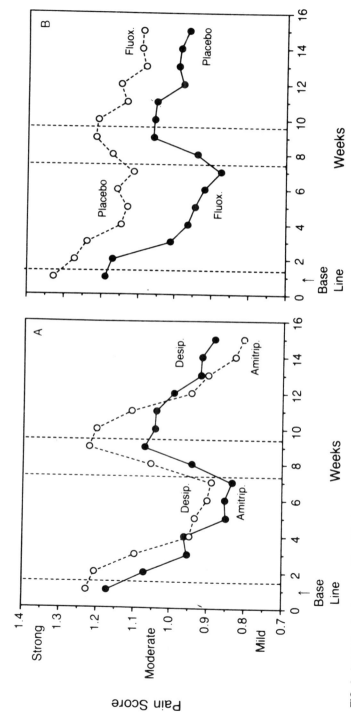

FIG. 2. Intensity of pain caused by diabetic neuropathy during treatment with amitriptyline and desipramine in 38 patients (**A**), and during treatment with fluoxetine and placebo in 46 patients (**B**). The mean weekly values of the descriptors of pain intensity are plotted; three of the actual descriptors used in the diary are shown in their equivalent positions on the ordinate. Each curve represents a single group receiving sequential treatments. The central vertical lines distinguish the two 6-week treatment periods from the intervening 2-week washout period. There was no statistically significant difference between the effects of amitriptyline and desipramine, but both were significantly more effective than placebo in the subgroup of patients who were randomized among all four possible treatments. There was no significant difference between the effects of fluoxetine and placebo, and the modest trend favoring fluoxetine was due entirely to the data from the 13 depressed patients. (From Max et al. 1992, with permission.)

TABLE 4. *Binding constants of amitriptyline, desipramine, and fluoxetine for inhibition of reuptake and receptor binding of various transmitters*

Drug[†]	Monoamine reuptake blockade K_i, nmol/L			Receptor blockade K_d, nmol/L			
	NE	5HT	DA	H_1	Musc	α_1	α_2
Amitriptyline [180 nmol/L]	24	66	2,300	1	18	27	940
Desipramine [190 nmol/L]	1	340	5,200	110	198	130	7,200
Fluoxetine [480 nmol/L]	280	12	1,600	6,200	2,000	5,900	13,000

Nortriptyline and 10-OH-nortriptyline, the major metabolites of amitriptyline (110 nmol/L and 150 nM in this study), are similar to desipramine in their potent NE and weak 5HT reuptake blockade. Effects of the desipramine metabolite 2-OH-desipramine (110 nmol/L), and the fluoxetine metabolite norfluoxetine [550 nmol/L] are similar to those of the parent compounds (Fuller and Wong 1977; Bertilsson et al. 1979; Potter et al. 1979).
[†]Drug name is followed in brackets by median serum concentration in the study by Max et al. (1992). Binding constants are from Richelson and Nelson (1984) and Richelson and Pfenning (1984). NE = norepinephrine; 5HT = serotonin; DA = dopamine; H_1 = histamine$_1$; musc = muscarinic cholinergic; α_1 and α_2 = adrenergic receptor subtypes.
(From Max et al. 1992, and Dubner and Max 1992, with permission.)

It is likely that the trend toward superiority of amitriptyline over desipramine was real, since other investigators have reported that blockers of both NE and 5HT reuptake were superior to selective NE reuptake blockers. Watson et al. (1992) reported that amitriptyline was more effective than the NE reuptake blocker maprotilene in postherpetic neuralgia. Sindrup et al., comparing drugs across studies of diabetic neuropathic pain, have found imipramine more frequently effective than desipramine (Table 3). Table 4 illustrates a number of possible mechanisms for this advantage of amitriptyline-like drugs. Amitriptyline is a better 5HT reuptake blocker than desipramine, and it is possible that while this action alone is not sufficient to relieve pain, it may enhance the pain-relieving effects of NE reuptake blockade. Other explanations for an advantage of amitriptyline suggested in Table 4 include its ability to antagonize histamine$_1$ (H_1), muscarinic cholinergic, or α_1-adrenergic receptors.

Sindrup et al. have reported results that agree in some respects with those of the Canadian and American groups, but differ regarding the effectiveness of selective 5HT reuptake blockers. Figure 3, from Sindrup et al. (1992a), combines the results from a number of their studies in patients with diabetic neuropathy (see Table 3 for references). In resemblance to the results described above, the tricyclic antidepressants with "balanced inhibition" of 5HT and NE reuptake, imipramine and clomipramine, appeared to be the most effective agents. The selective NE reuptake blocker desipramine, assessed in a single study, was also effective. Mianserin, a non-tricyclic antidepressant that does not block reuptake of either NE or 5HT but strongly antagonizes the H_1 receptor, did not relieve pain. This supports the monoamine hypothesis for antidepressant analgesia, and argues against an important contribution from antihistamine effects.

The perplexing difference between the findings of Sindrup et al. and those of the

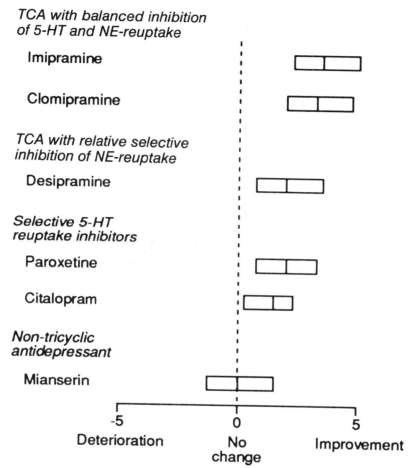

FIG. 3. Effectiveness of various antidepressants on symptoms of diabetic neuropathy. Medians (*vertical lines*) and 95% confidence intervals (*boxes*) describe the differences between different antidepressants and placebo as measured by physician scoring of symptoms of pain and discomfort on a 0 to 12 scale. Data are drawn from a number of the studies by Sindrup et al. listed in Table 3. As in the studies by Max et al. (Fig. 2) and Watson et al., a selective norepinephrine reuptake inhibitor was effective, and drugs that inhibit both norepinephrine and serotonin reuptake appeared even more effective. The results shown here differ from findings of Watson et al. and Max et al. in that the specific serotonin reuptake inhibitors paroxetine and citalopram showed a statistically significant analgesic effect. TCA = tricylic antidepressant; NE = norepinephrine. (From Sindrup et al. 1992a, with permission.)

Canadian and NIDR groups is that Sindrup found that two different selective 5HT reuptake inhibitors, paroxetine and citalopram, had analgesic effects in groups of 20 and 15 patients, respectively. Although the magnitude of the effects was less than Sindrup et al. and others found for mixed reuptake blockers, this contrasts with the flatly negative results in the 61 patients who were given fluoxetine or zimelidine in studies by the other two groups. There were no obvious differences between the populations of diabetic neuropathy patients studied by Sindrup et al. and by Max, and the spectrum of receptor actions of fluoxetine, paroxetine, and citalopram are similar (Leonard 1992). Larger studies of paroxetine and other 5HT reuptake blockers are needed because of the more favorable safety profile of these drugs than of amitriptyline and imipramine (Halper and Mann 1984; Blackwell 1987). These drugs, which cause no postural hypotension, cholinergic blockade, or heart block, will be valuable for elderly or medically unstable patients even if they are only modestly effective.

Other possible mechanisms for antidepressants' relief of neuropathic pain have been suggested. To take one example, patients who respond may have sympathetically maintained pain from NE-sensitive painful neuromas. This possibility has received little direct study, although Tsigos et al. (1993) found that in patients with diabetic neuropathy, severity of pain was significantly correlated with levels of plasma NE. Antidepressants might relieve this pain by directly blocking α_1-adrenergic receptors (Table 4) or by reducing sympathetic efferent activity; Esler et al. (1991) found that the acute intravenous infusion of desipramine in a dose of 0.5 mg/kg reduced peroneal nerve sympathetic impulses by 90%. Recent animal studies have also suggested that tricyclic antidepressants block the N-methyl-D-aspartate (NMDA) receptor (Cai and McCaslin 1992; McCaslin et al. 1992), but this relationship is complex (De Montis et al. 1993) and needs further clarification. Studies of antidepressants in animal models of chronic pain (Ardid and Guilbaud 1992) may clarify their site and mechanism of action. A challenging part of this task will be to explain the observation that amitriptyline relieved pain (in one small controlled study) caused by cerebral lesions (Leijon and Boivie 1989; and see Chapter 24).

CONCLUSIONS

At present, almost all of the scientific data about antidepressants and chronic pain come from human therapeutic trials, which provide at best only limited evidence about the neurochemical mechanism of drug action, and virtually no clues regarding site of action. It is clear that peripheral neuropathic pain responds to antidepressants, and there is some evidence for a benefit of these drugs in fibromyalgia, tension and migraine headache, and atypical facial pain. Response in back pain, chronic arthritis, and mixed groups of chronic-pain patients has been inconsistent.

The 16 published clinical trials of tricyclic antidepressants in neuropathic pain suggest that NE reuptake blockade may be the most important action of these drugs in mediating analgesia, but serotonin reuptake blockade, decreased sympathetic outflow, or antagonism of α_1-adrenergic or muscarinic cholinergic receptors may also contribute to pain relief. The program of studies of these effects would need to be replicated in at least one other model of chronic pain before one could conclude that these conclusions hold for chronic pain in general. The dissection of antidepressant pain mechanisms using animal models of chronic pain have just begun. Such studies are needed to assess the relative contribution of peripheral, spinal, and supraspinal mechanisms to the antidepressant drugs' relief of pain.

REFERENCES

Ansuategui M, Naharro L, Feria M. Noradrenergic and opioidergic influences on the antinociceptive effectiveness of clomipramine in the formalin test in rats. *Psychopharmacology* 1989;98:93–96.

Ardid D, Eschalier A, Laverenne J. Evidence for a central but not peripheral analgesic effect of clomipramine in rats. *Pain* 1991;45:95–100.

Ardid D, Guilbaud G. Antinociceptive effects of acute and "chronic" injections of tricyclic antidepressant drugs in a new model of mononeuropathy in rats. *Pain* 1992;49:279–287.

Basbaum AI, Fields HL. Endogenous pain control mechanisms: Review and hypothesis. *Ann Neurol* 1978;4:451–462.

Bertilsson L, Mellstrom B, Sjoqvist F. Pronounced inhibition of noradrenaline uptake by 10-hydroxy-metabolites of nortriptyline. *Life Sci* 1979;25:1285–1292.

Blackwell B. Side effects of antidepressant drugs. *Psychiatry Update* 1987;6:724–725.

Bromm B, Meier W, Scharein E. Imipramine reduces experimental pain. *Pain* 1986;25:245–257.

Cai Z, McCaslin PP. Amitriptyline, desipramine, cyproheptadine and carbamazepine, in concentrations used therapeutically, reduce kainate- and *N*-methyl-D-aspartate-induced intracellular Ca^{2+} levels in neuronal culture. *Eur J Pharmacol* 1992;219:53–57.

Coquoz D, Porchet HC, Dayer P. Central analgesic effects of desipramine, fluvoxamine, and moclobemide after single oral dosing: a study in healthy volunteers. *Clin Pharmacol Ther* 1993;54:339–344.

Davis JM, Glassman AH. Antidepressant drugs. In: Kaplan HI, Sadock BJ, eds. *Comprehensive textbook of psychiatry*, 5th ed. Baltimore: Williams & Wilkins, 1989;1627–1654.

De Montis MG, Gambarana C, Meloni D, Taddei I, Tagliamonte A. Long-term imipramine effects are prevented by NMDA receptor blockade. *Brain Res* 1993;606:63–67.

Dubner R, Bennett GJ. Spinal and trigeminal mechanisms of nociception. *Annu Rev Neurosci* 1983;6:381–418.

Dubner R, Max M. Antidepressants and relief of neuropathic pain: evidence for noradrenergic mechanisms. In: Besson J-M, Guilbaud G, eds. *Noradrenergic agonists for the treatment of pain*. Amsterdam: Excerpta Medica, 1992;211–218.

Dworkin RH, Gitlin MJ. Clinical aspects of depression in chronic pain patients. *Clin J Pain* 1991;7:79–94.

Esler MD, Wallin G, Dorward PK, et al. Effects of desipramine on sympathetic nerve firing and norepinephrine spillover to plasma in humans. *Am J Physiol* 1991;260:R817–R823.

Fasmer OB, Hunskaar S, Hole K. Antinociceptive effect of serotonergic reuptake inhibitors in mice. *Neuropharmacology* 1989;28:1363–1366.

Fuller RW, Wong DT. Inhibition of serotonin reuptake. *Fed Proc* 1977;36:2154–2158.

Gordon NC, Heller PH, Gear RW, Levine JD. Temporal factors in the enhancement of morphine analgesia by desipramine. *Pain* 1993;53:273–276.

Halper JP, Mann JJ. Cardiovascular effects of antidepressant medications. *Br J Psychiatry* 1988;153 (Suppl 3):87–98.

Kerrick JM, Fine PG, Lipman AG, Love G. Low dose amitriptyline as an adjunct to opioids for postoperative orthopedic pain: a placebo-controlled trial. *Pain* 1993;52:325–330.

Kishore-Kumar R, Max MB, Schafer SC, et al. Desipramine relieves postherpetic neuralgia. *Clin Pharmacol Ther* 1990;47:305–312.

Kishore-Kumar R, Schafer SC, Lawlor BA, Murphy DL, Max MB. Single doses of the serotonin agonists buspirone and m-chlorophenylpiperazine do not relieve neuropathic pain. *Pain* 1989;37: 223–227.

Kvinesdal B, Molin J, Froland A, Gram LF. Imipramine treatment of painful diabetic neuropathy. *JAMA* 1984;251:1727–1730.

Langohr HD, Stohr M, Petruch F. An open and double-blind cross-over study on the efficacy of clomipramine (Anafranil) in patients with painful mono- and polyneuropathies. *Eur Neurol* 1982; 21:309–317.

Leijon G, Boivie J. Central post-stroke pain: a controlled trial of amitriptyline and carbamazepine. *Pain* 1989;36:27–36.

Leonard BE. Pharmacological differences of serotonin reuptake inhibitors and possible clinical relevance. *Drugs* 1992;43(Suppl 2):3–10.

Levine JD, Gordon NC, Smith R, McBryde R. Desipramine enhances opiate postoperative analgesia. *Pain* 1986;27:45–49.

Magni G. The use of antidepressants in the treatment of chronic pain: a review of the current evidence. *Drugs* 1991;42:730–748.

Max MB. Antidepressants as analgesics. In: Fields HL, Liebeskind JC, eds. *Pharmacological approaches to the treatment of chronic pain: The Fourth Annual Bristol-Myers Squibb Symposium on Pain Research*. Seattle: IASP Publications, 1994;229–246.

Max MB, Culnane M, Schafer SC, et al. Amitriptyline relieves diabetic neuropathy pain in patients with normal or depressed mood. *Neurology* 1987;37:589–596.

Max MB, Kishore-Kumar R, Schafer SC, Meister B, Gracely RH, Smoller B, Dubner R. Efficacy of desipramine in painful diabetic neuropathy: a placebo-controlled trial. *Pain* 1991;45:3–9.

Max MB, Lynch SA, Muir J, Shoaf SE, Smoller B, Dubner R. Effects of desipramine, amitriptyline, and fluoxetine on pain in diabetic neuropathy. *N Engl J Med* 1992;326:1250–1256.

Max MB, Schafer SC, Culnane M, Smoller B, Dubner R, Gracely RH. Amitriptyline, but not lorazepam, relieves postherpetic neuralgia. *Neurology* 1988;38:1427–1432.

Max MB, Ziegler D, Shoaf SE, et al. Effects of a single oral dose of desipramine on postoperative morphine analgesia. *J Pain Symptom Management* 1992;7:454–462.

McCaslin PP, Yu XZ, Ho IK, Smith TG. Amitriptyline prevents N-methyl-D-aspartate (NMDA)-induced toxicity, does not prevent NMDA-induced elevations of extracellular glutamate, but augments kainate-induced elevations of glutamate. *J Neurochem* 1992;59:401–405.

Onghena P, Van Houdenhove B. Antidepressant-induced analgesia in chronic non-malignant pain: a meta-analysis of 39 placebo-controlled studies. *Pain* 1992;49:205–220.

Potter WZ, Scheinin M, Golden RN, et al. Selective antidepressants and cerebrospinal fluid: lack of specificity on norepinephrine and serotonin metabolites. *Arch Gen Psychiatry* 1985;42:1171–1177.

Potter WZ, Calil HM, Manian AA, Zavadil AP, Goodwin FK. Hydroxylated metabolites of tricyclic antidepressants: preclinical assessment of activity. *Biol Psychiatry* 1979;14:601–613.

Poulsen L, Arendt-Nielsen L, Brosen K, Nielsen KK, Gram LF, Sindrup SH. The hypoalgesic effect of imipramine in different human experimental pain models. *Pain* 1995;60:287–294.

Price DD. The affective-motivational dimension of pain: a two-stage model. *APS Journal* 1992;1:229–239.

Richelson E. Antidepressants: pharmacology and clinical use. In: Karasu TB, ed. *Treatments of psychiatric disorders*, vol. 3. Washington, DC: American Psychiatric Association, 1989;1773–1787.

Richelson E, Nelson A. Antagonism by antidepressants of neurotransmitter receptors of normal human brain *in vitro*. *J Pharmacol Exp Ther* 1984;230:94–102.

Richelson E, Pfenning M. Blockade by antidepressants and related compounds of biogenic amine uptake into rat brain synaptosomes: most antidepressants selectively block norepinephrine uptake. *Eur J Pharmacol* 1984;104:277–286.

Sindrup SH, Bjerre U, Dejgaard A, Brøsen K, Aes-Jørgensen T, Gram LF. The selective serotonin reuptake inhibitor citalopram relieves the symptoms of diabetic neuropathy. *Clin Pharmacol Ther* 1992a; 52:547–552.

Sindrup SH, Gram LF, Brøsen K, Eshøj O, Mogensen EF. The selective serotonin reuptake inhibitor paroxetine is effective in the treatment of diabetic neuropathy symptoms. *Pain* 1990b;42:135–144.

Sindrup SH, Gram LF, Skjold T, Frøland A, Beck-Nielsen H. Concentration-response relationship in imipramine treatment of diabetic neuropathy symptoms. *Clin Pharmacol Ther* 1990a;47:509–515.

Sindrup SH, Gram LF, Skjold T, Grodum E, Brøsen K, Beck-Nielsen H. Clomipramine vs desipramine vs placebo in the treatment of diabetic neuropathy symptoms: a double-blind cross-over study. *Br J Clin Pharmacol* 1990c;30:683–691.

Sindrup SH, Tuxen C, Gram LF, et al. Lack of effect of mianserin on the symptoms of diabetic neuropathy. *Eur J Clin Pharmacol* 1992b;43:251–255.

Sullivan M, Katon W. Somatization: the path between distress and somatic symptoms. *Am Pain Soc J* 1993;2:141–149.

Tsigos C, Reed P, Winkove C, White A, Young RJ. Plasma norepinephrine in sensory diabetic polyneuropathy. *Diabetes Care* 1993;16:1–6.

Watson CPN, Chipman M, Reed K, Evans RJ, Birkett N. Amitriptyline versus maprotiline in postherpetic neuralgia: a randomized, double-blind, crossover trial. *Pain* 1992;48:29–36.

Watson CPN, Evans RJ. A comparative trial of amitriptyline and zimelidine in post-herpetic neuralgia. *Pain* 1985;23:387–394.

Watson CPN, Evans RJ, Reed K, Merskey H, Goldsmith L, Warsh J. Amitriptyline versus placebo in postherpetic neuralgia. *Neurology* 1982;32:671–673.

Pain and the Brain: From
Nociception to Cognition,
edited by Burkhart Bromm and
John E. Desmedt, Advances in Pain
Research and Therapy Vol. 22.
Raven Press, Ltd., New York © 1995.

34

Opioids and Diffuse Noxious Inhibitory Control (DNIC) in the Rat

Daniel Le Bars, Didier Bouhassira, and Luis Villanueva

Department of Physiopharmacology, INSERM U-161, F-75014 Paris France

SUMMARY

Both spinally and supraspinally mediated systems modulate the spinal and trigeminal transmission of nociceptive signals. Spinal networks underlie the segmental inhibitions produced through large-diameter cutaneous afferent fibers and are naturally activated by mechanical non-noxious stimuli. In contrast, inhibitions triggered by heterosegmental stimuli are supraspinally mediated and depend on the activation of nociceptors connected to fine myelinated or unmyelinated afferent fibers. Thus, activities of convergent neurons, which play a major role in the transmission of nociceptive information, are selectively and powerfully inhibited by the application of noxious stimuli to any body areas distant from their excitatory receptive fields. Such inhibitory phenomena, termed diffuse noxious inhibitory controls (DNIC), were initially described in the rat and subsequently in other animal species. The main features of DNIC have been determined in the rat: these controls affect all convergent neurons, including those projecting to the thalamus, whether in the spinal cord or the trigeminal system; they affect all activities of these neurons and are exclusively triggered by noxious stimuli, whatever their type; and the inhibitions are correlated to the intensity of the conditioning stimuli. Such inhibitory effects are not observed in spinalized animals, which indicates that they are sustained by an anatomic loop involving supraspinal structures. Most of the peripheral and central elements of this loop have been determined in the rat, including: (a) the involvement of peripheral $A\delta$ and C fibers in the activation of DNIC; (b) localization of the ascending and descending spinal pathways in the anterolateral quadrant and dorsolateral funiculi, respectively; (c) the demonstration, in a series of studies aimed at determining the supraspinal structures of the loop, that they were entirely confined within the caudalmost part of the medulla. These last results also indicated that DNIC modulate nociception independently of the classically described descending systems, which involve midbrain structures such as the periaqueductal grey (PAG) or nucleus raphe magnus. With regard to the physiologic role of DNIC, it was proposed that they may facilitate the extraction of nociceptive information by an increase in the signal-to-noise ratio between a pool of neurons activated by a painful focus and the remaining silent population. Although differently organized, this mechanism is reminiscent of lateral inhibition described in various relays of other sensory systems, and could act in synergy with segmental processes for the amplification of nociceptive signals. According to this model, hypo- or hyperalgesia may result from a decrease or an increase in this contrast, respectively. One way of testing such a hypothesis was to investigate the effects of morphine on DNIC. DNIC were found to be extremely sensitive to the systemic or intracerebroventricular (ICV) administration of low doses of morphine. These effects are dose-dependent, stereospecific, and naloxone-reversible. Several lines of evidence suggested that these effects of morphine on DNIC are due to interaction with opioid receptors within the PAG. Among such evidence was that: (a) microinjections of morphine directly into the PAG induced a significant depression of DNIC; (b) autoradiographic controls with tritiated morphine performed after ICV morphine revealed a massive binding throughout the rostro-caudal extent of the PAG; (c) the lifting of DNIC by systemic morphine disappeared in animals with lesions of the PAG. The effects of morphine on DNIC were also tested in animals with lesions of the rostral ventromedial medulla (RVM) since this region, together with the PAG, has been suggested as one major supraspinal site involved in the supraspinal mechanisms of morphine analgesia. DNIC were found to be similarly reduced following systemic morphine in sham-operated animals and animals tested 1 week after lesioning of the RVM. In contrast, DNIC were not significantly altered in animals tested 3 weeks after lesioning. Interestingly, behavioral studies of the antinociceptive effects of morphine in RVM-lesioned animals have produced similar time-dependent effects. On the basis of the striking similarities between the effects of lesions of either the PAG or RVM on the pharmacologic responses in both behavioral and DNIC studies in animals, it was suggested that the blockade of DNIC has a role in the antinociceptive effects of low doses of morphine. Thus, in addition to its spinal action, a reduction of descending inhibitory controls may contribute to the antinociceptive effects of morphine. However, the participation of opioidergic systems in DNIC is complex, since systemic naloxone can also reduce these controls. Such effects of naloxone were observed in PAG-lesioned animals, indicating that more than one opioidergic system is involved in DNIC. Within the proposed theoretical framework, such an effect of naloxone may explain its paradoxical analgesic effects in humans, following its systemic administration in low doses. Data obtained in humans tend to reinforce these conclusions about opioid systems and DNIC (see Chapter 35).

INTRODUCTION

The transmission of nociceptive signals can be modulated by powerful controls at as early a stage as the first spinal relay. These controls include both segmental mechanisms and systems that involve supraspinal structures, and some of them can be triggered by somesthetic stimuli (see the references in Dubner and Bennett 1983; Le Bars et al. 1984, 1986, 1989; Besson and Chaouch, 1987; Wall 1989; Willis and Coggeshall 1991). This last point is true for segmental mechanisms that can be triggered by stimulation of the corresponding dermatome: the responses of dorsal-horn neurons to nociceptive stimuli can be inhibited by innocuous stimulation of large-diameter cutaneous fibers. It is generally thought that these phenomena are triggered by the activation of $A\alpha\beta$-fibers alone; however, numerous studies have demonstrated that the activation of $A\delta$-fibers produces the most powerful segmental inhibitions (Woolf et al. 1980; Kawakita and Funakoshi 1982; Chung et al. 1984; Lee et al. 1985; Sjölund 1985). Such effects are essentially restricted to dermatomes and are reflected in the properties of the receptive fields (RFs) of dorsal-horn neurons. They could explain the hypoalgesia that can be elicited by high-frequency, low-intensity stimulation of peripheral nerves (transcutaneous electric nerve stimulation, TENS) and by some forms of acupuncture or electro-acupuncture. It should be noted, however, that the time constants of these clinical effects and of the electrophysiologic phenomena are very different: patients can gain pain relief that lasts for hours after such stimulation, whereas the inhibition of neurons in animals or of nociceptive reflexes in humans can end as soon as the stimulation stops.

However, there is another category of somesthetic stimulus that can induce hypalgesic effects. Although it seems paradoxical at first sight, painful stimuli can diminish, or even mask, pain elicited by stimulation of a remote (extrasegmental) part of the body (see references in Le Bars et al. 1984, 1989; Melzack 1989). This phenomenon has been known since ancient times, and has even been used during surgical procedures on both humans and domesticated animals. In the latter category, two examples are the uses of the twitch in horses and of nasal forceps in cattle for performing caudectomies or castrations, both of which are potentially painful operations.

The nature of the controls that underlie these observations is different from that of the inhibitory phenomena described above, which are triggered by light stimuli and are essentially segmental. Accordingly, we have developed the working hypothesis that some of the neurons involved in the transmission of nociceptive signals can be inhibited by nociceptive stimulation of peripheral territories outside their own excitatory RFs. That this applies at as early a stage in sensory pathways as the spinal cord was revealed by the finding that some dorsal-horn neurons are strongly inhibited when a nociceptive stimulus is applied to any part of the body distinct from their excitatory RFs. For convenience, this phenomenon was termed diffuse noxious inhibitory control (DNIC).

DNIC affect all convergent neurons (i.e., those neurons activated both by a variety of nociceptive stimuli and by weak mechanical stimulation. The term "convergent neurons" summarizes quite well the main property of these cells (i.e., that they constitute a strategic site at which various types of excitatory and inhibitory influences converge). Various other names are used by different authors for these neurons (e.g., "common carriers," "trigger cells," "wide-dynamic-range cells," "lamina V type neurons," "class 2 neurons," and "multireceptive neurons") (see references in Melzack and Wall 1965; Dubner and Bennett 1983; Le Bars et al. 1986; Zieglgänsberger 1986; Besson and Chaouch 1987; Willis and Coggeshall 1991). These terms can be considered as being synonymous. The cutaneous excitatory RFs of these cells exhibit a gradient of sensitivity: in the center of the RF, any mechanical stimulus, including small hair movements or light touch, can activate the neuron, whereas at the periphery, only more intense stimuli elicit neuronal responses. In view of the fact that there is overlapping of their RFs, the spatial organization of the convergence on this class of neurons is likely to play an essential role in elaborating the signals they emit. Since they can also receive nociceptive signals of visceral and/or muscular origin, these neurons are adapted for a global processing of information from both the external environment, via the skin, and from the internal environment. The idea that convergent neurons may play an important role in the sensory perception of the "body scheme" cannot be excluded.

DIFFUSE NOXIOUS INHIBITORY CONTROLS IN ANIMALS

In the rat (see the references listed below), the cat (Morton et al. 1987), and probably the monkey (Gerhart et al. 1981; Brennan et al. 1989), the activity of certain dorsal-horn neurons can be strongly inhibited by noxious inputs applied outside their RFs. Such effects do not appear to be somatotopically organized, but apply to the whole body and affect all convergent neurons, including those projecting to the thalamus (Dickenson and Le Bars 1983), whether in the dorsal horn of various segments of the spinal cord (Le Bars et al. 1979a; Cadden et al. 1983; Tomlinson et al. 1983; Calvino et al. 1984; Schouenborg and Dickenson 1985; Fleischmann and Urca 1989; Sher and Mitchell 1990; Cadden and Morrison 1991) or in both the nucleus caudalis and nucleus oralis of the trigeminal system (Dickenson et al. 1980; Dallel et al. 1990; Hu 1990). By contrast, DNIC do not affect the other types of neurons found in these structures (i.e., lamina I noxious-specific, non-noxious-specific, cold-responsive, or proprioceptive neurons) (Le Bars et al. 1979b; Dickenson et al. 1980; Villanueva et al. 1984a, b). It should be noted that the inhibitions triggered by heterotopic noxious stimuli are highly sensitive to both type and dose of general anesthesia, an observation that could explain some reports of lesser inhibitory effects in studies of DNIC (Gerhart et al. 1981; Tomlinson et al. 1983; Cervero and Morales 1988; Alarcón and Cervero 1989; Ness and Gebhart 1991a,b).

The principal feature of DNIC is that they can be triggered by conditioning stimuli applied to any part of the body, including the viscera, that is distant from the excitatory RF of the neuron under study, provided that the stimuli are clearly noxious. Indeed, DNIC can be triggered by any heterotopic nociceptive stimulus whatever its type, whether mechanical, thermal, chemical, or electrical, whereas non-noxious stimuli are completely ineffective. With strong stimuli, the inhibitory effects are powerful and are followed by poststimulus effects that can last for several minutes.

When the general characteristics of DNIC are analyzed, one striking feature is their capacity to affect all kinds of activity of convergent neurons, no matter whether it is evoked by noxious or non-noxious, natural or electrical peripheral stimuli, or by the direct microelectrophoretic application of excitatory amino acids (EAAs) (Villanueva et al. 1984a,b). All noxious conditioning stimuli tested to date have markedly inhibited these responses (Fig. 1).

DNIC are not observed in anesthetized or decerebrate animals in which the spinal cord has been sectioned (Le Bars et al. 1979b; Cadden et al. 1983; Morton et al. 1987). It is therefore obvious that the mechanisms underlying DNIC are not confined to the spinal cord, and that they must involve supraspinal structures. Such a system is therefore completely different from segmental inhibitory systems, which work both in intact and in spinal animals, and can be triggered by the activation of low-threshold afferents. DNIC are also very different from the propriospinal inhibitory processes that can be triggered by noxious inputs (Gerhart et al. 1981; Fitzgerald 1982; Cadden et al. 1983).

Interestingly, a C-fiber reflex recorded from the biceps femoris muscle, elicited by electrical stimulation of the sural nerve, was reported to be strongly inhibited in

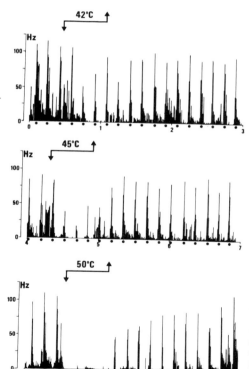

FIG. 1. Inhibitory effects of heating of the tail (temperatures as indicated between the *arrows*) on the responses of a convergent neuron, recorded in the lumbar dorsal horn of a rat, to regular tactile stimulation (stroking every 10 sec, as indicated by the *black circles*) of its peripheral receptive field located on the extremity of the ipsilateral hindpaw. Note that increasing the intensity of the noxious heat used for conditioning induced an increase in the degree of inhibition of the evoked activities, and prolonged the period of poststimulus effects. (From Le Bars et al. 1979, with permission.)

intact anesthetized rats by both mechanical and thermal noxious heterotopic stimuli, whether applied to the muzzle, a paw, or the tail, and by colorectal distention (Falinower et al. 1991, 1993). These inhibitory effects disappeared when the C-fiber reflex was recorded in spinal animals, or ipsilaterally to a rostral unilateral lesion of the dorsolateral funiculus (DLF). These observations are in keeping with several earlier reports in which the reflex discharge in the common peroneal nerve following electrical stimulation of the sural nerve in the rat was inhibited by pinching the muzzle or tail (Schouenborg and Dickenson 1985); that the gastrocnemious medialis reflex evoked by sural-nerve stimulation in the decerebrate rabbit was inhibited by electrical stimulation of the contralateral common peroneal or either the ipsi- or contralateral median nerves (Taylor et al. 1991); and that the digastric reflex evoked by tooth-pulp stimulation in the cat was inhibited by toe pinch, percutaneous electrical stimulation of a limb, or electrical stimulation of the saphenous nerve (Cadden 1985; Clarke and Matthews 1985; Banks et al. 1992).

In humans, exactly analogous results have been obtained by means of electrical stimulation of the sural nerve at the ankle, which elicits a nociceptive reflex in the biceps femoris muscle (the RIII reflex): painful heterotopic conditioning stimuli, whether thermal, mechanical, or chemical, depress such a reflex, with stronger effects being observed with more intense conditioning stimuli. By contrast, in tetraplegic patients, heterotopic nociceptive stimulation did not produce any depression of the RIII reflex (see Chapter 35).

The peripheral and central mechanisms involved in DNIC are considered below.

Peripheral Mechanisms

The relationship between the intensity of a stimulus and the strength of the resultant DNIC was investigated by studying the effects of various temperatures applied to the tail on the C-fiber responses of lumbar and trigeminal convergent neurons to transcutaneous electrical stimulation of these neurons' RFs on the hindpaw or face. A highly significant correlation existed between the conditioning temperature in the 44-52°C range and the extent of the inhibition, see in Fig. 4 (Le Bars et al., 1981a; Villanueva and Le Bars, 1985).

These data suggest that DNIC are triggered specifically by the activation of peripheral nociceptors whose signals are carried by Aδ- and C-fibers (Van Hees and Gybels 1972; Dubner and Beitel 1976; Adriansen et al. 1983, Torebjörk et al. 1984; Raja et al. 1988; Handwerker and Kobal 1993). In order to further investigate the types of peripheral fibers involved in DNIC, we took advantage of the facts that: (a) trigeminal and spinal dorsal-horn neurons respond with relatively steady discharges to the electrophoretic application of EAAs, and (b) DNIC act on convergent neurons by a final postsynaptic inhibitory mechanism involving hyperpolarization of the neuronal membrane (Villanueva et al. 1984a, b). It was found that when trigeminal convergent neurons were directly excited by the electrophoretic application of DL-

A

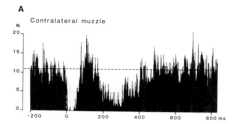

Contralateral muzzle

B

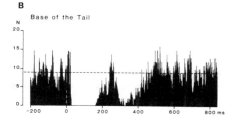

Base of the Tail

FIG. 2. Peristimulus histograms (bin width: 5 msec) prepared during the continuous electrophoretic application (15 nA) of DL-homocysteate onto the membrane of a convergent neuron recorded in the lumbar dorsal horn of a rat. Percutaneous electrical stimulation (10 mA; 2 msec duration; .66 Hz; 200 msec delay; 100 sweeps) applied either to the contralateral muzzle (upper histogram), the base (middle histogram), or the tip (lower histogram) of the tail induced a biphasic inhibition. The *broken white line* shows the time of stimulation, while the *broken black line* represents the mean firing calculated during the prestimulation control period (-200 to 0 msec). (Bouhassira, Villanueva and Le Bars, unpublished observations.)

C

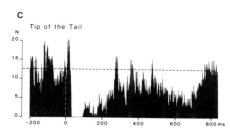

Tip of the Tail

homocysteate (DLH), the percutaneous application of single square-wave, electrical stimuli (10 mA; 2 msec) to the tail always induced a biphasic depression of the resultant activity (Bouhassira et al. 1987). Both the early and late components of this inhibition occurred with shorter latencies when the base rather than the tip of the tail was stimulated. Such differences in latency were used to estimate the mean conduction velocities of the peripheral fibers triggering the inhibitions: these were found to be 7.3 and 0.7 msec, which fall into the Aδ- and C-fiber ranges, respectively (Gasser and Erlanger 1927; Burgess and Perl 1973). Such biphasic inhibitions could be evoked from any part of the body recorded from any convergent neurons. Fig. 2 shows a recording from a lumbar convergent neuron with an excitatory RF located on the extremity of the ipsilateral hindpaw; the activity was evoked by DLH, and two components of inhibition were induced by the activation of Aδ- and C-fibers, respectively, when a single shock of 10 mA and 2-msec duration was applied to the muzzle, the base, or the tip of the tail.

Central Mechanisms

As already mentioned, DNIC are known to be sustained by a complex loop involving supraspinal structures since, unlike segmental inhibitions, they are not observed in animals in which the spinal cord has previously been transected at the cervical level (Le Bars et al. 1979b; Cadden et al. 1983; Morton et al. 1987). The ascending and descending limbs of this loop travel through the ventrolateral and dorsolateral funiculi, respectively (Villanueva et al. 1986a, b). Since thalamic lesions do not affect DNIC (Villanueva et al. 1986b), It has been proposed that they result from a physiologic activation of some of the brain-stem structures that produce descending inhibition. In this context, the more efficient structures exert their actions through bulbospinal inhibitory pathways that are confined to the dorsolateral funiculi (see the references in Basbaum and Fields 1984; Willis 1984; Fields and Besson 1988; Fields and Basbaum 1989; Willis and Coggeshall 1991).

Surprisingly, lesions of the following structures did not modify DNIC: periaqueductal grey (PAG), cuneiform nucleus, parabrachial area, locus coeruleus/subcoeruleus, rostral ventromedial medulla (RVM) including the nucleus raphe magnus, and gigantocellular and paragigantocellular nuclei (Bouhassira et al, 1990, 1992a, 1993). By contrast, lesions of the subnucleus reticularis dorsalis (SRD) in the caudal medulla strongly reduced DNIC (Bouhassira et al. 1992b). The SRD is located ventral to the cuneate nucleus, between the trigeminal nucleus caudalis and the nucleus of the solitary tract, and contains neurons with characteristics suggesting that they have a key role in processing specifically nociceptive information (Villanueva et al. 1988a,b, 1989, 1991; Bing et al. 1989, 1990a; Bernard et al. 1990; Roy et al. 1992). Indeed, these neurons are unresponsive to visual, auditory, or proprioceptive stimulation, but are preferentially or exclusively activated by nociceptive stimuli, and have "whole-body" RFs; they encode precisely the intensity of cutaneous and visceral stimulation within noxious ranges, and are activated exclusively by cutaneous Aδ- or Aδ- and C-fiber peripheral volleys; they send descending projections through the dorsolateral funiculus that terminate in the dorsal horn at all levels of the spinal cord. The fact that the supraspinal loop sustaining DNIC is confined within the caudal medulla was recently confirmed in a series of experiments in which the potency of DNIC was tested in animals with complete transections at different levels in the brain stem (Villanueva et al. 1993).

On the basis of these results, one can conclude that the most caudal part of the medulla, including at least the SRD, is involved in the loop sustaining DNIC in the rat. This conclusion is in agreement with data obtained in patients with unilateral caudal medullary lesions (see Chapter 35). In addition, it is suggested that DNIC (Fig. 3) are likely to constitute a system modulating the spinal transmission of nociceptive signals independently of the descending inhibitory controls originating from those midbrain and medullary structures that have been implicated in the postulated "endogenous pain inhibitory system(s)" (Liebeskind et al. 1976; Basbaum and Fields 1984; Fields and Basbaum 1989).

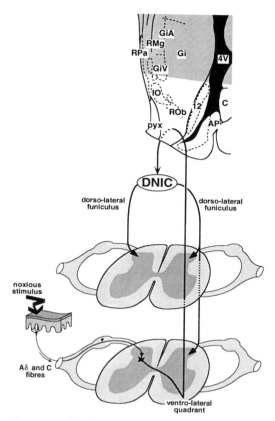

FIG. 3. Triggering of descending inhibitory controls by nociceptive stimulation. When a noxious focus appears in a region of the body, neurons in the dorsal horn are activated and send an excitatory signal through the ventrolateral quadrant toward higher centers, including the lower brain stem. This signal activates DNIC, which will inhibit spinal and trigeminal convergent neurons through the dorsolateral funiculus. The levels of transection that did not modify DNIC are shown as *shaded areas* in the upper drawing of a sagittal section of the brain stem. By contrast, transection caudal to this area blocked DNIC completely, suggesting that the open areas of the drawing correspond to the parts of the brain stem involved in the upper part of the DNIC circuit. Abbreviations: 12 = hypoglossal nucleus; AP = area postrema; C = cerebellum; Gi = gigantocellular nucleus; GiA = gigantocellular nucleus pars alpha; GiV = gigantocellular nucleus ventral; IO = inferior olive; pyx = pyramidal decussation; RMg = nucleus raphe magnus; RPa = nucleus raphe pallidus; ROb = nucleus raphe obscurus.

HYPOTHESES

Is Pain Triggered By a Gradient of Activity Between
Two Populations of Spinal Neurons?

The data presented in brief above indicate that nociceptive stimuli activate certain inhibitory controls that originate in the brain stem. Since all convergent neurons, including those projecting to the thalamus (Dickenson and Le Bars 1983), are subject to DNIC, one can assert that the transmission of nociceptive signals to higher centers is under the influence of these controls. This has actually been confirmed for nociceptive reticular neurons recorded in the caudal brain stem (Villanueva et al. 1994).

These descending inhibitory controls, which seemed to have a function directly related to analgesic phenomena, may in fact have a physiologic role in the detection of nociceptive signals. Such an interpretation seems to go against good sense, but perhaps this would not seem so if one were to take into account a paradoxical property of convergent neurons: that they do indeed respond, and sometimes very well, to non-nociceptive stimuli (e.g., rubbing, hair movements), and are therefore randomly and perpetually being activated by all of the somesthetic stimuli arising from the environment (Le Bars and Chitour 1983). Such activity, once transmitted toward higher centers, could constitute a basic somesthetic activity or "background noise" from which the brain's centers could extract a significant nociceptive signal only with difficulty. DNIC could constitute the filter by which a specific nociceptive signal would be extracted from this basic somesthetic activity. The basic somesthetic activity might have an essential role in the sensory perception of the "body picture," which is profoundly disorganized during clinical pain.

Indeed, when a noxious focus occurs in a region of the body, both convergent and specific nociceptive neurons are activated and send an excitatory signal toward higher centers. This signal will secondarily activate DNIC, which will inhibit all of those spinal and trigeminal convergent neurons that were not directly activated by the initial stimulus (Fig. 4B). Such a mechanism will improve the signal-to-noise (S/N) ratio by increasing the contrast between the activity of the segmental focus of excited neurons and the silence of the remaining population, by a mechanism reminiscent of, albeit more generalized than, the lateral inhibitions observed at various levels of most sensory systems (Kandel and Jessell 1991). The destination of such a "picture," its recognition, and its processing by cerebral centers remain unsolved problems. As a hypothesis, one can propose that the brain is able to recognize this picture, which would infer that DNIC constitute not only a filter that allows the extraction of the signal for pain, but also—and perhaps more importantly—an amplifier in the transmission system that increases the potential alarm function of the nociceptive signals. Fig. 4 illustrates the possible complementary action of both excitatory and inhibitory events in the encoding of noxious stimuli by convergent neurons. Consequently, it is conceivable that during clinical pain the global message sent by convergent neurons is polymorphic, or even complex, and that a large

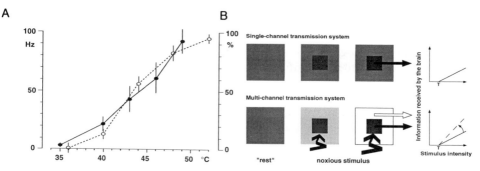

FIG. 4. Complementary action of excitatory and inhibitory events in the encoding of noxious stimuli by convergent neurons. **A:** *Solid line,* left ordinate, shows the relationship between radiant heat (abscissa = °C) applied to the excitatory receptive fields of lumbar convergent neurons, and the mean resultant firing rate (from Le Bars and Chitour 1983). *Dotted line,* right ordinate, shows the inhibitory effects (%) elicited by the application of various temperatures to the tail on neuronal responses of trigeminal convergent neurons (from Villanueva and Le Bars 1985, with permission). **B:** Hypothetical coding of the intensity of nociceptive stimuli by both excitatory responses and silencing of the remaining population of neurons. The global activity of all convergent neurons at all spinal and trigeminal levels is represented as *squares.* At "rest" (left squares), because of the properties of these neurons, such activity would not be negligible, and thus a basic somesthetic signal would be sent toward the brain. It is generally believed that there is a single-channel transmission system (upper drawings) in which the application of increasingly noxious stimuli to a part of the body (*arrows*) would result in an increase in the activity of the corresponding segmental pool of convergent and noxious-specific neurons (from left to right). In a multichannel transmission system (lower drawings), such a stimulus would also trigger the DNIC system (see Fig. 3), inducing a progressive decrease in the basic somesthetic activity of the convergent neuronal population (from left to right). The complementary action of excitatory and inhibitory events would produce a contrast picture for the brain, and could be the source of an amplification of the gain of the transmission system (right; T = threshold). (From Le Bars and Chitour 1983, with permission.)

variety of syndromes could result from this state of affairs. Interestingly, polyarthritis is associated with a reduction of the threshold for triggering DNIC in the rat (Calvino et al. 1987).

It will probably be difficult to demonstrate the validity of the proposed model in a formal fashion. However, one can argue about its theoretical implications and try to submit them to experimental testing. In this way the hypothesis is reinforced by two types of observation: the first related to the effects of opioids, and the second related to some behavioral and clinical observations.

Effects of Morphine on DNIC

According to the model, it should be possible to produce hypo- or hyperalgesic effects by manipulations that affect excitatory and/or inhibitory phenomena. An intensification of the contrast effect should facilitate the recognition of nociceptive signals by higher centers; in this respect we have already noted that in a model of chronic pain—the arthritic rat—hyperalgesic phenomena occur together with an exacerbation of DNIC (Calvino et al. 1987). Conversely, a reduction of the contrast should hinder the recognition of nociceptive signals and thus produce a hypo- or analgesic effect. In order to verify this hypothesis, one can ask whether or not an analgesic drug such as morphine can produce a recovery in the somesthetic background activity that would normally be depressed by DNIC. In fact, DNIC have been found to be extremely sensitive to the administration of low doses of morphine systemically or into the cerebral ventricles (Le Bars et al. 1981b; Bouhassira et al. 1988a; 1988b). These effects are dose-dependent, stereospecific, and naloxone-reversible. Descending inhibitory controls from the brain stem, at least those triggered by peripheral nociceptive stimuli, are therefore depressed by morphine. Interestingly, such effects of low doses of systemic morphine were confirmed upon the inhibitions triggered by heterotopic noxious stimuli on both the C-fiber reflex in the rat (Falinower et al. 1993) and on the RIII reflex in humans (see Chapter 35).

The PAG represents one of the major supraspinal sites for the action of morphine in producing analgesia (see the references in Yaksh and Rudy 1978). This region contains both terminals that are immunoreactive to endogenous opioids, including β-endorphin, enkephalins, and dynorphin, and opioid-binding sites, notably of the μ subtype (see references in Bouhassira et al. 1992c). Further electrophysiologic data support the hypothesis that the elimination of DNIC following systemic morphine is due at least in part to binding of the drug within the PAG, since: (a) microinjections of morphine (5μg) directly into the PAG produced a significant depression of DNIC (Dickenson and Le Bars 1987); (b) as already mentioned, DNIC were depressed in a dose-dependent fashion after microinjections of morphine into the third ventricle, and in these experiments autoradiographic controls with tritiated morphine indicated that the morphine reached the PAG throughout its rostrocaudal extension (Bouhassira et al. 1988a); and (c) as shown in Fig. 5, the effect of systemic morphine disappeared in PAG-lesioned animals (Bouhassira et al. 1992c). Coincidentally, these results also demonstrated that the elimination of DNIC in normal animals following a low systemic dose of morphine was not due to an action on the afferent pathways, notably those within the spinal cord activated by the conditioning stimulus. Thus, although the PAG is not directly involved in the loop subserving DNIC, it can modulate these controls indirectly. The relationship between DNIC and the other pain-modulatory systems is therefore more complex than expected. However, the neural network between the PAG and the DNIC circuit has yet to be determined.

The effects of systemic morphine on DNIC in animals with lesions of the rostral ventromedial medulla (RVM) were also tested. This region, which includes the nucleus raphe magnus and adjacent reticular nuclei, contains a large number of terminals and cell somata that are immunoreactive to endogenous opioids, and opioid-binding sites of the μ subtype (see references in Bouhassira et al. 1993). The RVM has been implicated in the antinociceptive effects of morphine by behavioral studies using local microinjections of opioids (see the references in Yaksh and Rudy 1978), and by electrophysiologic recordings from RVM neurons (see references in Fields et al. 1991). It was therefore possible that the depression of DNIC following

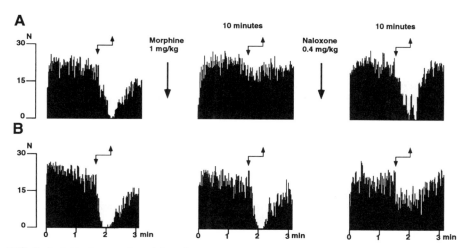

FIG. 5. Individual examples of the effects of 1 mg/kg morphine on the inhibitions triggered by heterotopic noxious stimulation. Each histogram corresponds to a sequence of 120 stimuli during which C-fiber-evoked responses of spinal dorsal-horn convergent neurons were inhibited by immersion of the muzzle in a 50°C water bath (*arrow*). Ordinate: N = number of spikes per stimulus; abscissa = time. **A:** Sham-operated animal. Note that the inhibition was blocked 10 min after the injection of morphine, and that this effect was reversed by an injection of naloxone (0.4 mg/kg; i.v.). **B:** Rat with a lesion of the PAG. Note that the inhibition triggered by the heterotopic stimulus was not modified by the injection of morphine but was reduced following naloxone (see comments in text). Note that in both animals the unconditioned C-fiber-evoked responses were not modified after morphine or naloxone. (From Bouhassira et al. 1992c, with permission.)

the systemic administration of morphine both involved the PAG and was mediated through the RVM. The effects of morphine on DNIC were compared in sham-operated rats and animals in which electrolytic lesions of the RVM had been made either 1 or 3 weeks earlier. DNIC were similarly reduced, again in a naloxone-reversible fashion, following morphine injections in sham-operated animals and animals tested one week after lesioning of the RVM. By contrast, DNIC were not significantly altered by morphine in animals tested 3 weeks after lesioning. This time-dependent attenuation of the effects of morphine indicates that the RVM is not directly involved in the reduction of DNIC induced by systemic morphine, but suggests that electrolytic lesions of the RVM induce long-term modifications of the opioidergic and/or other system(s) that mediate(s) the action of morphine. Interestingly, behavioral studies of the antinociceptive effects of morphine in RVM-lesioned animals have produced similar time-dependent effects (see references in Bouhassira et al. 1993).

On the basis of the striking similarities between the effects of electrolytic lesions of either the PAG or the RVM on the pharmacologic responses in both the behavioral and DNIC studies, it was suggested that the blockade of DNIC has a functional role in the behavioral effects of low doses of systemic morphine (see below and references in Bouhassira et al. 1993).

Taken together, these data are difficult to interpret within the framework of the hypotheses generally proposed to explain morphine analgesia. In fact, some authors claim that morphine, in addition to its indisputable spinal effect, acts by increasing the descending inhibitory controls from the brain stem (Basbaum and Fields 1984; Fields and Basbaum 1989), thus giving a second, indirect mechanism for blocking nociceptive inflow at the spinal level. The arguments that support this hypothesis are very controversial (see references in Le Bars et al. 1983; Duggan and North 1984; Advokat 1988; Bouhassira et al. 1988a).

On the other hand, the data reported herein come within the scope of the model according to which a contrast between two neuronal populations is fundamental to the triggering of pain (Fig. 6B). Indeed, morphine at a systemic dose low enough not to depress the excitatory signals from the spinal relay, or if given into the cerebral ventricles, can restore the background noise by decreasing DNIC and thus reducing the contrast (Fig. 6C); with larger doses, an additional mechanism for reducing the contrast is achieved by the direct spinal depressive effect of the drug (Fig. 6D); this effect can be mimicked by administering the drug intrathecally (Villanueva and Le Bars 1985).

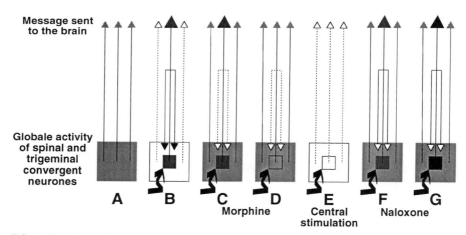

FIG. 6. Hypothetical interpretation of the global activity of all convergent neurons involved in nociception at spinal and trigeminal levels. At "rest," because of the properties of these neurons, such activity would not be negligible, and a basic somesthetic signal would therefore be sent toward the brain. A nociceptive focus will activate some convergent and nociceptive-specific (NS) neurons **(A)**, which in turn will transmit an excitatory signal toward supraspinal centers. This will trigger DNIC, which will inhibit those convergent neurons that were not directly affected by the initial stimulus, and thus the background noise that constitutes the basic somesthetic activity will be reduced or abolished **(B)**. Morphine, either systemically at low doses, intracerebrally, or intraventricularly, blocks DNIC and thus restores the background noise **(C)**. At high systemic doses or intrathecally, morphine blocks the spinal transmission of nociceptive information and therefore further reduces the contrast **(D)**. Electrical stimulation of some zones in the brain stem blocks the activities of the whole neuronal population and therefore elicits strong analgesia **(E)**. (Adapted from Le Bars et al. 1986, and from Le Bars and Villanueva, 1988.) In the case of naloxone, hyperalgesia might result from the facilitatory effect of naloxone on the spinal transmission of nociceptive signals **(F)**, while hypoalgesia might result from the lifting of DNIC **(G)**.

This interpretation does not attempt to question the fact that analgesia can be obtained by direct electrical stimulation of some supraspinal structures, such as the nucleus raphe magnus: in this case, all convergent and nociceptive-specific (NS) neurons are inhibited, the contrast is completely abolished, and the analgesia is indeed powerful (Fig. 6E).

In any case, our view is in accord with the findings in clinical and behavioral studies of the characteristics of morphine analgesia. In humans, morphine is analgesic at low doses (0.15 mg/kg) resembling those that lift DNIC ($ED_{50} = 0.6$ mg/kg) and almost identical to the doses that block the inhibitory poststimulus effect ($ED_{50} = 0.13$ mg/kg). It is interesting to note that these low doses are without effect on the behavioral tests in animals in which threshold measurements are made using acute cutaneous nociceptive stimuli, but are clearly effective against nociceptive reactions elicited either by prolonged stimuli from deep structures, such as experimentally induced arthritis (Pircio et al. 1975; Kayser and Guilbaud 1983), intraperitoneal injections of algogenic agents (Niemegeers et al. 1975), or vocalization elicited by the activation of C-fibers (Kraus and Le Bars, 1986; Ardid et al. 1993; and see Fig. 7). Additionally, the direct spinal action of morphine, far from counteracting its supraspinal action, tends to amplify it for two major reasons. It is generally agreed that morphine acts on the nociceptive-related activities of convergent cells without altering their responses to innocuous stimuli (Le Bars et al. 1976; Duggan and North 1984). This property would not have functional significance if the convergent neurons were able to discriminate the two types of information. In contrast, this observation is particularly significant in light of our hypothesis, since the spinal action of morphine will not hinder or counteract its supraspinal effect in restoring the "background somesthetic activity" from the sensory milieu. Furthermore, it is clear that the direct depression of activity in the spinal cord by morphine will lead to a reduced activation of the loop subserving DNIC, and so result in a recovery of the level of somesthetic activity. Our results, showing that intrathecal morphine can block DNIC (Villanueva and Le Bars 1986), provide evidence for this premise. Effects such as this will facilitate the supraspinal effect of eliminating DNIC and signify that the spinal and supraspinal actions of morphine will not simply be additive but will be synergistic. In accord with this hypothesis, behavioral studies have clearly demonstrated that the analgesia produced by the intracerebroventricular administration of morphine is potentiated by intrathecal injection of the drug (Yeung and Rudy 1980; Roerig and Fujimoto 1989; Miyamoto et al. 1991).

Effects of Naloxone on DNIC

The participation of opioidergic systems in the mechanisms of DNIC is complex, since systemic naloxone also reduces DNIC in both the rat (Le Bars et al. 1981c) and humans (see Chapter 35). Since systemic administration was used in both cases, we have no way of determining the target(s) of the drug. However, the injection of naloxone in PAG-lesioned animals (see Fig. 5) produced a significant reduction

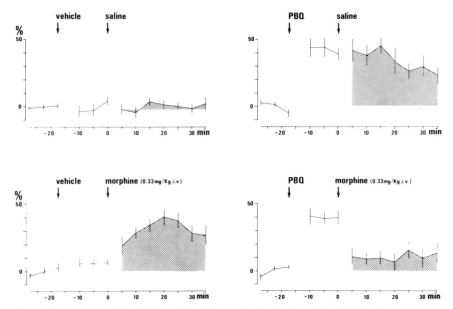

FIG. 7. Effects of morphine (0.33 mg/kg, i.v.) on a behavioral model of DNIC. Changes in pain reactivity were evaluated using the vocalization threshold elicited by electrical pulses (50 Hz, 2 msec, 500-msec duration). Upper left graph: control sequence with intraperitoneal injection of vehicle, followed by i.v. saline. Upper right graph: control sequence for the effects of intra-peritoneal phenylbenzoquinone (PBQ) followed by saline 15 min later. Note the sustained in-crease in vocalization threshold. Lower left graph: effects of 0.33 mg/kg morphine in the absence of the conditioning stimulus. Lower right graph: interaction between PBQ and morphine. Note the lifting of PBQ-induced blockade of nociception. A dose of 8 µg/kg naloxone blocked the effects of 0.33 mg/kg morphine shown in **C** and **D**. (From Kraus and Le Bars, 1986, with permission.)

in DNIC, although the lesions in these animals had abolished the effect of mor-phine (Bouhassira et al. 1992c). Such a result confirms that more than one opioidergic system can modulate DNIC, and suggests that removing the first, supra-spinal, "morphine-sensitive" mechanism unmasked a second, "naloxone-sensitive" one.

In any case, the finding of a blockade of DNIC by naloxone is in keeping with the paradoxical hypoalgesic effect of this drug (in low doses), which has been observed in both animals and humans. In fact, naloxone has been reported to elicit both hypo- and hyperalgesic effects, depending on its dose (Lasagna 1965; Sewell and Spencer 1976; Buchsbaum et al. 1977; Chesher and Chan 1977; Levine et al. 1978, 1979; Pinsky et al. 1978; Ferreira and Nakamura 1979; Kayser and Guilbaud 1981; Levine and Gordon 1986). While these experimental and clinical data do not support the idea of an unequivocal action of naloxone on nociception, they are compatible with the model we have proposed. Hyperalgesia (Jacob and Ramabadran 1978) might result from the facilitatory effect of naloxone on the spinal transmission of nociceptive signals (Fig. 6F), which has been described by various authors (see references in Willer et al. 1990), while hypoalgesia might result from the lifting of DNIC (Fig. 6G). Within this theoretical framework it is not easy to predict what the final sensation will be, and this could be the source of the apparent discrepancies in the literature on the effect of naloxone on pain thresholds.

Behavioral and Clinical Implications

If one accepts that convergent neurons have an important role in nociception, then a second direct implication of the model is that there are interactive phenomena between nociceptive signals from different areas of the body and, hence, between pains with distinct topographic origins. Evidence for such interactions has been reported in animals, but more convincing observations have been made in humans, with the common observation that "one pain can mask another." For centuries, a large number of popular medical practices for relieving pain, including some forms of acupuncture, have been based on this principle (see Mann 1974; Macdonald 1989; Melzack 1989; Bing et al. 1990b). These empirical observations have been confirmed under conditions of scientific objectivity, and such phenomena are often designated as "counterirritation" or "counterstimulation" (see the references in Le Bars et al. 1984, 1989). DNIC probably represent, at least in part, the functional substrate for these observations; the experiments in humans described in Chapter 35 support this hypothesis.

A behavioral model for counterstimulation was developed in the rat by the concomitant application of two noxious stimuli used in classical pharmacologic testing. It was found that the threshold for vocalization induced by electric shocks to the tail was increased by the intraperitoneal injection of algogenic agents such as phenylbenzoquinone (PBQ) or acetic acid (Kraus et al. 1981; Calvino et al. 1984; Kiyatkin 1989). Interestingly, a very close parallel was found after the administration of such algogenic agents between the time course of the (behavioral) hypoalgesic effect in the vocalization test and the temporal pattern of the (electrophysiologic) inhibition of coccygeal convergent neurons (Calvino et al. 1984). This paradoxical hypoalgesic effect was reversed by naloxone (Kraus et al. 1981; Kiyatkin 1989). The fact that a lifting of DNIC by morphine also has a functional, behavioral role in the rat is supported by the observation that the sharp and sustained increase that the intraperitoneal injection of PBQ induced in the threshold of vocalization in response to transcutaneous electrical stimulation of the tail was morphine sensitive (Kraus and Le Bars 1986). As shown in Fig. 7, the increase in the pain threshold was antagonized almost completely by the i.v. injection of 0.33 mg/kg morphine. While lower doses of morphine were completely or largely ineffective, increasing doses resulted first in a biphasic effect (1 mg/kg), and then, at the highest doses tested (3.3. mg/kg), in an immediate and overriding analgesia involving a very large increase in the pain threshold. This initially surprising observation is not really novel: as early as 1940, Wolff et al. reported that in humans, a heterotopic pain could block the morphine-induced increase in the pain threshold to radiant heat, and concluded that "the threshold-raising action of opium derivatives . . . was reduced or obliterated by pain." In any case, these experiments show a very significant negative interaction between the effect of morphine and the PBQ-induced effect on the threshold for vocalization. Note that this interaction was observed at low doses of morphine. Here again these paradoxical phenomena are difficult to explain in the light of classical hypotheses about morphine analgesia, but fit well with our proposal of a lifting of descending inhibitory controls when these are triggered by noxious input.

CONCLUSION

The results reported above indicate that the three routes of administration of morphine used for alleviating pain in humans—systemic, intrathecal, and intracerebroventricular—can be correlated with a reduction in DNIC. It could be rather disconcerting to think of two opposing manipulations—the activation of DNIC by counterirritation procedures and the blocking of DNIC by morphine—leading, in therapeutic terms, to the same end of hypoalgesia. We feel, however, that this apparent paradox reflects the complexity of the spinal transmission of nociceptive signals and provides an insight into the likely role of convergent neurons in the encoding of nociceptive and non-nociceptive sensory information. In this context, we believe that the existence of gradients of activity within a neuronal population should be taken into consideration in pharmacologic and biochemical studies of nociceptive transmission toward higher centers.

ACKNOWLEDGMENTS

This work was supported by l'Institut National de la Santé et de la Recherche Médicale (INSERM) and la Direction des Recherches et Etudes Techniques (DRET). The authors are very grateful to Dr. S. W. Cadden for advice in the preparation of the manuscript.

REFERENCES

Adriansen H, Gybels J, Handwerker HO, Van Hees J. Response properties of thin myelinated (Aδ) fibres in human skin nerves *J Neurophysiol* 1983;49:111–122.
Advokat C. The role of descending inhibition in morphine-induced analgesia. *Trends Pharmacol Sci* 1988;9:330–334.
Alarcón G, Cervero F. Effects of two anesthetic regimes on the heterotopic inhibition of rat dorsal horn neurones. *J Physiol* (Lond), 1989;416:19P.
Ardid D, Jourdan D, Eschalier A, Arabia C, Le Bars D. Vocalization elicited by activation of Aδ- and C-fibres in the rat. *Neuroreport* 1993;5:105–108.
Banks D, Kuriakose M, Matthews B. Modulation by peripheral conditioning stimuli of the responses of trigeminal brain stem neurones and of the jaw opening reflex to tooth pulp stimulation in chronically prepared, anaesthetized cats. *Exp Physiol* 1992;77:343–349.

Basbaum AI, Fields HL. Endogenous pain control system: Brainstem spinal pathways and endorphine circuitry. *Annu Rev Neurosci* 1984;7:309–398.

Bernard JF, Villanueva L, Carroué J, Le Bars D. Efferent projections from the subnucleus reticularis dorsalis (SRD) a *Phaseolus vulgaris* leucoagglutinin study in the rat. *Neurosci Lett* 1990;116: 257–262.

Besson JM, Chaouch A. Peripheral and spinal mechanisms of nociception. *Physiol Rev* 1987;67:67–186.

Bing Z, Villanueva L, Le Bars D. Effects of systemic morphine upon Aδ- and C-fibre evoked activities of subnucleus reticularis dorsalis neurones in the rat medulla. *Eur J Pharmacol* 1989;164:85–92.

Bing Z, Villanueva L, Le Bars D. Ascending pathways in the spinal cord involved in the activation of subnucleus reticularis dorsalis neurons in the medulla of the rat. *J Neurophysiol* 1990a;63:424–437.

Bing Z, Villanueva L, Le Bars D. Acupuncture and diffuse noxious inhibitory controls: naloxone reversible depression of activities of trigeminal convergent neurones. *Neuroscience* 1990b;37:809–818.

Bouhassira D, Bing Z, Le Bars D. Studies of the brain structures involved in diffuse noxious inhibitory controls: The mesencephalon. *J Neurophysiol* 1990;64:1713–1723.

Bouhassira D, Bing Z, Le Bars D. Effects of lesions of locus coeruleus/subcoeruleus on diffuse noxious inhibitory controls in the rat. *Brain Res* 1992a;571:140–144.

Bouhassira D, Bing Z, Le Bars D. Studies of the brain structures involved in diffuse noxious inhibitory controls: the rostral ventromedial medulla. *J Physiol* (Lond) 1993;463:667–687.

Bouhassira D, Chitour D, Villanueva L, Le Bars D. Morphine and diffuse noxious inhibitory controls: effects of lesions of the rostral ventromedial medulla. *Eur J Pharmacol* 1993;232:207–215.

Bouhassira D, Le Bars D, Villanueva L. Heterotopic activation of Aδ- and C-fibres triggers inhibition of trigeminal and spinal convergent neurones in the rat. *J Physiol* (Lond) 1987;389:301–317.

Bouhassira D, Villanueva L, Bing Z, Le Bars D. Involvement of the subnucleus reticularis dorsalis in diffuse noxious inhibitory controls. *Brain Res* 1992b;595:353–357.

Bouhassira D, Villanueva L, Le Bars D. Intracerebroventricular morphine decreases descending inhibitions acting on lumbar dorsal horn neuronal activities related to pain in the rat. *J Pharmacol Exp Ther* 1988a;247:332–342.

Bouhassira D, Villanueva L, Le Bars D. Intracerebroventricular morphine restores the basic somesthetic activity of dorsal horn convergent neurones in the rat. *Eur J Pharmacol* 1988b;148:273–277.

Bouhassira D, Villanueva L, Le Bars D. Effects of systemic morphine on diffuse noxious inhibitory controls: role of the periaqueductal grey. *Eur J Pharmacol* 1992c;216:149–156.

Brennan TJ, Oh UT, Hobbs SF, Garrison DW, Foreman RD. Urinary bladder and hindlimb afferent input inhibits activity of primate T2-T5 spinothalamic tract neurons. *J Neurophysiol* 1989;61: 573–588.

Buchsbaum MS, Davis GC, Bunney WE. Naloxone alters pain perception and somatosensory evoked potentials in normal subjects. *Nature* 1977;270:620–622.

Burgess PR, Perl ER. Cutaneous mechanoreceptors and nociceptors. In: Iggo A, ed. *Handbook of sensory physiology*. New York: Springer Verlag, 1973;29–78.

Cadden SW. The digastric reflex evoked by tooth-pulp stimulation in the cat and its modulation by stimuli applied to the limbs. *Brain Res* 1985;336:33–43.

Cadden SW, Morrison JFB. Effects of visceral distension on the activities of neurones receiving cutaneous inputs in the rat lumbar dorsal horn; comparison with effects of remote noxious somatic stimuli. *Brain Res* 1991;558:63–74.

Cadden SW, Villanueva L, Chitour D, Le Bars D. Depression of activities of dorsal horn convergent neurones by propriospinal mechanisms triggered by noxious inputs: comparison with diffuse noxious inhibitory controls (DNIC). *Brain Res* 1983;275:1–11.

Calvino B, Villanueva L, Le Bars D. The heterotopic effects of visceral pain: behavioural and electrophysiological approaches in the rat. *Pain* 1984;20:261–271.

Calvino B, Villanueva L, Le Bars D. Dorsal horn (convergent) neurones in the anaesthetized arthritic rat. II. Heterotopic inhibitory influences. *Pain* 1987;31:359–379.

Cervero F, Morales A. Heterotopic noxious heating of the skin inhibits dorsal-horn neurones in normal rats and in rats treated at birth with capsaicin. *J Physiol* (Lond) 1988;398:29P.

Chesher GB, Chan B. Footshock induced analgesia in mice: its reversal by naloxone and cross tolerance with morphine. *Life Sci* 1977;21:1569–1574.

Chung JM, Lee KH, Hori Y, Endo K, Willis WD. Factors influencing peripheral nerve stimulation produced inhibition of primate spinothalamic tract cells. *Pain* 1984;19:277–293.

Clarke RW, Matthews B. The effects of anaesthetics and remote noxious stimuli on the jaw-opening reflex evoked by tooth-pulp stimulation in the cat. *Brain Res* 1985;327:105–111.

Dallel R, Raboisson P, Woda A, Sessle B. Properties of nociceptive and non-nociceptive neurons in trigeminal subnucleus oralis of the rat. *Brain Res* 1990;521:95–106.

Dickenson AH, Le Bars D. Diffuse noxious inhibitory controls (DNIC) involve trigeminothalamic and spinothalamic neurones in the rat. *Exp Brain Res* 1983;49:174– 180.

Dickenson AH, Le Bars D. Supraspinal morphine and descending inhibitions acting on the dorsal horn of the rat. *J Physiol* (Lond) 1987;384:81–107.

Dickenson AH, Le Bars D, Besson JM. Diffuse noxious inhibitory controls (DNIC). Effects on trigeminal nucleus caudalis neurones in the rat brain. *Brain Res* 1980;200:293–305.

Dubner R, Beitel E. Peripheral neural correlates of escape behavior in rhesus monkey to noxious heat applied to the face. In: Bonica JJ, Albe-Fessard D, eds. *Advances in pain research and therapy*, vol.1, New York: Raven Press, 1976;155–160.

Dubner R, Bennett GJ. Spinal and trigeminal mechanisms of nociception. *Annu Rev Neurosci* 1983;6: 381–418.

Duggan AW, North A. Electrophysiology of opioids. *Pharmacol Rev* 1984;35:219–291.

Falinower S, Junien JL, Willer JC, Le Bars D. Inhibition of a hindlimb C-fibre reflex by colo-rectal distension in the rat: blockade by low doses of morphine. Proceedings of the 7th world congress on pain: Paris, 1993; 206.

Falinower S, Willer JC, Junien JL, Le Bars D. 1991: Diffuse noxious inhibitory controls (DNIC) on a C-fibre reflex in the rat. Abstr, 3rd IBRO World Congress: Montreal, Canada 28–3.

Ferreira SH, Nakamura M. Prostaglandin hyperalgesia: the peripheral analgesic activity of morphine, enkephalins and opioid antagonists. *Prostaglandins* 1979;18:191–200.

Fields HL, Basbaum AI. Endogenous pain control mechanisms. In: Wall PD, Melzack R, eds. *Textbook of pain*. Edinburgh: Churchill Livingstone, 1989;206–217.

Fields HL, Besson JM, eds. Pain modulation. *Progress in brain research*, vol. 77. Amsterdam: Elsevier, 1988;

Fields HL, Heinricher MM, Mason P. Neurotransmitters in nociceptive modulatory circuits. *Annu Rev Nerosci* 1991;14:219–245.

Fitzgerald M. The contralateral input to the dorsal horn of the spinal cord in the decerebrate spinal rat. *Brain Res* 1982;236:275–287.

Fleischmann A, Urca G. Clip-induced analgesia: noxious neck pinch supresses spinal and mesencephalic neural responses to noxious peripheral stimulation. *Physiol Behav* 1989;46:151–157.

Gasser HS, Erlanger J. The role played by the sizes of the constituent fibres of a nerve trunk in determining the form of its action potential wave. *Am J Physiol* 1927;80:522–547.

Gerhart KD, Yezierski RP, Giesler GJ, Willis WD. Inhibitory receptive fields of primate spinothalamic tract cells. *J Neurophysiol* 1981;46:1309–1325.

Gybels J, Handwerker JO, Van Hees J. Comparison between the discharges of human nociceptive nerve fibres and the subject's rating of his sensation. *J Physiol* (Lond) 1979;292:193–206.

Handwerker HO, Kobal G. Psychophysiology of experimentally induced pain. *Physiol Rev* 1993;73: 639–671.

Hardy JD, Wolff HG, Goodell H. Studies on pain. A new method for measuring pain threshold: observations on spatial summation of pain. *J Clin Invest* 1940;19:649–657.

Hu JW. Response properties of nociceptive and non-nociceptive neurons in the rat's trigeminal subnucleus caudalis (medullary dorsal horn) related to cutaneous and deep craniofacial afferent stimulation and modulation by diffuse noxious inhibitory controls. *Pain* 1990;41:331–345.

Jacob JJ, Ramabadran K. Enhancement of a nociceptive reaction by opioid antagonists in mice. *Br J Pharmacol* 1978;64:91–98.

Kandel ER, Jessell TM. Touch. In: Kandel ER, Schwartz JH, Jessell TM, eds. *Principles of neural science*. Amsterdam: Elsevier, 1991;367–384.

Kawakita K, Funakoshi M. Suppression of the jaw opening reflex by conditioning A-delta fibre stimulation and electroacupuncture in the rat. *Exp Neurol* 1982;78:461–465.

Kayser V, Guilbaud G. Dose-dependent analgesic and hyperalgesic effects of systemic naloxone in arthritic rats. *Brain Res* 1981;226:344–348.

Kayser V, Guilbaud G. The analgesic effect of morphine, but not those of the enkephalinase inhibitor thiorphan, are enhanced in arthritic rats. *Brain Res* 1983;267:131–138.

Kiyatkin EA. Nociceptive sensitivity/behavioral reactivity regulation in rats during aversive states of different nature: its mediation by opioid peptides. *Int J Neurosci* 1989;44:91–110.

Kraus E, Le Bars D. Morphine antagonizes inhibitory controls of nociceptive reactions, triggered by visceral pain in the rat. *Brain Res* 1986;379:151–156.

Kraus E, Le Bars D, Besson JM. Behavioral confirmation of "diffuse noxious inhibitory controls" (DNIC) and evidence for a role of endogenous opiates. *Brain Res* 1981;206:495–499.

Lasagna L. Drug interaction in the field of analgesic drugs. *Proc R Soc Med* 1965;58:978–983.

Le Bars D, Calvino B, Villanueva L, Cadden SW. Physiological approaches to counter-irritation phenomena. In: Tricklebank MD, Curzon G, eds. *Stress-induced analgesia*. Chichester: Wiley, 1984;67–101.

Le Bars D, Chitour D. Do convergent neurones in the spinal dorsal horn discriminate nociceptive from non-nociceptive information? *Pain* 1983;17:1–19.

Le Bars D, Chitour D, Clot AM. The encoding of thermal stimuli by diffuse noxious inhibitory controls (DNIC). *Brain Res* 1981a;230:394–399.

Le Bars D, Chitour D, Kraus E, Clot AM, Dickenson AH, Besson JM. The effect of systemic morphine upon diffuse noxious inhibitory controls (DNIC) in the rat: evidence for a lifting of certain descending inhibitory controls of dorsal horn convergent neurones. *Brain Res* 1981b;215:257–274.

Le Bars D, Chitour D, Kraus E, Dickenson AH, Besson JM. Effect of naloxone upon diffuse noxious inhibitory controls (DNIC) in the rat. *Brain Res* 1981c;204:387–402.

Le Bars D, Dickenson AH, Besson JM. Diffuse noxious inhibitory controls (DNIC): I. Effects on dorsal horn convergent neurones in the rat. *Pain* 1979a;6:283–304.

Le Bars D, Dickenson AH, Besson JM. Diffuse noxious inhibitory controls (DNIC): II. Lack of effect on non-convergent neurones, supraspinal involvement and theoretical implications. *Pain* 1979b;6: 305–327.

Le Bars D, Dickenson AH, Besson JM. Opiate analgesia and descending control systems. *Adv Pain Res Ther* 1983;5:341–372.

Le Bars D, Dickenson AH, Besson JM, Villanueva L. Aspects of sensory processing through convergent neurons. In: Yaksh TL, ed. *Spinal afferent processing*. New York: Plenum, 1986;467–504.

Le Bars D, Guilbaud G, Jurna I, Besson JM. Differential effects of morphine on responses of dorsal horn lamina V type cells elicited by A and C fibre stimulation in the spinal cat. *Brain Res* 1976;115: 518–521.

Le Bars D, Villanueva L. Electrophysiological evidence for the activation of descending inhibitory controls by nociceptive afferent pathways. In: Fields HL, Besson JM, eds. *Pain modulation. Progress in brain research*, vol. 77. Amsterdam: Elsevier, 1988;275–299.

Le Bars D, Willer JC, De Broucker T, Villanueva L. Neurophysiological mechanisms involved in the pain-relieving effects of counter-irritation and related techniques. In: Pomerantz, B, Stüx G, eds. *Scientific basis of acupuncture*. Berlin: Springer Verlag, 1989;79–112.

Lee HK, Chung JM, Willis WD. Inhibition of primate spinothalamic tract cells by TENS. *J Neurosurg* 1985;2:276–287.

Levine JD, Gordon NC. Method of administration determines the effects of naloxone on pain. *Brain Res* 1986;365:377–378.

Levine JD, Gordon NC, Fields HL. Naloxone dose-dependently produces analgesia and hyperalgesia in post-operative pain. *Nature* 1979;278:740–741.

Levine JD, Gordon NC, Jones RT, Fields HL. The narcotic antagonist naloxone enhances clinical pain. *Nature* 1978;272:826–827.

Liebeskind JC, Giesler GJ Jr, Urca G. Evidence pertaining to an endogenous mechanism of pain inhibition in the central nervous system. In: Zotterman I, ed. *Sensory functions of the skin in primates*. Oxford: Pergamon Press, 1976;561–573.

Macdonald AJR. Acupuncture analgesia and therapy. In: Wall PD, Melzack R, eds. *Textbook of pain*. Edinburgh: Churchill Livingstone, 1989;906–919.

Mann F. Acupuncture analgesia, report of 100 experiments. *Br J Anaesth* 1974;46:361–364.

Melzack R. Folk medicine and the sensory modulation of pain. In: Wall PD, Melzack R, eds. *Textbook of pain*. Edinburgh: Churchill Livingstone, 1989;897–905.

Melzack R, Wall PD. Pain mechanisms: a new theory. *Science* 1965;150:971–979.

Miyamoto Y, Morita N, Kitabata Y, Yamanishi T, Kishioka S, Ozaki M, Yamamoto H. Antinociceptive synergism between supraspinal and spinal sites after subcutaneous morphine evidenced by CNS morphine content. *Brain Res* 1991;552:136–140.

Morton CR, Maisch B, Zimmermann M. Diffuse noxious inhibitory controls of lumbar spinal neurons involve a supraspinal loop in the cat. *Brain Res* 1987;410:347–352.

Ness TJ, Gebhart GF. Interactions between visceral and cutaneous nociception in the rat. I. Noxious cutaneous stimuli inhibit visceral nociceptive neurones and reflexes. *J Neurophysiol* 1991a;66:20–28.

Ness TJ, Gebhart GF. Interactions between visceral and cutaneous noiception in the rat. II. Noxious visceral stimuli inhibit cutaneous nociceptive neurones and reflexes. *J Neurophysiol* 1991b;66:29–39.

Niemegeers CJE, Van Bruggen JAA, Janssen PAJ. Suprofen, a potent antagonist of acetic acid-induced writhing in the rat. *Arzeim Forsch* 1975;25:1505–1509.

Pinsky C, Labella FS, Havlicek V, Dua AK. Apparent central agonists actions of naloxone in the unrestrained rat. In: Van Ree JM, Terenius L, eds. *Characteristics and functions of opioids*. Amsterdam: Elsevier, 1978;439–440.

Pircio AW, Fedele CT, Bierwagen ME. A new method for the evaluation of analgesic activity using adjuvant-induced arthritis in the rat. *Eur J Pharmacol* 1975;31:207–215.

Raja SN, Meyer RA, Campbell JN. Peripheral mechanisms of somatic pain. *Anesthesiology* 1988;68: 571–590.

Roerig SC, Fujimoto JM. Multiplicative interaction between intrathecally and intracerebroventricularly administered mu opioid agonists but limited interaction between delta and kappa agonists for antinociception in mice. *J Pharmacol Exp Ther* 1989;249:762–768.

Roy JC, Bing Z, Villanueva L, Le Bars D. Convergence of visceral and somatic inputs onto subnucleus reticularis dorsalis neurones in the rat medulla. *J Physiol* (Lond) 1992;452:235–246.

Schouenborg J, Dickenson AH. The effects of a distant noxious stimulation on A and C fibre evoked flexion reflexes and neuronal activity in dorsal horn of the rat. *Brain Res* 1985;328:23–32.

Sewell RDE, Spencer PSJ. Antinociceptive activity of narcotic agonist and partial agonist analgesics and other agents in the tail-immersion test in mice and rats. *Neuropharmacology* 1976;15:683–688.

Sher GD, Mitchell D. Intrathecal N-Methyl-D-aspartate induces hyperexcitability in rat dorsal horn convergent neurones. *Neurosci Lett* 1990;119:199–202.

Sjölund BH. Peripheral nerve suppression of C-fibre evoked flexion reflex in rats. Part 1: parameters of continuous stimulation. *J Neurosurg* 1985;63:612–616.

Taylor JS, Neal RI, Harris J, Ford TW, Clarke RW. Prolonged inhibition of a spinal reflex after intense stimulation of distant peripheral nerves in the decerebrated rabbit. *J Physiol* (Lond) 1991;437:71–83.

Tomlinson RWW, Gray BG, Dostrovsky JO. Inhibition of rat spinal cord dorsal horn neurons by non-segmental, noxious cutaneous stimuli. *Brain Res* 1983;279:291–294.

Torebjörk HE, Lamotte RH, Robinson C. Peripheral neural correlates of magnitude of cutaneous pain and hyperalgesia: simultaneous recordings in humans of sensory judgements of pain and evoked responses in nociceptors with C-fibres. *J Neurophysiol* 1984;51:325–329.

Van Hees J, Gybels JM. Pain related to single afferent C fibres from human skin. *Brain Res* 1972;48: 397–400.

Villanueva L, Le Bars D. The encoding of thermal stimuli applied to the tail of the rat by lowering the excitability of trigeminal convergent neurones. *Brain Res* 1985;330:245–251.

Villanueva L, Le Bars D. Indirect effects of intrathecal morphine upon diffuse noxious inhibitory controls (DNICs) in the rat. *Pain* 1986;26:233–243.

Villanueva L, Bing Z, Le Bars D. Effects of heterotopic noxious stimuli on activity of neurones in subnucleus reticularis dorsalis in the rat medulla. *J Physiol* (Lond) 1994;475:255–266.

Villanueva L, Bing Z, Bouhassira D, Le Bars D. Encoding of electrical, thermal and mechanical noxious stimuli by subnucleus reticularis dorsalis neurons in the rat medulla. *J Neurophysiol* 1989;61: 391–402.

Villanueva L, Bouhassira D, Bing Z, Le Bars D. Convergence d'informations nociceptives hétérotopiques sur des neurones du subnucleus reticularis dorsalis chez le rat. *CR Acad Sci* 1988;306:25–30.

Villanueva L, Bouhassira D, Bing Z, Le Bars D. Convergence of heterotopic nociceptive information onto subnucleus reticularis dorsalis neurons in the rat medulla. *J Neurophysiol* 1988b;60:980–1009.

Villanueva L, Cadden SW, Le Bars D. Evidence that diffuse noxious inhibitory controls (DNIC) are mediated by a final post-synaptic inhibitory mechanism. *Brain Res* 1984a;298:67–74.

Villanueva L, Cadden SW, Le Bars D. Diffuse noxious inhibitory controls (DNIC): evidence for postsynaptic inhibition of trigeminal nucleus caudalis convergent neurones. *Brain Res* 1984b;321:165–168.

Villanueva L, Chitour D, Le Bars D. Involvement of the dorsolateral funiculus in the descending spinal projections responsible for diffuse noxious inhibitory controls in the rat. *J Neurophysiol* 1986a;56: 1185–1195.

Villanueva L, Chitour D, Bouhassira D, Le Bars D. Effects of brain stem transections on diffuse noxious inhibitory controls (DNIC) in the rat. *Proceedings of the 7th world congress on pain* Paris, 1993;270.

Villanueva L, De Pommery J, Menétrey D, Le Bars D. Spinal afferent projections to subnucleus reticularis dorsalis in the rat. *Neurosci Lett* 1991;134:98–102.

Villanueva L, Peschanski M, Calvino B, Le Bars D. Ascending pathways in the spinal cord involved in triggering of diffuse noxious inhibitory controls (DNIC) in the rat. *J Neurophysiol* 1986b;55:34–55.

Wall PD. The dorsal horn. In: Wall PD, Melzack R, eds. *Textbook of pain*. Edinburgh: Churchill Livingstone, 1989;102–111.

Willer JC, De Broucker T, Le Bars D. Diffuse noxious inhibitory controls (DNIC) in man: involvement of an opioidergic link. *Eur J Pharmacol* 1990;182:347–355.

Willis WD. The raphé-spinal system. In: Barnes CD, ed. Brainstem control of spinal cord function. Orlando FL: Academic Press, 1984;141–214.

Willis WD, Coggeshall RE. *Sensory mechanisms of the spinal cord*. New York: Plenum Press, 1991.

Wolff HG, Hardy JD, Goodell H. Studies on pain. Measurement of the effect of morphine, codeine and other related opiates on the pain threshold, and an analysis of their relation to the pain experience. *J Clin Invest* 1940;19:659–680.

Woolf CJ, Mitchell D, Barrett GD. Antinociceptive effect of peripheral segmental electrical stimulation in the rat. *Pain* 1980;8:237–252.

Yaksh TL, Rudy TA. Narcotic analgetics, CNS sites and mechanisms of action as revealed by intracerebral injection techniques. *Pain* 1978;4:299–360.

Yeung JC, Rudy TA. Multiplicative interaction between narcotic agonisms expressed at spinal and supraspinal sites of antinociceptive action as revealed by concurrent intrathecal and intracerebroventricular injections of morphine. *J Pharmacol Exp Ther* 1980;215:633–642.

Zieglgänsberger W. Central control of nociception. In: Mountcastle VB, Bloom FE, Geiger SR, eds. *Handbook of physiology*, vol. 4. *The nervous system*. Baltimore: Williams & Wilkins, 1986;581–645.

*Pain and the Brain: From
Nociception to Cognition,*
edited by Burkhart Bromm and
John E. Desmedt, Advances in Pain
Research and Therapy Vol. 22.
Raven Press, Ltd., New York © 1995.

35

Electrophysiologic Studies of Morphine Analgesia in Humans

*Jean Claude Willer and †Daniel Le Bars

*Laboratory of Neurophysiology, Medical Faculty of Pitié-Salpêtrière, University Pierre et Marie Curie, F-75634 Paris, France, and †Department of Physiopharmacology, INSERM-U 161, F-75014 Paris, France

SUMMARY

Psychophysiologic and clinical studies have shown that analgesia produced by morphine or other related narcotics is associated with an increase in the threshold of experimentally induced pain elicited either by radiant heat, mechanical pressure, or electrical stimulation (Wolff et al., 1940; Gaensler 1951; Lee and Pfeiffer 1951). For instance, Wolff et al. (1940), in their pioneer study, reported that intramuscular morphine produced a dose-dependent increase in the threshold for cutaneous pain elicited by radiant heat. On the other hand, our knowledge of both opioid receptors and pain mechanisms has made great strides in recent years. It is therefore paradoxical that the neural substrates involved in the mechanisms of morphine-induced analgesia in humans are largely unknown. This is probably due to the ubiquitous properties of the opioid receptors and, as a consequence, to the numerous pharmacologic effects of morphine. One mechanism of the analgesic action of morphine, however, is well documented. In animals, morphine is known to cause a potent depression of the transmission of nociceptive signals at the level of the first relays in the central nervous system (CNS) (i.e., in the dorsal horn of the spinal cord) (Le Bars and Besson 1981; Duggan and North 1984; Yaksh and Noueihed 1985). Clinically, the administration of morphine over the lumbar spinal cord via the epidural or intrathecal route is widely used to relieve pain emanating from the lower part of the body (Cousins and Mather 1984). The human spinal cord contains opioid receptors (Czlonkowski et al. 1983; Gouardères et al. 1986; Faull and Villiger 1987) and neurons containing endogenous opioids, mainly in the most superficial layers of the gray matter (De Lanerolle and LaMotte 1982; Przewlocki et al. 1983; Schoenen et al. 1985; Chung et al. 1989). It is a matter of fact that the direct spinal effect of morphine is a cornerstone in the understanding of pain mechanisms. A second, indirect and complementary mechanism has been proposed for explaining the analgesic properties of morphine: the drug is supposed to act at some brain-stem sites, mainly the periaqueductal grey matter (PAG), to reinforce descending inhibitory influences that are involved in modulating pain. This would be another means of depressing the spinal transmission of nociceptive signals through dorsal-horn neurons (Irwin et al. 1951; Takagi et al. 1955; Mayer and Price 1976; Fields and Basbaum 1978). However, this idea is controversial, since attempts to demonstrate that supraspinal administration of morphine decreases the activity of dorsal-horn neurons have been inconclusive (Le Bars et al. 1983; Duggan and North 1984; Advokat 1988). We have previously shown a close relationship between a nociceptive flexion reflex from a knee-flexor muscle and the sensation of pain elicited by stimulating the ipsilateral sural nerve at the ankle (Willer 1977). On the basis of studies of this reflex, we will show herein that in humans, morphine may have different mechanisms of action, depending on its dose and site of administration. We will first present evidence for a direct spinal depressive effect as one of the main mechanisms of morphine-induced analgesia. We then describe the supraspinal sites of action of morphine and its consequences for descending controls; it will be seen that morphine depresses descending inhibitory controls. All data presented herein were obtained in experiments approved either by national or local committees. According to the ethical principles of the Helsinki Convention, signed informed consent was always obtained from subjects (normal or patients) who participated in the studies.

MORPHINE DECREASES NOCICEPTIVE SIGNALS DIRECTLY AT THE SPINAL LEVEL

In the following sections we will describe in succession the effects of i.v. morphine in normal subjects, the effects of i.v. morphine in paraplegic patients, and the effects of epidural administration of morphine in patients with postoperative pain.

Effects of Intravenous Morphine in Normal Volunteers

The experiments were done on healthy volunteers from the medical staff and on the investigators themselves, with all being carefully informed of the goals of the study and the procedures involved, particularly regarding the i.v. administration of morphine and naloxone. Polysynaptic nociceptive flexion reflexes (RIII reflexes) in the lower limb were elicited by stimulating the ipsilateral sural nerve by means of a pair of needle electrodes inserted through the skin at the ankle, at the retromalleolar path of the nerve. Recordings were made from the tibialis anterior muscle (TA) using a couple of surface electrodes placed on the scratched and degreased skin overlying the muscle. The subjective quality (tactile or painful) and intensity of the sensation elicited by the sural-nerve stimulus were estimated by the subjects on a ten-level visual scale consisting of 10 switches, with the pain threshold being arbitrarily defined as level 3. Before the administration of drugs, there was a significant correlation between the recruitment curves of the reflex and the pain score as functions of stimulus intensity. Consequently, the reflex (Tr) and the pain (Tp) thresholds were found to be almost identical (mean: 10.6 and 10.3 mA, respectively), while the threshold of the maximal reflex response (Tmr) was very close to that for tolerance to pain (Tip): 37.1 and 38.8 mA, respectively.

The effect of four different doses of morphine chlorhydrate (0.05, 0.1, 0.2, and 0.3 mg/kg, i.v.) were studied in each subject in a random order during four different experiments. At the end of each experiment, the specificity of the effects of morphine was tested with naloxone hydrochloride (0.005 mg/kg, i.v.). For a given subject, the interval between two successive sessions was deliberately set at 6 to 8 months in order to avoid any phenomenon of tolerance. For a given session, the general experimental procedure consisted of studying the parameters described above (Tr, Tmr, Tp, Tip) in a control period, after the administration of morphine and after the subsequent administration of naloxone. However, just before and during drug injections, the sural-nerve stimulus was kept constant at 1.2 to 1.3 times the reflex threshold, in order to study the time course of the drug effect on a nociceptive reflex response elicited by a constant stimulus. In addition, blood pressure and respiratory activity were clinically monitored at regular 5- to 6-min intervals throughout the session.

Morphine injections resulted in a depression of both nociceptive reflex activity and related sensations of pain in a dose-dependent fashion. In every case, naloxone hydrochloride i.v. reversed these effects. While 0.05 mg/kg morphine did not significantly modify the four parameters being considered, higher doses increased the four thresholds in a dose-dependent fashion; this relationship was significantly linear in the 0.05 to 0.3 mg/kg range. For each dose of morphine studied, there was no significant difference between the percentage increase in Tr compared to that in Tp, or between the percentage increase in Tmr compared to that in Tip (Fig. 1). In the same way, morphine depressed, in a dose-dependent fashion, the nociceptive reflex activity elicited by a constant intensity of stimulation. These depressive effects appeared within the first minute following morphine injection, reached their maximum within 3 to 5 minutes, and then remained stable at this level for the rest of the experimental period (30–40 min).

Since flexion reflexes involve activation of alpha-motoneurons by nociceptive afferent volleys, there was an *a priori* possibility that morphine was exerting a direct postsynaptic effect on the motoneurons. To test this hypothesis, the H-reflex from the soleus muscle was studied, since it involves a monosynaptic arc via large-diameter myelinated afferent fibers; the reflex was elicited and recorded using an established method (Hugon 1973). The administration of morphine at the highest dose used for the RIII reflex did not significantly affect the monosynaptic H-reflex.

The classical side-effects of narcotics on mood were reported by the subjects, and appeared within the first minute following the injection, reached their maximum at 5 minutes, and then decreased slowly toward a state of drowsiness and laziness. There was no clear relationship between the dose of morphine administered and the

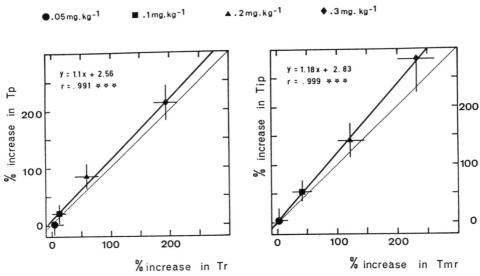

FIG. 1. Effects of intravenous morphine in normal volunteers: relationships between the percentage increase in the thresholds for RIII reflex (abscissae) and pain (ordinates) following four doses of morphine (0.05; 0.01; 0.2; 0.3 mg/kg). Left: relationship between increases in reflex (Tr) and pain (Tp) thresholds. Right: relationship between increases of the thresholds for the maximal reflex response (Tmr) and tolerance to pain (Tip). *Dotted lines* show the 45° lines that were very similar to the experimental regression curves. (From Willer 1985, with permission.)

extent of the subjective side-effects, but intersubject variations in sensitivity were obvious: the same dose of morphine could produce minor side effects in some subjects and stronger effects in others. There was no correlation between the subjective reactions and the effects observed on either the nociceptive reflex or the pain sensation. At any dose used, morphine did not produce major changes in either blood pressure or respiratory rate. In two subjects we observed a small, transient change in the systolic blood pressure, which increased, with all of the doses administered, from 130 to 150 to 160 mm Hg within 2 min after morphine injection. Such short-lasting (3–4 min) increases could result from nonspecific, anxiogenic reactions to morphine in these individuals. However, these subjects did not want to stop the experiment when the investigator asked them if they wished to do so. All of the effects of morphine described herein were completely and immediately reversed by naloxone.

   This study demonstrated that intravenous morphine can elicit a dose-dependent analgesic effect on experimentally induced pain, in association with the simultaneous depression of a spinal nociceptive flexion reflex. Both threshold and supra-threshold sensations and reflexes were affected. The methodology used for investigating the experimentally induced pain was derived from earlier studies (Willer 1977; Willer and Bussell 1980; Willer et al. 1984) showing a close relationship between the threshold of the nociceptive flexion reflex from the biceps femoris muscle and the threshold of pain elicited by stimulation of the ipsilateral sural nerve. Of special interest was the observation of a linear relationship for both the reflex response and the pain sensation within a limited range of stimulus intensities. As a consequence, the response thresholds (Tr and Tp) and the maximal response thresholds (Tmr and Tip) were very similar in the control situations and following morphine. These observations suggest a common spinal mechanism in the triggering of both nociceptive reflex activity and pain sensations, including the maximal responses under our experimental conditions.

Effects of Intravenous Morphine in Paraplegic Patients

The aim of this study was to gauge, in humans with chronic spinal injury, the direct spinal depressive action of morphine on nociceptive flexion reflexes as compared to its effects on monosynaptic reflexes. Four young adults volunteered for this study: all had chronic paraplegia of traumatic origin, and according to careful neurologic investigations, all were clinically complete spinal subjects.

Polysynaptic nociceptive flexion reflexes (RIII reflexes) in the lower limb were elicited as described above. The intensity of stimulation was then chosen at four to five times the threshold of the reflex. The H reflex from the soleus muscle was elicited and recorded as described above. Since we had previously verified the absence of interaction between the mono- and polysynaptic reflexes, they were elicited synchronously at a rate of 0.2 Hz, in different legs.

When naloxone hydrochloride (0.005 mg/kg) was injected alone, no significant change could be observed in either the RIII or the H reflex. By contrast, morphine induced a rapid and very significant depression of the nociceptive flexion reflex without significantly affecting the monosynaptic reflex. A dose-dependent relationship was seen: following 0.2 mg/kg morphine chlorhydrate, there was a 70% depression of the reflex, which reached 90 and 95% with 0.3 and 0.35 mg/kg of the drug, respectively. This depressive effect was stable during the 30-min observation period following the administration of morphine (Fig. 2). During the same period, classical side effects were reported by the subjects at 4 to 5 min after the injections, including a transient sweating and redness of the face and a certain degree of drowsiness. The classical opiate-induced respiratory depression was never observed, even following larger doses (0.43 mg/kg) of morphine, and the blood pressure was not significantly modified during these periods. All of the effects were reversed by administration of naloxone (0.005 mg/kg).

One can conclude that in humans as in animals, morphine selectively depresses nociceptive spinal reflexes by a direct spinal mechanism. This depressive effect is specific, since it is completely reversed by naloxone, and seems to play an important role in the modulation of nociceptive signals at the spinal level, because morphine in its usual therapeutic doses can markedly depress nociceptive flexion reflexes without affecting monosynaptic ones.

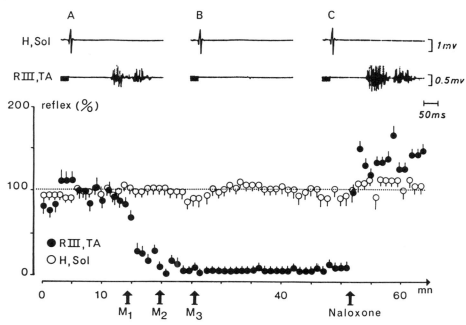

FIG. 2. Effects of intravenous morphine in paraplegic patients. Upper recordings: monosynaptic (H,Sol) and polysynaptic nociceptive (RIII,TA) reflexes recorded during: **(A)** control periods, **(B)** following injection of 0.35 mg/kg morphine, and **(C)** following injection of 0.02 mg/kg naloxone. Each trace is a superimposition of 10 responses. Note the large depression (in **B**) and the enhancement (in **C**) of RIII,TA while H,Sol is not changed in **(B)** and is slightly increased in **(C)**. Lower graph: time course of the effects of morphine and naloxone on RIII,TA and H,Sol. The results are expressed as percentages of the rectified reflex amplitude (100% represents the mean of all the control values, i.e., 100 responses). Each point is the mean of 10 averaged successive values with one SE. M_1 corresponds to injection of 0.2 mg/kg morphine, M_2 and M_3 indicate additional doses of 0.1 and 0.05 mg/kg morphine, respectively. Naloxone was given at a dose of 0.02 mg/kg. (From Willer and Bussel 1980, with permission.)

Effects of Epidural Morphine in Patients with Postoperative Pain

The spinal administration of opiates for the relief of pain is becoming a classical technique (see references in Willer et al. 1985). In normal subjects with acute postoperative pain following orthopedic surgery of the knee, we observed that epidural administration of low doses of morphine (0.03–0.04 mg/kg) resulted in pain relief and a parallel powerful depression of lower-limb nociceptive flexion reflexes.

The control values for the thresholds of the reflex responses were $16.3 + 1.2$ and $52.5 + 6.1$ mA for Tr and Tmr, respectively, which are higher than in normal healthy volunteers. Epidural morphine produced a progressive increase in both Tr (87%) and Tmr (84%) over the 60-min period of study. The onset of pain relief occurred by 25 to 30 min after morphine administration, when the increased thresholds for both Tr and Tmr reached 40%.

With supraliminal responses, epidural morphine resulted in a strong progressive depression of the nociceptive reflex (Fig.3A). This effect became statistically significant by 20 min after dosing and reached a 90% maximum by 50 min (Fig. 3A). Correspondingly, morphine induced segmental pain relief, which was obvious by 25 to 30 min and increased progressively until there was almost total relief of both postoperative and electrically induced pain. These depressive and pain-relieving effects were not associated with the classical opiate side effects reported by subjects following intravenous morphine. During the experimental sessions, the subjects did not describe the adverse effects of spinal morphine (e.g., itching or urinary retention) observed with higher doses of epidural morphine (6–9 mg). Neurologic testing did not reveal any motor deficiency in the tendon-jerk reflexes or in the strength of the voluntary contraction of the normal lower limb at the end of each experimental session. There was no significant change in heart rate, blood pressure, or respiration during the course of the 60-min session.

The finding that epidural morphine elicits a powerful depression of the transmission of nociceptive spinal reflexes that parallels the relief of acute postoperative pain agrees with animal experiments showing that morphine selectively depresses nociceptive reflexes in chronic spinal cats and dogs (Wikler 1944; Koll 1962). In our study, there was no clinical evidence for a supraspinal involvement of morphine in the mechanisms of pain relief, since side effects were not reported by the subjects and no vegetative depressions (respiration, heart rate, blood pressure) were found. The pain-relieving action of epidural morphine can therefore be explained by a direct depressive effect on spinal nociceptive transmission, at least for the initial 60-

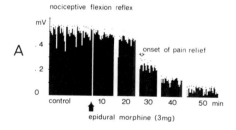

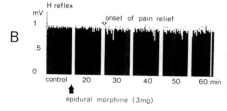

FIG. 3. Effects of epidural morphine in patients with postoperative pain. The example shows the effects of morphine, administered at the time indicated by the *arrows*, on the RIII reflex (upper part) and on the monosynaptic H reflex (lower part). Each bar corresponds to a single response plotted against time. (From Willer et al. 1985, with permission.)

min postinjection period. Note that intravenous injections of 0.05 mg/kg morphine in normal subjects modified neither the nociceptive reflexes nor the associated sensation of pain, but elicited the classical side effects of opiates. Thus, in the present study, even if vascular absorption of epidural morphine had occurred, its blood levels must have been lower than 0.05 mg/kg.

Because flexion reflexes involve the activation of alpha-motoneurons by the nociceptive afferent volleys, it was possible that epidural morphine depressed these reflexes by a direct postsynaptic effect on the motoneuronal membrane. This was certainly not the case, however, since the H reflex from the soleus muscle was not modified by epidural morphine in these patients (Fig. 3B).

These data are in keeping with animal studies showing that morphine selectively depresses the responses of dorsal-horn cells to Aδ- and C-fiber inputs, whereas responses to large-diameter fibers (A$\alpha\beta$) inputs are unchanged or only weakly affected (Le Bars et al. 1976; Duggan and North 1984).

In sum, the data presented above provide clear evidence that one of the most important mechanisms in morphine-induced analgesia is a selective and direct depressive effect on the transmission of nociceptive signals at the spinal level.

MORPHINE DEPRESSES SUPRASPINAL DESCENDING INHIBITORY CONTROLS

Effects of a Low Dose of Intravenous Morphine in Normal Subjects

This section of the chapter describes the effects of morphine on descending inhibitory controls involved in the modulation of pain in humans. Such inhibitory processes can be activated in normal subjects: we have demonstrated that painful heterotopic conditioning stimuli inhibit both a nociceptive flexion reflex (RIII reflex) and the corresponding sensation of pain elicited by sural-nerve stimulation (Willer et al. 1984, 1989). While nonpainful conditioning stimuli have no effect, the extent of the inhibition is related directly to the intensity of the painful conditioning stimuli. This is exemplified in Fig. 4, in which electrical stimulation of the sural nerve at regular intervals elicited an RIII reflex that was recorded over the ipsilateral biceps femoris muscle. The subject was then asked to immerse his contralateral hand in a thermoregulated and agitated water bath. At 44°C and below (nonpainful temperatures), the RIII reflex activity did not exhibit any change during or after this conditioning procedure; in contrast, at the higher temperatures of 45°C (becoming painful), 46°C, and 47°C, a clear-cut inhibition of the RIII reflex was observed during and for several minutes after the conditioning procedure, the maximal effects and longest lasting after-effects being obtained with the highest temperature. Such inhibitions of the RIII reflex were not observed in tetraplegic patients suffering from clinically complete spinal-cord transections of traumatic origin (Roby-Brami et al. 1987). Observations were also made (De Broucker et al. 1990) on patients with cerebral lesions, consisting either of a unilateral thalamic lesion or a lesion of the

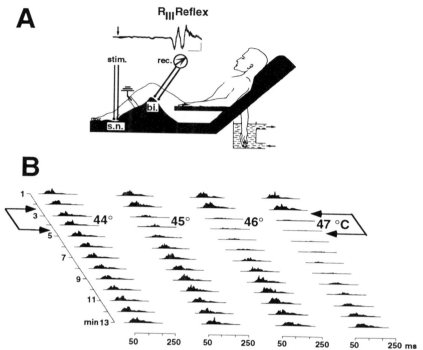

FIG. 4. Evidence for DNIC in humans. **A:** Experimental set-up used for eliciting a nociceptive reflex (RIII) by stimulation (stim.) of the sural nerve (s.n.) and recording (rec.) from over the left biceps femoris muscle (bi.). An example of the (RIII) reflex is shown at the top of the diagram (calibrations: horizontal 25 msec; vertical 100 mV). The reflex evoked by juxtathreshold (1.2 times threshold) stimulation was studied before, during, and after a 2-min period of immersion of the right hand in a thermoregulated waterbath. **B:** Examples of the effects of heterotopic thermal conditioning stimulation on the RIII reflex. Each trace represents the average of 10 successive full-wave-rectified responses recorded during a 1-min period. For each experimental sequence, the temporal evolution is shown from back to front, the 2-min conditioning period (indicated by *arrows*) being in the third and fourth minutes. The nonpainful temperature (44°C, left) did not modify the reflex. By contrast, the painful temperatures (45,46,47°C) depressed the reflex during and after the application of the conditioning stimuli. The magnitudes of these depressions were temperature-dependent. Note the long duration (around 10 min) of the inhibitory post-effects following the application of the highest temperature (47°C, right). (From Le Bars et al. 1992, with permission.)

retro-olivary part of the medulla (Wallenberg's syndrome), that caused contralateral hemianalgesia. In the thalamic lesion group, the RIII reflex was strongly depressed, as in normal subjects, by nociceptive conditioning stimuli applied to the affected side, although these stimuli were not felt as painful. By contrast, in the patients with Wallenberg's syndrome, no inhibitions were observed when the nociceptive conditioning stimuli were applied to the affected side, whereas if they were applied to the normal side they triggered inhibitory effects and after-effects very similar to those seen in normal subjects. Thus, the brain stem is the site of a key neuronal link in a loop subserving such inhibitory effects. We concluded that painful heat triggers descending impulses which, in turn, elicit an inhibition of a spinal nociceptive flexion reflex. We then sought to investigate the effects of a supraspinally acting dose of morphine on such inhibitory processes.

We studied the effects of noxious thermal conditioning stimuli applied to the left hand on the RIII reflex elicited by stimulation of the right sural nerve. As described previously (Willer et al. 1984, 1989), the subjects were required to dip the hand to a depth of 5 cm above the wrist in a 46°C thermoregulated and agitated waterbath for a period of 2 min. This conditioning temperature was selected because it produces a frank but bearable sensation of pain and elicits clear-cut inhibitions of the RIII reflex and associated pain, both during and for 6 to 8 min after the end of its application. Measured with planimetric methods, the total surface area of the skin exposed to the thermal conditioning stimulus was found to be close to 500 cm^2.

Heart and respiratory rates were recorded continuously, since both are sensitive parameters of vegetative responses to emotion or stress (Porges and Raskin 1969; Gautier 1972). The electrocardiogram was recorded via the VI international derivation. The respiratory rate was measured from the ventilatory movements detected by a pneumograph placed around the thorax.

At the beginning of a session, the intensity of the test stimulus was adjusted so as to elicit a supraliminal RIII reflex response that fluctuated minimally from one stimulus to the next. The organization of each experimental sequence was as follows: a 2-min control period followed by a 2-min period during which the conditioning procedure (CP) was applied, and finally a period of 7 min during which any aftereffects were studied. The duration of an entire sequence was therefore 11 min. Identical sequences were repeated 15 min after the intravenous administration of morphine hydrochloride (0.05 mg/kg) and 5 min after an intravenous injection of naloxone hydrochloride (0.006 mg/kg), which was administered 30 min after the morphine.

Under control conditions, the mean stimulus intensity for eliciting a liminal RIII reflex was 10.1 mA ± 0.5 mA. Stimulation at 1.2 times threshold (i.e., about 12 mA) elicited a slightly supraliminal RIII reflex response with minimal spontaneous fluctuations under control conditions. Such an intensity simultaneously produced a pinprick type of pain that the subjects reported as originating from the stimulating electrodes and projecting into the receptive field (RF) of the sural nerve. This painful sensation was well tolerated by all of the subjects, and was reported to be constant under resting conditions. The reflex responses were depressed during and after the application of the 46°C conditioning stimulus to the contralateral hand. The depressive effects appeared rapidly (within 15–20 sec), had their maximum effect during the second minute of the conditioning procedure, and outlasted the conditioning period by 6 to 7 minutes. Simultaneously and in parallel with these electrophysiologic effects, the noxious heating of the hand also produced a decrease or abolition of the sensation of pain elicited by the 12-mA sural-nerve stimulus. These effects were observed unequivocally in all of the subjects.

Administration of morphine at 0.05 mg/kg resulted in a complete abolition of these inhibitions without any modification of the reflex itself (Fig. 5). At 5 to 6 min after the injection of morphine, the conditioning procedure failed to produce any inhibitory effect or aftereffect; at 5 to 16 min after the naloxone injection, the inhibitions had recovered, and were in fact even more pronounced, especially in terms of poststimulus effects. It is noteworthy that 5 min after the injection of morphine, the sensations of pain produced by the 12-mA stimuli to the sural nerve were not modified by the conditioning stimulation, whereas these sensations were again decreased or abolished, along with the RIII reflex, 5 min after the administration of naloxone (Fig. 5). No significant changes were observed in the heart or respiratory rates during any of the situations described above.

These results demonstrate that a low i.v. dose of morphine completely blocks the inhibitory effects of heterotopic nociceptive thermal-conditioning stimuli on a nociceptive flexion reflex. This blockade occurred without any change in the electrophysiologic characteristics (latency, duration, and magnitude) of the RIII reflex itself, and disappeared after subsequent naloxone administration. Stress-induced analgesia has been reported repeatedly in both animals and humans (Tricklebank and Curzon 1984; Kelly 1986). In humans, a progressive increase in the thresholds for both pain and the RIII reflex was observed during repetitive stressing by the anticipation of intolerable pain; this increasing analgesia was associated with progressive tachycardia and polypnea (Willer and Albe-Fessard 1980). Although in the present study we deliberately excluded intolerable levels of conditioning stimuli that would produce obviously stressful reactions, the depressive effects elicited by the 46°C conditioning stimulus could have been produced by discrete emotional and/or stressful reactions to the nature of the conditioning stimulus. However, this hypothesis seems unlikely, since the most sensitive parameters for these reactions, namely heart and respiration rates (Porges and Raskin 1969; Willer 1975), remained stable before, during, and after the conditioning procedures. Moreover, the values of these parameters were very similar to those recorded during studies of the RIII reflex in normal relaxed subjects who did not receive any additional noxious stimuli (Willer and Albe-Fessard 1980; Willer 1975). That such factors, together with others such as attentional processes, were not involved in the inhibitions described herein is further emphasized by observations made in patients with unilateral thalamic or parietal ischemic lesions (De Broucker et al. 1990): a highly noxious conditioning stimulus applied to the anaesthetic hand (contralateral to the lesion) produced a strong inhibitory effect on the RIII reflex. In this case, the spinal transmission of nociceptive signals was clearly impaired by heterotopic noxious but nonpainful stimuli, without any change in attentional or vegetative processes. Identical observations were made during the pharmacologic tests: following morphine and naloxone, the conditioning stimulus did not elicit any detectable state of stress or emotion that might in itself have introduced a bias to our results.

Interestingly, although injected in a low dose, morphine elicited a complete blockade of the inhibitory effects produced by the noxious thermal-conditioning stimulus. This observation can be easily explained by our exclusive use of supra-

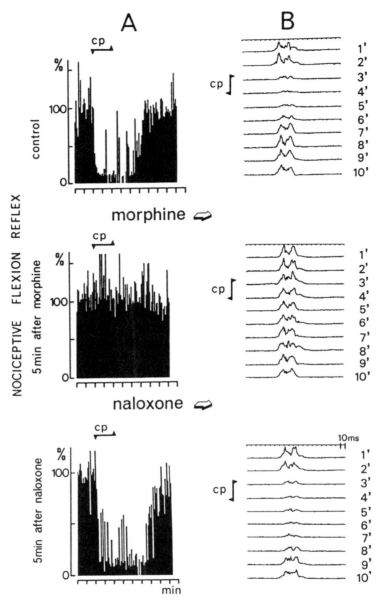

FIG. 5. Example of the effects of i.v. injections (at *arrows*) of 0.05 mg/kg morphine and subsequent injections of 0.006 mg/kg naloxone on the inhibitions of the RIII reflex produced by a noxious conditioning temperature (cp): immersion of the right hand for 2 min in a 46°C waterbath. The individual example shows the effects of the conditioning procedure on the RIII relfex before treatment (control); 5 min after morphine, and 5 min after a subsequent injection of naloxone (30 min after morphine). **A:** Each bar corresponds to a single response plotted against time. **B:** From top to bottom, each trace is an average of 10 successive reflex responses. In the control situation, note the clear depression of the RIII reflex both during and after the 2-min conditioning period, its complete blockade after morphine, and its complete recovery following naloxone.

threshold stimulation parameters for both the conditioned and the conditioning stimulus (i.e., 1.2 times the threshold for the RIII reflex response, and 46°C as the heterotopic conditioning stimulus, which is 1°C higher than the threshold for pain produced by heating the skin) (Hardy et al. 1951; Lamotte and Campbell 1978). Such juxtathreshold stimuli might have optimized the pharmacologic effects of morphine.

We are thus dealing in humans with an inhibitory process sustained by a spinobulbospinal loop (Roby-Brami et al. 1987; De Broucker et al. 1990), which is completely blocked by morphine. Since the effect of the drug was completely reversed by naloxone, one can conclude that opioid receptors were involved. Interestingly, the inhibitory processes were even more pronounced in terms of poststimulus effects, following subsequent administration of naloxone. This observation is reminiscent of many electrophysiologic data in animals and humans, which show that for several minutes after the administration of naloxone following morphine, the responses were greater than in controls (Le Bars et al. 1976; Duggan and North 1984; Willer 1985).

These results are very much in keeping with observations in the rat. Indeed, the supraspinally mediated inhibition of dorsal-horn neurons by heterotopic noxious stimuli, which have been termed diffuse noxious inhibitory controls (DNIC), are blocked by morphine administered either in low systemic doses, intracerebrally within the nucleus raphe dorsalis, intracerebroventricularly, or intrathecally (see Chapter 34). The low dose of morphine used in the present study (0.05 mg/kg) precludes the possibility that the signals emanating from the upper-limb nociceptors were blocked at the spinal level; indeed, a higher dose of morphine, in the 0.1 to 0.3-mg/kg range, is required before a direct spinal depressive effect can be observed (see above). An effect of morphine is therefore to be found at supraspinal sites. Thus, there is a growing body of evidence in both animals and humans that morphine clearly impairs descending inhibitory systems modulating pain, at least when they are activated by nociceptive afferents. We have previously discussed the possibility that DNIC may offer a possible neuronal mechanism for analgesia based on the counter-irritation principle (i.e., pain relief produced by painful or unpleasant stimuli, such as hyperstimulation, acupuncture, or transcutaneous electric nerve stimulation [TENS] with acupuncture-like stimuli (see Chapter 34). If such a proposition is correct, then the present results strongly suggest a negative interaction between analgesia elicited by morphine and that produced with the use of the physical techniques described above. Some behavioral experiments in the rat (Kraus and Le Bars 1986) support this assertion, which should be tested in clinical situations. Interestingly, the data described herein could represent the neural basis for the initially surprising observation made by Wolff et al. (1940) that in humans, a heterotopic pain could block the morphine-induced increase in the pain threshold to radiant heat. Wolff et al. came to the conclusion that the "threshold-raising action of opium derivatives . . . was reduced or obliterated by pain."

Effects of Intracerebroventricular Morphine in Patients With Cancer Pain

Guieu et al. (1993) evaluated the effect of intracerebroventricular morphine on RIII reflexes in patients with cancer pain in order to test the current hypothesis that morphine given in this way reinforces descending inhibitory controls that modulate the spinal transmission of nociceptive signals. The investigations were done on patients suffering intractable pain from squamous-cell carcinomata of the head and neck who were treated with intracerebroventricular morphine (0.7–1 mg, total dose). Both RIII reflexes and associated sensations of pain elicited by sural-nerve stimulation were studied before and after (1–4 hours) morphine injections. In all of the patients the treatment relieved clinical cancer pain. Similarly, the threshold for the experimental pain was increased from 9.04 ± 0.56 mA to 10.18 ± 0.89 mA. By contrast, not only was the RIII reflex not depressed, it was slightly enhanced, with its threshold falling from 8.76 ± 0.78 mA to 7.43 ± 0.54 mA. These data clearly show that morphine administered into the cerebral ventricles depresses the descending inhibitory control of nociceptive transmission at the spinal level in humans. They do not support the hypothesis that supraspinal morphine reinforces descending inhibitory controls. These results are very similar to those of Bouhassira et al. (1988a), which showed that intracerebroventricular morphine decreased descending inhibitions acting on lumbar dorsal-horn neuronal activities related to pain in the rat.

Several other electrophysiologic studies support this hypothesis. For example, the depressive effects of i.v. morphine on C-fiber-evoked responses were found to be remarkably similar in the 1 to 10-mg/kg dose range in intact and spinal rats (Le Bars et al. 1980). The results of three studies (LeBars et al. 1976; Duggan et al. 1980; Soja and Sinclair 1983) are consistent with the hypothesis that morphine decreases tonic descending inhibitions. Four studies using microinjection techniques in the rat, the first two within the nucleus raphe magnus (NRM) (Le Bars et al. 1980; Llewelyn et al. 1987) and the other two within the PAG (Dickenson and Le Bars 1987a,b) have shown that morphine can increase the responses evoked in dorsal-horn neurons by noxious stimulation of their RFs. Finally, Sinclair (1986) reported that perfusion of the cat ventricular system with morphine also resulted in a facilitation of dorsal-horn neuronal activities evoked by noxious stimuli.

When these findings are added to the present results, it appears that the evidence for an increase in descending inhibition by morphine is at least highly controversial. By contrast, the reduction in DNIC produced by low doses of intracerebroventricular morphine and microinjections of the drug into the medioventral PAG, including the nucleus raphe dorsalis (Dickenson and Le Bars 1987a), shows that supraspinal morphine blocks descending inhibitions triggered by noxious stimuli.

The present data, added to previous reports in animals showing that both systemic (Le Bars et al. 1981) and intrathecal (Villanueva and Le Bars 1986) morphine reduces DNIC, thus indicate that the three routes of administration of this drug that are used for alleviating pain in humans can be correlated with a reduction in these inhibitory controls. Taking account of this decrease in descending inhibitory controls, what could be the mechanism for supraspinal morphine analgesia? This question is specifically addressed in this volume in Chapter 34 which deals with diffuse noxious inhibitory controls in the rat, and is summarized below.

Because convergent neurons respond to both noxious and non-noxious stimuli, their activities in the absence of any noxious stimulation can be interpreted as a basic somesthetic activity from which a significant nociceptive signal could not easily emerge. A local, restricted noxious stimulus induces two related phenomena at the level of the spinal cord: (a) a segmental excitation of nociceptive neurones, and (b) as a result of the activation of the DNIC system, a reduction in the activity of all of the (other) spinal and trigeminal convergent neurons not concerned with the segmental activation. The contrast signal between the excited segmental and larger, inhibited extrasegmental pools of neurons could indicate to higher centers that a nociceptive event was occurring. In this hypothesis, hypoalgesia could be induced by a decrease in DNIC that would restore the background somesthetic activity. If the responses to innocuous stimuli are facilitated, one could envisage this phenomenon as being able to induce a further increase in "background spinal noise," and could thus envision its participation in the mechanism of analgesia. To verify such a premise, it would be essential to know whether morphine introduced into the cerebral ventricles can also depress DNIC-mediated inhibitions when convergent neurons are activated by innocuous stimuli; in fact, further data in animals are consistent with such an hypothesis (Bouhassira et al. 1988b).

ACKNOWLEDGMENTS

This work was supported by INSERM, CRC AP-HP, and by la Fondation pour la Recherche Médicale. The authors are very grateful to Dr. Sam Cadden for advice in the preparation of the manuscript.

REFERENCES

Advokat C. The role of descending inhibition in morphine-induced analgesia. *Trends Pharmacol Sci* 1988;9:330–334.

Bouhassira D, Villanueva L, Le Bars D. Intracerebroventricular morphine decreases descending inhibitions acting on lumbar dorsal horn neuronal activities related to pain in the rat. *J Pharmacol Exp Ther* 1988a;247:332–342.

Bouhassira D, Villanueva L, Le Bars D. Intracerebroventricular morphine restores the basic somesthetic activity of dorsal horn convergent neurones in the rat. *Eur J Pharmacol* 1988b;148:273–277.

Chung K, Briner RP, Carlton SM, Westlund KN. Immunohistochemical localization of seven different peptides in the human spinal cord. *J Comp Neurol* 1989;280:158–170.

Cousins MJ, Mather LE. Intrathecal and epidural administration of opioids. *Anesthesiology* 1984;61: 276–310.

Czlonkowski A, Costa T, Przewlocki R, Pasi A, Herz A. Opiate receptor binding sites in human spinal cord. *Brain Res* 1983;267:392–396.

De Broucker T, Cesaro P, Willer JC, Le Bars D. Diffuse noxious inhibitory controls (DNIC) in man: involvement of the spinoreticular tract. *Brain* 1990;113:1223–1234.

De Lanerolle NC, LaMotte CC. The human spinal cord: substance P and methionine-enkephalin immunoreactivity. *J Neurosci* 1982;10:1369–1386.

Dickenson AH, Le Bars D. Supraspinal morphine and descending inhibitions acting on the dorsal horn in the rat. *J Physiol (Lond)* 1987a;384:81–107.

Dickenson AH, Le Bars D. Lack of evidence for increased descending inhibition on the dorsal horn of the rat following periacqueductal grey morphine microinjections. *Br J Pharmacol* 1987b;92:271–280.

Duggan AW, Griersmith BT, North RA. Morphine and supraspinal inhibition of spinal neurones: Evidence that morphine decreases tonic descending inhibition in the anaesthetized cat. *Br J Pharmacol* 1980;69:461–466.

Duggan AW, North RA. Electrophysiology of opioids. *Pharmacol Rev* 1984;35:219–281.

Faull RLM, Villiger JW. Opiate receptors in the human spinal cord: a detailed anatomic study comparing the autoradiographic localization of [3H]diprenorphine binding sites with the laminar pattern of substance P, myelin and Nissl staining. *Neuroscience* 1987;20:395–407.

Fields HL, Basbaum AI. Brainstem control of spinal transmission neurons. *Annu Rev Physiol* 1978; 40:193–221.

Gaensler EA. Quantitative determination of the visceral pain threshold in man. Characteristics of visceral pain, effect of inflammation and analgesics on the threshold and relationship of analgesia to visceral spasm. *J Clin Invest* 1951;30:406–420.

Gautier H. Respiratory and heart rate responses to auditory stimulations. *Physiol Behav* 1972;8: 327–332.

Gouarderes C, Kopp N, Cros J, Quirion R. Kappa opioid receptors in human lumbo-sacral spinal cord. *Brain Res Bull* 1986;16:355–361.

Guieu JD, Blond S, Meynadier J, Le Bars D, Willer JC. Intracerebroventricular (ICV) morphine depresses descending inhibitory controls in patients with cancer pain. *Proceedings of the 7th world congress on pain.* Paris, 1993, 209.

Hardy JD, Goodell H, Wolff HG. The influence of skin temperature upon the pain threshold as evoked by thermal radiation. *Science* 1951;114:149–150.

Hugon M. Methodology of the Hoffmann reflex in man. In: Desmedt JE, ed. *New developments in electromyography and clinical neurophysiology*, vol. 3. Basel: Karger, 1973;227–293.

Irwin S, Houde RW, Bennett DR, Hendershot LC, Seevers MH. The effects of morphine, methadone and meperidine on some reflex responses of spinal animals to nociceptive stimulations. *J Pharmacol Exp Ther* 1951;101:132–143.

Kelly DD. Stress-induced analgesia. *Ann NY Acad Sci* 1986;46–47.

Koll W. Physiological observations and pharmacological actions on nociceptive spinal reflexes. In: Keele CA, Smith R, eds. *The assessment of pain in man and animals*. Edinburgh and London: Churchill Livingstone, 1962;92–103.

Kraus E, Le Bars D. Morphine antagonizes inhibitory controls of nociceptive reactions, triggered by visceral pain in the rat. *Brain Res* 1986;379:151–156.

Lamotte RH, Campbell JN. Comparison of responses of warm and nociceptive C-fibre afferents in monkey with human judgment of thermal pain. *J Neurophysiol* 1978;41:509–528.

Le Bars D, Besson JM. The spinal site of action of morphine in pain relief: from basic research to clinical application. *Trends Pharmacol Sci* 1981;2:323–325.

Le Bars D, Chitour D, Kraus E, Clot AM, Dickenson AH, Besson JM. The effect of systemic morphine upon diffuse noxious inhibitory controls (DNIC) in the rat: Evidence for a lifting of certain descending inhibitory controls of dorsal horn convergent neurones. *Brain Res* 1981;215:257–274.

Le Bars D, De Broucker T, Willer JC. Morphine blocks pain inhibitory controls in humans. *Pain* 1992;48:13–20.

Le Bars D, Dickenson AH, Besson JM. Microinjection of morphine within nucleus raphé magnus and dorsal horn neurone activities related to nociception in the rat. *Brain Res* 1980;189:467–481.

Le Bars D, Dickenson AH, Besson JM. Opiate analgesia and descending control system. *Advances in pain research and therapy*, vol. 5. New York: Raven Press, 1983;341–372.

Le Bars D, Guilbaud G, Chitour D, Besson JM. Does systemic morphine increase descending inhibitory controls of dorsal horn neurones involved in nociception? *Brain Res* 1980;202:223–228.

Le Bars D, Guilbaud G, Jurna I, Besson JM. Differential effects of morphine on responses of dorsal horn lamina V type cells elicited by A and C fibre stimulation in the spinal cat. *Brain Res* 1976;115: 518–524.

Le Bars D, Ménetrey D, Besson JM. Effects of morphine upon the lamina V type cells activities in the dorsal horn of the decerebrate cat. *Brain Res* 1976;113:293–310.

Lee RE, Pfeiffer CC. Influence of analgesics, dromoran, nisentil and morphine, on pain thresholds in man. *J Appl Physiol* 1951:193–198.

Llewelyn MB, Azami J, Roberts MHT. Brainstem mechanisms of antinociception: Effects of electrical stimulation and microinjection of morphine into nucleus raphe magnus. *Neuropharmacology* 1987;25: 727–735.

Mayer DJ, Price DD. Central nervous system of analgesia. *Pain* 1976;2:379–404.

Porges SW, Raskin DC. Respiratory and heart rate components of attention. *J Exp Psychol* 1969;81: 497–503.

Przewlocki R, Gramsch C, Pasi A, Herz A. Characterization and localization of immunoreactive dynorphin and a-neo-endorphin, met-enkephalin and substance P in human spinal cord. *Brain Res* 1983;280: 95–103.

Roby A, Bussel B, Willer JC. Morphine reinforces post-discharge inhibition of a-motoneurones in man. *Brain Res* 1981;222:209–212.

Roby-Brami A, Bussel B, Willer JC, Le Bars D. An electrophysiological investigation into the pain relieving effects of heterotopic nociceptive stimuli: probable involvement of a supraspinal loop. *Brain* 1987;110:1497–1508.

Schoenen J, Lotstra F, Vierendeels G, Reznik M, Vanderhaegen JJ. Substance P, enkephalins, somatostatin, cholecystokinin, oxytocin and vasopressin in human spinal cord. *Neurology* 1985;35:881–890.

Sinclair JG. The failure of morphine to attenuate spinal cord nociceptive transmission through supraspinal actions in the cat. *Gen Pharmacol* 1986;17:351–354.

Soja PJ, Sinclair JG. Spinal vs supraspinal actions of morphine on cat spinal cord multireceptive neurons. *Brain Res* 1983;273:1–7.

Takagi H, Matsunara M, Yanai A, Ogiu K. The effects of analgesics on the spinal reflex activity of the cat. *Jpn J Pharmacol* 1955;4:176–187.

Tricklebank MD, Curzon G. *Mechanisms of stress-induced analgesia.* Chicester, UK: Wiley, 1984.

Villanueva L, Le Bars D. Indirect effects of intrathecal morphine upon diffuse noxious inhibitory controls (DNICs) in the rat. *Pain* 1986;26:233–243.

Wikler A. Studies on the action of morphine on the central nervous system of the cat. *J Pharmacol Exp Ther* 1944;80:176–187.

Willer JC. Influence de l'anticipation de la douleur sur les frequences cardiaque et respiratoire et sur le reflexe nociceptif chez l'homme. *Physiol Behav* 1975;15:411–415.

Willer JC. Comparative study of perceived pain and nociceptive flexion reflex in man. *Pain* 1977;3: 69–80.

Willer JC. Studies on pain. Effects of morphine on a spinal nociceptive flexion reflex and related pain sensation in man. *Brain Res* 1985;331:105–114.

Willer JC, Albe-Fessard D. Electrophysiological evidence for a release of endogenous opiates in stress-induced "analgesia" in man. *Brain Res* 1980;198:419–426.

Willer JC, Bergeret S, Gaudy JH. Epidural morphine strongly depresses nociceptive flexion reflexes in patients with postoperative pain. *Anesthesiology* 1985;63:675–680.

Willer JC, Bussel B. Evidence for a direct spinal mechanism in morphine-induced inhibition of nociceptive reflexes in humans. *Brain Res* 1980;187:212–215.

Willer JC, De Broucker T, Le Bars D. Encoding of nociceptive thermal stimuli by diffuse noxious inhibitory controls in humans. *J Neurophysiol* 1989;62:1028–1038.

Willer JC, Roby A, Le Bars D. Psychophysical and electrophysiological approaches to the pain-relieving effects of heterotopic nociceptive stimuli. *Brain* 1984;107:1095–1112.

Wolff HG, Hardy JD, Goodell H. Studies on pain. Measurement of the effect of morphine, codeine and other opiates on the pain threshold and an analysis of their relation to the pain experiences. *J Clin Invest* 1940;19:659–680.

Yaksh TL, Noueihed R. The physiology and pharmacology of spinal opiates. *Annu Rev Pharmacol Toxicol* 1985;25:433–462.

Pain and the Brain: From
Nociception to Cognition,
edited by Burkhart Bromm and
John E. Desmedt, Advances in Pain
Research and Therapy Vol. 22.
Raven Press, Ltd., New York © 1995.

36

The Effects of Analgesics on Mood in Patients with Pain of Different Etiologies

*Stanley L. Wallenstein,[1] †George Heidrich, III, ‡Robert F. Kaiko,
and *Raymond W. Houde

*Memorial Sloan-Kettering Cancer Center, New York, New York, 10021 USA, and
†Global Pharma Services, Inc., Madison, Wisconsin 53704, and
‡The Purdue Frederick Company, Norwalk, Connecticut 06850-3590, USA

SUMMARY

A self-administered questionnaire consisting of 15 pairs of descriptors representing mood opposites (i.e., shaky–serene, blue–cheerful, etc.) was developed to
evaluate various aspects of mood in patients with pain. In cancer-pain patients who
completed the questionnaire before and after receiving a narcotic for pain, factor
analysis of the items in the questionnaire developed four main factors: I, agitation–
serenity; II, euphoria–dysphoria; III, optimism–pessimism; and IV, apathy–enthusiasm. Factor I accounted for 70% of the variation and factor II for 15%. The factors
correlated highly with mood measurements on a visual analogue scale (VAS), and
the patients showed significant improvement in mood measurements for factors I
and IV after receiving narcotics. Factor II, consisting of items related to euphoria–
dysphoria commonly associated with the effects of narcotics in addicts, was only
minimally affected in these patients. The questionnaire has been employed in volunteer subjects without pain and in a variety of patient populations (chronic cancer
pain, postoperative cancer pain, and postoperative orthopedic pain) in studies involving narcotics (morphine and heroin), a nonsteroidal antiinflammatory drug
(NSAID) (zomepirac), and a partial narcotic agonist/antagonist (buprenorphine).
Patients with chronic cancer pain had measurably poorer mood than patients with
postoperative pain. Improvements in mood correlated well with analgesia after the
use of all analgesics in the postoperative-pain patients. However, in patients with
chronic cancer pain, significantly greater mood changes occurred after the narcotics
than after the non-narcotics, even when degrees of analgesia were similar. While
mood in postoperative-pain patients would appear to directly reflect the degree of

---

[1]Send all correspondence to: Stanley L. Wallenstein, 198-04 53 Avenue, Flushing, NY 11365.

pain, the relationship is more complex in chronic-pain patients. The interactions of mood, pain severity, and pain etiology merit further study.

INTRODUCTION

Pain is recognized as a significant subjective aspect of the illness experience. It is the complaint that most often leads people to seek medical help, and more often than not is treated aggressively with medications and/or other therapies. Varieties of subjective scales, numerical, categorical, and analog, have been developed to measure the severity of pain or the degree of relief provided by its treatment, and the effects of analgesics have been quantified and compared utilizing sophisticated statistical procedures. Drugs are compared in terms of onset, duration, peak action, and area under the time–effect curve in studies involving patients with a wide variety of painful conditions (Lasagna 1980; Wallenstein 1984a).

Nevertheless, despite often sophisticated tools for measuring pain, much of the pain experience remains unexplained. We observe that patients with essentially similar physical problems may report widely different pain experiences. These differences may involve both the severity and quality of pain, and may well affect the quality of the patient's life. That placebo is capable of modifying pain is *per se* evidence that other subjective states can affect the pain experience, and these states may in turn be modified by pain. The problems of analysis are compounded when active analgesics are evaluated. For example, narcotics are commonly known to be capable of inducing euphoria, but the effects of these drugs can also be modified by the conditions and populations in which they are employed.

Early investigators of both clinical and experimental pain attempted to distinguish between the pure sensation of pain and a subsequent reaction component of the pain experience (Beecher 1957). More recently, psychologists have attempted to analyze the pain experience by the application of signal-detection theory to the measurement of experimentally induced pain (Jones 1979). The McGill Pain Questionnaire, in which patients rate pain in terms of a variety of sensory, affective, and evaluative descriptors, has been successful in distinguishing patients with a variety of pain syndromes. The various components of the questionnaire, however, have been somewhat less sensitive to the effects of analgesics (Melzack 1975).

In our own studies at the Memorial Sloan-Kettering Cancer Center, a global measure of mood employing a 10-cm VAS, anchored on the left with the statement "Worst I Could Feel" and on the right with "Best I Could Feel," was found to be sensitive to narcotics with results that correlate well with the effects of these drugs on pain (Fishman et al. 1987). These results, however, remained difficult to interpret, since the VAS scale for mood is not only global but vague. What particular aspects of mood may be affected, or indeed whether the patients interpreted "Worst I could feel" and "Best I could feel" as including or exclusive of the pain experience, cannot be readily determined from the results. On a practical level, the question of whether particular narcotics such as heroin or morphine have different or similar mood-elevating effects, whether these effects may be greater than those of other narcotics in a variety of patient populations, and the degree to which mood influences reports of pain or are in turn influenced by pain are issues that cannot be answered solely with data from the VAS Mood scale.

A more comprehensive and detailed measure of mood, sensitive to the effects of analgesics and capable of being readily and easily employed by patients with pain in studies done in a variety of clinical pain populations, is requisite for a meaningful analysis of these questions. This paper reports on our efforts to develop such a scale, and on some of the more interesting results we have obtained.

METHODS

A self-scoring mood questionnaire was developed for use in conjunction with clinical studies of analgesic drugs in hospitalized patients with pain (Wallenstein 1984). The questionnaire consisted of 15 pairs of word opposites (i.e., "Shaky–Serene," "Cheerful–Got the blues," etc.). The design of the questionnaire is illustrated in Fig. 1. The order of word pairs, and the left or right placement of the words in each pair (in terms of better or worse mood), were randomized to insure as well as possible that the patients would rate each pair of descriptors individually and on its own merits. Patients were instructed to circle either the neutral value, 0, or 1, 2, or 3 in the direction of either word in the pair for "slight," "moderate," or "strong,"

Feeling of Heaviness	3	2	1	0	1	2	3	Buoyant
I Feel Sociable	3	2	1	0	1	2	3	I Want to be Alone
Very Uneasy	3	2	1	0	1	2	3	Very Much At Ease
Cheerful	3	2	1	0	1	2	3	Got the Blues
Happy	3	2	1	0	1	2	3	Sad
I'm Very Interested in What's Going On	3	2	1	0	1	2	3	I Don't Give A Damn About Anything
Lethargic	3	2	1	0	1	2	3	Peppy
Angry	3	2	1	0	1	2	3	Contented and Friendly
Apathetic	3	2	1	0	1	2	3	Enthusiastic
Confident	3	2	1	0	1	2	3	Apprehensive
Amused	3	2	1	0	1	2	3	Very Serious
Calm	3	2	1	0	1	2	3	Very Nervous
I Feel Pessimistic	3	2	1	0	1	2	3	I Feel Optimistic
Restless	3	2	1	0	1	2	3	Peaceful
Shaky	3	2	1	0	1	2	3	Serene

FIG. 1. The 15-item mood questionnaire. Subjects are instructed to circle appropriate number: 0 for neutral, or 1, 2, or 3 for "slight," "moderate," or "strong" in the direction of one of the words in a pair. The ordering of the words within each pair is randomized so that the direction of the words is not related to better or worse mood.

as dictated by their feelings at the moment. The questionnaire is a modification of a mood and physiologic questionnaire developed by Lasagna et al. (1955).

Each of the 15 items on the mood questionnaire was scored on an arithmetic scale of 1 to 7, from poorest to best mood. Factor analysis of the 15 word-pair scores was done employing Varimax rotation with Kaiser normalization (Norusis 1993). Where appropriate, in studies involving analgesics, drug effects on mood as measured by the questionnaire were evaluated in terms of score changes from before to after drug, in terms of the 15 word-pairs, and in terms of the mood factors that were developed from the 15 items.

VAS scales for mood, pain, and relief were also employed in these studies. These analog scales were scored in terms of the number of centimeters from the left edge to the point at which the patients marked the scales. In cases in which verbal reports of pain and/or relief were obtained, each category of pain or relief was scored arithmetically in ascending order of degree of severity, from no pain to most severe pain, and from no relief to complete relief (Wallenstein 1984b).

RESULTS

Preliminary Observations

A pilot evaluation of the mood questionnaire was undertaken at Memorial Hospital in conjunction with analgesic relative potency studies of heroin and morphine in adult, hospitalized cancer patients who had either postoperative pain or chronic pain from their cancers (Kaiko et al. 1981). A global estimate of mood was also obtained in these patients, using the VAS Mood scale, and subjective pain severity and pain relief were evaluated employing both verbal categorical measures and VAS scales.

In these studies, both morphine and heroin were effective analgesics, and were observed to improve mood as measured on both the VAS scale and the questionnaire. These two mood measures correlated well in the postoperative patient group ($R^2 = 0.62$). A positive relationship was also obtained in the chronic cancer-pain patients, but the correlation was weaker ($R^2 = 0.36$), possibly because, at least in part, of the smaller number of patients in this group. Analysis of the word pairs indicated that patients were significantly more peaceful, serene, at ease, calm, happy, cheerful, buoyant, content, and friendly after receiving either drug. They were more confident, enthusiastic, sociable, and amused after morphine, and more interested after heroin. The results in chronic-pain and postoperative-pain patients were qualitatively similar, but the mood improvements were smaller in the patients with chronic pain, despite the fact that this group of patients began the study with poorer pretreatment moods (Kaiko et al. 1981).

Factor analysis of the questionnaire items developed four main factors. Factor I is primarily associated with items relating to an "agitation–serenity" dichotomy, and accounts for 70% of the variability; Factor II relates to "euphoria–dysphoria," with 15% of the variability; Factor III is an "optimism–pessimism" factor; and factor IV an "apathy–enthusiasm" factor. Only factors I and IV were significantly affected by the narcotics, and these in the direction of improved mood. Interestingly, the "dys-phoria–euphoria" factor, commonly associated with the effects of narcotic drugs, was only minimally affected in these patients.

These results demonstrated that it is feasible to obtain a moderately detailed questionnaire of subjective mood states in hospitalized patients with relatively severe pain, and that measurable changes in responses to selected items on the questionnaire can be obtained after analgesic medication. These positive results encouraged further investigation of the questionnaire in different pain populations and employing a variety of analgesic drugs, as well as studies of responses to the questionnaire by normal subjects.

Validation Studies

Using both the mood questionnaire and the VAS Mood scale, subjective mood data were obtained in a group of 31 pain-free volunteer subjects, mostly from the professional staff at Memorial Hospital. These data were intended to serve as a baseline for comparison with the subjective mood data obtained from patients with pain. Validation studies in patients, incorporating the mood questionnaire in clinical analgesic drug studies, were also undertaken. These studies were undertaken in three hospitalized patient populations: at Memorial Hospital in cancer patients with chronic pain from their disease and in cancer patients with postoperative pain after abdominal surgery, and at the University of Wisconsin in orthopedic postoperative patients with postoperative pain. The 15-item mood questionnaire was incorporated into analgesic drug studies involving these patients, along with standard subjective measures of analgesia.

Baseline measurements for the word pairs in the mood questionnaire were obtained in the volunteer subjects without pain and in the three hospitalized patient groups. Mean scores on the 15 mood items in these subjects are summarized in Table 1. Not unexpectedly, the mean scores for the volunteer subjects were measurably higher than those of any of the patient groups. Among the patient groups, the patients with chronic cancer pain had the lowest mood scores on the 15 items. The patients with postoperative pain had slightly better mood scores than the postoperative cancer patients, but the differences between the two groups were not significant. These results are graphically illustrated in the radar plot in Fig. 2.

Factor analysis of questionnaire items in normal subjects produced four factors that were essentially similar to those for chronic cancer pain in the initial study reported above. However, in contrast with the results in the latter group of patients, for whom the factor relating to "agitation–serenity" accounted for most of the variation, with the "optimism–pessimism" factor second, the "euphoria–dysphoria" factor was predominant in the normal subjects and accounted for 42% of the variation, while the "agitation–serenity" factor was second with 15%.

The Mood VAS correlated highly with the four mood factors ($R^2 = 0.81$) in the volunteers, and accounted for about two-thirds of the variability in the factors ($R^2 = 0.66$). This relationship is illustrated in Fig. 3. The two measures of mood thus bear

TABLE 1. *Mood descriptors in normal volunteers and in patients with pains of varying etiologies. Scores are means on a scale of 1 for worst mood to 7 for best mood in each item*

Mood descriptors	Normal volunteers	Chronic cancer	Cancer postoperative	Orthopedic postoperative
Alone–Sociable	5.6	2.8	2.8	3.1
Angry–Friendly	5.6	3.0	3.4	3.7
Apathetic–Enthusiastic	5.5	2.7	3.4	3.3
Apprehensive–Confident	5.6	2.8	3.8	3.9
Blue–Cheerful	5.7	2.7	3.3	3.4
Disinterested–Interested	6.0	3.8	4.5	4.5
Heavy–Buoyant	4.7	2.0	2.0	2.0
Lethargic–Peppy	4.8	2.2	2.1	2.4
Nervous–Calm	5.4	2.7	3.3	3.7
Pessimistic–Optimistic	5.2	3.0	4.1	4.1
Restless–Peaceful	4.7	2.2	2.6	2.6
Sad–Happy	5.6	2.6	3.3	3.5
Serious–Amused	4.8	2.0	2.4	2.7
Shaky–Serene	4.8	2.2	2.6	2.7
Uneasy–At Ease	5.5	2.3	2.7	2.9

a significant relationship to each other; however, 34% of the variation in the questionnaire is unaccounted for in the VAS scale.

The relative moods of the three patient groups and the volunteers, in terms of both the individual items and the four factors in the questionnaire, followed a predictable pattern (Fig. 4). The best mood was reflected in the scores for the volun-

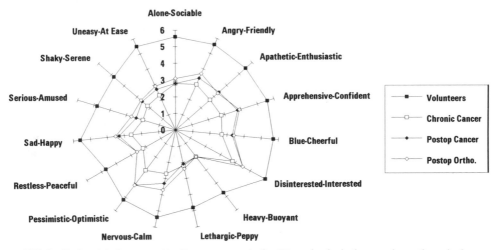

MOOD DESCRIPTORS IN NORMALS AND PAIN PATIENTS

FIG. 2. Radar plot of mean subjective responses to the 15 word pairs in the mood questionnaire by normal volunteers without pain, cancer patients with chronic pain and postoperative pain, and orthopedic patients with postoperative pain. Higher values on the scale respresent improved mood.

N = 31 Normal Volunteers

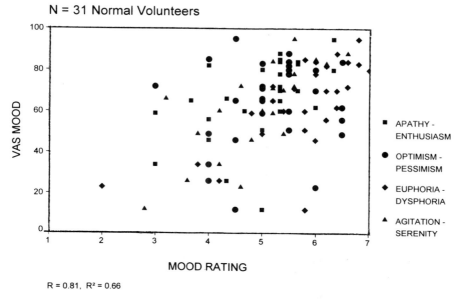

R = 0.81, R^2 = 0.66

FIG. 3. Scatter plot for normal volunteers without pain of their subjective scores on the Mood VAS versus mean values for the four factor clusters "agitation–serenity," "euphoria–dysphoria," "optimism–pessimism," and "apathy–enthusiasm" derived from the 15-item questionnaire.

teers, followed at some distance by the orthopedic surgery patients, with the cancer surgery patients close behind. The patients with chronic cancer pain understandably had the poorest mood. This ordering was consistent for each of the four factors and also for all of the individual items.

Analgesic Drug Studies

The mood questionnaire has been incorporated into studies of analgesic drugs in the three populations of hospitalized pain patients, and subjective mood measurements have been obtained before and after treatment with a variety of analgesic medications. Table 2 summarizes some of the more interesting findings after treatment with a variety of selected analgesics in the three clinical pain groups. The drugs described include potent and mild narcotics (morphine and codeine), nonsteroidal antiinflammatory analgesics (zomepirac and ibuprofen), and a partial narcotic agonist/antagonist (buprenorphine [Wallenstein et al. 1980]), and a placebo. Changes in mood for the questionnaire items were measured at 2 hours after medication. Significant changes are indicated by appropriate asterisks in the table. We have not observed any significant worsening of mood after treatment. All significant effects in the table are in the direction of improved mood.

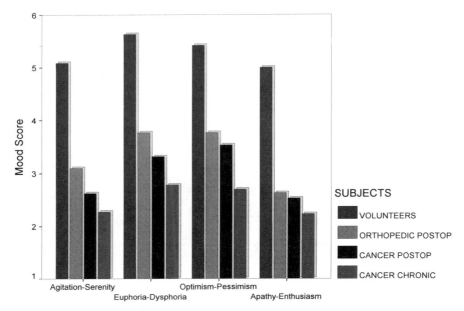

FIG. 4. Bar plot of mean responses to the four factor clusters "agitation–serenity," "euphoria–dysphoria," "optimism–pessimism," and "apathy–enthusiasm" by normal volunteers without pain, cancer patients with chronic pain and postoperative pain, and orthopedic patients with postoperative pain.

As measured by the questionnaire items, mood was relatively unaffected by placebo. In the postoperative patients, improvement in mood paralleled reduction in pain, regardless of the etiology of their pain or the type of analgesic employed, and the mood changes after drug treatment are essentially similar for the two postoperative patient groups. Greater mood improvement after drug treatment was observed in the postoperative patients than in the patients with chronic cancer pain, despite the chronic cancer patients' significantly lower mood scores before receiving medication.

Changes in mood in chronic cancer patients appear to be more dependent on the type of analgesic drug used to treat them than on the degree of relief they experience. These patients report significantly improved mood after potent narcotics on a number of items in the questionnaire. They were more interested, sociable, happy, peaceful, serene, calm, friendly, and amused after receiving morphine, and these results are consistent with what was observed in the morphine-heroin study in a similar population with chronic cancer pain, reported above (Kaiko et al. 1981). The factors for "euphoria–dysphoria," "agitation–serenity," and "apathy-enthusiasm" all show significant positive improvement after morphine and other potent narcotics.

In contrast, little in the way of significant mood improvement was observed after

TABLE 2. Rotated factor loadings for the self-scoring mood questionnaire in normal volunteers and signifant mood improvement in patients with pain after the following analgesic medications: zomepirac (ZOM), morphine (MOR), buprenorphine (BUP), ibuprofen (IBU), codeine (COD), and placebo (PLA)

Factor	Mood descriptors	Load	Cancer, chronic			Cancer, postoperative			Orthopedic, postoperative		
			ZOM, PO	MOR, IM	BUP, SL	MOR, IM	BUP, SL	IBU, PO	COD, PO	IBU + COD	PLA, PO
Euphoria–Dysphoria Eigenvalue: 6.355 % Variation: 42.4	Disinterested–interested	0.928	*	*			*	*	**	**	
	Alone–sociable	0.895	*	*		*	*	*	**	**	
	Apathetic–enthusiastic	0.824			*	*	*		**	**	
	Blue–cheerful	0.823							*	**	
	Sad–happy	0.816		**		*	**	**	*	**	
Agitation–Serenity Eigenvalue: 2.192 % Variation: 14.5	Restless–peaceful	0.896		**		**	*	**		**	
	Shaky–serene	0.809		*		**	*	**		**	
	Nervous–calm	0.707	*	**		*	*	**		**	
	Angry–friendly	0.670		**		**	*			**	
	Uneasy–at ease	0.492			**	**	*	**	**		
Optimism–Pessimism Eigenvalue: 1.643 % Variation: 11.0	Heavy–buoyant	0.758			*	*	**	**		**	
	Lethargic–peppy	0.741			*	*	**	**		**	
	Pessimistic–optimistic	0.646				*	**	**		**	**
Apathy–Enthusiasm Eigenvalue: 1.224 % Variation: 8.2	Serious–amused	0.868		*		*				**	
	Apprehensive–confident	0.704									

Asterisks show significant drug effects (*$p < 0.05$., **$p < 0.01$). All significant changes were in the direction of improved mood.

use of the nonsteroidal antiinflammatory agent zomepirac in the chronic pain patients, despite the fact that the drug was at least as effective an analgesic as morphine in these patients (Wallenstein et al. 1980). The lack of significant mood effects after zomepirac in patients with chronic pain contrasts with the dramatic improvement in mood observed in postoperative orthopedic pain patients after ibuprofen, another nonsteroidal antiinflammatory agent.

A similar pattern of mood responses can be seen with buprenorphine, a potent partial narcotic agonist/antagonist. This drug, also an effective analgesic in both chronic and postoperative pain (Wallenstein et al. 1986), produced little in the way of mood improvement in patients with chronic pain, but in postoperative pain, observed changes in mood were comparable to those seen after morphine.

DISCUSSION

The mood questionnaire provides supplemental information not available in the Mood VAS. Although mood measures using a VAS scale and the questionnaire are highly correlated, roughly one-third of the variability in the questionnaire items cannot be accounted for in terms of the VAS alone. The questionnaire is comparatively simple and easy to administer, and hospitalized patients with relatively severe pain had little problem in filling it out. Repeated measures before and after receiving analgesic drugs are readily obtainable while making other observations during clinical analgesic studies. The questionnaire is sensitive to patients' changes in mood following the administration of analgesic drugs. Baseline measures in normal subjects without pain are consistent with results in patients, and factor analysis produces four distinct factors useful in evaluating mood and changes in mood after drug administration.

Results obtained with the questionnaire in the volunteers and in the three patient populations are generally in the expected direction. As measured by the questionnaire, volunteers evinced the best mood and the chronic cancer-pain patients the worst. Narcotic drugs produced improvements in mood that corresponded well with changes in pain in all of the pain populations studied. In the postoperative patients, all analgesics, narcotics, partial narcotic agonists, and nonsteroidal antiinflammatory drugs produced mood changes that paralleled reductions in pain.

Perhaps the most challenging results occurred in patients with chronic cancer pain. In this population narcotics such as heroin and morphine consistently produced positive mood changes that paralleled their analgesic effects, while the nonsteroidal agent zomepirac and the partial narcotic agonist buprenorphine produced only minimal mood effects, despite the fact that both drugs are highly effective analgesics in these patients. These results contrast with the significant positive mood changes in postoperative patients observed after treatment with all analgesics. Whether the differences between zomepirac and ibuprofen result from differences in the two drugs or differences in reaction of the two pain groups is a matter for conjecture. However, buprenorphine, which was studied in both chronic and postoperative cancer-pain populations, also produced dramatically different mood changes in these two patient groups, providing a strong argument that the differences are attributable to differences between the patient groups.

Major differences in the determinants for mood are likely to exist in the chronic- and postoperative-pain patients. Moods in the postoperative-pain patients is apparently directly linked to the degree of the patients' pain, with changes in pain reflected directly in corresponding changes in mood. Mood in chronic cancer-pain patients would appear to be a more complex phenomenon, and is more likely to center around their concept of their illness and its consequences. Pain, while part of this overall picture, may influence mood, but is likely to be less of a determinant of mood than in postoperative-pain patients. Powerful mood-altering drugs such as morphine and heroin will indeed improve mood in chronic cancer-pain patients, while drugs with a lesser mood-altering potential may not. The interactions of mood, pain severity, pain etiology, and type of analgesic drug are a complex network of interacting relationships, and merit additional study. The picture at this point remains incomplete, and to advance our understanding, mood effects of a variety of analgesics should be studied in pain of different etiologies.

ACKNOWLEDGMENT

This research was supported in part by Grant DA-01707 from the U.S. National Institute of Drug Abuse.

REFERENCES

Beecher HK. The measurement of pain. *Pharmacol Rev* 1957;9:59–209.
Fishman B, Pasternak S, Wallenstein SL, Houde RW, Holland JC, Foley KM. The Memorial Pain Assessment Card. A valid instrument for the evaluation of cancer pain. *Cancer* 1987;60:1151–1158.
Jones B. Signal detection theory and pain research. *Pain* 1979;7:305–312.
Kaiko RF, Wallenstein SL, Rogers AG, Grabinsky PY, Houde RW. Analgesic effects of heroin and morphine in cancer patients with postoperative pain. *N Engl J Med* 1981;304:1501–1505.
Lasagna L. Analgesic methodology: a brief history and commentary. *J Clin Pharmacol* 1980; 20:373–376.
Lasagna L, von Felsinger JM, Beecher HK. Drug induced mood changes in man. 1. Observations on healthy subjects, chronically ill patients and "postaddicts." *JAMA* 1955;157:1006–1020.
Melzack, R. The McGill pain questionnaire: Major properties and scoring methods. *Pain* 1975; 1:277–299.
Norusis MJ. *SPSS for Windows. Professional Statistics. Release 6.0.* Chicago: SPSS Inc., 1993; 47–81.
Wallenstein SL. The evaluation of analgesics in man. In: Kuhar M, Pasternak G, eds. *Analgesics: Neurochemical, behavioral and clinical perspectives.* New York: Raven Press, 1984a;235–255.
Wallenstein SL. Measurement of pain and analgesia in cancer patients. *Cancer* 1984b;53:2260–2266.
Wallenstein SL, Kaiko RF, Rogers AG, Houde RW. Crossover trials in clinical analgesic assays: Studies of buprenorphine and morphine. *Pharmacotherapy* 1986;6:228–235.
Wallenstein SL, Rogers A, Kaiko RF, Heidrich III G, Houde RW. Relative analgesic potency of oral zomepirac and intramuscular morphine in cancer patients with postoperative pain. *J Clin Pharmacol* 1980;250–258.

Subject Index